THE HUMAN NERVOUS SYSTEM

THE HUMAN NERVOUS SYSTEM
BASIC PRINCIPLES OF NEUROBIOLOGY

SECOND EDITION

Text by **Charles R. Noback, Ph.D.**
Department of Anatomy
College of Physicians and Surgeons
Columbia University

Illustrated by **Robert J. Demarest**
Department of Anatomy
College of Physicians and Surgeons
Columbia University

McGRAW-HILL BOOK COMPANY
A Blakiston Publication

New York St. Louis San Francisco Auckland
Düsseldorf Johannesburg Kuala Lumpur London
Mexico Montreal New Delhi Panama Paris
São Paulo Singapore Sydney Tokyo Toronto

This book was set in Optima by York Graphic Services, Inc.
The editors were J. Dereck Jeffers, Stuart D. Boynton, and Richard S. Laufer;
the designer was Barbara Ellwood;
the production supervisor was Leroy A. Young.
Von Hoffmann Press, Inc., was printer and binder.

Library of Congress Cataloging in Publication Data

Noback, Charles Robert, date
  The human nervous system: basic principles of
neurobiology.

  "A Blakiston publication."
  1. Neurobiology. I. Demarest, Robert J., illus.
II. Title. [DNLM: 1. Nervous system—Anatomy &
histology. 2. Neurophysiology. WL101 N744h]
QP361.N58 1975   612'.8   74-12411
ISBN 0-07-046848-6

THE HUMAN NERVOUS SYSTEM
Basic Principles of Neurobiology

5 6 7 8 9 0 VHVH 7 9

To Eleanor and TEPP

CONTENTS

Preface to the Second Edition ix

Preface to the First Edition x

On Terminology xii

1 The brain: gross anatomy, blood
  supply, and meninges 1

2 Basic microscopic anatomy 44

3 Basic neurophysiology 77

4 Development and growth of the
  nervous system 109

5 The spinal cord 133

6 The autonomic nervous system 191

7 The cranial nerves 217

8 The brainstem: medulla, pons,
  and midbrain 241

9 Cerebellum 289

10 The ear, auditory system, and
   vestibular system 305

11 Hypothalamus 327

12 The optic system 345

13 The sensory systems and the
   thalamus 385

14 The somatic motor systems and
   the basal ganglia 407

15 The olfactory system and the
   limbic system 427

16 The cerebral cortex 443

Atlas 1 The brainstem 481

Atlas 2 The brainstem in Nissl preparations 491

Index 509

PREFACE TO THE SECOND EDITION

This second edition is the culmination of the efforts of a neuro-anatomist and a medical illustrator to incorporate many of the recent significant advances in basic neurobiology into the general format of the first edition. Special attention has been directed to the organization of a concise account of the subject matter. Thus the information contained in the current explosive expansion of the neurobiologic literature cannot be presented comprehensively. New drawings illustrate many recent findings and modern concepts. An atlas of Nissl-stained sections of the human brain has been added. For the photographs comprising this atlas, we are indebted to Dr. Sven O. E. Ebbesson and Miss Linda Small of the University of Virginia at Charlottesville.

Only a sampling of the articles of the hundreds of investigators whose researches have contributed important data and concepts to this discipline are included in the bibliographies accompanying each chapter. The cited literature has been selected to include handbooks, monographs, reviews, and general sources as well as a few original research papers. Many of the references contain informative articles on topics discussed in chapters in addition to the one in which they are included. Many of the books listed in Chapter 1 contain comprehensive bibliographies. Valuable sources with articles on a broad spectrum of subjects are *The Neurosciences* (1967, 1970, 1974) and *Neurosciences Research Program* (1966 to date). These are cited in Chapter 3.

We especially appreciate Mrs. Ruth Gutmann's valuable editorial advice and assistance during the preparation of the manuscript. For their help and suggestions, we wish to thank Drs. Elizabeth Taber-Pierce, Malcolm B. Carpenter, Fred A. Mettler, and Manuel Rivera-Dominguez. For their constructive and detailed comments, we are most grateful to Professors Maurice Arnold and Colin Hinrichsen of the University of New South Wales, Australia. In addition, we are thankful for the efforts of Miss Jean Walsh, Mrs. Eileen McEvoy, and Mrs. Maureen Keigher. For permission to reprint some of the illustrations, we wish to thank Academic Press, Inc., American Physiological Society, Elsevier Publishing Company, S. Karger A. G., Prentice-Hall, Inc., and The Readers Digest Association.

Charles R. Noback
Robert J. Demarest

PREFACE TO THE FIRST EDITION

This textbook is the product of the combined efforts of a neuro-anatomist and a medical illustrator to present the basic elements of the structure and function of the human nervous system. All the illustrations are original although some ideas incorporated in the drawings have come from others. Among the features of this book which the authors regard as particularly valuable are the following:

1 Descriptions of the brain emphasize those structural relationships leading to a three-dimensional visualization of the brain.

2 Fundamentals of neurophysiology, neural processing, and feedback circuits are outlined.

3 Significant tracts and pathways are illustrated in variations of the same basic drawing, permitting the reader to orient himself more rapidly.

4 The neuroanatomy of the lower brainstem (medulla, pons, and midbrain) is described and analyzed as a unit in one chapter.

5 The ascending "sensory" pathways are reviewed in conjunction with the discussion of the thalamus (Chapter 13); the descending "motor" pathways are reviewed with the presentation of the basal ganglia (Chapter 14).

To produce a volume of the desired limited length, the material was organized to stress fundamental principles and the more significant aspects of this complex subject. Because a complete analysis of some topics is beyond the scope of this text, they are developed from a specific point of view. The author assumes the responsibility for what some may consider to be important omissions. This is not a reference book; therefore the bibliography was selected to include only a few pertinent references from diverse sources. Many of these references, however, contain exhaustive bibliographies.

Both the subject matter and the illustrations were selected to be of value to *1* the medical specialist who wishes to refresh his knowledge of modern neuroanatomy, *2* the medical student who needs an introduction to this seemingly elusive subject, and *3* the psychologist, paramedical specialist, or biologist who wants to familiarize himself with those topics in the fields of neuroanatomy and neurophysiology of specific interest to him. We hope that others will find the book helpful in their particular areas of study.

For their valuable suggestions, we wish to thank Drs. Malcolm B. Carpenter, Dominick P. Purpura, Joyce E. Shriver, Richard Bunge, and Norman Strominger. We are grateful for the help of Mrs. Marie Kelly, Mrs. Charlotte Breitung, Mrs. Caroline Malinowski, Mrs. Jean Kelly, and Miss Joyce Thomas. We also wish to thank the publisher for whole-hearted support and constructive efforts toward the realization of this book.

Charles R. Noback
Robert J. Demarest

ON TERMINOLOGY

The long axis through the brain and spinal cord is called the *neur-axis*. It takes the form of a T, the vertical axis being a line passing through the entire spinal cord and brainstem (medulla, pons, and midbrain) and the horizontal axis being a line extending from the frontal pole to the occipital pole of the cerebrum (Chap. 1, Fig. 1-1). In essence, the cerebral axis is oriented at a right angle to the long axis of the brainstem-spinal cord axis. The bend in the axis occurs at the junction of the midbrain and the diencephalon (Chap. 1).

The term *rostral* ("toward the beak") means in the direction of the cerebrum. *Caudal* means in the direction of the coccygeal region. These terms are used in relation to the neuraxis, not the body. In this usage, the cerebrum is rostral to the brainstem and the frontal pole of the cerebrum is rostral to the diencephalon.

Coronal sections are those cut at right angles to the neuraxis; thus a coronal section of the cerebrum is at right angles to a coronal section of the brainstem or spinal cord. *Horizontal sections* are those cut parallel to the neuraxis. Horizontal sections through the cerebrum are cut from the frontal pole to the occipital pole, parallel to a plane passing through both eyes. Horizontal sections through the brainstem and spinal cord are cut rostrocaudally parallel to the front and back of the neuraxis. A *sagittal section* is cut in a vertical plane along the midline; it divides the central nervous system into two symmetric right and left halves. Midsagittal is sometimes used for sagittal. Parasagittal sections, then, are also in the vertical plane but lateral to the sagittal section.

Within the central nervous system, a group or column of cell bodies and dendrites of neurons is variously known as a *nucleus, ganglion, lamina, body, cortex,* or *center. Afferent* (or *-petal,* as in centripetal) refers to bringing to or into a structure such as a nucleus; afferent is often used for sensory. *Efferent* (or *-fugal,* as in centrifugal) refers to going away from a structure such as a nucleus; efferent is often used for motor.

Bundles of nerve fibers in the central nervous system which are characterized by anatomic or functional criteria are called by such terms as *tract, fasciculus, brachium, peduncle, column, lemniscus, commissure, ansa,* or *capsule.* A *commissure* is a bundle of fibers crossing the midline at right angle to the neuraxis, often interconnecting similar structures on each side. A *decussation* refers to fibers crossing the midline either at right angles or obliquely. *Contralateral* refers to the opposite side; it is used primarily to indicate, for example, that pain is lost or paralysis occurs on the side opposite to that of the lesion. *Ipsilateral* refers to the same side; it is used primarily to indicate, for example, that pain is lost or paralysis occurs on the same side as that of the lesion.

A *modality* refers to the quality of a stimulus and the resulting forms of sensation (e.g., touch, pain, sounds, vision). Some pathways (tracts, nuclei, or areas of cortex) are *somatotopically* (*topographically*) organized; specific portions of these structures are associated with restricted regions of the body. For example, *1* fibers conveying position sense from the hand are in definite locations within the posterior columns (ascending sensory pathway), and *2* certain areas of the motor cortex regulate movements of the thumb. Some structures of the visual pathways are topographically related to specific regions within the retina (retinotopic organization), and similarly some structures of the auditory pathways are organized functionally with respect to different frequencies or tones (tonotopic organization).

THE HUMAN NERVOUS SYSTEM

CHAPTER 1
THE BRAIN: GROSS ANATOMY,
BLOOD SUPPLY, AND MENINGES

The average adult brain weighs about 1,400 Gm (3 lb), or approximately 2 percent of the total body weight. This semisolid, pinkish-gray organ is invested by a succession of three membranes called *meninges* and is protected by an outer rigid capsule, the bony skull. The meninges are, from the brain outward, the *pia mater, arachnoid,* and *dura mater.* The brain floats in a fluid; this *cerebrospinal fluid* (*CSF*) supports the soft delicate brain and acts as a shock absorber against external blows on the head. The CSF is located within the subarachnoid space (between the pia mater and the arachnoid) and within the ventricular cavities deep in the brain. The major arteries and veins which supply the brain are associated with the meninges.

The brain has a gelatinous consistency because its soft nervous tissues are held together and supported by only a meager connective tissue matrix. Because of the paucity of connective tissue, brain tissue cannot be sutured. As a result, neurosurgeons generally use an aspirator instead of a scalpel to excise pieces of damaged brain tissue, and an electric cautery or inert silver clips instead of surgical sutures to control bleeding.

Neurosurgery may be performed under local anesthesia, in part, because the brain is insensitive when directly stimulated; it has no sensory receptors. In contrast, the meninges and the blood vessels, which are innervated by sensory nerves, are sensitive to "pain" stimuli.

Basic subdivisions of the brain

The brain, or *encephalon,* is conventionally divided into five major divisions: telencephalon or endbrain, diencephalon or inter- (twixt-) brain, mesencephalon or midbrain, metencephalon or afterbrain, and myelencephalon or medulla oblongata. The *telencephalon* and the *diencephalon* form the *prosencephalon,* or forebrain. The *metencephalon* and *myelencephalon* form the *rhombencephalon,* or hindbrain. The *metencephalon* comprises the pons and cerebellum. The *cerebrum* includes the telencephalon, diencephalon, and upper midbrain.

The cerebrum is partially divided into two halves—the cerebral hemispheres—by the deep vertical *longitudinal fissure.* A *cerebral hemisphere* is one-half of the forebrain (Table 4-1). The cerebral hemispheres include such telencephalic structures as the cerebral cortex, white matter deep to the cortex, the basal ganglia, and the corpus callosum. A cerebral hemisphere is less than half the cerebrum, for it does not include the diencephalon and the midbrain. The *ventricular system* is a continuum of cavities within the brain filled with cerebrospinal fluid. It is subdivided as follows: the lateral ventricles are the cavities of the cerebral hemispheres, the third ventricle is the cavity of the diencephalon, the cerebral aqueduct (iter or aqueduct of Sylvius) is the cavity of the mesencephalon, and the fourth ventricle is the cavity of the rhombencephalon. The *cerebellum* is the expanded dorsal portion of the metencephalon.

The *brainstem* is a collective term for the diencephalon, mesencephalon, and rhombencephalon exclusive of the cerebellum. (The diencephalon is sometimes not included with the brainstem.) The brainstem is the part of the brain which remains after the cerebral hemispheres and the cerebellum are removed. The brainstem is subdivided by its topographic relation to the tentorium (Figs. 1-2 and 1-29) into the *supratentorial* and *infratentorial divisions.*

The diencephalon is the supratentorial division, and the midbrain, pons, and medulla oblongata form the infratentorial division. All the cranial nerves, except the olfactory and optic nerves, emerge from the infratentorial brainstem. The pons and the medulla are also called the *bulb*. Often, the infratentorial division is called the brainstem.

Topography of the outer surface of the brain and of the medial surface of the midsagittally sectioned brain

Each *cerebral hemisphere* is conventionally divided into six lobes: frontal, parietal, occipital, temporal, central (insula or island of Reil), and limbic. The cerebral cortex, or the gray matter on the surface of the cerebrum, is marked by slitlike incisures called *sulci*. The raised ridges are called *gyri*. The patterns formed by the sulci and gyri are variable, with no two brains having precisely identical patterns; not even the two hemispheres of one brain have the same pattern. Gyri and sulci are a manifestation of the great size and complexity of the cerebral cortex, whose surface area, including that exposed to the sulcal depressions, totals over 2 sq ft. A cerebral cortex with gyri and sulci is called a *gyrencephalic cortex*. Two-thirds of the cortical surface area faces the sulcal spaces. In primate evolution, the tremendous increase in the volume of the cortex was accompanied not by a proportional increase in the thickness of the cortex but rather by an increase in the cortical area (two-dimensional expansion). The resulting "buckling" produces gyri and sulci. These surface markings are useful descriptive landmarks but are of limited functional significance.

LATERAL ASPECT OF THE CEREBRAL HEMISPHERE (Fig. 1-1)

Several major sulci are boundaries which divide the cerebral cortex into lobes. In turn, the lobes are subdivided by secondary and tertiary sulci into gyri. The "end" of each of three lobes is called a pole, viz., *frontal pole, temporal pole,* and *occipital pole.*

The boundaries of the frontal, parietal, temporal, and occipital lobes on the lateral surface of the cerebral hemispheres are the *lateral sulcus (lateral fissure of Sylvius), central sulcus of Rolando,* and the *parieto-occipital line.* The lateral sulcus comprises a short stem and the horizontal, ascending, and posterior rami (Fig. 16-1). The *stem of the lateral sulcus* is located between the frontal and temporal lobes and reaches the basal surface of the hemisphere. The stem continues as the *posterior ramus,* which is located between the frontal and parietal lobes above and the temporal lobe below. The *horizontal* and *ascending rami* of the lateral sulcus extend for a short distance into the frontal lobe. Deep in the lateral sulcus is the *central lobe (insula)*; it is hidden from a surface view.

The central sulcus extends from the medial surface with a forward slope to just short of the lateral sulcus.

The parieto-occipital line parallels the parieto-occipital sulcus, a prominent landmark on the medial surface.

The *frontal lobe* is located rostral to the central sulcus. The *parietal lobe* lies between the central sulcus and the parieto-occipital line. The *occipital lobe* is located posterior to the parieto-occipital line and sulcus. The *temporal lobe* lies below the lateral sulcus and rostral to the parieto-occipital line. The boundaries separating the parietal, occipital, and temporal lobes on the lateral surface of the hemisphere are not precise or meaningful.

The large frontal lobe is indented by three major sulci: the *precentral sulcus* and the *superior and inferior frontal sulci.* These sulci divide the frontal lobe into the *precentral gyrus* (known as the *motor cortex*) and the *superior, middle,* and *inferior frontal gyri.* These gyri extend onto the medial aspect of the hemisphere. The ascending and horizontal rami of the lateral sulcus subdivide the inferior frontal gyrus into the *pars opercularis, pars triangularis,* and *pars orbitalis.* The opercular and triangular parts are called *Broca's speech area.*

The parietal lobe has two major sulci—the *postcentral sulcus* and the *intraparietal sulcus.* These divide the lobe into the postcentral gyrus and two lobules, called the *superior and inferior parietal lobules.* The inferior parietal lobule is

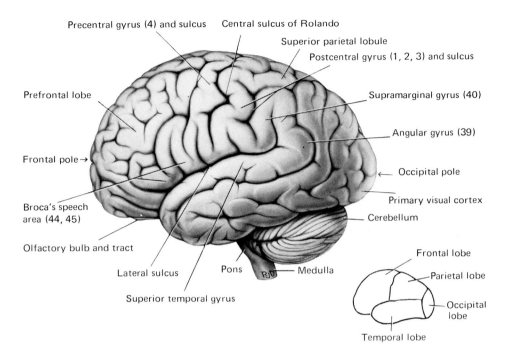

Precentral gyrus (4) and sulcus

Central sulcus of Rolando

Superior parietal lobule

Postcentral gyrus (1, 2, 3) and sulcus

Prefrontal lobe

Supramarginal gyrus (40)

Angular gyrus (39)

Frontal pole →

← Occipital pole

Primary visual cortex

Broca's speech area (44, 45)

Cerebellum

Olfactory bulb and tract

Lateral sulcus

Pons

Medulla

Superior temporal gyrus

Frontal lobe

Parietal lobe

Occipital lobe

Temporal lobe

FIGURE 1-1
Lateral surface of the brain.

Numbers refer to Brodmann's areas.

further subdivided into a *supramarginal gyrus* and an *angular gyrus*. The occipital lobe is divided by secondary occipital sulci into several unnamed gyri.

The temporal lobe has two sulci which form boundaries of three gyri. These include the *superior and inferior sulci* and the *superior, middle, and inferior gyri*. On the upper face of the temporal lobe facing the lateral sulcus are the *transverse temporal gyri of Heschl*, which extend medially toward the central lobe.

Buried deep in the lateral sulcus is the *central lobe*. It is surrounded by a *circular sulcus*. Oblique, short (in the rostral insula), and long (in the posterior insula) gyri subdivide the insular cortex. A tongue of insula extends medially to the anterior perforated substance; it is called the *limen insula*.

MEDIAL ASPECT OF THE CEREBRAL HEMISPHERE

The medial aspect of the cerebral hemisphere can be subdivided into the limbic lobe and portions of the frontal, parietal, and occipital lobes (Figs. 1-2 to 1-4). The *limbic lobe* is the ring of cortex and associated structures surrounding the central core of the cerebrum. It comprises the

septal cortex (paraterminal body and parolfactory area), cingulate gyrus, indusium griseum, fasciolar gyrus, parahippocampal gyrus, dentate gyrus, and hippocampal formation (Figs. 1-4, 15-2). The limbic cortex is significant, for it is the old cortex which has its evolutional rudiment in the reptiles, amphibians, and fish. The *cortex* of the *limbic lobe* comprises the *archicortex, paleocortex,* and *mesocortex* (Chap. 15). The *neocortex,* which is the cerebral cortex exclusive of the limbic cortex, is the phylogenetically new cortex (Chap. 16). It is the exclusive possession of the mammals, though there is a rudimentary neocortex in reptiles.

The line of the cingulate sulcus, the anterior portion of the collateral sulcus, and the rhinal sulcus, is roughly the border between neocortex and limbic cortex. The parahippocampal sulcus is a fissure of the limbic lobe located within the temporal lobe (Fig. 1-4). The central sulcus (of Rolando) partially divides the paracentral

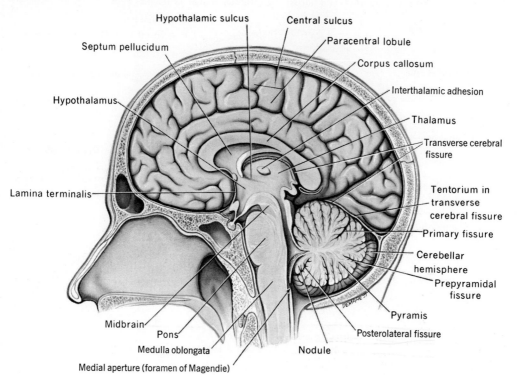

FIGURE 1-2
Median sagittal section of the brain and part of
the head.

lobule, which is continuous with the precentral
gyrus and the postcentral gyrus on the lateral surface. The parieto-occipital sulcus is the boundary
between the occipital and the parietal lobes.
The calcarine sulcus marks the boundary between the cuneus and the lingual gyrus. The taut
extension of the inner dura mater, called the
tentorium, is located between the occipital lobe
(which it helps to support) and the cerebellum.

TELENCEPHALIC STRUCTURES VISIBLE FROM
MIDSAGITTAL ASPECT

The *corpus callosum* is a bundle of nerve fibers
that traverses the midplane (commissure), interconnecting the neocortex of one hemisphere

with that of the other hemisphere (Fig. 1-2). The
corpus callosum is divided into the *rostrum,
genu, body,* and *splenium* (Fig. 15-2). The genu
and the U-shaped bundles of callosal fibers
radiating to the frontal lobe form the forceps
minor. The splenium and the callosal fibers radiating to the occipital lobe form the forceps
major. The genu blends into the rostrum, which
is continuous with the lamina terminalis. Some
callosal fibers, called the tapetum, radiate laterally and inferiorly to form a thin sheet on the
outer border of the inferior and posterior horns
of the lateral ventricle. On the upper surface of
the corpus callosum is a vestigial thin layer of
gray matter called the *indusium griseum,* in
which are two bilateral pairs of fiber strands,
called the *medial and lateral longitudinal striae*
(Fig. 15-4). These structures are continuous rostrally with the septal region and caudally with
the fasciolar gyrus; the latter extends into the
dentate gyrus (Chap. 15).

The *anterior commissure* is a bundle of the

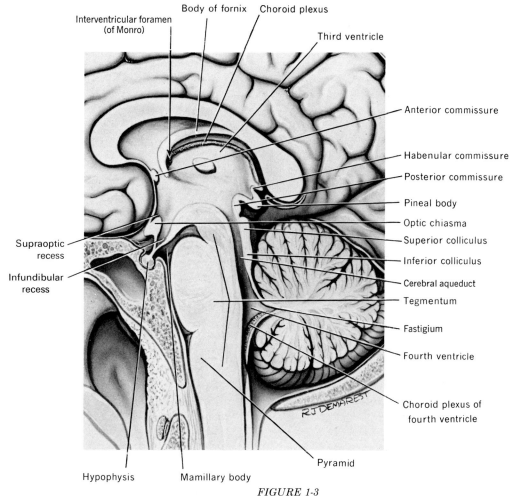

Interventricular foramen
(of Monro)

Body of fornix

Choroid plexus

Third ventricle

Anterior commissure

Habenular commissure

Posterior commissure

Pineal body

Optic chiasma

Superior colliculus

Inferior colliculus

Cerebral aqueduct

Tegmentum

Fastigium

Fourth ventricle

Supraoptic
recess

Infundibular
recess

RJDEMAREST

Choroid plexus of
fourth ventricle

Pyramid

Hypophysis

Mamillary body

FIGURE 1-3
Median sagittal section of the brainstem.

limbic lobe and of part of the temporal lobe neocortex.

The lamina terminalis is a thin plate of neural tissue that forms the anterior boundary of the third ventricle. The median telencephalon includes the anterior commissure, the lamina terminalis, and the neural tissue in front of a line from the interventricular foramen (of Monro) to the optic chiasma. (The interventricular foramen is for the passage of cerebrospinal fluid from the lateral ventricle of a cerebral hemisphere to the third ventricle.)

The fornix (seen only in part) is a bundle of fibers forming an arc from the hippocampus (archicortex) to the mamillary body of the diencephalon (Fig. 1-3).

The septum pellucidum consists of paired thin plates in the midplane extending from the corpus callosum to the fornix. The midline slit between the two septa of the septum pellucidum is the self-contained cavum septum pellucidum; it is not connected to the ventricular system or to a subarachnoid space.

The transverse cerebral fissure separates the

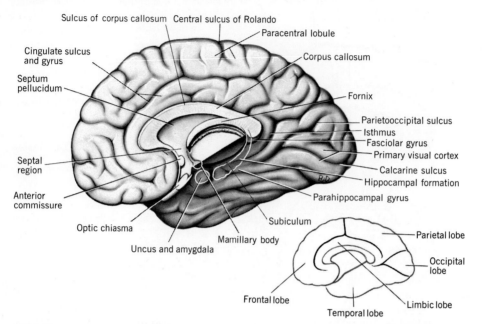

FIGURE 1-4
Median surface of the cerebral hemispheres.

The amygdaloid body and the hippocampus are outlined by white lines. The subcortical amygdaloid body is located within the uncus. The hippocampus and dentate gyrus are located in the floor of the temporal horn of the lateral ventricle (see Fig. 1-5).

thalamus, midbrain, and cerebellum, located below, from the cerebral hemispheres (Fig. 1-2).

The *tentorium* is primarily located between the cerebellum and the occipital lobes (see Fig. 1-2 and "Meninges," further on in this chapter).

The *velum interpositum* is the fold of pia mater occupying the transverse cerebral fissure between the diencephalon and corpus callosum (caudal to the interventricular foramen; see Fig. 1-29 and "Meninges").

BASAL VIEW OF THE CEREBRAL HEMISPHERE

The *frontal lobe* is demarcated by the olfactory sulcus, which extends parallel to the medial border, and an irregular group called the *orbital sulci*. The *gyrus rectus* is located medial to the

olfactory sulcus; the orbital gyri are located among the orbital sulci.

The rhinal sulcus and the collateral sulcus may be discontinuous or continuous. The *rhinal sulcus* separates the neocortex, located laterally, from the older paleocortex, located medially. The *collateral sulcus* forms the boundary between the parahippocampal gyrus and the occipitotemporal gyrus. The latter gyri may be further divided into a medial and lateral occipitotemporal gyrus by the occipitotemporal sulcus. The medial bulge in the most anterior portion of the parahippocampal gyrus is the *uncus*, which is located near the incisura of the tentorium.

FUNCTIONAL SUBDIVISIONS OF THE NEOCORTEX

The general functional significance of various portions of the cerebral neocortex is schematically outlined in Chap. 16. The frontal lobe is subdivided into (1) the precentral gyrus (including part of the paracentral lobule), (2) the cortical area in front of the precentral gyrus, and (3) the prefrontal "lobe" (most anterior expansion).

The precentral gyrus has a motor function and hence is called the *motor cortex*. If it is stimulated electrically, precise movements can be elicited in the conscious patient. For example, a patient responds to cortical stimulation by moving his finger because he says he had to move it.

The area in front of the precentral gyrus, also associated with motor activities, is called the *premotor area*. The portion of the premotor area in the vicinity of the ascending ramus (the inferior frontal gyrus) of the lateral sulcus, known as *Broca's speech area*, has a role in the motor aspects of vocalization.

The *prefrontal lobe* has a role in such subtle expressions as anxiety, placidity, drive, and concern with social attitudes. The prefrontal lobe is structurally and functionally integrated with the anterior temporal lobe. Intractable visceral pain may be alleviated by bilateral prefrontal lobotomy (disconnection of the prefrontal cortex by surgical transection of its nerve fibers).

The parietal, occipital, and temporal lobes may be functionally subdivided into primary receptive and association areas. The postcentral gyrus and the posterior portion of the paracentral lobule are known as the primary receptive area for the general senses, including touch, pressure, and others. The *transverse gyri of Heschl*, located in the upper part of the temporal lobe in the depth of the lateral cerebral sulcus, constitute the primary receptive area for audition. The cortex on either side of the calcarine fissure (including portions of the cuneus and lingual gyrus) is known as the primary receptive area for vision. The remaining parts of the neocortex in these lobes are called the association areas. These association areas are essential to such general sensations as the recognition and comprehension of weight, shape, texture, and form, and to the elaboration of the sensations of vision and audition (e.g., recognition of the written and spoken word). No solid evidence exists relating specific regions of the cortex with learning or creative ability. The temporal lobe is associated with memory.

The cerebral cortex has been subdivided into areas by the use of microscopic anatomic criteria (cytoarchitecture). The numbered areas proposed by Brodmann are often used (Figs. 16-3, 16-4): precentral gyrus or motor cortex as area 4, premotor cortex as areas 6 and 8, precentral gyrus or general sensory cortex as areas 1, 2, and 3, the primary receptive area for vision as area 17, and the primary receptive area for audition as comprising areas 41 and 42.

Medial aspect of the diencephalon, mesencephalon, metencephalon, and myelencephalon

DIENCEPHALON

The *diencephalon* is surrounded laterally and dorsally by the cerebral hemispheres. Its ventral aspect is exposed (Fig. 1-5). It is continuous caudally with the midbrain. In the median view (Fig. 1-3), the perimeter of the diencephalon includes, in order, the choroid plexus of the third ventricle, habenular commissure, pineal body, posterior commissure (roof), a hypothetic line from the posterior commissure to the mamillary bodies (caudal margin), mamillary bodies, tuber cinereum, hypophysis (pituitary gland), and optic chiasma (floor), and the line from the optic chiasma to the interventricular foramen (anterior margin). The midsagittal plane of the diencephalon is occupied by the slitlike third ventricle, which is the central canal of the diencephalon. Note that the choroid plexus of the third ventricle is continuous through each interventricular foramen with the choroid plexus of each lateral ventricle of the cerebral hemispheres. Each choroid plexus is composed of extensions of the pia mater and its vascular network which are covered by the cuboidal epithelial cells of the ependyma lining the ventricular cavity.

Three of the four subdivisions of the diencephalon are visible in a midsagittal view of the brain: epithalamus, thalamus (dorsal thalamus), and hypothalamus. The subthalamus is not visible in this view.

The *epithalamus* is the narrow band on the roof of the diencephalon, including the stria medullaris thalami (which parallels the entire attachment of the choroid plexus), habenula, habenular commissure, pineal body, and poste-

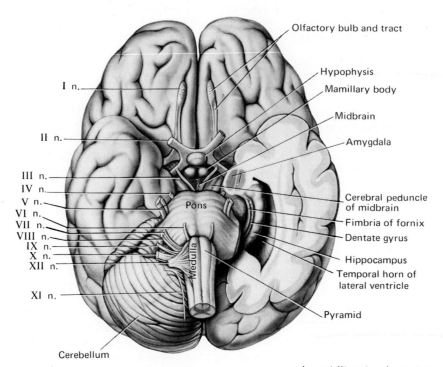

Olfactory bulb and tract
Hypophysis
Mamillary body
Midbrain
Amygdala
Cerebral peduncle of midbrain
Fimbria of fornix
Dentate gyrus
Hippocampus
Temporal horn of lateral ventricle
Pyramid

I n.
II n.
III n.
IV n.
V n.
VI n.
VII n.
VIII n.
IX n.
X n.
XII n.
XI n.

Pons
Medulla
Cerebellum

FIGURE 1-5
Basal surface of the brain.

A horizontal section has been made through the right temporal and occipital lobes, exposing the hippocampus, dentate gyrus, fornix, and temporal horn of the lateral ventricle. n., cranial nerve.

rior commissure; the first three are associated with the limbic system (Chap. 15). The function of the pineal body is discussed in Chap. 11. The posterior commissure is associated with reflexes of the optic system.

The *thalamus,* the largest subdivision of the diencephalon, is located above the hypothalamic sulcus. The thalamus is the major integrative station that is intercalated between many subcortical structures and the cerebral cortex. For example, all sensory impulses, except those of olfaction, are relayed to the thalamus before reaching the cerebral cortex. The interthalamic adhesion is merely a site of secondary fusion (soft commissure) of the dorsal thalamus across

the midline in about 70 percent of brains. The *hypothalamus* is located below the hypothalamic sulcus and includes the floor structures. Through the optic chiasma pass the fibers from the eyes to the brain. The hypothalamus contains the highest integrative centers of the autonomic nervous system; it is involved in such functional activities as the regulation of body temperature, emotional expressions, and endocrine gland activities. The hypophysis, or pituitary gland, is the master endocrine gland.

The *subthalamus,* which flanks the hypothalamus laterally and hence is not visible, is a significant subcortical station in the motor activities of voluntary muscles.

MESENCEPHALON, METENCEPHALON, AND MYELENCEPHALON

These segments of the brainstem have similar basic features; each has a roof, a central canal (ventricular system), a tegmental portion, and a basilar portion. The *tegmentum* of the brainstem comprises some structures functionally integrated into somatic and visceral reflex activities, into ascending systems associated with conscious and unconscious afferent pathways, and into descending systems associated with autonomic and somatic motor activities. The *basilar portion of the brainstem* consists of descending pathways originating in the cerebral cortex, including the corticospinal, corticobulbar, and corticopontine-pontocerebellar pathways. Thus the basilar portion consists of cortically derived structures.

Mesencephalon (Midbrain)   The roof consists of the *lamina quadrigemina* (*tectum*), which includes a pair of *superior colliculi* (*optic system*) and a pair of *inferior colliculi* (*auditory system*). Caudal to the inferior colliculus is the exit for the fourth cranial nerve (trochlear nerve). Rostral to the superior colliculus is a small region called the pretectum. The *posterior commissure*, located at the junction between the midbrain (pretectum) and the diencephalon, is composed of fibers interconnecting several tectal nuclei. A small *intercollicular commissure*, located at the level of the inferior colliculi, interconnects the nuclei of the inferior colliculus. The central canal is the *cerebral aqueduct* which extends from the third ventricle to the fourth ventricle. The midbrain tegmentum is prominent. The basilar portion comprises paired crura cerebri. The tegmentum and crura form the cerebral peduncles. Between the two peduncles is the interpeduncular fossa; the rootlets of the oculomotor (third) cranial nerve emerge from the base of the midbrain into the *interpeduncular fossa*. The *substantia nigra* is located between the tegmentum and the crura cerebri. The *cerebral peduncle* is composed of the midbrain tegmentum, substantia nigra, and crus cerebri (Fig. 8-10); stated otherwise, the cerebral peduncle is one-half of the midbrain, excluding the tectum.

Metencephalon (Pons)   The roof is basically the cerebellum and the part of the choroid plexus of the fourth ventricle. The canal is the rostral half of the fourth ventricle. The tegmentum is continuous with that of the midbrain and the medulla. The basilar portion is the *pons proper*.

Myelencephalon (Medulla oblongata)   The roof consists of the rest of the choroid plexus of the fourth ventricle. The apex of the roof of the fourth ventricle extending into the cerebellum is called the *fastigium*. The canal is the caudal half of the fourth ventricle and its caudal continuation is the central canal of the medulla and spinal cord. The tegmentum comprises the bulk of the medulla. The basilar portion is the pyramids.

The boundaries between any two divisions of the brainstem are not defined precisely. The boundary between the diencephalon and the mesencephalon is a plane passing through the posterior commissure and the caudal aspect of the mamillary bodies; that between the mesencephalon and the metencephalon is a plane passing caudal to the fourth cranial nerve and the rostral border of the pons; that between the metencephalon and the myelencephalon is a plane passing through the eighth cranial nerve and the caudal border of the pons; and that between the myelencephalon and the spinal cord is roughly a transverse plane in the region between the caudal end of the twelfth cranial nerve and the first cervical nerve in the vicinity of the foramen magnum.

Basal aspect of the brain

The telencephalic structures, visible in a basal view, are portions of the frontal, temporal, and occipital lobes (Figs. 1-5 and 1-6). Significant landmarks are the *rhinal sulcus* and the *collateral sulcus* (sulci delineating the limbic lobe from the neocortex, Fig. 1-4). Elements of the olfactory pathways include the olfactory nerve (first cranial nerve), olfactory bulb, olfactory tract, and the three olfactory striae (lateral, medial, and intermediate). In the region of the olfactory trigone lateral to the optic tract is the *anterior perforated substance;* it is indented and stippled by small arterial branches of the middle cerebral artery.

The diencephalic structures include the optic nerve (second cranial nerve) and optic tract of the visual system; and the hypophysis, tuber cinereum, and mamillary bodies of the hypothalamus. Two areas on the base of the brain— the *anterior perforated substance* and *posterior perforated substance*—are perforated by numerous small blood vessels (Fig. 1-5). The former is located behind the olfactory trigone adjacent to

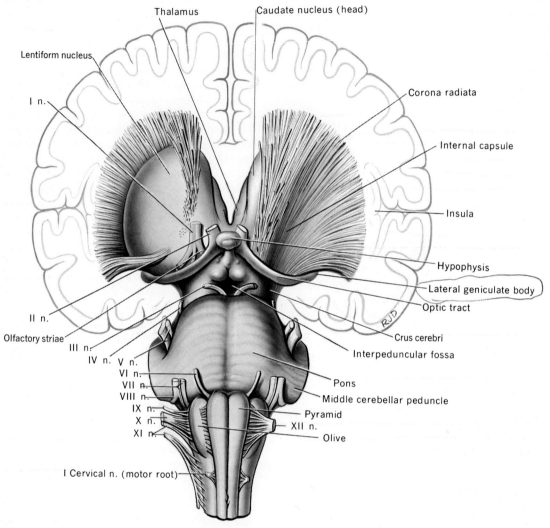

FIGURE 1-6
Basal surface of the brainstem and roots of cranial nerves.

the optic tract, and the latter is in the floor of the interpeduncular fossa of the midbrain.

The mesencephalic structures include the crura cerebri, the third cranial nerve (oculomotor nerve) emerging in the interpeduncular fossa, and the fourth (trochlear) cranial nerve.

The metencephalic structures include the pons proper, cerebellum, and fifth (trigeminal) cranial nerve. This nerve emerges on the lateral aspect of the pons. Note the sensory ganglion, sensory root, and motor root of the trigeminal nerve.

The myelencephalic (medullary) structures include the pyramids, olives, and roots of seven cranial nerves. The pyramids are formed by the fibers of the motor pyramidal tract that crosses the midline at the pyramidal decussation in the lower medulla. The *olive* is a protuberance formed by the inferior olivary nucleus (Chap. 8). The sixth (abducent), seventh (facial), and eighth (vestibulocochlear) cranial nerves emerge at the pontomedullary junction. The ninth (glossopharyngeal) and tenth (vagus) nerves emerge as a series of rootlets from the postero-lateral (postolivary) sulcus on the posterior margin of the olive. The eleventh (spinal accessory) cranial nerve emerges in the form of rootlets from the medulla (posterolateral) and from the spinal cord (between the dorsal and ventral roots of the first six cervical spinal nerves). The twelfth (hypoglossal) cranial nerve emerges from the preolivary sulcus on the anterior margin of the olive.

Note that the third, sixth, and twelfth cranial nerves emerge from the anterior aspect of the brainstem in a longitudinal line just lateral to the midsagittal plane; the fifth, seventh, ninth, tenth, and eleventh cranial nerves emerge from the lateral aspect of the brainstem.

Lateral aspect of the brainstem

Of the subdivisions of the diencephalon, only the dorsal thalamus and subthalamus extend to the lateral surface of the diencephalon adjacent to the internal capsule (Fig. 1-7). The epithalamus and hypothalamus are not visible from this view because they are medial structures bordering the third ventricle. The thalamus is the only diencephalic subdivision which extends throughout the width of the diencephalon from the internal capsule to the third ventricle.

Note the pulvinar, a posterior extension of the thalamus proper. The optic nerve, optic chiasma, optic tract, and lateral geniculate body are structures of the visual pathways (Fig. 1-7). The lateral geniculate body is a thalamic nucleus located below the pulvinar. Each *internal capsule,* which flanks the diencephalon laterally, is continuous with the crus cerebri of the midbrain and the corona radiata of the white matter of the cerebral hemisphere (see further on in this chapter, "The Brain as a Three-dimensional Structure: Solid Geometry of the Brain").

The mesencephalic structures viewed (Fig. 1-7) include the superior and inferior colliculi (or the corpora quadrigemina) and the fourth

cranial nerve (all roof structures), tegmentum, and crus cerebri of the basilar portion (see "Solid Geometry of the Brain," further on). The brachium of the superior colliculus, which extends from the lateral geniculate body of the thalamus to the superior colliculus, consists of fibers of the optic pathways. The brachium of the inferior colliculus, which extends from the inferior colliculus to the medial geniculate body of the thalamus, consists of fibers of the auditory pathways. The fourth cranial nerve is the only cranial nerve that emerges from the posterior aspect of the brainstem.

The metencephalic structures viewed include the cerebellum, pons, three brachia of the cerebellum, and fifth cranial nerve. The *superior cerebellar peduncle* (brachium conjunctivum) consists of fibers that project mainly from the cerebellum to the upper brainstem. The *middle cerebellar peduncle* (brachium pontis) of fibers that project from the pons proper to the cerebellum. The *inferior cerebellar peduncle* (restiform body) consists of a bundle that extends from the lower brainstem to the cerebellum.

The myelencephalic structures viewed include the choroid plexus, tuberculum gracilis, tuberculum cuneatus, eminentia trigemini, olive, and pyramids. The *tuberculum gracilis* and *tuberculum cuneatus* are hillocks produced by nuclei associated with ascending sensory pathways from the spinal cord. The *eminentia trigemini* (tuberculum cinereum) is a ridge produced by the spinal (descending) nucleus and tract of the fifth cranial nerve (Chap. 8).

Posterior aspect of the brainstem

The diencephalic structures viewed include the epithalamus, which is flanked laterally by the thalamus proper. The mesencephalic structures viewed include the superior and inferior colliculi and their brachia, fourth cranial nerves, and the lateral surfaces of the tegmentum and the crura cerebri (Figs. 1-8, 1-9).

The metencephalic and myelencephalic structures viewed include the three cerebellar

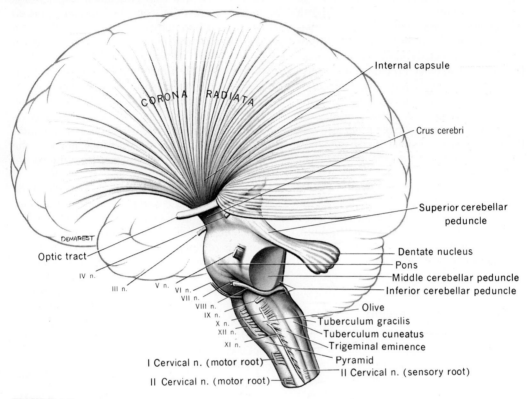

FIGURE 1-7
Lateral surface of the brainstem and roots of
cranial nerves.

peduncles and some landmarks on the floor of
the fourth ventricle. The floor is marked by a
groove, the sulcus limitans. Medial to this
groove are located the trigonum vagi and trigonum hypoglossi, and lateral to it is the area
vestibularis. The *trigonum hypoglossi* is a short
ridge formed by the underlying hypoglossal nucleus; the *trigonum vagi* is formed by the underlying motor (parasympathetic) nucleus of the
vagus nerve (Chap. 8). The *area vestibularis* is
the region of the vestibular nuclei. The *facial
(or abducent) colliculus* is a hillock formed by
the genu (Chap. 8) of the facial nerve and the
nucleus of the abducent nerve.

On the dorsal surface of the inferior medulla
are the tuberculum gracilis and tuberculum

cuneatus. Note the diamond-shaped fourth
ventricle (rhomboid fossa). The lateral recesses
of the ventricle extend laterally at the level of
the upper medulla. The eminence formed by the
dorsal cochlear nucleus lateral to the vestibular
area is the *acoustic tubercle* (Fig. 1-9). The *taenia
of the fourth ventricle* is the line of attachment
of the tela choroidea to the medulla (Fig. 1-9).
The *obex* is a fold of tissue overhanging the site
at the apex where the fourth ventricle funnels
into the central canal of the medulla; it is used
as a landmark by neurosurgeons.

Cerebellum

The cerebellum is a fissured and lobated structure which is a modulator and coordinator of
motor activities (Chap. 9). The cerebellar surface

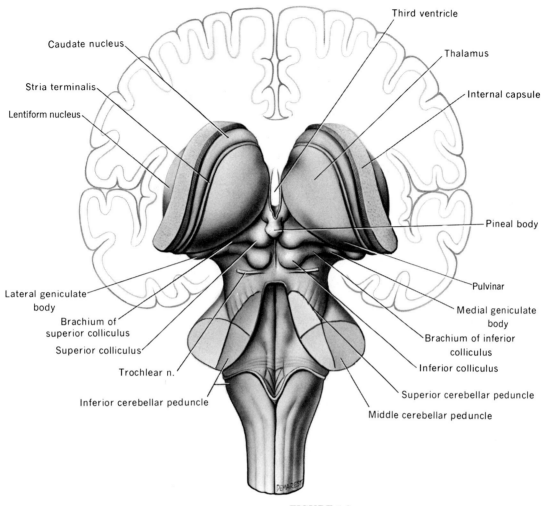

FIGURE 1-8
Dorsal surface of the brainstem.

is marked by numerous fissures separating long narrow folds called *folia.* Only one-sixth of the cerebellar cortex is exposed to the surface; five-sixths face the fissural clefts.

The contours of the lobes, lobules, and fissures of the cerebellum have been colorfully named and subdivided. Most of them have no special functional significance. Three schemas for grossly subdividing the cerebellum are helpful (Fig. 9-1).

1 The centrally placed median subdivision is the wormlike *vermis,* which is flanked laterally by the expansive cerebellar hemispheres.

2 The cerebellum consists of an anterior lobe, a middle (posterior) lobe, and a flocculonodular lobe. Each of these lobes includes portions of the vermis and the hemispheres. The *anterior lobe* is the rostral segment of the cerebellum, delineated from the posterior lobe by the primary fissure (fissura prima). The *middle lobe* consists of the rest of the cerebellum except for the small flocculonodular lobe located on the underside of the cerebellum near the brainstem.

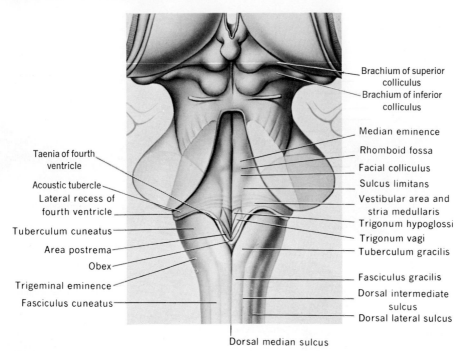

Taenia of fourth
ventricle

Acoustic tubercle

Lateral recess of
fourth ventricle

Tuberculum cuneatus

Area postrema

Obex

Trigeminal eminence

Fasciculus cuneatus

Brachium of superior
colliculus

Brachium of inferior
colliculus

Median eminence

Rhomboid fossa

Facial colliculus

Sulcus limitans

Vestibular area and
stria medullaris

Trigonum hypoglossi

Trigonum vagi

Tuberculum gracilis

Fasciculus gracilis

Dorsal intermediate
sulcus

Dorsal lateral sulcus

Dorsal median sulcus

FIGURE 1-9
Dorsal surface of the lower brainstem.

The *flocculonodular lobe* (vestibulocerebellum) consists of a small median lobule, called the *nodule of the vermis,* and of the laterally extended lobule, called the *flocculus,* of each hemisphere. The fissure delineating the middle lobe from the flocculonodular lobe is the posterolateral fissure; its medial extension was called the prenodular fissure.

3 A phylogenetically based schema subdivides the cerebellum into archicerebellum, paleocerebellum, and neocerebellum. The archicerebellum is the flocculonodular lobe. It is phylogenetically the oldest lobe of the cerebellum and is functionally associated with the vestibular system. The paleocerebellum is roughly the vermis less the nodule.

This lobe, too, is old phylogenetically; it is associated generally with fibers from the spinal cord and lower brainstem. The neocerebellum includes the cerebellar hemispheres less the flocculi. These lobes are new phylogenetically, and they are functionally associated largely with the upper brainstem and cerebrum, including the cerebral cortex.

The precise boundaries of these various divisions of the cerebellum are not defined similarly by all authorities. The surface of the cerebellum is covered by the cerebellar cortex. The *tonsil* is a lobule located on the medial inferior aspect of the cerebellum (Fig. 9-1). On the inferior surface of the cerebellum between the tonsils is a medial subarachnoid space called the *vallecula.* Deep to the cortex is a mass of nerve fibers forming the white matter (corpus medullare) of the cerebellum. Within this white matter are the four pairs of deep cerebellar nuclei, from medial to lateral: the nuclei fastigii, globosus, emboliformis, and dentatus (Chap. 9). The cerebellum is connected with the brainstem by the three cerebellar peduncles (brachia or pillars) previously noted.

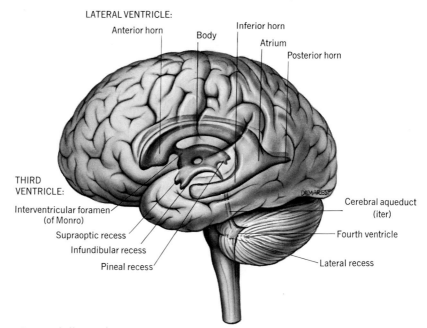

LATERAL VENTRICLE:
Anterior horn
Body
Inferior horn
Atrium
Posterior horn

THIRD VENTRICLE:
Interventricular foramen (of Monro)
Supraoptic recess
Infundibular recess
Pineal recess

Cerebral aqueduct (iter)
Fourth ventricle
Lateral recess

FIGURE 1-10
Lateral view of the ventricles of the brain.

A thin lamina—the superior medullary velum—extends rostrally from the cerebellum to the midbrain tectum; another lamina—the inferior medullary velum—extends caudally from the cerebellum to the choroid plexus of the fourth ventricle. These veli roof the fourth ventricle.

Ventricular system

The ventricular system (Figs. 1-10, 1-11) is the series of cavities within the brain, lined by the ependyma and filled with cerebrospinal fluid. Each cerebral hemisphere contains a *lateral ventricle,* each of which is connected through one of the paired interventricular foramina (of Monro) with the third ventricle of the diencephalon. The *third ventricle* is continuous with the tubelike cerebral aqueduct of the midbrain, and the latter with the large *fourth ventricle* of the pons and medulla. The *central canal* of the spinal cord joins the fourth ventricle slightly rostral to the junction of medulla and spinal cord.

The lateral ventricle is subdivided into four parts: the anterior horn, located rostral to the interventricular foramen, is in the frontal lobe;

the body, located posterior to the interventricular foramen is in the parietal lobe; the inferior or temporal horn is in the temporal lobe; and the occipital horn is in the occipital lobe. The *atrium,* or *trigone,* of the lateral ventricle is located at the junction of the temporal horn, occipital horn, and body of the ventricle.

The pia mater, which is in direct apposition with the ependymal lining of the ventricles, is known as the *tela choroidea.* The vascular cores of the choroid plexuses are located within the tela choroidea.

Each ventricle contains a *choroid plexus,* a rich network of blood vessels of the pia mater which are in contact with the ependymal lining of a ventricle. These plexuses have a role in the elaboration of the cerebrospinal fluid. The choroid plexus of each lateral ventricle is located in the body and temporal horn; it is continuous through an interventricular foramen with the choroid plexus of the third ventricle. The choroid plexus of the fourth ventricle is a T-shaped structure located in the roof of the medulla. In this roof are three foramina through which the cerebrospinal fluid escapes from the fourth ventricle into the subarachnoid space. One of these three apertures is located at one of the ends of the T. The two lateral openings are the lateral apertures (Luschka); the probable midline opening is the medial aperture (Magendie). Some choroid plexus extends through the lateral aperture into the subarachnoid space.

The brain as a three-dimensional structure: solid geometry of the brain

AXES OF THE BRAIN (Fig. 1-12)

The brain may be visualized as a geometric figure with two main axes: vertical and horizontal (Fig. 1-12). Description of the relation of the major structures of the brain to these axes is the purpose of the following schema, which outlines some pertinent aspects of the topographic anatomy of the brain. The vertical axis is the line which extends caudally from the region of the pre- and postcentral gyri through the brainstem and spinal cord. The horizontal axis extends from the frontal pole toward the occipital pole of the cerebrum; this axis bifurcates in the region deep to the angular gyrus into *1* an extension which reaches the occipital pole and *2* a recurved arc which is directed toward the temporal pole. The latter is illustrated by the broken line in Fig. 1-12.

A major pathway which parallels the vertical axis is the corticospinal (pyramidal) tract. This motor pathway originates largely from the pre- and postcentral gyri and descends successively through portions of the corona radiata, internal capsule, crus of the midbrain, pons, pyramid of the medulla, and spinal cord (Figs. 1-7, 1-16, and 5-25).

The visual pathway from the eyes to the primary visual cortex in the vicinity of the calcarine sulcus (Fig. 12-13) is oriented parallel to the horizontal axis from the frontal pole to the occipital pole. The long axis of the diencephalon

[from the interventricular foramen (of Monro) to the pineal body] is also parallel to this axis (Fig. 1-2). The lateral ventricle of the cerebral hemisphere parallels the horizontal axis and its arc into the temporal lobe (Figs. 1-10 and 1-16). The sequence of frontal lobe, parietal lobe, and temporal lobe also follows this curve. Other structures oriented to this curve are outlined below as arc structures. The archiform shape of the cerebral hemispheres and their arc structures is formed during early ontogeny. The cerebral hemispheres develop from the region in the vicinity of the interventricular foramen. From this region cells migrate rostrally to develop into the frontal lobe and caudally along the horizontal axis to the occipital pole and to the temporal pole.

The junctional region between the midbrain and diencephalon forms an angle between the infratentorial brainstem, which is oriented parallel to the vertical axis, and the diencephalon, which is oriented parallel to the horizontal axis. This is illustrated in Fig. 1-3; note that the long axis of the third ventricle and its choroid plexus are oriented approximately at a right angle to the long axis of the cerebral aqueduct and fourth ventricle and to the sequence of superior colliculus, inferior colliculus, cerebellum, and choroid plexus of the fourth ventricle.

CORE STRUCTURES AND ARC STRUCTURES

Anatomically the cerebrum may be subdivided into a group of central or core structures and a group of arc structures. The diencephalon and the lentiform nucleus are considered to be core structures located centrally in the cerebrum. Each cerebral hemisphere forms an arc, which flanks the core structures.

Knowledge of the anatomic relation of the core structures to one another is useful in identifying them in sections of the brain. In the following sequence, the core structures are listed, in order, from the most medially located third ventricle to the most laterally located cortex of the central lobe (insula). The sequence is third ventricle, diencephalon, internal capsule, lentiform nucleus (globus pallidus and putamen), external capsule, claustrum, extreme capsule, and cortex of central lobe (Figs. 1-6, 1-8, and 1-24).

The arc structures of the cerebral hemi-

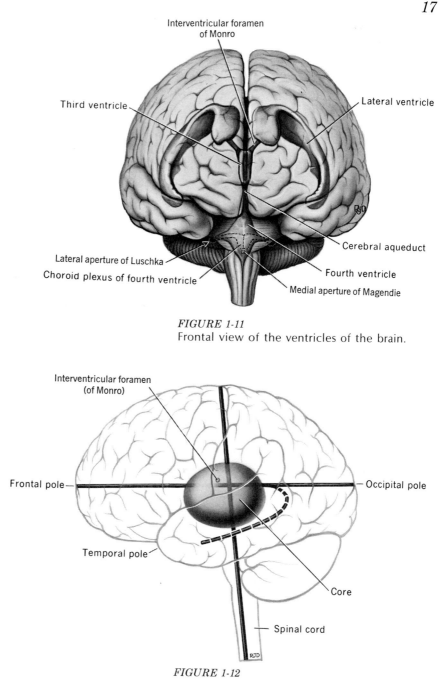

FIGURE 1-11
Frontal view of the ventricles of the brain.

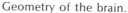

FIGURE 1-12
Geometry of the brain.

Vertical axis is parallel to the long axis of the brainstem and spinal cord. Horizontal axis is parallel to the long axis of cerebrum from frontal pole to occipital pole. For explanation of broken line, see p. 16.

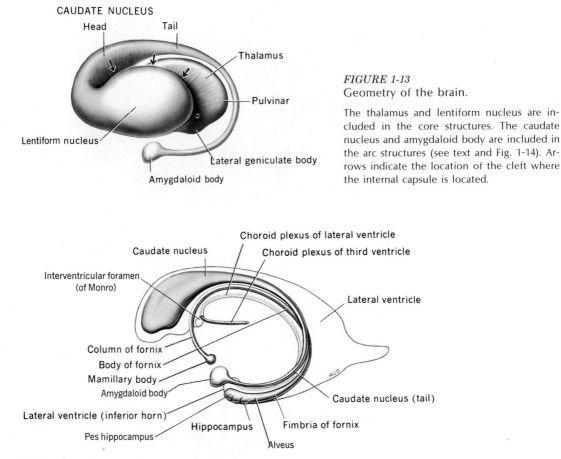

CAUDATE NUCLEUS

FIGURE 1-13
Geometry of the brain.

The thalamus and lentiform nucleus are included in the core structures. The caudate nucleus and amygdaloid body are included in the arc structures (see text and Fig. 1-14). Arrows indicate the location of the cleft where the internal capsule is located.

FIGURE 1-14
Geometry of the brain.

The horizontal axis is modified into an arc by the curved extension into the temporal lobe. Structures of the cerebral hemisphere which parallel this arc (arc structures) include the lateral ventricle, fornix-hippocampus complex, stria terminalis (not illustrated)—amygdaloid body, caudate nucleus, and choroid plexus of lateral ventricle.

spheres are illustrated in Figs. 1-10, 1-13, and 1-14. These include the *1* lateral ventricle, *2* choroid plexus of the lateral ventricle, *3* caudate nucleus, *4* sequence of hippocampus, fimbria, body, and column of the fornix and mamillary body, *5* sequence of amygdaloid body, stria terminalis, and hypothalamus (Fig. 15-3), and *6* corpus callosum (Fig. 1-2). Many of these structures form boundaries of the lateral ventricles. Because these structures curve and extend into the temporal lobe, each arc structure may be viewed twice in some sections through the cerebrum (Figs. 1-15, 1-20, 1-21, and 1-24).

Note that the anterior horn and body of the lateral ventricle and its associated arc structures are located in a sagittal plane which is medial to the internal capsule (Figs. 1-6, 1-8, 1-16, 1-20, and 1-21).

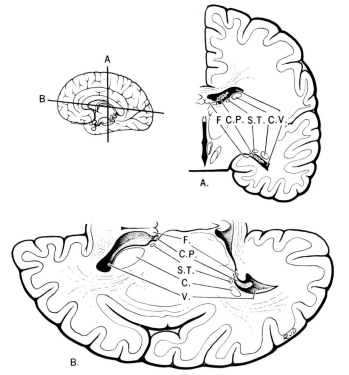

FIGURE 1-15
Sections illustrating that the arc structures may be visualized twice in a section through the cerebrum (see Fig. 1-14).

A Coronal section (see Figs. 1-20 through 1-22 for other details).

B Horizontal section (see Fig. 1-24 for other details). F., fornix; C.P., choroid plexus; S.T., stria terminalis; C., caudate nucleus; V., lateral ventricle.

The cerebrum peripheral to the core structures just noted includes the white matter deep to the cortex (subcortical white matter) and the cerebral cortex. Three general categories of fibers are present in this white matter: *1* the *projection fibers,* which project from (and to) the cortex to (and from) deep cerebral structures, brainstem, and spinal cord (most of them passing through the internal capsule); *2* the major *commissural fibers,* which originate in the cortex of one cerebral hemisphere and terminate in the cortex of the contralateral hemisphere [these are the *corpus callosum, anterior commissure,* and *fornical (hippocampal) commissure*]; and *3* the *association fibers,* which arise in the cortex of one hemisphere and terminate in the cortex of the same hemisphere.

The *corpus callosum* is the largest commissure in the brain; it interconnects most of the neocortical areas of one hemisphere with those of the other hemisphere (refer to Chap. 16). The corpus callosum comprises several portions called the rostrum, genu, body, and splenium (Fig. 15-2).

The *anterior commissure* consists of two portions. The smaller anterior portion interconnects olfactory structures of the two sides. The larger posterior portion interconnects the neocortex of the anterior aspects of the temporal lobe (neocortical areas not interconnected by the corpus callosum). In a midsagittal section of the brain the anterior commissure is seen to be located just behind the upper part of the lamina terminalis and in a plane rostral to the interventricular foramen and the column of the fornix (Fig. 1-3). As viewed from above, the anterior commissure has the form of an arc with a slight posterior curve extending laterally. It extends laterally along the inferior aspect of the globus pallidus and putamen to the inferior border of the claustrum.

The *fornical (hippocampal) commissure* consists of a few fibers interconnecting the hippocampus of both sides. They pass from the hippocampus successively through the fimbria and crus of the fornix, cross the midline as the fornical commissure, and continue through the crus and fimbria to the opposite hippocampus (archicortex).

Cerebrum as viewed in coronal sections and horizontal sections

The topographic relations of the major cerebral structures can be understood by examining the selected series of coronal sections and horizontal sections of the cerebrum (Figs. 1-15, 1-17 through 1-24). The analysis of these sections, accompanied by reference to the following five topics, should prove helpful.

BOUNDARIES OF LATERAL VENTRICLE AS VIEWED IN CORONAL SECTIONS

The *anterior horn* has a triangular outline, with the superior border formed by the corpus callosum, the medial wall by the septum pellucidum, and the posterolateral floor by the head of the caudate nucleus (Fig. 1-18).

The *body* of this ventricle has a transverse slitlike outline, with the superior border formed by the corpus callosum, the medial wall by the narrow septum pellucidum and body of the fornix, the ventral floor by the superior aspect of the thalamus, the stria and vena terminalis, and the tail of the caudate nucleus (Fig. 1-21). The choroid plexus, which is attached medially to the fornix and the tissue over the thalamus, extends into the cavity of the ventricle.

The *temporal horn* has a comma-like outline, with the superior border formed by the tail of the caudate nucleus, stria terminalis, and white matter, and the floor and medial border formed by the fimbria of the fornix, the hippocampal formation, and white matter (Fig. 1-20). The choroid plexus extends into the ventricle from

the medial aspect. The amygdaloid body forms a bulge into the rostral tip of the inferior horn.

The *posterior horn* is bordered laterally by the corpus callosum, called the *tapetum* in this region, and the white matter (Fig. 1-23).

BASAL GANGLIA

The term *basal ganglia* refers to several masses of subcortical gray matter deep in the cerebral hemispheres. These basal ganglia (telencephalic nuclei) are functionally integrated into motor activities (Chap. 14).

The basal ganglia include the caudate nucleus and the lentiform (lenticular) nucleus and, according to some authorities, the amygdaloid body (amygdaloid complex, corpus amygdaloideum) and the claustrum. The *caudate nucleus* consists of a head (floor of the anterior horn of the lateral ventricle) and a tail. The tail is long and attenuated (commencing at the level of the interventricular foramen), forming a boundary of the body and the temporal horn of the lateral ventricle (Fig. 1-14). The *lentiform* nucleus is subdivided into a medial nucleus, called the *globus pallidus* (pallidum), and a lateral nucleus called the *putamen.*

The *amygdaloid body* is located deep in the uncus rostral to the temporal horn, where it is more or less fused with the tip of the tail of the caudate nucleus.

The claustrum is a thin plate of gray matter located between the cortex of the central lobule (insula) and the putamen.

The *lentiform (lenticular) nucleus* and the *caudate nucleus* are collectively called the *corpus striatum.* The globus pallidus is referred to as the *paleostriatum,* the amygdaloid body as the *archistriatum,* and the caudate nucleus and the putamen as the *neostriatum* or *striatum.*

INTERNAL CAPSULE

The internal capsule, so named because it is internal (or medial) to the lentiform nucleus, is divided into an anterior limb, a genu, a posterior limb, a retrolentiform (postlentiform) part, and a sublentiform part (Fig. 1-24). The *anterior limb* (caudato-lenticular limb) is located between the head of the caudate nucleus and the lentiform nucleus (Fig. 1-18). The *genu* (knee) is located between the anterior and the posterior limbs—

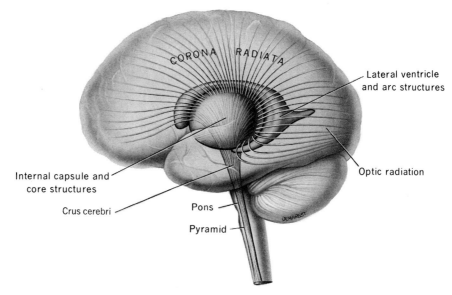

FIGURE 1-16
Geometry of the brain.

The internal capsule passes through the central core and fans out to the cerebral cortex as the corona radiata.

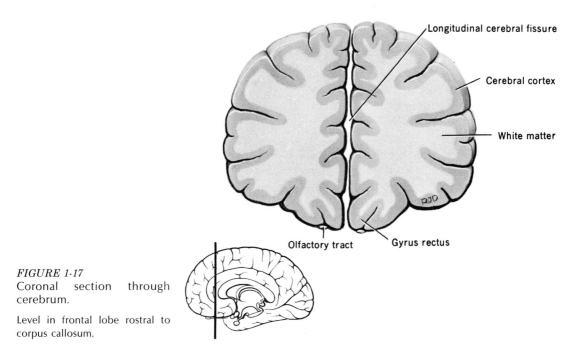

FIGURE 1-17
Coronal section through cerebrum.

Level in frontal lobe rostral to corpus callosum.

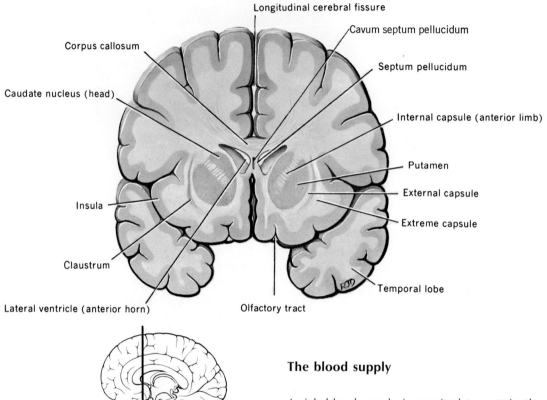

FIGURE 1-18
Coronal section through cerebrum.

Level of anterior horn of lateral ventricle and anterior
limb of internal capsule.

medial to the lentiform nucleus, posterior to the
head of the caudate nucleus, and anterior to the
thalamus (Fig. 1-19). The *posterior limb* (thalamolenticular limb) is located between the lentiform nucleus, located laterally, and the thalamus
and tail of the caudate nucleus, located medially
(Fig. 1-20). The *postlentiform part* is lateral to
the thalamus and posterior to the lentiform nucleus. The *sublentiform part* is the portion
below the lentiform nucleus. The locations of
the fiber tracts that pass through the internal
capsule are outlined in Chap. 16 (Figs. 16-9,
16-10).

The blood supply

A rich blood supply is required to sustain the
ever-active brain. The blood flow is not absolutely uniform, but it is invariably ample. Irreversible damage to the brain results when it
is deprived of its circulation for more than a few
minutes. Paradoxically the blood circulation
provides such a slight margin of physiologic
safety that consciousness is lost if the supply is
cut off for about 5 sec.

The brain requires about one-fifth of the
blood pumped by the heart (one-third of the
output of the left side of the heart), for the brain
consumes approximately 20 percent of the oxygen utilized by the body (as much as 50 percent
in the young infant). It takes about 7 sec for a
drop of blood to flow through the brain from
the internal carotid artery to the internal jugular
vein. Roughly 800 ml of blood flows through the
brain each minute, with 75 ml being present in
the brain at any moment. Approximately 50 ml

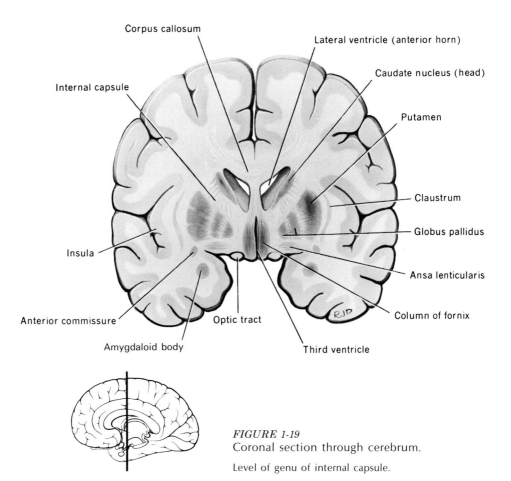

Corpus callosum

Lateral ventricle (anterior horn)

Caudate nucleus (head)

Internal capsule

Putamen

Claustrum

Globus pallidus

Insula

Ansa lenticularis

Anterior commissure

Optic tract

Column of fornix

Amygdaloid body

Third ventricle

FIGURE 1-19
Coronal section through cerebrum.

Level of genu of internal capsule.

of blood flows through 100 Gm of brain each minute. The necessity for this copious blood flow is that the brain possesses little metabolic reserve and derives its energy almost exclusively from sugar glucose. The brain utilizes about 400 Kcal a day, or about one-fifth of a 2,000-Kcal diet. Because the normal brain is never at rest, the availability of oxygen and glucose must be maintained by a constant blood flow, for the demand is the same whether one is resting, sleeping, thinking, or daydreaming.

The blood flow to the brain is largely regulated by the effect of metabolic products in the bloodstream on the vascular (arteriolar) tone of the cerebral blood vessels. For example, carbon dioxide is not only the prime physiologic driver of respiration; it is, in addition, a potent relaxant and dilator of the arterioles of the brain. In man, the role of the autonomic nervous system proper in cerebral vasodilatation is relatively minor. The delicate adjustments of the blood flow by CO_2 and other metabolites are the means by which the brain ensures that its blood flow is adequate and sufficient with respect to the normal blood pressure. The vascularity and blood flow vary in different regions of the brain. The gray matter, with its higher metabolic activity, has a richer blood supply than the white matter.

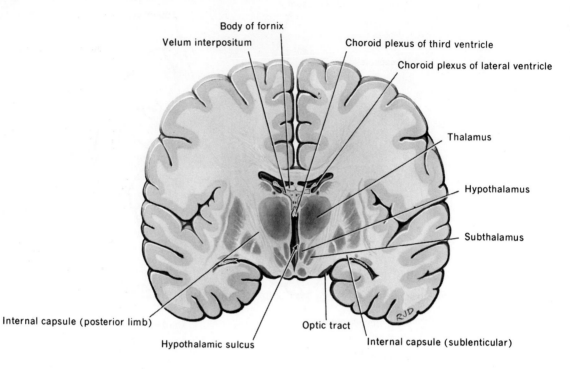

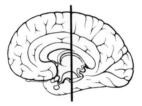

FIGURE 1-20
Coronal section through cerebrum.

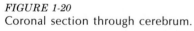

Level of body of lateral ventricle and posterior limb of
internal capsule (see Fig. 1-15).

The organism has several lines of defense so
that the brain can obtain its required oxygen:

1 Pressure receptors in the carotid sinus and
chemoreceptors in the carotid body at the bifurcation of the common carotid artery are integrated into reflexes through the respiratory and
cardiovascular centers in the medulla; these
function to maintain a constant blood flow to
the brain. Pressure (baro-) receptors are also
located in the aortic arch.

2 Autoregulatory control of the blood flow to
the brain is achieved through the response of
the smooth muscles within the cerebral vessels
to the blood pressure exerted by these vessels.
When the pressure drops, the smooth muscles
relax, the vessels dilate, and resistance to blood
flow decreases. When the pressure increases,
the smooth muscles contract, the vessels constrict, and the resistance to blood flow increases.
When the intracranial pressure increases (rise in
cerebrospinal fluid pressure), the vessels respond by dilating.

3 Metabolic control of blood flow to the brain
is most important. Cerebral vessels dilate when
the blood levels of CO_2 are high and of O_2 are
low. They constrict when the levels of CO_2 are
low and of O_2 are high.

4 When the blood flow through the brain is reduced, the brain compensates by extracting more O_2 from the available O_2 in the blood than otherwise.

5 A severe pressure drop evokes the *cerebral ischemic reflex.* Neurons in the medulla respond by stimulating the sympathetic nervous system outflow to the heart, which, in turn, increases the blood flow from the heart to the brain.

ARTERIAL SUPPLY OF THE BRAIN

The arterial blood supply to the brain is basically derived from two pairs of trunk arteries, located at the base of the brain: the *vertebral arteries* (*vertebral arterial system*) and the *internal corotid arteries* (*carotid arterial system*) (Fig. 1-25). The vertebral arteries enter the cranial cavity through the foramen magnum and become located on the anterolateral aspect of the medulla. The blood flowing through the vertebral arterial system supplies the medulla, pons, midbrain, caudal portion of the diencephalon, cerebellum, medial and inferior regions of the temporal and occipital lobes, and small variable portions of the lateral regions of the temporal, parietal, and occipital lobes. The internal carotid arteries enter the base of the cranial cavity and become located just lateral to the hypophysis of the hypothalamus. The blood flowing through the carotid arterial system will supply most of the cerebrum (including most of the diencephalon) except for that supplied by the vertebral arterial system (Fig. 1-25).

The vertebral arteries unite at the pontomedullary junction to form the basilar artery, which continues to the midbrain level, where it bifurcates into the two posterior cerebral arteries. The intracranial portion of each *vertebral artery* gives rise to the *anterior spinal artery,* the *posterior spinal artery,* the *posterior inferior cerebellar artery,* and a small meningeal branch. The branches of the basilar artery include the *labyrinthine (internal auditory) arteries,* the *anterior inferior cerebellar arteries,* small pontine branches, and the *superior cerebellar arteries.* Each posterior cerebral artery gives off a number of blood vessels to the midbrain, diencephalon, and cerebrum (temporal, occipital, and parieto-occipital branches) and a *posterior*

choroidal artery. The branches of the vertebral, basilar, and posterior cerebral arteries supply the medulla, pons, and midbrain in patterns which may be conceptually summarized as follows: the *paramedian branches* are distributed to a medial zone on either side of the midsagittal plane, the *short circumferential branches* to an anterolateral zone, and the *long circumferential branches* to a posterolateral zone and to the cerebellum (Fig. 8-21). The superior cerebellar, anterior inferior cerebellar, and posterior inferior cerebellar arteries may be considered to be long circumferential arteries.

Two small vessels from the vertebral arteries join to form the anterior spinal artery. It supplies the median zone, in which are located the pyramids, medial lemniscus, medial longitudinal fasciculus, hypoglossal nucleus and nerve, caudal portions of the dorsal motor nucleus of the vagus nerve, and solitary nucleus (Fig. 8-21). Each *posterior spinal artery* supplies the posterior region of the lower medulla, in which are located the nuclei and fasciculi gracilis and cuneatus. Each *posterior inferior cerebellar artery* supplies the lateral zone dorsal to the inferior olive in which are located the spinothalamic tract, spinal trigeminal nucleus and tract, nucleus ambiguus, dorsal motor nucleus of the vagus nerve, and roots of cranial nerves XI, IX, and X (Fig. 8-21). Each *vertebral artery* has branches which supply portions of the anterolateral zone of the medulla; in this zone are located portions of the pyramid, hypoglossal nucleus, inferior olive, reticular formation, solitary nucleus, and dorsal motor nucleus of the vagus nerve (Fig. 8-21).

The *paramedian branches of the basilar artery* supply the medial pons (excluding most of the tegmentum), in which are located the corticospinal, corticobulbar, and corticopontine tracts and the pontine nuclei (Fig. 8-21). The *short* and *long circumferential arteries* supply the anterolateral, lateral, and posterior regions of the pons, respectively; the anterior inferior cerebellar and superior cerebellar arteries also supply vessels (Fig. 8-21). Structures located in this region include the medial lemniscus, medial longitudinal fasciculus, spinothalamic and pos-

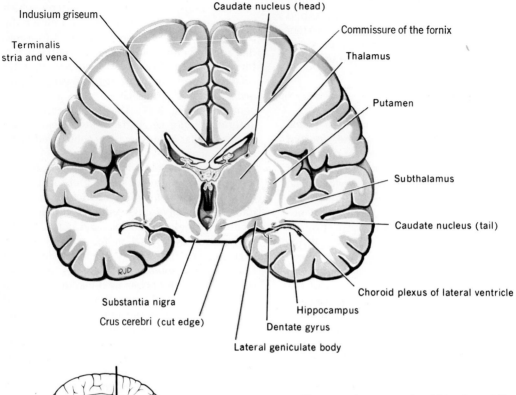

Caudate nucleus (head)
Indusium griseum
Commissure of the fornix
Terminalis stria and vena
Thalamus
Putamen
Subthalamus
Caudate nucleus (tail)
Choroid plexus of lateral ventricle
Substantia nigra
Hippocampus
Crus cerebri (cut edge)
Dentate gyrus
Lateral geniculate body

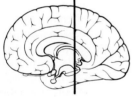

FIGURE 1-21
Coronal section through cerebrum.

Level of occipital aspect of posterior limb of internal capsule (see Fig. 1-15).

terior spinocerebellar tracts, middle and superior cerebellar peduncles, reticular formation, and some cranial nerve nuclei. The *labyrinthine arteries* join cranial nerves VII and VIII and are distributed to the internal ear.

The cerebellum is supplied by the posterior inferior cerebellar, anterior inferior cerebellar, and superior cerebellar arteries.

The vascular network within the midbrain is organized with the basic brainstem pattern of paramedian, short circumferential, and long circumferential branches. The blood vessels include the *posterior cerebral, posterior communicating,* and *superior cerebellar arteries.*

In its proximal postion, the *posterior cerebral artery* has branches which, after penetrating through the posterior perforating substance, supply the upper midbrain and posterior thalamus. The *posterior choroidal artery* is a branch to the choroid plexus of the lateral ventricle. Its distal branches supply the cortex and white matter on the medial aspect and small portions on the lateral aspect of the occipital and temporal lobes.

Each *internal carotid artery* ascends to the base of the skull, passes through the carotid canal, and then curves as a sigmoid-shaped vessel (curving upward, backward, and upward)

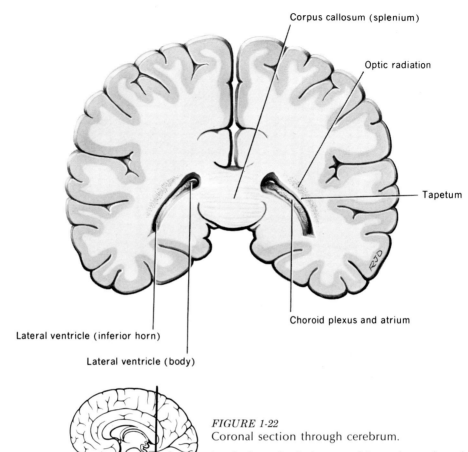

Corpus callosum (splenium)

Optic radiation

Tapetum

Choroid plexus and atrium

Lateral ventricle (inferior horn)

Lateral ventricle (body)

FIGURE 1-22
Coronal section through cerebrum.

Level of retrolenticular part of internal capsule and splenium of corpus callosum (see Fig. 1-15).

close to the medial wall of the cavernous sinus. After passing through the sinus, it bifurcates in the region of the anterior perforating substance into the anterior and middle cerebral arteries. The sigmoid contour of the artery within the sinus—known as the *carotid siphon*—probably accounts for the resilience of the artery.

After emerging from the cavernous sinus, the internal carotid artery gives off the ophthalmic, posterior communicating, and anterior choroidal arteries. Just beyond this, lateral to the optic chiasma, it bifurcates into the anterior cerebral artery and the large middle cerebral artery. The latter is considered to be the continuation of

the internal carotid artery. The *ophthalmic artery* has an important branch, the *central retinal artery;* this end artery runs along the optic nerve and then in the center of the nerve to the retina. Some other branches of the ophthalmic artery are components of the *ophthalmic anastomoses* with branches of the external carotid artery. The *anterior choroidal artery* supplies the choroidal plexus of the lateral ventricle and a number of cerebral structures along its course (including the optic tract, cerebral peduncle, lateral geniculate body, and posterior limb and retrolenticular portion of the internal capsule).

A ring of blood vessels is present on the base

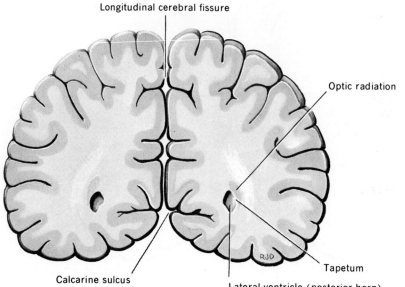

Longitudinal cerebral fissure

Optic radiation

Tapetum

Calcarine sulcus

Lateral ventricle (posterior horn)

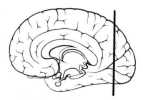

FIGURE 1-23
Coronal section through cerebrum.

Level of posterior horn of lateral ventricle.

of the brain which is known as the *cerebral arterial circle* (*of Willis*) and which includes the part of the posterior cerebral arteries, posterior communicating branches between the posterior cerebral arteries and the internal carotid artery, part of the internal carotid arteries, anterior cerebral arteries, and a short anterior communicating branch between the two anterior cerebral arteries. The "classic" cerebral arterial circle is bilaterally symmetric with well-developed communicating branches in only about 20 percent of individuals. The right vertebral artery is often

hypoplastic. Absence of a portion of the circle is not uncommon. Generally the circle is unsymmetric; a communicating branch may be narrow or absent. The cerebral arterial circle does not act as a circle for blood flow, but it may act as a safety valve when differential pressures are present in these arteries. Numerous small arteries (striate, ganglionic, and thalamic) from the circle and the proximal portions of its branches penetrate into the base of the brain, supplying the diencephalon, internal capsule, basal ganglia, and surrounding deep structures.

The *anterior cerebral artery* gives off *1* the medial (recurrent) striate artery, which supplies portions of many structures including the head of the caudate nucleus, internal capsule, putamen, globus pallidus, and septal nuclei; and *2* the orbital branches, frontal branches, pericallosal artery, and callosomarginal artery to portions of the frontal and parietal lobes (Fig. 1-25).

The *middle cerebral artery* runs laterally on a transverse course along the base of the cerebrum and depths of the lateral sulcus before

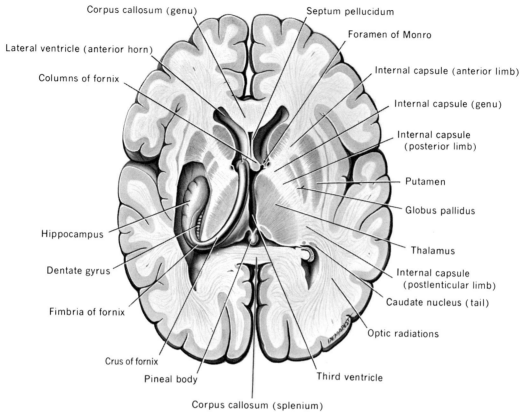

Corpus callosum (genu)

Lateral ventricle (anterior horn)

Columns of fornix

Septum pellucidum

Foramen of Monro

Internal capsule (anterior limb)

Internal capsule (genu)

Internal capsule (posterior limb)

Putamen

Globus pallidus

Hippocampus

Dentate gyrus

Thalamus

Internal capsule (postlenticular limb)

Caudate nucleus (tail)

Fimbria of fornix

Optic radiations

Crus of fornix

Pineal body

Third ventricle

Corpus callosum (splenium)

FIGURE 1-24
Horizontal section through cerebrum.

On the left side, note that the hippocampus, dentate gyrus, inferior horn of the lateral ventricle, and the fimbria of the fornix are below the plane of the section, and the crus of the fornix is above the plane of the section (see Fig. 1-15).

dividing into branches which supply the insular lobe and large regions of the frontal, parietal, temporal, and occipital lobes on the surface of the cerebrum. The *lenticulostriate (striate) arteries* of the transverse course supply large segments of the globus pallidus, putamen, caudate nucleus, thalamus, and internal capsule. Occlusion or rupture of the striate arteries of the middle cerebral artery may interrupt the motor pathways of the internal capsule, and this may result in the paralysis associated with the classical stroke (Chap. 14).

The large arteries and their branches on the surface of the brain are known as *superficial or conducting arteries.* The branches of these arteries that penetrate into the substance of the brain are small vessels known as *penetrating or nutrient arteries.* These vessels branch roughly

at right angles from the superficial arteries and continue through the brain as graceful curves resembling the silhouette of an elm tree. The nutrient arteries branch into extensive capillary networks, which anastomose with each other. The gray matter, with its high metabolic rate, is more vascular than the white matter. One cc of gray matter may have more than 1,000 mm of capillaries.

Anastomotic connections are extensive in the brain. The anastomoses among the large

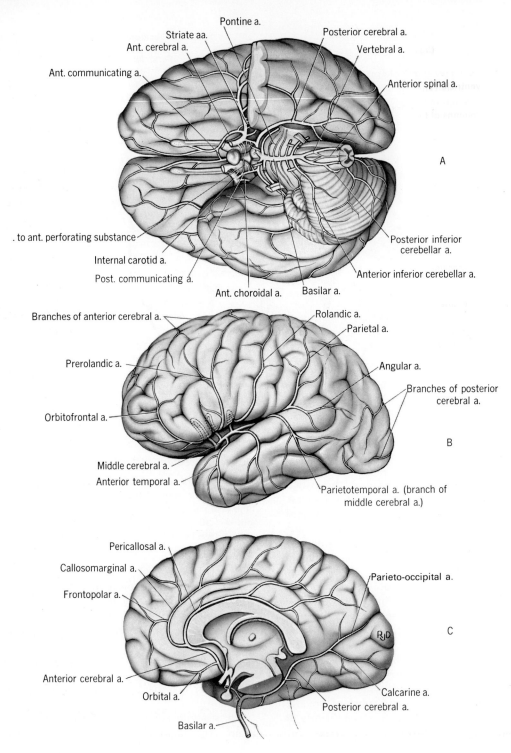

Pontine a.

Striate aa.

Ant. cerebral a.

Ant. communicating a.

Posterior cerebral a.

Vertebral a.

Anterior spinal a.

. to ant. perforating substance

Posterior inferior cerebellar a.

Internal carotid a.

Post. communicating a.

Ant. choroidal a.

Basilar a.

Anterior inferior cerebellar a.

A

Branches of anterior cerebral a.

Rolandic a.

Parietal a.

Prerolandic a.

Angular a.

Branches of posterior cerebral a.

Orbitofrontal a.

B

Middle cerebral a.

Anterior temporal a.

Parietotemporal a. (branch of middle cerebral a.)

Pericallosal a.

Callosomarginal a.

Frontopolar a.

Parieto-occipital a.

C

RJD

Anterior cerebral a.

Orbital a.

Calcarine a.

Posterior cerebral a.

Basilar a.

branches of the superficial arteries are usually physiologically effective, so that occlusion of a vessel need not result in any impairment of the blood supply to the neural tissues. Rich anastomoses exist among the capillary beds of adjacent nutrient arteries and between the deep and superficial circulation. In all probability, true end arteries are not present in the human brain. However, occlusion of the large nutrient vessels often results in neural damage, because the anastomotic connections are not sufficient to allow enough blood to reach the deprived region rapidly enough to meet the high metabolic requirements of the region.

In general, the occlusion of an artery results in a brain lesion which is usually less extensive than the region supplied by that artery. This occurs because the peripheral regions normally supplied by the occluded artery are adequately supplied by collateral circulation from bordering arteries. The anterior communicating artery of the cerebral arterial circle acts as an anastomotic channel between the two cerebral hemispheres. This anastomosis is utilized by neuroradiologists in order to compare the arterial patterns of both middle cerebral arteries by angiography. When the carotid flow to the brain is blocked (by pressure applied in the neck) on the side opposite the site of the carotid puncture for the injection of radiopaque substance, cross filling of the middle cerebral artery on the blocked side with radiopaque substance takes place through the anterior communicating artery. Unlike the cerebrum, the two sides of the brainstem have poor anastomotic connections. As a consequence the occlusion of a brainstem artery results in a lesion restricted to one side.

The *ophthalmic artery* may serve as an anastomotic channel between the internal carotid circulation to the brain and the external carotid circulation to the face and scalp. This so-called *ophthalmic anastomosis* can help to furnish

FIGURE 1-25
Distribution of the arteries on the surface of the brain.

A Basal surface.

B Lateral surface.

C Medial surface.

*Superior cerebellar artery.

blood from the external carotid circulation of the facial region to the brain via the sequence of ophthalmic artery, anterior cerebral artery, and cerebral arterial circle in the course of obstructive diseases of the internal carotid artery system. An entire hemisphere can be adequately supplied through the ophthalmic anastomosis following the gradual occlusion of an internal carotid artery.

Considerably more blood to the brain flows through the internal carotid system than through the vertebral arterial system. Although the arterial trees formed by these two systems are basically similar in the brains of most individuals, many variations of these basic patterns exist. In fact, variation may be the rule. For example, a posterior cerebral artery may be a branch of the middle cerebral artery in one in five brains; in this situation the cerebral arterial circle is incomplete. The anterior cerebral arteries of both sides may be supplied with blood from only one internal carotid artery; in this case, the anterior communicating artery continues as the contralateral anterior cerebral artery.

VENOUS DRAINAGE OF THE BRAIN

The venous drainage of the brainstem and cerebellum roughly parallels the arterial supply. On the other hand the venous trees in the cerebrum do not usually parallel the arterial trees. In general the venous trees have short stocky branches that come off at right angles, resembling the silhouette of an oak tree. Venous anastomoses of the deep veins and the superficial veins are *extensive* and *effective*. The veins of the brain drain into superficial venous plexuses and the dural sinuses (Fig. 1-26). The dural (venous) sinuses are valveless channels located between two layers of the dura mater, the outer meningeal layers. Most of the venous blood of the brain ultimately drains to the base of the skull and into the internal jugular veins of the neck.

The cerebral veins are classified as a *superficial (external surface) cerebral group* and a *deep cerebral group.* Rich anastomoses between the two groups occur through the vascular networks within the brain substance (Fig. 1-27). The

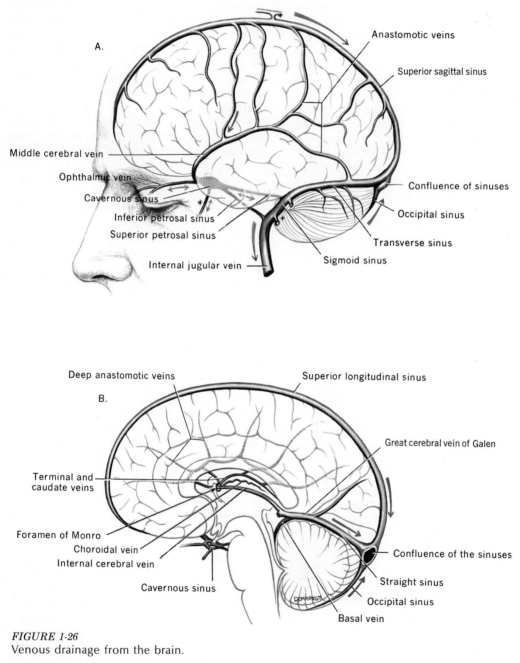

A.

Anastomotic veins

Superior sagittal sinus

Middle cerebral vein

Ophthalmic vein

Cavernous sinus

Inferior petrosal sinus

Superior petrosal sinus

Internal jugular vein

Confluence of sinuses

Occipital sinus

Transverse sinus

Sigmoid sinus

Deep anastomotic veins

Superior longitudinal sinus

B.

Great cerebral vein of Galen

Terminal and
caudate veins

Foramen of Monro

Choroidal vein

Internal cerebral vein

Cavernous sinus

Confluence of the sinuses

Straight sinus

Occipital sinus

Basal vein

DEMAREST

FIGURE 1-26

Venous drainage from the brain.

A Lateral view of the brain.

B Medial view of the brain.

*Emissary veins.

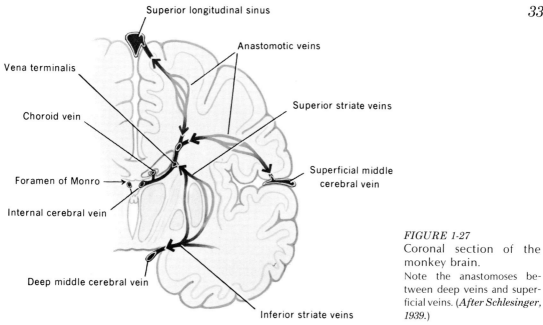

Superior longitudinal sinus

Anastomotic veins

Vena terminalis

Choroid vein

Superior striate veins

Foramen of Monro

Superficial middle
cerebral vein

Internal cerebral vein

Deep middle cerebral vein

Inferior striate veins

FIGURE 1-27
Coronal section of the
monkey brain.
Note the anastomoses be-
tween deep veins and superficial veins. (*After Schlesinger,
1939.*)

blood from the cortex on the upper lateral and medial aspects of the cerebrum drains to the *superior sagittal (dural) sinus,* which drains blood to the occipital region (*confluence of the sinuses*) and then to the *right transverse* and *sigmoid sinuses* into the *right internal jugular vein.* Blood from the other regions of the cerebral cortex drains into the other dural sinuses in the vicinity of the veins and finally into the internal jugular veins. The deep cerebral veins drain toward the regions of the interventricular foramina to form the two internal cerebral veins located within the velum interpositum just above the choroid plexus of the third ventricle. These vessels join in the vicinity of the pineal body to form the *great cerebral vein of Galen.* Blood then flows in order through the straight dural sinus, confluence of sinuses, left lateral sinus, and sigmoid sinuses to the *left internal jugular vein. Note:* Blood from the superficial veins tends to drain through the right jugular vein, and blood from the deep cerebral veins tends to drain through the left jugular vein in the neck.

Some venous sinuses are located in the basal region of the cranial cavity. The spongelike *cavernous sinuses* are a bilateral network of venous

channels on either side of the sphenoid body next to the sella turcica. *Intercavernous sinuses* surrounding the hypophysis and the *basilar venous plexus* behind the sella turcica interconnect the two cavernous sinuses across the midline. A number of venous channels communicate with the cavernous sinuses. Although the blood may flow in either direction in these venous channels, there is a general pattern of drainage. The *ophthalmic vein* from the orbit, the *sphenoparietal sinus* (connected with the meningeal veins), and the middle cerebral vein drain into the cavernous sinus. Each *superior petrosal sinus* and *inferior petrosal sinus* drains posteriorly from the cavernous sinus to the transverse sinus and bulb of the internal jugular vein, respectively. Anastomotic connections via *emissary veins* are made with the *pterygoid* and *pharyngeal venous plexuses.*

Several important structures are associated with the cavernous sinuses. The *internal carotid artery,* its accompanying sympathetic plexus and the abducent nerve pass through the cavernous sinus; the oculomotor, trochlear, ophthalmic, and maxillary nerves course within the lateral wall of the cavernous sinus in which they are embedded.

Some of the dural sinuses connect with the veins superficial to the skull by emissary veins (Figs. 1-28). These veins act as pressure valves when intracranial pressure is raised, and also as pathways for the spread of infection into the brain case (infection in the nose may spread via an emissary vein high in the nose into the meninges and may result in meningitis).

The blood may flow in either direction through the *emissary veins,* depending upon the differential venous pressure within the cranial cavity as compared to that outside the skull. Some emissary veins are *1* a frontal vein interconnecting the superior sagittal sinus with the veins in the nasal cavity, *2* parietal veins interconnecting the superior sagittal sinus with the occipital veins of the scalp, *3* the mastoid veins interconnecting the sigmoid sinus with the postauricular and occipital veins of the scalp, *4* condylar and hypoglossal veins interconnecting the sigmoid sinus with the suboccipital plexus of veins, and *5* veins interconnecting the cavernous sinus with the ophthalmic vein and pharyngeal veins.

Meninges and cerebrospinal fluid

MENINGES

The *meninges* are the three layers of nonneural (connective tissue) membrane that surround and protect the soft brain and spinal cord (Figs. 1-28, 1-29). Each of these layers—pia mater, arachnoid, and dura mater—is a separate continuous sheet. The pia mater and arachnoid are collectively called the *leptomeninges,* and the dura mater is the *pachymeninx.*

The *pia mater* is intimately attached to the brain and the spinal cord, following every sulcus and fissure. It is a vascular layer of delicate connective tissue through which pass the blood vessels that nourish the neural tissues. Astrocytes of the central nervous system have processes that terminate as end feet in the pia mater to form the pia-glial membrane (Chap. 2, Fig. 2-15). This membrane apparently prevents the entrance of harmful materials into the central nervous system.

The *arachnoid* (from the Greek *arachnes,* "spider") is a thin delicate layer, so named because of the numerous fine trabeculae that extend from it to the pia mater. The arachnoid layer does not follow each indentation of the central nervous system, but rather skips from crest to crest. The subarachnoid space between the pia mater and the arachnoid contains the cerebrospinal fluid.

The *velum interpositum* is a triangular fold of pia mater interposed between the corpus callosum and fornix above and the roof of the third ventricle and thalamus below (Fig. 1-29). The subarachnoid space between these two laminae is filled with cerebrospinal fluid and blood vessels; it is continuous posteriorly with the superior cistern. This side forms the base of the triangle. The apex of the triangle is located rostrally at the two interventricular foramina, while the two sides of the triangle extend laterally into each lateral ventricle. The pial vascular bed of the apex and two sides combines with the ependyma of the lateral ventricles and interventricular foramina to form the choroid plexuses of the lateral ventricle and interventricular foramina. After passing through these foramina, the choroid plexus continues as a single midline structure extending from the apex to the middle of the base of the triangle. This is the choroid plexus of the third ventricle, formed by the union of the vascular plexus of the pia with the ependyma in the roof of the third ventricle of the diencephalon.

Several large spaces, called *cisterns,* are located in the subarachnoid space. Cisterns are located in regions where indentations are present on the surface of the brain; at these sites the pia hugs closely to the surface of the brain and a large subarachnoid space is formed because the arachnoid skips from promontory to promontory.

Three cisterns are located on the anterior aspect of the brainstem and hypothalamus: the *pontine cistern,* located at the medullary-pontine junction; the *interpeduncular cistern,* in the interpeduncular fossa of the midbrain; and the chiasmatic cistern, in the region of the optic chiasm (Fig. 1-28). Two cisterns are located on the posterior aspect of the brainstem. *The cerebellomedullary (magna) cistern* is located between the choroid plexus of the medulla and the cerebellum. The *superior cistern* of the great cerebral vein is found posterior to the midbrain

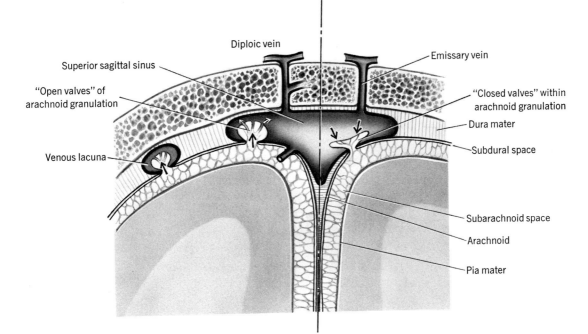

Diploic vein

Superior sagittal sinus

"Open valves" of
arachnoid granulation

Venous lacuna

Emissary vein

"Closed valves" within
arachnoid granulation

Dura mater

Subdural space

Subarachnoid space

Arachnoid

Pia mater

Falx cerebri

FIGURE 1-28
Coronal section through superior sagittal sinus and associated structures.

The arachnoid granulation (left of the vertical line) expands and its "valves" open when the cerebrospinal fluid in the subarachnoid space exceeds venous pressure in the sinus. The arachnoid granulation (right of the vertical line) collapses and its "valves" close when the venous pressure in the sinus exceeds the pressure of the cerebrospinal fluid within the subarachnoid space.

tectum. The *cistern of the lateral cerebral fossa* is located in the region of the lateral cerebral sulcus.

The *spinal cistern* is located in the lumbar and upper sacral regions caudal to the spinal cord (second lumbar to sacral vertebral levels). This cistern is formed because the spinal cord and its pia mater terminate at the second lumbar level (except for the filamentous filum terminale —a hairlike extension of the pia mater to the sacral region) and the arachnoid layer continues as a membrane sac to the sacral levels. The spinal cistern contains the cauda equina (roots of the lower spinal nerves) and the cerebrospinal fluid (CSF). The CSF can be aspirated from the spinal cistern by a lumbar puncture (tap). Many blood vessels are present in the subarachnoid space.

The tough nonstretchable *dura mater* consists of two layers in the head—the outer and inner dura mater. The dura, skull, and vertebral column act as an inelastic case enclosing the brain, spinal cord, cerebrospinal fluid, and blood vessels. The outer dura mater is actually the membrane of the skull bones (periosteum).

The inner dura mater is reflected from the surface of the skull to form the falx cerebri, tentorium cerebelli, and diaphragma sellae.

The sickle-shaped *falx cerebri* is a midline partition located in the longitudinal fissure between the cerebral hemispheres. This falx extends from the rostrally located crista galli of the ethmoid bone posteriorly to the internal occipital protuberance and the tentorium cerebelli. Its free border roughly follows the corpus callosum.

The *tentorium* is a partition located within the transverse fissure between the occipital lobe

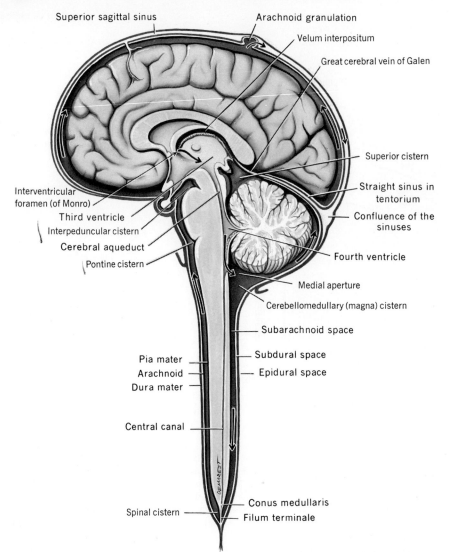

Superior sagittal sinus

Arachnoid granulation

Velum interpositum

Great cerebral vein of Galen

Superior cistern

Straight sinus in tentorium

Confluence of the sinuses

Interventricular foramen (of Monro)

Third ventricle

Interpeduncular cistern

Cerebral aqueduct

Pontine cistern

Fourth ventricle

Medial aperture

Cerebellomedullary (magna) cistern

Subarachnoid space

Subdural space

Epidural space

Pia mater

Arachnoid

Dura mater

Central canal

Conus medullaris

Spinal cistern

Filum terminale

FIGURE 1-29
Meninges, brain ventricles, subarachnoid spaces, and ventricles.

The arrows indicate the normal direction of flow of the cerebrospinal fluid.

of the cerebrum and the cerebellum. The tentorium is attached to the upper edges of the petrous bone and to the ridges along the occipital bones. Within the attachments to the petrous bones are the superior petrosal dural sinuses, and within those to the occipital bones are the transverse dural sinuses. The tentorium resembles a tent with its medial ridge drawn upward and taut by its attachment to the falx cerebri. Within this attachment is the straight dural sinus. The inner free border of the tentorium is called the tentorial incisure; this incisure rings a space which is occupied by the midbrain near its junction with the diencephalon.

The *diaphragma sellae* forms the roof of the pituitary fossa (sella turcia); it is a dural reflection with a perforation through which passes the infundibular stalk of the hypophysis.

The falx cerebri and tentorium cerebelli create three cavities, each of two above the tentorium enclosing a cerebral hemisphere, and the one below the tentorium enclosing the cerebellum and infratentorial brainstem. These compartments act to restrict movement of the brain from side to side and from fore to aft.

The *subdural space* is the potential thin space located between the inner dura mater and the arachnoid. The film of fluid in the subdural space is *not* cerebrospinal fluid. The *epidural space* surrounding the spinal cord is the space between the dura mater and the periosteum of the vertebral column, occupied by blood vessels and fat. The epidural space is not present in the head because the inner dura and outer dura are fused together, except where they form the walls of the dural venous sinuses, which drain the venous blood from the brain. The dura mater is continuous over the cranial and spinal nerves as a dural sleeve that is actually continuous with the epineurium of the peripheral nerves (Chap. 2). The epidural space in the sacral region of the vertebral column is utilized clinically as a site for the injection of anesthetics to block sensory input from the periphery (in painless childbirth).

In head injuries, bleeding may occur into the subarachnoid space (*subarachnoid hemorrhage*), into the subdural space (*subdural hemorrhage*), between the outer dura and the skull (*extradural hemorrhage*), or into the brain substance itself. The common cause of a subarachnoid hemorrhage is arterial bleeding following the rupture of an aneurysm, which is a congenital weakness of a main branch of the internal carotid or vertebral arteries. Such bleeding into the leptomeningeal space can be confirmed by obtaining blood-stained cerebrospinal fluid from the lumbar cistern (lumbar puncture). Subdural hemorrhage is usually caused by the tearing of veins at the sites where they pass through the subdural space. An abrupt fore-and-aft movement of the brain relative to the dura may occur following a blow which does not fracture the skull. Extradural hemorrhages result from torn meningeal vessels, which usually result from a fracture of the skull. Bleeding within the substance of the brain itself is often caused by hypertension. This tends to be rapidly fatal because of the destruction of brain tissue.

INNERVATION OF THE DURA MATER

The dura mater is supplied with a rich innervation by branches of the trigeminal and vagus nerves and by sympathetic nerves (Fig. 1-30). The sympathetic fibers accompany the middle meningeal arteries which supply the skull and dura mater but not the blood vessels to the brain. The ethmoidal nerves of the ophthalmic nerve innervate the anterior cranial fossa and rostral part of the falx cerebri. Recurrent tentorial branches of the ophthalmic nerve course close to the tentorial incisure and then spread out to supply the tentorium cerebelli and the posterior part of the falx cerebri. Branches of the maxillary and mandibular nerves supply the innervation to the middle cranial fossa. A recurrent meningeal branch of the vagus nerve supplies the innervation to the posterior cranial fossa. Recurrent branches of the spinal nerves innervate the dura mater surrounding the spinal cord. The large blood vessels of the brain also have a rich sensory innervation. Irritation of these sensory nerves from the distention or constriction of these arteries is the source of many common *headaches*. The ophthalmic branch of the trigeminal nerve is reported to be the one most frequently involved. The brain is actually insensitive to pain; it has no sensory receptors.

CEREBROSPINAL FLUID (CSF)

The *cerebrospinal fluid* is a crystal-clear, colorless, almost protein-free solution, which looks like water and is found in the ventricular system and the subarachnoid space. The brain and spinal cord are shock-mounted against injury, for they literally float in this medium (like a log submerged in water); the 1,400-Gm brain has a net weight of about 50 to 100 Gm while suspended in the cerebrospinal fluid. The specific gravities of the brain and CSF are 1.040 and 1.007, respectively. The soft nonrigid brain, which is 80 percent water, is able to stand the stresses incurred during movements of the head because of the buoyancy of this fluid jacket and of the protection of the meninges, and the rigid bony skull. In addition, the CSF prevents the brain from tugging on the meninges, nerve roots, and blood vessels, which are innervated by sensory nerves. Should some fluid be removed, as in certain diagnostic procedures, the patient suffers from intense pain and excruciating headaches with every shift of the brain resulting from a

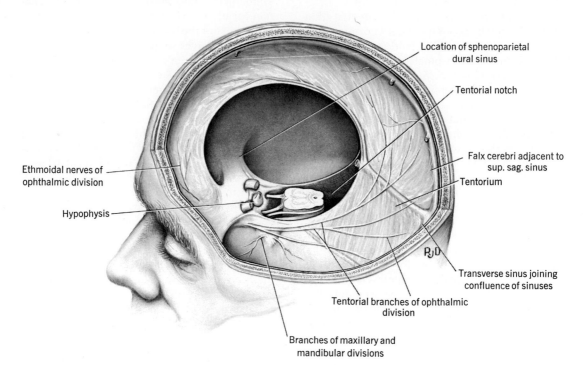

Location of sphenoparietal
dural sinus

Tentorial notch

Falx cerebri adjacent to
sup. sag. sinus

Tentorium

Ethmoidal nerves of
ophthalmic division

Hypophysis

Transverse sinus joining
confluence of sinuses

Tentorial branches of ophthalmic
division

Branches of maxillary and
mandibular divisions

FIGURE 1-30
Innervation of the dura mater and the cranial
fossae.

Branches of the ophthalmic division of the trigeminal
nerve innervate the anterior cranial fossa, falx cerebri,
and tentorium. Branches of the maxillary and mandibular divisions innervate the middle cranial fossa.
Branches of the vagus nerve innervate the posterior
cranial fossa.

movement of the head. These painful symptoms
last until the CSF is naturally replaced.

The pressure of the fluid is lower than that
of the blood pressure. In the individual lying on
his side the pressure varies from about 60 to
180 mm of water (not mercury) throughout the
subarachnoid space. In the seated individual the
pressure may reach 400 mm of water in the lumbar cistern, may be zero in the cisterna magna,
and is below atmospheric pressure in the ventricles of the brain. Fluctuations in the pressure
of this fluid are directly related and synchronous
to changes associated with the heartbeat and

the respiratory cycle. High abdominal and thoracic pressures that result during the lifting of
a heavy object can raise the pressure in the
subarachnoid space to such a level that the
venous drainage of blood from the spinal cord
is impeded. The reason for these shifts in pressure is that the rigid skull box (dura and bone)
does not yield and therefore any addition to or
subtraction from inside the cranial box results
in a change in the internal pressure.

The volume of CSF in the average adult is
estimated to be about 135 ml (75 to 150 ml), of
which roughly 80 ml is in the ventricles and
55 ml is in the subarachnoid space. Daily production is roughly estimated at about 300 ml. In
all probability most of the fluid is produced at
the choroid plexuses and significant amounts by
the brain. The latter diffuses through the ependyma and pia mater (Chap. 2).

The CSF fluid consists of water, a small
amount of protein, gases in solution (oxygen
and carbon dioxide), sodium, potassium, cal-

cium, magnesium, and chloride ions, glucose, a few white blood cells (mostly lymphocytes and some monocytes), and many other organic constituents. Because the CSF is essentially isotonic to blood plasma, with minimal amounts of protein and cells, it has been characterized as a cell-free, protein-free ultrafiltrate of blood. This is not an accurate description, because the composition of nascent CSF from the choroid plexus, where it is primarily formed, differs significantly from an ultrafiltrate of blood (Cserr).

Although some CSF is probably the product of extrachoroidal tissues (the brain itself), most CSF is elaborated at the choroid plexus of the lateral, third, and fourth ventricles. The choroid plexus is large; its surface area ranges from 150 to 300 sq cm. Its structural organization is illustrated in Fig. 2-16 and outlined in Chap. 2, under "Blood-Brain Barrier." The *choroid plexus* is a functionally complex structure specialized to secrete, to dialyze, and to absorb; some of these roles are performed by active transport acting bidirectionally. The epithelial layer of the choroid plexus is a key structure for the transcellular transport of solvents and solutes from the choroidal vessels to the ventricular CSF. Some substances are known to "flow" in the opposite direction from the CSF to the choroidal blood vessels.

Following its formation by the choroid plexuses, the composition of the CSF becomes modified during its passage through the ventricular system and subarachnoid space. The active transport and diffusion of the molecular and ionic constituents take place in both directions—between the blood plasma and the CSF, and between the CSF and the brain tissues. The capillaries and associated tissues of the choroid plexuses and pia mater are the sites for the exchange between the blood vascular system and the CSF. The pia-ependymal membrane lining the ventricular system and the pia-glial membrane lining the subarachnoid space are the sites for the exchange between the brain tissues and the CSF. In general, those substances with high lipid solubility (such as CO_2, volatile anesthetics, and barbiturates) shift from the blood stream to the brain to the CSF. Hydrophilic substances of limited lipid solubility (such as electrolytes, sugars, and amino acids) shift from the bloodstream to the CSF to the brain.

The cycle of formation, flow, and disposal of CSF follows the pressure gradient from the ar-

terial stream, where the pressure is highest, to the ventricles and subarachnoid space, where the pressure is less, to the venous blood of the dural sinuses, where the pressure is least. The classical concept of the "faucet" system, although not necessarily correct in detail, has utility. The CSF formed at the choroid plexus (which acts as a faucet) of each ventricle enters the ventricles and flows from the lateral ventricles through the interventricular foramina into the third ventricle, through the aqueduct, and into the fourth ventricle. The CSF passes through the lateral and medial apertures in the roof of the fourth ventricle into the cisterna cerebellomedullaris and slowly circulates rostrally through the subarachnoid space to the region of the superior sagittal sinus at the top of the skull, where the CSF percolates through the channels of the arachnoid granulations to join the venous blood of the superior sagittal sinus.

The *arachnoid granulations* are extensive tufts of piarachnoid which, along with the thinned-out inner dura, project into the superior sagittal sinus and some of its outpockets, called lateral lacunae. A *granulation* (Pacchionian body) comprises a number of arachnoid villi, each of which is composed of loose connective tissue permeated by a meshwork of channels 10 to 20 μ in diameter. This meshwork has a valve-like role; it permits the one-way bulk flow of CSF from the subarachnoid space into the venous blood of the superior sagittal sinus, and it prevents the regurgitation of blood from the sinus into the subarachnoid space (Fig. 1-28). When the CSF pressure exceeds the venous pressure, the "valves" open and CSF flows to the dural sinus. When the venous pressure is elevated (as in coughing or lifting a heavy object), the arachnoid villi are compressed and the channel meshwork becomes occluded (the "valve" closes). The unidirectional flow is, in a sense, regulated by the pressure of the CSF.

The ventricular system and the subarachnoid space, when they contain air, can be visualized on an x-ray plate. This is accomplished after some CSF is withdrawn and replaced by air. The air may be introduced by passing a needle *1* through a small hole drilled in the skull and then through the brain into a lateral ventricle; or *2* between two lower lumbar vertebrae (*spinal tap*) into the *spinal cistern* (caudal to the spinal cord). The air in the lumbar region can ascend and outline the subarachnoid space of the spinal and cranial cavities (by *pneumoencephalography*); it can also pass through the medial and lateral apertures (foramina of Magendie and Luschka) to outline the ventricular system (*ventriculogram*).

By adjusting the position of the head to manipulate the air into particular locations, desired x-ray films can be made. Many topographic details are revealed. In the subarachnoid space, the following are a sample of some structures visualized: proximal portions of cranial nerves V through X, internal auditory meatus, all cisterns, valleculae, subarachnoid space of velum interpositum, and the pineal gland. The following ventricular structures can be outlined: medial aperture, lateral recess and choroid plexus of fourth ventricle, fastigium, aqueduct in the midbrain, supraoptic recess, infundibular recess, lamina terminalis, anterior commissure of the third ventricle, interventricular foramen, and many structures in the walls of the lateral ventricles.

Bibliography

Anson, B.: *Morris' Human Anatomy*. McGraw-Hill Book Company, New York, 1966.

Barr, M. L.: *The Human Nervous System*. Harper & Row, Publishers, Incorporated, New York, 1972.

Brightman, M. W., and T. S. Reese: Junctions between intimately opposed cell membranes in the vertebrate brain. J. Cell Biol., 40:648–677, 1969.

Carpenter, M. B.: *Core Text of Neuroanatomy*. The Williams & Wilkins Company, Baltimore, 1972.

Crosby, E. C., T. Humphrey, and E. Lauer: *Correlative Anatomy of the Nervous System*. The Macmillan Company, New York, 1962.

Cserr, H. F.: Physiology of the choroid plexus. Physiol. Rev., 51:273–311, 1971.

Curtis, B. A., S. Jacobson, and E. M. Marcus: *An Introduction to the Neurosciences*. W. B. Saunders Company, Philadelphia, 1972.

Davson, H.: *Physiology of the Cerebrospinal Fluid*. Little, Brown and Company, Boston, 1967.

Everett, N. B.: *Functional Neuroanatomy*. Lea & Febiger, Philadelphia, 1971.

Ford, D. H., and J. P. Schadé: *Atlas of the Human Brain*. Elsevier Publishing Company, Amsterdam, 1966.

Krieg, W. J. S.: *Functional Neuroanatomy*. Brain Books, Evanston, Ill., 1966.

Manter, J. T., and A. J. Gatz: *Essentials of Clinical Neuroanatomy and Neurophysiology*. F. A. Davis Company, Philadelphia, 1970.

Matzke, H. A., and F. M. Foltz: *Synopsis of Neuroanatomy*. Oxford University Press, New York and London, 1967.

Mettler, G. A.: *Neuroanatomy*. The C. V. Mosby Company, St. Louis, 1948.

Miller, R. A., and E. Burack: *Atlas of the Central Nervous System in Man*. The Williams & Wilkins Company, Baltimore, 1968.

Minckler, J. (ed.): *Introduction to Neuroscience*. The C. V. Mosby Company, St. Louis, 1972.

Netter, F. H.: *Nervous System*. Ciba Pharmaceutical Products, Summit, N.J., 1958.

Noback, C. R., and R. J. Demarest: *The Nervous System: Introduction and Review*. McGraw-Hill Book Company, New York, 1972.

Peele, T. L.: *The Neuroanatomic Basis for Clinical Neurology*. McGraw-Hill Book Company, New York, 1968.

Rasmussen, A. T.: *The Principal Nervous Pathways*. The Macmillan Company, New York, 1957.

Roberts, M., and J. Hanaway: *Atlas of the Human Brain in Section*. Lea & Febiger, Philadelphia, 1970.

Sidman, R. L., and M. Sidman: *Neuroanatomy: A Programmed Text*. Little, Brown and Company, Boston, 1965.

Singer, M., and P. I. Yakovlev: *The Human Brain in Sagittal Section*. Charles C Thomas, Publisher, Springfield, Ill., 1954.

Sobotta, J.: *Atlas of Descriptive Human Anatomy*. Hafner Publishing Company, New York, 1954.

Stephans, R. B., and D. L. Stilwell: *Arteries and Veins of the Human Brain*. Charles C Thomas, Publisher, Springfield, Ill., 1969.

Truex, R. C., and M. B. Carpenter: *Human Neuroanatomy*. The Williams & Wilkins Company, Baltimore, 1969.

Villiger, E., E. Ludwig, and A. T. Rasmussen: *Atlas of Cross Section Anatomy of the Brain*. McGraw-Hill Book Company, New York, 1951.

Willis, W. D., and R. G. Grossman: *Medical Neurobiology*. The C. V. Mosby Company, St. Louis, 1973.

CHAPTER 2
BASIC MICROSCOPIC ANATOMY

The structural elements

The nervous system is composed of three basic elements: *1* nerve cells called *neurons* (Fig. 2-1), *2* interstitial cells, including neuroglia cells, neurolemma cells, and satellite cells, and *3* connective tissue elements, including fibroblast cells and their fibrous products (collagenous fibers and reticular fibers), microglia, blood vessels, and extracellular fluids.

The *neuron* is the keystone; it is the *morphologic* unit, the *functional* unit, and the *ontogenetic* unit of the nervous system. Morphologically, each neuron is in contact (synapse) through its processes with other neurons, so that each neuron is an interconnecting segment in the network of the entire nervous system. Functionally, each neuron is an integrator, conductor, and transmitter of coded information. Ontogenetically, all neurons develop from one primordial cell type, the neuroblast.

The *interstitial cells* are in intimate contact with the neurons and their processes. Actually, the entire surface of each neuron, with a few exceptions (synapses and nerve endings), is enveloped and insulated from other tissues by the interstitial cells. These cells are interposed between each neuron and the immediate blood capillaries and adjacent neurons. The interstitial cells of the central nervous system are the two glial cell types (astroglia and oligodendroglia); those of the peripheral nervous system are the neurolemma cells (Schwann cells) of the peripheral nerves and the inner satellite cells of the peripheral ganglia.

The *connective tissue elements* are similar to the connective tissue proper present in other regions of the body. They have several ancillary roles in the functional economy of the nervous system. The fibroblasts and their collagenous and reticular fiber products are the supporting and structural binding elements of the nervous system. For example, the meninges surrounding the central nervous system and the capsules of some of the peripheral sense organs are connective tissues. Blood vessels transport and exchange gases, nutrients, and numerous metabolic products. The microglia of the central nervous system and the histiocytes of the peripheral nervous system are the scavenger cells, capable of ingesting particulate matter.

The neurons and interstitial cells are embryologically derived from ectoderm; the connective tissue elements are of mesodermal origin. The central nervous system develops from a pseudostratified epithelium, called the ventricular zone (Chap. 4). This "epithelial" origin is expressed later by similarities between the central nervous system and structures composed of epithelium (e.g., epidermis). Both are composed of closely packed cells with a minimal amount of extracellular space intercalated among their cellular elements. No connective tissue cells and fibers are located in these spaces. In addition, the cells of both are joined by cell-to-cell junctions.

Neuron

The diversity of form and size of neurons is probably greater than for any other cell type in the body (Figs. 2-1 and 2-2). However diverse, all neurons have common qualities designed to express the three fundamental properties of nerve cells, viz., the specialized capacity to react to stimuli, to transmit the resulting excitation

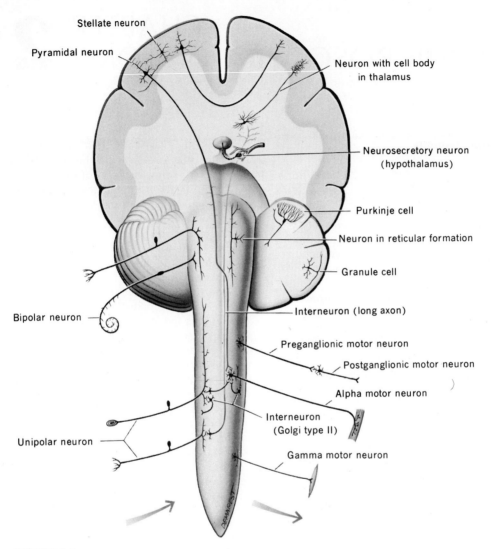

FIGURE 2-1
Typical neurons.

Left, afferent (sensory) neurons projecting to the central nervous system.

Right, efferent (motor neurons) and hypothalamic neurosecretory neurons (Chap. 11) projecting from the central nervous system.

rapidly to other portions of the cell, and to influence other neurons, muscle cells, and glandular cells.

The typical neuron consists of a *cell body* (*soma, perikaryon,* and *nerve cell*) and thin, threadlike processes—one axon and several dendrites (Figs. 2-3 and 2-4). *Soma* is often used in its combining form, "somatic," i.e., an axosomatic synapse is a synapse between an axon and a cell body. *Perikaryon* refers to the region around the nucleus. The cell body, the portion of the neuron essential to the life of the neuron, is usually just beyond the range of visibility of the unaided eye. In man, cell bodies vary in size from 4 to 135 μm in diameter; the cell size is roughly correlated with the length of the axonal process. A neuron with a cell body of less than 25 μm in diameter generally has a short unmyelinated axon, while that with a cell body of over 25 μm in diameter has a myelinated axon. The axonal and dendritic processes are from 0.1 to 3 μm thick (many are below the resolution of the light microscope) and range from a fraction of an inch to several feet in length. The fine processes can attain a sizable bulk. In a large neuron, the total volume of the processes may be from 100 to over 1,000 times that of the cell body. The entire neuron—cell body and processes—is surrounded by the *plasma membrane.* The axon and its plasma membrane are often called the *axis cylinder* and *axolemma,* respectively.

Some idea of the relative proportions of various parts of a neuron can be gained from this well-known comparison. If the cell body of a motor neuron is enlarged to the size of a baseball, the axon could be about 1 mile long and the dendrites and their branches would arborize throughout a large amphitheater.

PLASMA MEMBRANE (Cell membrane)

The *plasma membrane* is the continuous outer layer of the cell body and its processes. Estimates indicate that about 10 percent of the surface area of a large neuron is located on the cell body and the remaining 90 percent on the processes. This thin cell membrane, about 80 to 100 Å thick, is a highly organized, dynamic structure composed of three layers, called the unit membrane. This trilaminar membrane comprises a bimolecular leaflet of lipid between two monolayers of proteins. Each of the three layers is about 25 to 30 Å wide. On the external surface is an outer coat of glycoproteins adjacent to the intercellular space. The so-called greater neuronal membrane consists of the plasma membrane, the cell coat, and the immediately surrounding intercellular space. The precise molecular organization is not known; it possibly varies in different regions (e.g., receptor sites of

a postsynaptic membrane at a synapse may differ from a membrane adjacent to a node of Ranvier) and in different physiologic states. A cell membrane is a dynamic structure, not a static one. This membrane hypothesis accounts for the electrical properties and permeability of the plasma membrane. It acts as a sievelike barrier between the neuronal cytoplasm, which is negatively charged, and the extracellular fluid, which is positively charged. In one sense the functional activity of the neuron is channeled to maintain the plasma membrane, which has a significant role in the generation and conduction of nerve impulses. In some neurons and muscle fibers (smooth muscle and cardiac muscle), the plasma membranes of two cells abut against each other, leaving a gap of but 20 Å between them (*electrical synapse, gap junction*). These junctions are zones of diminished resistance to current and are thus sites of electrical continuity (action potential).

CELL BODY

Within the cell body are located the nucleus and a number of cytoplasmic structures, including neuroplasm, mitochondria, Nissl substance, Golgi apparatus, lysosomes, lipofuscin granules, microtubules, neurofilaments, and, at times, cilia (Figs. 2-3 through 2-5).

The nucleus is spherical and proportional to the neuron it occupies. Its clear vesicular appearance with widely dispersed fine chromatin material is indicative of active transcriptional activity. The *chromatin* is composed of deoxyribonucleic acid (DNA), the chemical carrier of hereditary characteristics. Some neurons carry twice the normal amount of DNA (tetraploid). The nucleus is characteristically located in the center of the cell body. Exceptions to this rule include the neurons of the dorsal nucleus of Clarke, cells of the sympathetic ganglia, and injured neurons; in these cells the nuclei are in an eccentric location.

The prominent *nucleolus* is composed largely of ribonucleic acid (RNA) and associated proteins, the chemical substances involved with the synthesis of proteins. Adjacent to the nucleolus is a small DNA-containing body, called the *nu-*

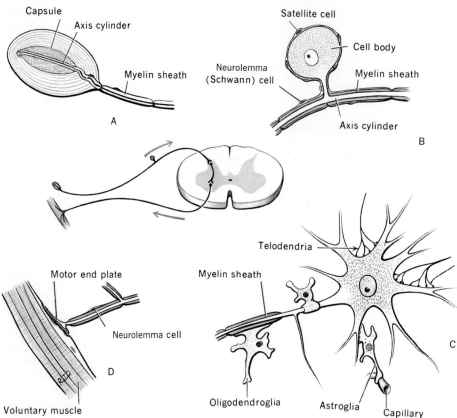

FIGURE 2-2
Structures associated with a three-neuron spinal reflex include the sensory neuron, interneuron, and alpha motor neuron.

A Pacinian corpuscle contains an unmyelinated axis cylinder with the corpuscle.

B The cell body and its processes of the unipolar spinal neuron within a spinal ganglion are associated with the neurolemma (Schwann) cells and the satellite cells.

C Alpha motor neuron (multipolar neuron) within the anterior horn. Note *1* the telodendritic endings of the interneuron synapsing with the dendrites (axodendritic synapses) and with the cell body (axosomatic synapses) of the motor neuron, *2* astrocyte with a process extending to a blood capillary and another process to the neuron, and *3* oligodendroglia with process extending to myelin sheath of axon within spinal cord.

D Motor end plate is a neuromuscular synapse between the nerve terminal and a voluntary muscle.

cleolar satellite, sex chromatin, paranucleolar body, or *Barr body*—named after the neuroanatomist who first described it. This Barr body, present in the female but seldom seen in the male, represents one of the paired X chromosomes. By noting the presence or absence of this satellite in various cells of the body, medical geneticists can determine the genetic sex in the intersexual state and in patients with certain sex-linked congenital diseases.

The *nuclear envelope* is the boundary structure between the nucleus and the cytoplasm; it is a double membrane which is separated by a single narrow space, called a perinuclear cisterna. The envelope is considered to be a specialization of the endoplasmic reticulum with which it is continuous in some places. *Nuclear pores,* with a fine diaphragm spanning each "opening," are located in the nuclear envelope. These pores may act as channels of communication between the nucleus and the cytoplasm.

The *neuroplasm* is the microscopic structureless cytoplasm in which are located the Nissl substance, mitochondria, and other inclusions. In the axon the neuroplasm is called axoplasm. In the neuroplasm are found the potassium ions and other chemical entities so critical to impulse transmission and to the metabolism of the cell.

The *mitochondria* are small slender rodlets and spherical granules, of about 0.1 μm in diameter, located randomly throughout the cell body, in the vicinity of nodes of Ranvier and nerve terminals and varicosities. Their structure and metabolic role are basically the same as in other cells. Each organelle is bounded by an outer membrane, which has a smooth contour, and by an inner membrane, which has numerous infoldings, called cristae, projecting in an internal cavity. This cavity is homogeneous. Mitochondria are rich in oxidative and hydrolytic enzymes. The inner layer contains the respiratory and energy-transferring enzymes and coenzymes involved with the Krebs cycle. Energy is stored in the form of energy-rich adenosine triphosphate (ATP); hence mitochondria are associated with those organelles which utilize the ATP as an energy source for their metabolic activities. In this respect mitochondria are the powerhouses of all cells, including neurons, because they are the main suppliers of energy. The outer membrane contains *monoamine oxidase (MAO),* which is important in the degradation of catecholamines (Chap. 6).

The *Nissl substance* (chromophilic or chromidial substance) comprises the intensely basophilic aggregates located in the cell bodies and dendrites of all neurons. It is absent in the axon and in that portion of the cell body, called the axon hillock, near the site of emergence of the axon (Figs. 2-3 through 2-5). As viewed under the light microscope, the Nissl substance ranges in appearance from small rhomboid blocks (Nissl bodies) in the lower motor neurons to dustlike particles in the cell bodies in the dorsal root ganglia. Electron micrographs indicate that the Nissl bodies are nodal points in the *endoplasmic reticulum (ER),* which permeates the cell body and dendrites. Each Nissl body comprises *1* broad sheets of *granular ER* (so-called *rough ER,* with ribosomes attached on the outer surface of the cisternae) piled up one upon the other in a regular pattern, and *2* free ribosomes arranged in clusters or rosettes of five or six granules surrounding a central granule (*polyribosomes*) located in the neuroplasm between the ER cisternae. Ribosomes are RNA-rich granules. The granular ER is continuous with the agranular ER (so-called smooth ER, without ribosomes).

The ER system of cisternae is continuous with the plasma membrane, nuclear envelope, and Golgi apparatus. In general, the Nissl aggregates are larger near the nucleus and smaller near the periphery of the cell and the dendrites. The Nissl substance is the principal protein-synthesizing organelle; it manufactures in 1 to 3 days an amount of protein equal to the protein content in the cell at one time. Much of it is transported down the axon by axoplasmic flow or transport. Among the cells of the body, large neurons rank among those with the highest concentrations of protein-synthesizing RNA, even exceeding those prodigious protein enzyme–producing cells of the pancreas. Neurons are actually glandular cells synthesizing proteins, including "trophic substances" and enzymes essential to the formation of neurotransmitters (Chap. 6). Nerve cells require large amounts of protein to maintain their integrity and to perform their functional activities.

When a neuron is injured (e.g., the axon is cut), the Nissl substance seems to disappear in a process known as *chromatolysis.* Actually the total amount of RNA within the cell body is the same. Its concentration decreases because the cell imbibes water and may triple its volume. Within a few days, the RNA responds by synthesizing protein to reconstitute the neuron (see "Degeneration" and "Regeneration" at the end of this chapter). After the neuron is reformed, the cell body and the Nissl substance return to their original form.

The quality of the stainability of the Nissl substance is related to the physiologic status of the neuron. The Nissl substance stains well in "physiologically inactive" neurons, moderately well in neurons stimulated to fire frequently, and poorly in neurons stimulated excessively for prolonged periods of time.

The *Golgi apparatus* is an organelle dispersed widely in the cytoplasm, especially as a reticulum surrounding the nucleus (Fig. 2-5). It is located in the proximal portions of the dendrites but is absent in the axon. At any locale, it consists of stacks of five to seven broad-flattened cisternae without granules, oriented roughly parallel to the nuclear envelope. The cisternae are interconnected by agranular ER, which in turn is continuous with granular ER. Some of the protein manufactured by the Nissl bodies is transported via the channels within the cisternae of the rough ER and smooth ER to the cisternae of the Golgi apparatus, where the protein product is concentrated and packaged. However, a substantial amount of the protein synthesized by the neuron is not conveyed to the Golgi apparatus. At present the reason for the prominence of this organelle in neurons is unknown. Small granules within its cisternae may possibly be immature neurosecretory granules or the enzymes associated with the lysosomal system. In an injured neuron the Golgi apparatus undergoes a dissolution; by the time the neuron recovers, the Golgi apparatus is reconstructed.

Numerous *lysosomes* are present in all neurons. These spherical or oval bodies (0.3 to 0.5 μ in diameter) are membrane-bound vesicles containing hydrolytic enzymes. The lysosomal system is an intracellular digestive system designed to ensure the removal of injured organelles and other "waste products." Its enzymes can break down proteins, RNA, and DNA. As long as the lysosomes are intact, access of their enzymes to the cytoplasmic substrates is prevented. At the death of a neuron, these lysosomes, acting as "suicide bags," release enzymes that can autolyze the cell.

Pigmented inclusions are present in some neurons. *Lipofuscin* pigment is first found ontogenetically in some neurons of young adults and continues to accumulate throughout life. Because the yellow-to-brown granules accumulate during aging, they are considered to be "wear-and-tear" pigments; they may be either the products of the degradation of neuronal cytoplasm by lysosomal activity, or a form of lysosome. These pigments are probably not injurious to the neuron; they are readily found in the aging but viable motor neurons of the spinal cord and cells of the inferior olivary nucleus. Almost all neurons of senile animals contain lipofuscin pigment in varying amounts. *Melanin* is present in certain cells as a dark brown pigment. These include certain neurons of the olfactory bulb, pars compacta of the substantia nigra, locus ceruleus, dorsal motor nucleus of the vagus nerve, spinal ganglia, and sympathetic ganglia. These cells begin to accumulate such pigment at about the fourth or fifth year of life. *Iron-containing granules* are found in nerve cells of the pars reticularis of the substantia nigra and the globus pallidus. Cells containing melanin pigment show very little lipofuscin pigment.

Microtubules (neurotubules) and *neurofilaments* (microfilaments) are filamentous, fibrous protein structures found in the cell body, dendrites, and axon of all neurons. They are oriented parallel to the long axis of each cell process. The neurofibrils observed in living neurons and in silver-stained preparations may be

FIGURE 2-3
A motor neuron (lower motor neuron, alpha motor neuron) of the anterior horn of the spinal cord.

A The neuron includes a cell body and its processes (dendrites and axons). Note the axon collateral process branching at a node of Ranvier.

B Axons terminate as telodendria; each telodendritic terminal has a bulbous ending, forming either an axosomatic or an axodendritic synapse.

C The synapse as reconstructed from electron micrographs. Note similarities between synapse and motor end plate in *E*.

D Motor end plate as visualized with the light microscope. The sarcolemma (plasma membrane of muscle cell) is the postsynaptic membrane of the motor end plate.

E Section through motor end plate as based on electron micrographs. Portion of terminal ending fits into synaptic gutter of muscle fiber. Neurolemma cells cover portion of axon not in the gutter. The secondary clefts (junctional folds) are modifications of the sarcolemma.

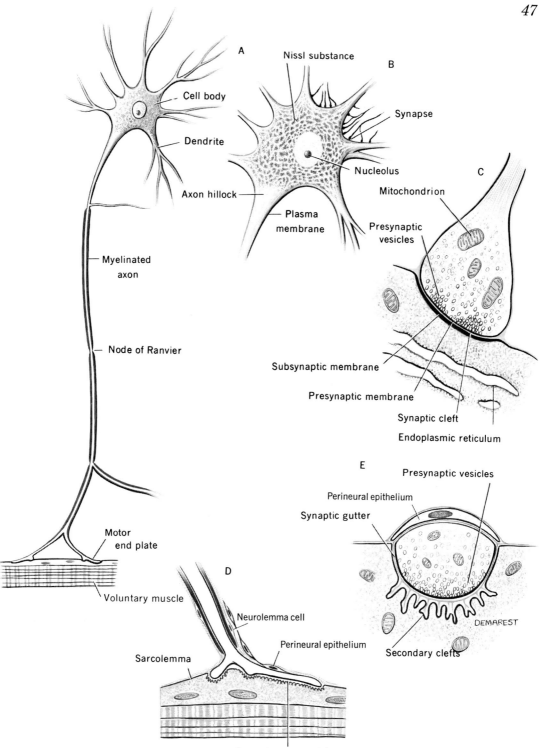

A

Nissl substance

B

Cell body

Dendrite

Synapse

Axon hillock

Nucleolus

Plasma
membrane

Mitochondrion

C

Presynaptic
vesicles

Myelinated
axon

Node of Ranvier

Subsynaptic membrane

Presynaptic membrane

Synaptic cleft

Endoplasmic reticulum

E

Presynaptic vesicles

Perineural epithelium

Synaptic gutter

Motor
end plate

Voluntary muscle

D

Neurolemma cell

Perineural epithelium

Sarcolemma

DEMAREST

Secondary clefts

Synaptic gutter (cleft)

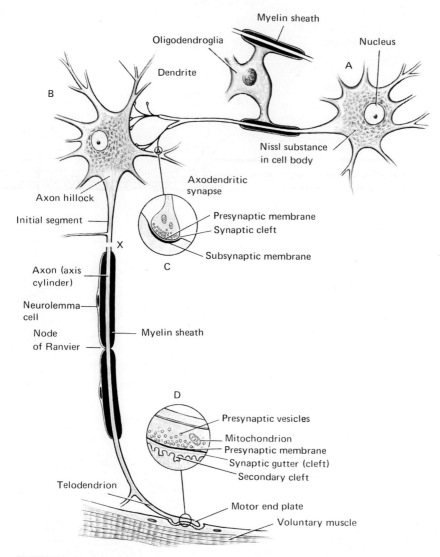

FIGURE 2-4

A A neuron located within the central nervous system.

B A lower motor neuron located in both the central and peripheral nervous systems. This synapses with a voluntary muscle cell to form a motor end plate. The hiatus in the nerve at X represents the border between the central nervous system above and the peripheral nervous system below.

microtubules and, in addition, neurofilaments. The microtubules are straight, long, unbranched structures of about 200- to 260-Å diameter with a central cylindrical core (or canal) of 100- to 140-Å diameter. They appear to be rigid structures extending as a continuum in the axons and dendrites. The neurofilaments with a diameter of 100 Å are finer filaments than the microtubules. These structures, especially the micro-

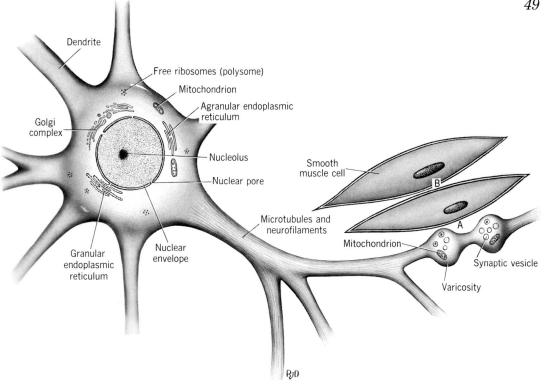

Dendrite

Free ribosomes (polysome)

Mitochondrion

Agranular endoplasmic reticulum

Golgi complex

Nucleolus

Nuclear pore

Smooth muscle cell

B

Microtubules and neurofilaments

Mitochondrion

A

Synaptic vesicle

Granular endoplasmic reticulum

Nuclear envelope

Varicosity

RjD

FIGURE 2-5
Some of the cytoplasmic organelles and associated structures of a postganglionic neuron of the autonomic nervous system.

The junction between the varicosity and smooth muscle cell (*A*) is a typical synapse. The junction between two smooth muscle cells (*B*) is an electrical synapse (gap junction, nexus).

tubules, are probably associated with the fast transport (axoplasmic flow) from cell body to nerve terminal. The microtubules may confer mechanical strength and rigidity to the long slender dendrites and axons. In general, there seems to be a reciprocal quantitative relation between these structures; some neurons have relatively equal numbers of both these structures, others have many microtubules and few neurofilaments, and others have many neurofilaments and few microtubules.

Cilia are often found in the ependymal cells and in the neurons from many regions of the central nervous system. They are probably vestigial and functionless remnants associated with the epithelial origin of neurons.

DENDRITES AND AXONS

Neurons have two types of processes, viz., *dendrites (dendrons)* and *axons*. The typical neuron has two or more branching dendrites extending out from the cell body and only one axon (*axis cylinder, neuraxon*). In these neurons, the cell

body and its dendrites form the receptor, or dendritic, zone of the neuron and the axon is the conducting zone. The receptor zone receives and processes input which evokes a graded, decremental (not all-or-none) response (Chap. 3). The conducting zone conveys influences from the receptor zone via nondecremental (all-or-none) action potentials (Chap. 3). Some specialized neurons lack an axon; an *anaxonic neuron* consists of a cell body and dendrites. Such neurons are the bipolar amacrine and horizontal neurons of the retina and the granule cells of the olfactory bulb. Functionally these neurons are dendritic zones. The primary sensory neurons conveying information from the sensory receptors in the body to the central nervous system are organized in a different manner. The receptor zone of a primary sensory neuron is the ending of the nerve associated with a sensory receptor (e.g., Meissner's touch receptor), while the rest of the neuron is essentially the conducting zone. The structural-functional characterization of neurons is illustrated in Fig. 3-10.

Dendrites are actually protoplasmic extensions of the cell body; they have the same structural and functional features as the cell body. In a sense, dendrites are the structural expression by which the neuron attains a large surface area for the receptor zone. In contrast, the axon is a process of the neuron.

Dendrites The dendrites are relatively short branched extensions which rarely extend more than 700 μm from the perikaryon. From thick bases of from 5 to 10 μm in diameter, the dendritic trunks taper and then divide. The trunks and their branches divide several times. Two daughter branches diverge at an acute angle, with the fork of the angle located on the side distal to the cell body. Small excrescences of various sizes and shapes—called *dendritic spines, thorns,* or *gemmules*—are present on many dendrites. They are synaptic structures. Spines are absent at the bases of large trunks and on cell bodies. Some spines consist of a threadlike segment with a bulbous ending; these "musical note" spines are the most common. Other spines are thick, stubby segments with bulbous endings of various sizes (Fig. 2-10). Many pyramidal neurons of the cerebral cortex have about 4,000 spines per cell. In such a neuron, the surface area of the spines accounts for about 40 percent of the total surface area of dendrites and cell body. In effect, the spines and the dendrites serve the role of increasing the area of the receptor zone of the neuron, which is usually greater than that of the axon. Most neurons are multipolar because many dendrites emerge and spread out from their cell bodies. Dendrites have the same organelles as the cell body. They are never myelinated.

Neurons have been classified into three groups, on the basis of their dendritic patterns (Ramón-Moliner): generalized, or isodendritic, neurons; specialized, or allodendritic neurons; and highly specialized, or idiodendritic, neurons (Fig. 2-6).

1 Isodendritic neurons are characterized by long straight dendrites which spread out either from the cell body in all directions or along a given plane. The dendrites show a medium degree of branching, with daughter branches longer than trunk branches. Only a moderate number of spines are present. These cells are the basic neuron of the reticular core of the brain (Chap. 8).

2 Allodendritic neurons have a heterogeneous configuration of various types; they have a few main dendritic trunks which branch. Examples of these neurons include the pyramidal cells of the cerebral cortex and neurons of many of the processing (relay) nuclei within the brainstem.

3 Idiodendritic neurons have dendrites which branch to form arbors. These specialized neurons include mitral neurons of the olfactory bulb, Purkinje cells of the cerebellum, and bipolar cells of the retina and auditory nerve (Fig. 2-6).

Axons (Figs. 2-12 through 2-14) The axon of a typical multipolar neuron arises from a cone-shaped region of the cell body, called the *axon hillock,* attains a small diameter within $\frac{1}{10}$ mm from the hillock to form the *initial segment,* and then usually enlarges slightly to the diameter that is, in general, maintained throughout most of the length of the axon. The diameter may be reduced in size in the terminal branches of the axon. The axon is usually ensheathed by a segmented, discontinuous layer called the myelin sheath, which is interrupted at regular intervals by the nodes of Ranvier (described further on under "Peripheral Nerves"). Along its course, side or collateral branches may emerge from the axon at nodes of Ranvier. Distally, each axon branches profusely and in an irregular manner into terminal arborizations known as telodendria. The initial, or proximal, branches of the telodendria are *preterminal (nonsynaptic) segments,* and the distal branches are *terminal (synaptic) segments.* The final tip of each branch is called *the terminal.*

In large neurons the axon hillock is deficient in Nissl substance, but in small neurons the

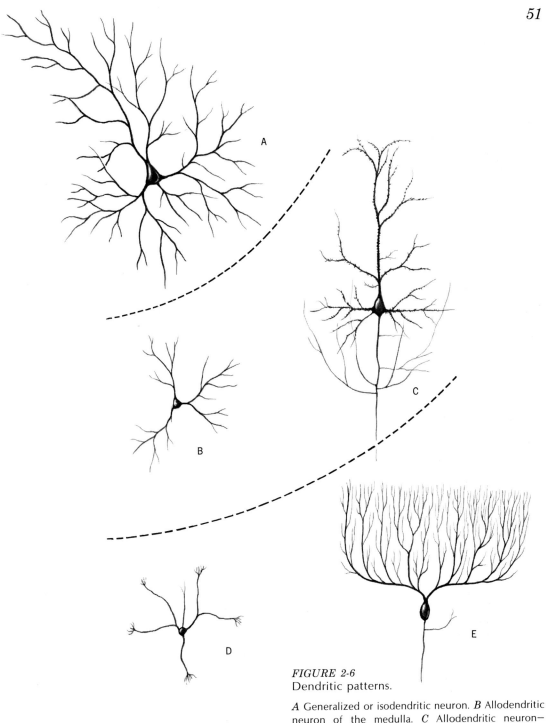

FIGURE 2-6
Dendritic patterns.

A Generalized or isodendritic neuron. *B* Allodendritic neuron of the medulla. *C* Allodendritic neuron—pyramidal cell of cerebral cortex. *D* Idiodendritic neuron—tufted neuron of a sensory nucleus. *E* Idiodendritic neuron—Purkinje cell of the cerebellum.

ribosomal content is essentially the same as in the cytoplasm of the cell body. A diagnostic feature of the axon hillock is the funnel arrangement of fascicles of microtubules which extend into and are oriented parallel to the long axis of the initial segment. In some cells the axon may arise from a dendrite. The unmyelinated initial segment (axon neck) is the nodal site, or trigger zone, associated with the initiation of the nerve impulse (action potential). Ribosomes are usually absent in this axon neck, as well as in the entire axon. In myelinated fibers the myelin sheath commences just distal to the initial segment. The axoplasm of an axon contains longitudinally oriented neurofilaments, microtubules, and agranular endoplasmic reticulum. The myelin sheath may extend along the preterminal segments but not necessarily along the terminal segments. Internodal distances are shorter in the telodendria than on the axon. The terminal segment has beaded dilatations (varicosities), or bulbous knobs, along its course before it terminates in an enlargement. These dilatations, or knobs, are called *boutons en passant* (*boutons de passage, end feet, synaptic knobs*), and the terminal enlargement is the bouton terminal (terminal *bouton, end bulb, terminal*). Each bouton is the presynaptic element of a synapse. Boutons en passant may be located at the node of Ranvier of a myelinated presynaptic segment. In the extensive axonal network of each postganglionic sympathetic fiber, the varicosities have diameters of 1 μm, the axon between varicosities is 0.1 μm in diameter, and the distance between two varicosities may average about 3 μm. Mitochondria are present especially in the vicinity of each node of Ranvier and in the boutons en passant and terminal bouton of the synaptic segments. Some neurons may have as many as 25,000 varicosities (Fig. 2-5).

Collateral and axonal branches emerge from a node of Ranvier at approximately right angles to the axon. A *recurrent collateral branch* may bifurcate at the first node of Ranvier, recurve, and arborize before synapsing with neurons other than the parent neuron.

Neurons with long axons (up to 3 ft in length)

are known as Golgi type I cells, and those small neurons with short axons are known as Golgi type II cells.

NEUROPIL

Within the gray matter of the nervous system are complex, highly organized entanglements of dendritic, axonal, and glial processes which act as the structural substrate where neural processing of organized physiologic activity takes place. This ordered meshwork of processes is called the *neuropil*. The high concentration of synaptic junctions among the plethora of neuronal processes is associated with the many sophisticated, subtle nuances processed through the functional interactions within this fiber matrix.

AXOPLASMIC TRANSPORT AND FLOW

A neuron is an actively secreting cell which has all the biosynthetic organization and high RNA content needed for the manufacture of enzymes, neurosecretions, and neurotransmitters. The products of the cell body are distributed to the axon terminals via unidirectional flow of axoplasm (bulk flow) and transport (not bulk flow). This process of *axoplasmic flow and transport* occurs at two general rates: *1* a *slow rate* of 1 to 10 mm per day, and *2 fast rates* of about 100 to 2,800 mm per day. The slow rate may be accounted for by "peristaltic-like waves" of the axon by which the axoplasm is "massaged forward" like a slug toward the nerve endings. Evidence indicates that fast rates are associated with transport along the microtubules and neurofilaments. Many microtubules are present in postganglionic sympathetic motor neurons, in which dense core vesicles are transported down the axon at the rate of 100 to 200 mm per day; and also in hypothalamic neurons, in which the transport of secretion granules occurs at rates of 2,800 mm per day. The microtubules have two possible roles in neurotransmitter granule transport: *1* they may have a passive role as the structural element along which granule movement takes place, or *2* they may have an active role in the granule movement.

Somatofugal axoplasmic flow from cell body through axon may serve several functions:

1 maintenance of neural integrity, *2* distribution of neurosecretory granules, *3* transport of enzymes and chemicals involved with the formation of neurotransmitters, and *4* distribution of substances associated with trophic activity.

Evidence indicates that some chemical substances may move up the axon somatopetally to the cell body. This suggests that *bidirectional flow* from and to the cell body occurs within an axon.

SYNAPSE

Synapses (*synaptic junctions*) are regions of specialized contact between neurons, between neurons and effector organs, or between two muscle fibers. According to one estimate, the human brain may have as many as 10^{14} synapses. They are one means by which cell-to-cell communication takes place. Many varieties of synapse are recognized (Figs. 2-7, 2-8).

Synapse may utilize chemicals or electrical currents as vehicles for communication. In a *chemical synapse*, a chemical neurotransmitter is released by the presynaptic neuron and this substance is capable of evoking a response in the postsynaptic cell. In this type of synapse the presynaptic cell is always a neuron; the postsynaptic cell may be a neuron, a muscle cell, or a glandular cell. In an *electrical synapse*, two cells are electrically coupled so that an electronic spread of nerve impulses directly crosses the synapse from the presynaptic cell to the postsynaptic cell. In this type of synapse, the presynaptic cell to postsynaptic cell linkage may be a neuron to neuron synapse, a cardiac muscle cell to cardiac muscle cell synapse (*intercalated disk*), or a smooth muscle cell to smooth muscle cell synapse (*nexus*).

In all synapses a small gap of from 20 to over 200 Å is present between the two cells. Hence these cells are in contiguity, not in continuity with other cells. The axon of a neuron may terminate in only a few synapses or in up to 50,000 synapses. A thousand synaptic boutons, or varicosities, may be considered to be a rough average. On the other hand, the dendrites and cell body of a single neuron may receive synaptic contacts from many neurons—from several hundred to as many as 100,000 separate axon terminals. In some neurons, as much as 40 per-

cent of the surface of the cell body is covered with synapses.

On the basis of the linkage of a neuron with some other cell, there are three types of synapse: *1* an interneuronal synapse, between two neurons; *2* a neuromuscular junction, between a neuron and a muscle cell; and *3* a neuroglandular junction, between a neuron and a glandular cell.

Interneuronal synapse (Figs. 2-7, 2-8, 2-9) These synapses are named on the basis of the parts of the neuron associated with the presynaptic and postsynaptic elements. Three of these synapses are numerous: *1* the *axosomatic synapse*, between an axon and a cell body; *2* the *axodendritic synapse*, between an axon and a dendrite; and *3* the *axoaxonic synapse*, between an axon and an axon. Other, less numerous synapses include *4* the *dendrodendritic synapse*, between a dendrite and a dendrite; *5* the *somatosomatic synapse*, between one cell body and another; *6* the *somatoaxonic synapse*, between a cell body and an axon; and *7* *somatodendritic synapse*, between a cell body and a dendrite.

These junctional complexes are identified as chemical synapses because two closely apposed parallel plasma membranes of the two structures are separated by a synaptic cleft, and synaptic vesicles are concentrated near the plasma membrane of the presynaptic element. Dendrodendritic synapses have been noted in the posterior horn of the spinal cord, lateral geniculate body, ventral posterior and ventral lateral thalamic nuclei, superior colliculus, retina (amacrine cells), and olfactory bulb. Reciprocal dendrodendritic synapses (Figs. 2-7, 2-8) are present in the olfactory bulb, retina, lateral geniculate body, and ventral lateral thalamic nucleus. Their possible functional roles are discussed under "The Olfactory System," in Chap. 15.

Chemical synapses (Figs. 2-4, 2-8) *Chemical synapses* are the classic synapses. They comprise three components: a *presynaptic element*, a *postsynaptic element*, and a *synaptic cleft* of about 200-Å width between the two elements. In the central nervous system the presynaptic element

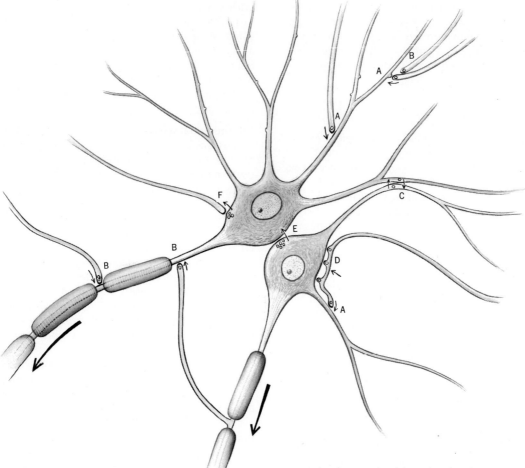

FIGURE 2-7
Several types of synapses.

A Axodendritic synapses. *B* Axoaxonic synapse. *C* Reciprocal dendrodendritic synapses (refer to Fig. 2-8). *D En passant* axosomatic synapses. *E* Somatosomatic synapse. *F* Somatoaxonic synapse.

of an axon is either a bouton en passant or a bouton terminal. Within the boutons are microvesicles, called synaptic vesicles, which contain putative neurotransmitter chemicals. These vesicles are clustered close to the presynaptic membrane. Mitochondria are present. The post-

synaptic element is either the dendritic spine or the smooth segment of a dendrite, a cell body, or an axon. The plasma membrane of the bouton is the *presynaptic membrane,* and that of the postsynaptic cell at the synapse is the *subsynaptic membrane.* This subsynaptic membrane is that region of the postsynaptic membrane that is juxtaposed against the presynaptic membrane at the synapse. In general usage, the subsynaptic membrane is referred to as the postsynaptic membrane. No concentration of synaptic vesicles is present in the postsynaptic cytoplasm near the subsynaptic membrane.

In some dendritic spines, there is a specialized postsynaptic structure called the spine apparatus; it comprises several flattened sacs separated by dense material. The presynaptic and subsynaptic membranes may have variable amounts of dense material apposed to the inner surface of one or both of the membranes. It may be present as irregular patches on the presynaptic membrane. Some dense material is also present in the synaptic clefts.

Chemical synapses are called *asymmetric synapses* because synaptic vesicles are present only in the presynaptic element; this is correlated with the fact that the transmission of the neural signals occurs unidirectionally from presynaptic to postsynaptic cell. On the basis of their sizes and shapes in electron micrographs, several types of synaptic vesicles are recognized. Among these are *1 spherical (or agranular) vesicles,* of about 400 to 600 Å in diameter, with clear centers; *2 dense-core (or granular) vesicles,* of from 500 to 800 Å in diameter, with a dense granule of about 280 Å in diameter; and *3 flat vesicles,* of from 200 to 400 Å. Some spherical vesicles and flattened vesicles are associated with the neurotransmitter acetylcholine; such associations are called "cholinergic synapses." The dense-core vesicles are associated with such biogenic amine neurotransmitters as norepinephrine or serotonin; these are called "adrenergic synapses." The small dense-core vesicles are found in the peripheral postganglionic sympathetic neurons, and the large dense-core vesicles may be associated with adrenergic endings in the central nervous system. The motor end plate "synapse" is described below in this chapter, and the synapse associated with postganglionic autonomic fibers is discussed in Chap. 6, The Autonomic Nervous System.

The combined presynaptic and subsynaptic membrane is called the *synaptolemma.* Following the disruption of the brain tissue by homogenization, the detached presynaptic nerve terminals can be fractionated; these pinched-off nerve endings are called "synaptosomes." They are useful in experimental studies for the analysis of neurotransmitters and synaptic activity.

Electric (Electronic) synapse (Fig. 2-8) An *electric synapse* is composed of three components: a presynaptic element, a postsynaptic element, and a narrow gap of 20 Å between the two elements. Because these plasma membranes are so closely apposed to each other, they form a *gap junction.* Formerly this was called a "tight junc-

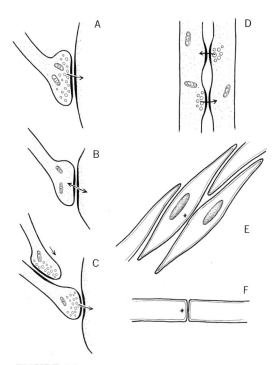

FIGURE 2-8
Several types of synapses.

A An asymmetric chemical synapse in which transmission occurs across a 200-Å-wide synaptic cleft in one direction (arrow).
B A symmetric electrical synapse in which transmission occurs across a 20-Å-wide cleft in either direction (arrow).
C Serial chemical synapses ("nests" or "glomeruli") in which transmission occurs serially across 200-Å-wide synaptic clefts in one direction.
D Reciprocal dendrodendritic asymmetric chemical synapses across 200-Å synapses (arrows).
E Symmetric electrical synapse (*) with a 20-Å-wide cleft between two smooth muscle cells.
F Symmetric electrical synapse (*) with a 20-Å-wide cleft between two cardiac muscle cells.

tion," because the outer leaflets of the plasma membranes of the pre- and postsynaptic membranes were thought to be in common; hence no gap was thought to exist. These synapses are called *symmetric synapses* because neither the presynaptic nor the postsynaptic element has

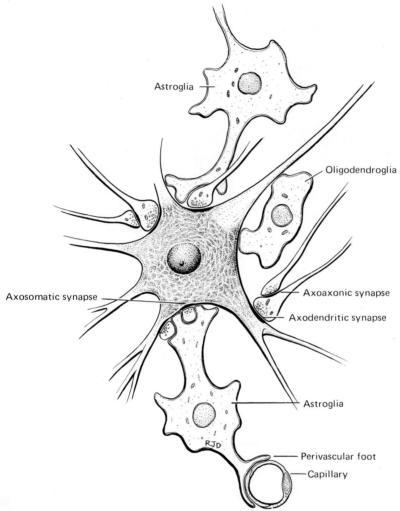

Astroglia

Oligodendroglia

Axosomatic synapse

Axoaxonic synapse

Axodendritic synapse

Astroglia

RJD

Perivascular foot

Capillary

FIGURE 2-9
Relation of a neuron, astrocyte, oligodendroglia, and
nerve terminals.

The axosomatic synapse, axodendritic synapse, and axoaxonic synapse in the central
nervous system have thickened subsynaptic membranes.
Astrocytes are glial cells with
thin processes extending to
the walls of the capillaries as
perivascular feet, and others
to neurons. The perineuronal
oligodendroglia are glial cells
with thick, stubby processes.

any synaptic vesicles and, in addition, the two junctional membranes are similar. The two cells are *"electrically coupled" ion resistance bridges;* the ionic flow from the presynaptic cell readily spreads to the postsynaptic cell. As a result there is no synaptic delay in electrical transmission. In mammals, electrical synapses are known to be present in a few places—in the lateral vestibular nucleus, the mesencephalic nucleus of the fifth nerve, and the bipolar cell–ganglion cell

junction in the primate retina. The junction (nexus) between two smooth muscle cells and that between two cardiac muscle cells (inter-calated disks) are gap junctions which function as electrical synapses.

Two morphologic types of synapses have been described in the pyramidal cells of the cerebral cortex. The *type I synapse* is present in the axodendritic synapses on the spines of the pyramidal cells (Fig. 2-10). The *type II synapse* is formed at the axodendritic synapses of the dendritic trunk and mainly at the axosomatic synapses on the pyramidal cells (Fig. 2-10). The type I synapse is characterized by thick, dense, and extensive subsynaptic membranes separated by a synaptic cleft 300 Å wide. The type II synapse is characterized by thin, dense patches on the presynaptic and subsynaptic membranes separated by a 200-Å synaptic cleft. In these pyramidal cells, the spines always have type I synapses; cell bodies always have type II synapses; and the dendritic membranes between spines have both type I and type II synapses. Intermediate types of synapses between type I and type II are present in the central nervous system.

A specific synapse need not be a permanent structure; it may be replaced by a new synapse. The degree to which this occurs normally is not known. For example, synapses are lost and new synapses are formed at the junctions between the sensory neurons and the neuroepithelial cells in the taste buds; neuroepithelial taste cells are replaced every few days, necessitating the formation of new synapses to maintain a functional end organ (Chap. 8).

FORMS OF NEURONS

Neurons assume a vast array of forms (Fig. 2-1). The cell bodies have a variety of shapes, with ovoid, pyramidal, stellate, spherical, bulbous, or irregular contours. The axons and dendrites exhibit an apparently endless number of arborization patterns. Some common neuron types will be described.

The *bipolar neuron* is a nerve cell with one axon and one dendrite. Bipolar cells are found in the retina of the eye and in the cochlear, vestibular, and olfactory nerves. In each of these examples the dendrite commences peripherally as a terminal arborization and the axon usually extends centrally.

The *unipolar neuron* (or *pseudounipolar neuron*) is a nerve cell with one short process that divides into two long processes. Basically this is a modified bipolar cell in which the axon and the dendrite are in common for a short distance from the cell body; hence the term "pseudounipolar neuron." The cell body of this neuron type is located in the spinal ganglia of the spinal nerves or in some sensory ganglia of the cranial

nerves (Chap. 7). The nominal "dendrite" in this neuron is the long process that extends to the sensory endings. Because nerve impulses are conducted via this process to the cell body, the process warrants the term "dendrite." The length, the relatively constant diameter, and the all-or-none conducting property (Chap. 3) of this long process account for its being called an axon. In brief, the distal process of a unipolar cell may be called either an axon or a dendrite. The other branch that terminates in the central nervous system is an axon.

The *Golgi type II* neuron has branching dendrites and one short arborizing axon. These neurons are multipolar cells because of the many processes extending from each cell body.

The *multipolar cells* have many short dendrites and one long axon. Examples of this neuron type include the motor neurons (motoneuron) that directly innervate the voluntary muscles, and the motor neurons of the autonomic nervous system that innervate the involuntary muscles and glands. A collateral branch emerges from the axon in the vicinity of the cell body.

The *Purkinje cell* is a neuron located in the cortex of the cerebellum. It has a dendrite with an extensive arborization in one plane, resembling the branches of a vine on a trellis. Its axon has a recurrent collateral branch.

The *pyramidal cell* of the cerebral cortex is a neuron named from the shape of its cell body. Each cell has a number of dendrites. The one apical dendrite extends from the apex of the pyramid to arborize in several branches; many collateral branches extend from one *apical dendritic* process. The other branched dendrites that extend from the cell body are called *"basilar dendrites"* (Chap. 16). The axons of some pyramidal cells may exceed 3 ft in length. Axon collateral branches are present.

Peripheral nervous system

The peripheral nerves are the cranial and spinal nerves, including their branches. The peripheral ganglia are the collections of cell bodies associ-

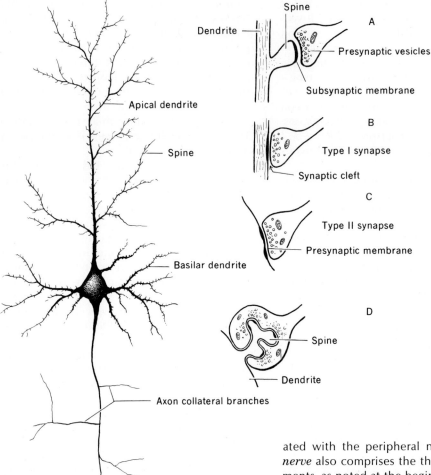

FIGURE 2-10
Synapses on a pyramidal neuron of the neo-cortex.

In a type I synapse, the entire subsynaptic membrane is thick. In a type II synapse the synaptic membrane has several small thick patches.

A Type I axodendritic synapse between an axon terminal and a dendritic spine.

B Type I axodendritic synapse between an axon terminal and a dendritic trunk.

C Type II axodendritic synapse between an axon terminal and a cell body (axosomatic synapse).

D A complex axodendritic synapse between an axon terminal and a dendritic spine on a pyramidal cell of the hippocampus with several thickened subsynaptic patches.

ated with the peripheral nerves. A *peripheral nerve* also comprises the three basic tissue elements, as noted at the beginning of the chapter (Fig. 2-11): *1* axons (neuron); *2* neurolemma (Schwann) cells and the myelin sheaths (interstitial elements); and *3* the endoneurium, perineurium, and epineurium (connective tissue elements). A *peripheral ganglion* also comprises the three basic elements: *1* cell bodies, proximal portions of axons and dendrites (of the neuron); *2* the inner satellite cells (interstitial elements); and *3* the outer satellite cells (connective tissue elements).

PERIPHERAL NERVES

A *peripheral nerve* with its numerous nerve fibers is comparable to a telephone cable (Fig. 2-11). The axons are analogous to the wires, and the neurolemma cells and the endoneurium to the insulation encapsulating each wire. Groups of the insulated nerve fibers are bound into fascicles by the perineurium. Groups of fascicles are in turn encapsulated by the epineurium. Each of these layers is continuous with a counterpart in most peripheral ganglia.

The *nerve fiber* includes an axon (axis cylinder), its neurolemma sheath, and its endoneural connective tissue sheath. The neurolemma sheath may elaborate myelin, a fatty layer surrounding an axis cylinder. A nerve fiber with a myelin sheath is called a myelinated or medullated nerve fiber, and that with little or no myelin is called an unmyelinated or nonmyelinated nerve fiber (Fig. 2-11). Nearly all nerve fibers over 2 μm in diameter are myelinated, and those under 2 μm are unmyelinated.

The *myelin sheath* is a segmented, discontinuous layer, interrupted at regular intervals by the *nodes of Ranvier* (Fig. 2-11). The distance from one node to the next is an internode, whose length is roughly proportional to the diameter of the axon. The length of the internodes varies from 50 to 1,500 μm. The diameters and lengths of internodes of the various fibers are directly related to the speed of conduction of the nerve impulse (Chap. 3). Each internode is formed by and surrounded by one neurolemma (Schwann) cell. Between the neurolemma cell proper and the axis cylinder is the myelin sheath, which consists of fine concentric layers. These myelin sheath lamellae are submicroscopic structures consisting of protein and lipid layers that are the repeating units of the myelin sheath (Fig. 2-11*C*). Each layer is actually derived from the cell membrane of the neurolemma cell. The spiral wrapping ("jelly roll") of these cell membranes encapsulates the axon (Fig. 2-11*C*). In effect, the myelin sheath is a helical arrangement of successive double cell membranes of the neurolemma cell from a few to 100 spirals per internode; the fused lamellae remain after the neurolemma cell cytoplasm is squeezed out, and the membranes fuse. The *clefts of Schmidt-Lantermann* are present in living nerves (Fig. 2-11*B*). These clefts are small pockets of cytoplasm formed by local separations of the myelin lamellae. The axon is almost naked at each node of Ranvier, for the myelin sheath is absent at each node. Only the finger-like processes of the adjacent neurolemma cells interdigitate over the nodal area (Fig. 2-12).

Four features of the nodes are important: *1* nerve fibers branch at a node; *2* concentrations of mitochondria in the axis cylinder at these sites suggest local high metabolic activity; *3* the close proximity of extracellular fluids to the axon at each node is critical to saltatory conduction (Chap. 3); and *4* the possible isolation of the periaxonal space of the internode from the node of Ranvier by the close apposition of the terminal loops of the myelin sheath to the axolemma (Fig. 2-12) may be critical to saltatory conduction.

Whereas a myelinated fiber is ensheathed by its private layer of neurolemma cells, a group of *unmyelinated fibers* share a common neurolemma cell (Fig. 2-13). As many as 15 or more unmyelinated fibers may share one neurolemma cell. These fibers are separated from one another, for each is embedded in a private sleeve of the surface of the neurolemma cell's plasma membrane. The fibers are not within the cytoplasm of the neurolemma cell, for the cell membrane of the neurolemma cell is intact everywhere. In effect, a theoretical myelin sheath is represented by the cell membrane of the neurolemma cell. The axons comprising the olfactory nerve present an unusual arrangement. Up to several dozens of axons are organized into a fascicle surrounded by one neurolemma cell; the axons in each fascicle are essentially in direct contact with each other (axons are separated by spaces 100 Å wide). The olfactory nerve comprises many fascicles (Chap. 15).

The *peripheral nerves and ganglia* of both the somatic and autonomic nervous system consist of myelinated and unmyelinated fibers bound together by several layers composed of connective tissue elements and by a layer of epithelium (Fig. 2-11). The *endoneurium* (*sheath of Henle*) surrounds each neurolemma cell as a private sheath; it comprises the basal lamina associated with the neurolemma cell, some scattered mesenchymal cells, fibroblasts, histiocytes, and a few delicate connective tissue fibers. The *perineurium* surrounds nerve fibers grouped into fascicles; it comprises an *outer lamina of connective tissue* and an *inner lamina of epithelium*. The inner lamina is a thin, continuous, multilayered sheet of squamous epithelial cells—called the *perineural epithelium* (Shantha

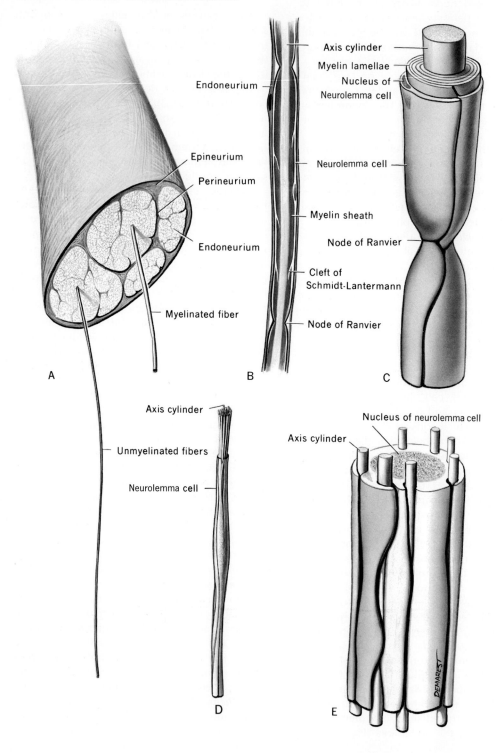

Endoneurium

Epineurium
Perineurium

Endoneurium

Myelinated fiber

A

Axis cylinder
Myelin lamellae
Nucleus of
Neurolemma cell

Neurolemma cell

Myelin sheath

Node of Ranvier

Cleft of
Schmidt-Lantermann

Node of Ranvier

B   C

Axis cylinder

Unmyelinated fibers

Neurolemma cell

D

Nucleus of neurolemma cell
Axis cylinder

E

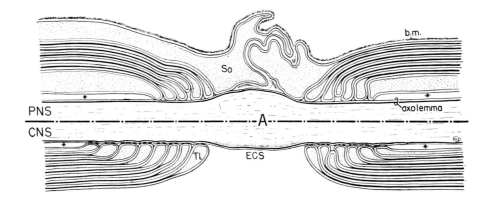

FIGURE 2-12
Regions of the nodes of Ranvier in the peripheral nervous system (PNS) compared with those in the central nervous system (CNS).

In the PNS, the neurolemma cell has an outer collar (So.) of cytoplasm which loosely interdigitates in the nodal region with the outer collar of the adjacent neurolemma cell. In the CNS, the axis cylinder (A) in the nodal region is exposed directly to the extracellular space (E.C.S.). In both the PNS and CNS the compact layered myelin surrounding the axis cylinder forms terminal loops (T.L.), which are in close apposition to the axolemma; this apposition may form a "seal," preventing ready movement of materials between the periaxonal space (*) and the nodal region. The neurolemma cell is covered by a basement lamina (b.m.). (*Courtesy of Dr. R. P. Bunge and the American Physiological Society.*)

FIGURE 2-11
Peripheral nerve as visualized under light microscope and under electron microscope magnifications.

A A myelinated nerve fiber and several unmyelinated nerve fibers extending out of the peripheral nerve trunk.
B Myelinated nerve fiber as visualized with light microscope.
C Myelinated nerve fiber as reconstructed from electron micrographs. The helically laminated myelin sheath (jelly roll) is continuous with the cell membrane of the neurolemma cell.
D Several unmyelinated nerve fibers as viewed with the light microscope. One neurolemma cell ensheaths several nerve fibers.
E Several unmyelinated nerve fibers ensheathed by one neurolemma cell, as reconstructed from electron micrographs.

and Bourne). It extends centrally along the dorsal and ventral roots, where it is continuous with the piarachnoid layers, and peripherally to form the capsules of the sensory receptors (e.g., Pacinian and Meissner's corpuscles and neuromuscular spindles) and motor end plates (Fig. 2-3). The perineural epithelium is thought to provide a barrier to the passage of many substances from the connective tissue of the epineurium and perineurium to the nerve fibers. The *epineurium* binds together large numbers of fascicles into the named peripheral nerves of gross anatomy. The connective tissue lamina of the perineurium of these layers are continuous with the dura mater. The connective tissue serves several useful purposes: a supportive role, a nutritive role by providing a network of blood vessels, and a role in the conductile activity of the nerve fiber through the electrolytes in the interstitial fluids.

According to the above description, the entire central nervous system and the peripheral nervous sytem are ensheathed by a *sleeve of epithelium* (*piarachnoid and perineural epithelium*), surrounded in turn by connective tissue (*dura mater and perineural-epineural layer*).

Of the peripheral motor nerves, *1* the thick, heavily myelinated fibers are the alpha motor

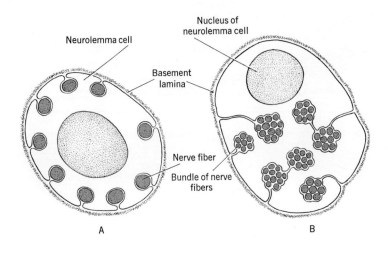

FIGURE 2-13
Unmyelinated fibers of peripheral nervous system.

A Nine myelinated fibers enclosed in individual troughs of a neurolemma cell. *B* Clusters of groups of fine fibers enclosed in troughs of a neurolemma cell as in the olfactory nerve. (*After Dr. R. P. Bunge.*)

fibers to the voluntary muscles; *2* the thin, lightly myelinated fibers are the gamma motor fibers to the neuromuscular spindles and the preganglionic autonomic fibers; and *3* the unmyelinated fibers are the postganglionic autonomic fibers to smooth muscles and glands. Of the peripheral sensory nerves, *1* the medium-sized, moderately myelinated fibers are generally associated with tactile and proprioceptive senses; *2* the thin to unmyelinated fibers with pain, temperature, taste, and visceral senses; and *3* the unmyelinated fibers with the olfactory sense.

PERIPHERAL GANGLIA

The *ganglia* of the peripheral nervous system are the structures consisting of the cell bodies and their adjacent cell processes. Two types of ganglia are present: *1* the sensory (afferent) ganglia of the cranial nerves and the spinal ganglia of the spinal nerves, and *2* the motor ganglia of the autonomic nervous system.

The *sensory ganglia,* located close to the central nervous system, are usually aggregations of unipolar cells (Chap. 5). No synapses are found in these ganglia. One process of these unipolar cells extends distally through a peripheral nerve to a sensory ending; the other process projects into the central nervous system (Fig. 2-2).

The *autonomic motor ganglia,* located at a distance from the central nervous system, are aggregations of multipolar (postganglionic) neurons of the autonomic nervous system (Chap. 6). The dendrites and cell bodies of these multipolar neurons, which are located wholly within a ganglion, make synaptic connections with the axons of preganglionic neurons (Chap. 6).

Each cell body of each ganglion is encapsulated by a single layer of inner satellite cells which is continuous with the neurolemma cell layer of a peripheral nerve fiber. No myelin sheath is associated with the cell bodies. There are two exceptions. The cell bodies of the vestibular and spiral ganglia of the eighth cranial nerve are myelinated. Surrounding the layer of the inner satellite cells is the layer of outer satellite cells, which is continuous with the endoneurium surrounding the peripheral nerve fiber. The connective tissue binding the ganglia is continuous with the perineurium and epineurium of the peripheral nerve. These layers are often absent in the small ganglia (parasympathetic ganglia) in smooth muscle.

The central nervous system is composed of the same three basic elements as the peripheral nervous system: neurons, neuroglia (astroglia, oligodendroglia, and ependymal cells) of the interstitial elements, and microglia and blood vessels of the connective tissue elements.

NEURONS

Fundamentally, the neurons of the central nervous system have the same structure as those of the peripheral nervous system (Fig. 2-1). The neurons of the brain and spinal cord are organized into interacting networks and pathways which are more complex than in the peripheral nervous system. To unravel the neuronal organization of the nervous system is the basic function of neuroanatomy and neurophysiology.

NEUROGLIA AND OTHER ELEMENTS (Fig. 2-9)

The neuroglial (glial) cells outnumber the neurons from five to ten times and comprise about half the total volume of the brain and spinal cord. Literally the neurons are in a sea of glial cells (Figs. 2-9 and 2-14 through 2-16).

The neuroglia cells—"nerve-glue"—are metabolically supportive cells of the nervous system, assisting the neurons to perform their roles. Glial cells do not form synapses or generate action potentials. They do form and sustain the myelin sheaths, which increase the speed of nerve impulse conduction. In ways not fully defined, the glial cells have significant roles in regulating the ionic concentrations within the extracellular space so critical to the electrophysiologic activity of neurons. In addition, they may provide high-energy compounds to neurons and may act as intermediary stations for conveying nutrients, gases, and waste products between the neurons and the vascular system and cerebrospinal fluid. Most tumors originating within the central nervous system arise from neuroglial elements.

Neuroglia are classified into the following types: *1 oligodendrocytes, 2 astrocytes, 3 microglia,* and *4 ependyma.* The oligodendrocytes and astrocytes are called *macroglia.*

Oligodendrocytes (Oligodendroglia) Three general types of oligodendrocytes are recognized: *perineuronal (satellite) oligodendrocytes,* adjacent to the cell bodies of neurons; *interfascicular oligodendrocytes,* associated with the myelin sheaths; and *perivascular oligodendrocytes,* in the vicinity of blood vessels.

The *perineuronal (satellite) oligodendrocytes* are found in gray matter, whereas the *interfascicular oligodendrocytes* are located between nerve fibers of the white matter and with groups of myelinated fibers located in the gray matter (Figs. 2-9, 2-12). An oligodendrocyte can be distinguished from an astrocyte by several criteria. It has a smaller, rounder, denser nucleus; only a few delicate processes extend from its cell body. Within their denser cytoplasm are many microtubules, mitochondria, and ribosomes but no filaments nor glycogen. Except for the form of their processes, these types of oligodendrocytes are morphologically similar.

Oligodendrocytes are presumed to perform two roles: forming and maintaining the myelin in the central nervous system; and sustaining neurons by supplying nutrition and possibly some unknown factors. A symbiotic association between these cells and neurons is an intriguing possibility.

The perineuronal oligodendrocytes that encapsulate the cell bodies are equivalent to the satellite cells of the spinal ganglia and autonomic peripheral ganglia. The interfascicular oligodendroglia surrounding the nerve fibers are the equivalent of the neurolemma (Schwann) cells of the peripheral nerves. All these cells are derived from ectoderm.

The myelin sheaths of the axons in the central nervous system are the products of layers of the plasma membranes of oligodendrocytes. Each oligodendroglial cell forms and maintains as many as 50 internodal segments of many axons (Fig. 2-14). Extending from each of these glial cells are several cytoplasmic tongues surrounded by the plasma membrane; each tongue extends to an axon, where it spreads out as a flat, thin sheath and a myelin membrane spiral. This is the myelinated internode. In brief, myelin sheaths of the central nervous system and pe-

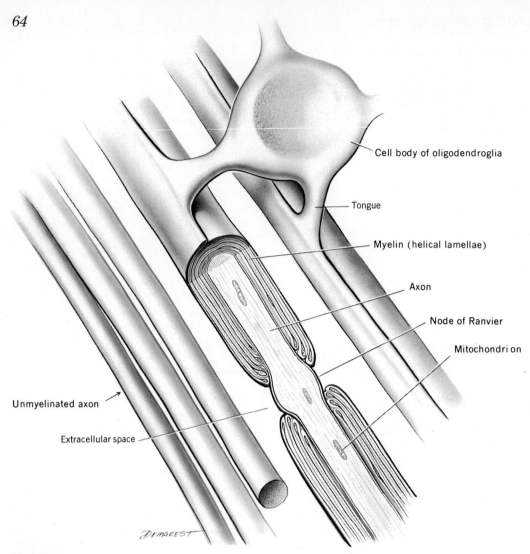

Cell body of oligodendroglia

Tongue

Myelin (helical lamellae)

Axon

Node of Ranvier

Mitochondrion

Unmyelinated axon

Extracellular space

DEMAREST

FIGURE 2-14
Relation of oligodendroglia to the axons of the central nervous system, as reconstructed from electron micrographs.

The three unmyelinated axons on the left are naked. The two myelinated axons on the right share one oligodendroglial cell. The myelin sheaths of each of the myelinated fibers are continuous through the protoplasmic tongue with the glial cell body. This glial tongue spreads out as a ridge, which extends throughout the entire length of an internode. The loop of the cell membrane at the ridge makes the site where the glial cell membrane is doubled (myelin unit of two plasma cell membranes) and is continuous as the laminated myelin sheath. (*Adapted from Bunge, Bunge, and Ris.*)

ripheral nervous system are similar; both are compacted layers of plasma membranes. The nodes of Ranvier in the central nervous system are exposed directly to the extracellular space; the node is not ensheathed by the plasma membrane of the glial cell. The tongue probably serves as the route through which material from the cell body passes to sustain the myelin sheath. The precise function of the perineuronal and perivascular oligodendrocytes is unknown.

Astrocytes (Astroglia) Two types of astrocytes include *protoplasmic astrocytes,* located primarily in the gray matter of the brain and spinal cord; and *fibrous astrocytes,* found chiefly in the white matter. As compared to an oligodendrocyte, an astrocyte has a larger, irregular ovoid nucleus, which is less compact; many cytoplasmic processes extend from its cell body. Cytoplasmic filaments and glycogen are characteristic.

The processes of the glial cells may extend to the blood capillaries to form *vascular feet, end feet,* or "sucker feet"; the *pia-glial membrane (external limiting gliosal membrane)* adjacent to the subarachnoid space (Fig. 2-15); and the nonsynaptic surface of a neuron (Fig. 2-16). In some regions of the brain, gap junctions interconnect two glial cells (refer to "Blood-Brain Barrier," further on).

Four general roles for astrocytes have been proposed.

1 Structural support. The astrocytes and their processes are insinuated throughout the spaces among the neurons and their processes and thereby embrace groups of neuronal fibers. In this sense they may act as a supporting network.

2 Repair following damage from injury. The fibrous astrocytes are considered to be the scarring cells of the nervous system which repair the gaps lost following destruction of neural tissues from a variety of insults. Connective tissue may also contribute to the central nervous system scarring, which is called sclerosis.

3 Isolation of the junctional surfaces of a synapse (Fig. 2-9). The astrocytic processes form junctional contacts with the plasma membrane of the neuronal surface; these contacts are conceived as being organized in a variety of structural patterns, in order to segregate certain regions of the postsynaptic receptor surface of the neuron from other regions. These ordered patterns could have a significant role in the processing taking place in the dendritic zone of each neuron.

4 Blood-brain barrier. The astrocytes and their specialized contacts with the blood vessels, pia-glial membrane, neuronal surface, and between themselves are thought to be critical in the blood-brain barrier concept (Fig. 2-16).

The *ependymal cells* are the glial cells which line the ventricular system and the choroid plexuses. The *microglia* are phagocytic cells which are related to the macrophages of the connective tissues. The microglia are found throughout the central nervous system; under proper stresses, as in an injury, they function to phagocytize, transform, and remove disintegration products of the neurons. They act as scavengers. The numerous blood vessels are accompanied, once they enter within the substance of the central nervous system, with a minimal amount of perivascular connective tissue. The pia mater, arachnoid, and dura mater, which envelop the central nervous system, are formed of connective tissue elements.

The glial elements have been implicated in information storage processes, in memory mechanisms, and in maintenance of bioelectric potentials (Chap. 3).

The freshly cut brain has areas that are grayish in appearance (gray matter) and others that are whitish (white matter). Gray matter is composed mainly of cell bodies of neurons and dendrites; white matter is made up largely of myelinated and unmyelinated axons. Glial cells and blood vessels are located in both white matter and gray matter.

BLOOD-BRAIN BARRIER (Brain barriers)

The concept of the *blood-brain barrier (hematoencephalic barrier)* was originally based on observations that many chemical substances which readily pass out of the bloodstream into the interstitial fluid and parenchyma of many organs do not do so in the brain and spinal cord. Thus a barrier was said to exist between the vascular system and the brain. The concept has since been modified to include the various anatomic features and physiologic and biochemical systems which operate to subdivide the central nervous system and associated structures into a number of compartments; hence, the existence of *brain barriers* which demarcate these compartments. Among these are *1* the *blood-brain barrier* between the vascular and the brain compartments, *2* the *blood–cerebrospinal fluid (CSF) barrier* between the vascular and the CSF compartments, and *3* the *brain-CSF barrier* between the brain and CSF compartments. Furthermore, the central nervous system has been divided into a *neuronal compartment,* a *neuro-*

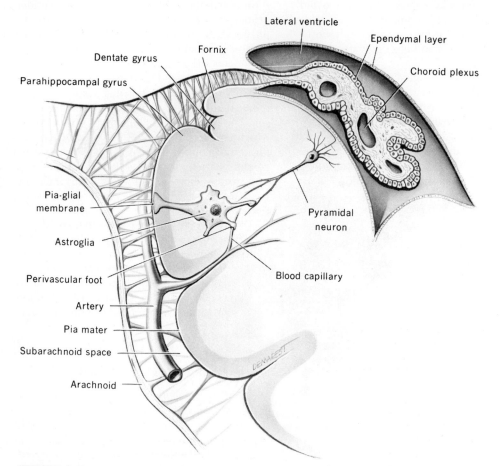

FIGURE 2-15
Relations of the leptomeninges, subarachnoid, choroid plexus, ventricle, astroglia, and neurons of the central nervous system.

The subarachnoid space is located between the arachnoid and pia mater. The choroid plexus is composed of an ependymal layer and a highly vascularized connective tissue core. Subarachnoid blood vessels and subarachnoid space are continuous with the core of the choroid plexus. The astrocyte has several processes: one extends to a blood capillary and terminates as a perivascular foot; another process extends to and contacts the pyramidal neuron; and another extends to the pia mater.

FIGURE 2-16
Some ultrastructural features in the brain, choroid plexus, piaarachnoid layer, and ventricle.

The continuous extracellular space of the central nervous system is located among the glial cells (G.) and neurons or their processes (N.). Many of these features are basic to modern concepts of the blood-brain barrier. See the text for details. (*After Brightman and Reese.*)

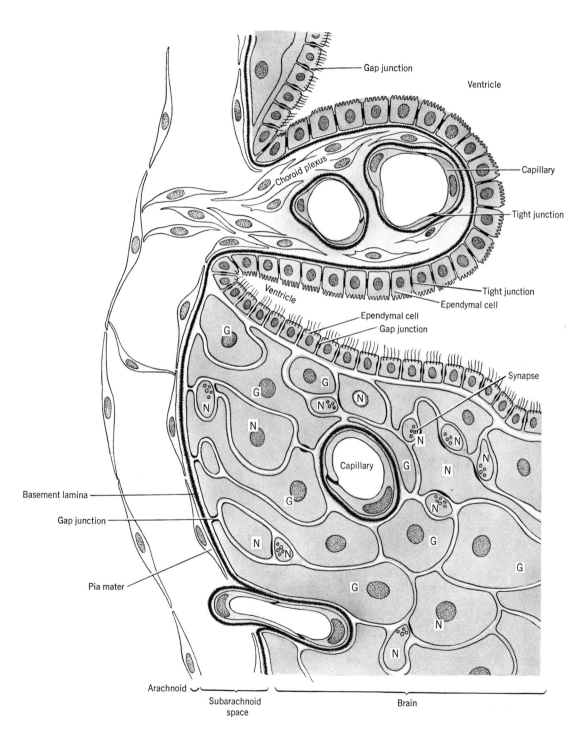

Gap junction

Ventricle

Choroid plexus

Capillary

Tight junction

Tight junction

Ependymal cell

Ventricle

Ependymal cell

Gap junction

Synapse

G

N

N

N

N

N

N

N

G

G

G

Capillary

G

N

G

N

N

G

G

Basement lamina

Gap junction

N

N

N

Pia mater

G

N

N

Arachnoid

Subarachnoid
space

Brain

glial compartment, and an *intercellular (ex-tracellular) fluid compartment* (Fig. 2-16). Some authorities think of the "barrier" as comprising both the structural entities and the physiologic processes that slow down rather than stop the movement of certain substances from one compartment into another compartment. The movement of these substances takes place by diffusion and/or active transport.

Recent studies on the ultrastructure of the brain, meninges, and choroid plexus (Fig. 2-16) illustrate some of the morphologic features associated with the brain-barrier concepts (Brightman and Reese). The capillaries of the brain (parenchymal vessels) and choroid plexuses and those entering the brain through the pia-glial membrane (leptomeningeal vessels) are surrounded by a perivascular basement lamina (membrane) composed of a mucopolysaccharide matrix. The endothelial cells of these capillaries are joined together throughout by tight junctions (in a tight junction, there is an actual fusion between the outer protein leaflets of the plasma membranes of the adjoining cells). The choroid plexus is characterized by having *fenestrated capillaries;* the endothelial cells have fenestrations, or pores, closed by diaphragms thinner than the plasma membrane. Fenestrated capillaries are located in structures noted for fluid transport. The capillaries in the brain are not fenestrated. The *basement lamina* is also found adjacent to the epithelial cells of the choroid plexus and continuous with the pia-glial membrane, where it is intercalated between the pial cells and the glial cells.

The *choroid plexus* consists of two layers: *1* The fenestrated capillaries are located within a connective tissue stromal layer. Its interface with the subarachnoid space is formed by a thin layer of flattened connective tissue cells joined together by gap junctions. *2* The single layer of cuboidal epithelium has a continuous basement lamina on its basal side. These cells are joined to adjacent cells by tight junctions. These junctions act to restrict intercellular movement of material. Microvilli are present on the free border of the cells facing the ventricles. The fenestrated capillaries, adequate stromal space, and active transport systems within the cuboidal

epithelial cells are geared to enhance the passage of materials from the vascular system to the CSF of the ventricles (and vice versa). The belts of tight junctions between the endothelial cells and cuboidal choroidal cells form limiting sheets which are barriers to the intercellular movement of proteins. Passage across the epithelial cells may take place by active transport and by pinocytosis. In the latter, the cell "drinks" a small quantity of fluid, forms a vesicle, transports it across the cell, and discharges the vesicle into the ventricle (or vice versa).

The brain and spinal cord contain an extracellular space located among nonfenestrated capillaries, glial cells, and neurons. They are surrounded by a pia-glial membrane and other meninges. The extracellular space probably occupies about 15 percent of the brain volume (depending upon the method used to obtain data, other estimates range from about 5 to 25 percent). These extracellular spaces are open and act as channels for the rapid diffusion of ions (e.g., Na^+ and K^+) and certain small molecules among the cells or to the CSF in the ventricles or subarachnoid space (Fig. 2-16). These substances in these extracellular spaces have an outlet to the CSF of the ventricular cavities; this is the intercellular space among the discontinuous gap junctions between adjacent ependymal cells lining the ventricles. Another outlet to the CSF of the subarachnoid space is through the intercellular spaces and basement lamina at the pia-glial membrane. The flattened pial cells, like the ependymal cells, are also joined together by discontinuous gap junctions (Fig. 2-16).

The capillaries of the central nervous system consist of a continuous endothelial lining surrounded by a continuous basement lamina. Physiologic evidence indicates that the basement lamina is not a barrier to diffusion. About 85 to 99 percent of the perivascular surface is covered with the end feet of astrocytes. These end feet are linked to one another by discontinuous gap junctions (unobstructed intercellular clefts are present between some portions of the end feet). Transport across the capillaries may occur by diffusion or by pinocytosis. All neurons and glial cells are no farther than 25 to 50 μm away from a blood capillary, but many are considerably farther away from the CSF. Evidence indicates that the exchange of materials between the CSF and the brain is considerably more rapid than between the capillaries and the brain.

The astrocytes have a significant location. They form a special compartment or pool *1* between the capillaries and the neurons, *2* between the capillaries and the pia-glial membrane, and *3* between the neurons and the pia-glial membrane. Discontinuous gap junctions join two astrocytes *1* at their end feet adjacent to a capillary, *2* at the glial processes of the pia-glial membrane, and *3* between their cell bodies or processes. Glial cells are similar to neurons in that they have high resting potentials, a high concentration of potassium ions, and a low concentration of sodium ions. In contrast to neurons, glial cells do not generate propagated impulses. Some substances probably pass from the astroglial compartment to the other compartments and the extracellular space.

The primary role of the brain barriers is to provide the control systems which regulate and maintain the optimal stable chemical environment for the neurons of the central nervous system. Homeostatic mechanisms utilize the molecular transport systems and various physical constraints (e.g., gap junctions) to regulate the ion fluxes between the blood plasma, extracellular space within the brain, and the CSF. The exquisite control of the chemical environment of the central nervous system is essential to minimize the effects of any potential variations, because neurons are most sensitive to their chemical milieu. Information on these mechanisms is incomplete.

The choroid plexuses, capillary beds of the central nervous system, and the CSF are the media which furnish, exchange, and eliminate the nutrients, ions, metabolites, and waste products. Apparently the extracellular space within the central nervous system is sufficient for ion flow associated with neuronal activity.

Recent studies suggest that certain substances are discharged into the CSF and transported within the ventricle to other sites. Hormones of the posterior lobe of the hypophysis, hypothalamic hormones, and melatonin of the pineal body may be discharged into the CSF and transported to other sites by intracerebral transport.

In summary, the CSF performs several functional roles: *1* its buoyancy protects the brain, *2* it is a link in the control of the chemical environment of the central nervous system, *3* it acts as a medium for the exchange of nutrients and waste products with the central nervous system, and *4* it may serve as a channel for intracerebral transport. In general, it seems that neuroglia function primarily as regulating systems rather than as indispensable adjuncts to the neuronal elements.

Nerve endings of the peripheral nerves

The nerve endings in the peripheral tissues may be characterized by functional and structural criteria. The afferent, or sensory, endings are those nerve terminals that transduce stimuli. The efferent, or motor, endings are those nerve terminals that stimulate muscles or glands (a form of synapse between a nerve fiber and an effector). One sensory neuron, its branches, and its sensory endings constitute a unit known as a *sensory unit*. One motor neuron, its branches, and the muscles innervated by its endings constitute a unit known as a *motor unit*.

Structurally the nerve endings may be classified as *free (nonencapsulated) nerve endings* and *encapsulated nerve endings*. The free nerve endings are the endings of the axis cylinders without any apparent structural modification of the adjacent tissues. The encapsulated endings are the endings of axis cylinders which are surrounded by organized connective tissue capsules. All nerve endings are naked in the sense that they are devoid of a neurolemmal sheath.

AFFERENT (SENSORY) ENDINGS

The *free nerve endings* are the branched terminations of myelinated and unmyelinated fibers that finally lose their neurolemma (Schwann) sheaths and terminate as naked axis cylinders. These simple endings are found in the epithelium of the skin, cornea of the eye, mucous membranes, intermuscular connective tissues, and pulp of the tooth. The unmyelinated nerves to the viscera (heart, intestinal tract) ramify and terminate in the same way (details of the junctional endings are controversial). Cold, warmth, touch, and pain are probably the subjective effects that follow the stimulation of these end-

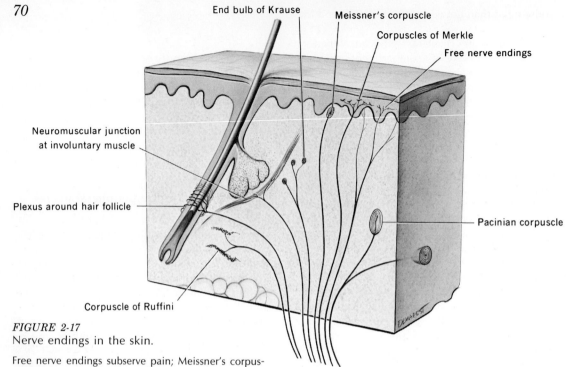

End bulb of Krause

Meissner's corpuscle

Corpuscles of Merkle

Free nerve endings

Neuromuscular junction at involuntary muscle

Plexus around hair follicle

Pacinian corpuscle

Corpuscle of Ruffini

FIGURE 2-17
Nerve endings in the skin.

Free nerve endings subserve pain; Meissner's corpuscles, Merkel's corpuscles, and plexus around hair follicle subserve the tactile sense; Pacinian corpuscles subserve pressure and vibratory sense; corpuscles of Ruffini subserve warmth; and end bulbs of Krause subserve cold. Free nerve endings form the motor innervation of involuntary (smooth) muscle.

ings. Some of these naked fibers end in the skin as disklike expansions of the tactile corpuscles of Merkel. Axons that terminate as a plexus around the hair follicle act as sensitive tactile receptors when a hair is moved. Those endings known as interoceptors are free nerve endings in the wall of viscus, as in the stomach (where they may give rise to discomfort and pains of distention, hunger sensations, and cramps of contraction), the bronchi of the lungs (where they monitor the tension in the lungs during respiration), and the aorta, other large arteries, and the right atrium of the heart (where they are sensitive to changes in blood pressure).

The afferent encapsulated nerve endings are found in the skin, muscles, tendons, joints, and the deep tissues of the body. The afferent endings include the neuromuscular spindles within the voluntary muscles, the neurotendinous spindles (organs of Golgi) in tendons, Meissner's

corpuscles in the skin, end bulbs of Krause, and corpuscles of Ruffini, among others. This classification is unsatisfactory because transitional forms are common (Figs. 2-17, 2-18).

Neuromuscular spindles are encapsulated, elongated fusiform sensory receptors of several millimeters in length. A spindle contains both nervous and muscular elements. To perform its functional role, not only is each spindle mounted within a voluntary muscle, but its long axis is oriented *in parallel* to the muscle fibers of the voluntary muscle. The capsule of the spindle is continuous at its two tapered ends with the connective tissue surrounding the normal muscle fibers. Within this structural orientation to the voluntary muscle, the spindle will stretch when the muscle relaxes (lengthens). It will shorten when the voluntary muscle contracts (Fig. 2-18). On this basis it performs its role as a stretch receptor monitoring tension (Chap. 5).

Two afferent nerve endings innervate the muscle fibers of each spindle. The *primary sensory ending (annulospiral ending)* terminates as a spiral around the *central region (bag region)* of a nuclear bag fiber and nuclear chain fiber. The *secondary sensory ending (flower-spray ending)* terminates on the polar segment of a nuclear bag fiber and nuclear chain fiber. Each spindle has one and only one primary nerve fiber innervating the central region of all intrafusal fibers, and from none to five secondary nerve fibers. The secondary fibers may terminate in the form of spirals, as a spray of fine branches, or as both (Fig. 2-18).

Motor nerves, called *gamma efferent fibers,* innervate each intrafusal muscle fiber in the polar regions (not in or near the bag region). From 1 to 25 gamma efferent fibers innervate a spindle. One gamma efferent fiber may branch and innervate several spindles within the same muscle. These gamma efferent fibers terminate as plate endings or as diffuse multiterminal endings. The plate endings are similar to the motor plate endings on the voluntary muscles. The multiterminal endings—also called *"trail endings"* or *"en grappe"* endings—have a number of varicose-like enlargements making the nerve-muscle synaptic junctions. Several motor endings may be located on each intrafusal fiber.

The miniature striated muscle cells of the spindle are called *intrafusal fibers,* and those of the voluntary muscles are called *extrafusal fibers.* From 2 to 20 (average 6) long intrafusal fibers are located within the enveloping connective tissue capsule of each spindle. Two types of intrafusal fibers are recognized: nuclear bag fibers and nuclear chain fibers. The *nuclear bag muscle fibers* extend the entire length of the neuromuscular spindle. In the thickened equatorial region of each intrafusal fiber is the noncontractile *nuclear bag,* so called because of its large concentration of cell nuclei. This bag is separated from the spindle capsule by a tissue fluid—filled space transversed by nerve fibers. The two ends of the nuclear bag are continuous with the polar segments of the intrafusal muscle fibers; the polar segments are striated and contractile. When active, the pull from the intrafusal fibers is on the bag. The *nuclear chain muscle fibers* do not extend the length of the spindle; they are shorter and thinner than nuclear bag fibers. The thin equatorial region of each fiber is the noncontractile region, with muscle nuclei arranged in a single-file chain. This region is continuous with the polar segments.

The number of spindles per gram of muscle is high in those small muscles subserving fine delicate movements (e.g., muscles of hand, eye, and deep muscles of the neck). There is considerable variation between the relative number of bag and chain fibers per spindle. Physiologic evidence indicates that the central nervous system control of the bag fibers is largely independent of the chain fibers.

The functional significance of this end organ is described in Chap. 5.

Neurotendinous endings of Golgi (Golgi tendon organs, GTOs) are branched endings terminating as numerous leaflike expansions in a tendon, at the junction of a muscle and tendon, or within a muscle sheath (Fig. 2-18).

Meissner's corpuscles (tactile) are ovoid bodies found just beneath the epidermis of the skin (Fig. 2-17). They are mainly in the hairless portions of the skin (toes, fingers, palms, and soles). The terminal branches of from one to seven nerve fibers end as a spiral of naked nerve endings among the perineural epithelium cells of the corpuscle. From 20 to 30 corpuscles may be concentrated in a square millimeter.

Pacinian corpuscles are the largest encapsulated receptors (from 1 to 4 by 2 mm), large enough to be visible to the naked eye (Figs. 2-2A, 2-17). They resemble miniature onions for they are formed by a large number of concentric lamellae or flattened perineural epithelium cells enclosing a cylindric central core in which is found a nerve fiber.

The evidence that a specific ending is associated with a specific modality is not firmly established. However, specificity of function is still ascribed by some investigators to many endings. The attempts to relate physiologically mapped touch spots, pain spots, heat spots, and cold spots with anatomically localized endings have not been conclusive. For example, a Ruffini corpuscle is a receptor for warmth (or of position sense of a joint), and an end bulb of Krause is a receptor for cold. Other endings are involved; the thermal sense is present in the skin of the ear, which has only unmyelinated free endings. Touch, warmth, cold, and pain can be readily felt in several regions of the body in which the only endings are free nerve endings.

The afferent nerves from the sensory endings are also classified into several groups, as follows: The "primary sensory endings" (annulospinal

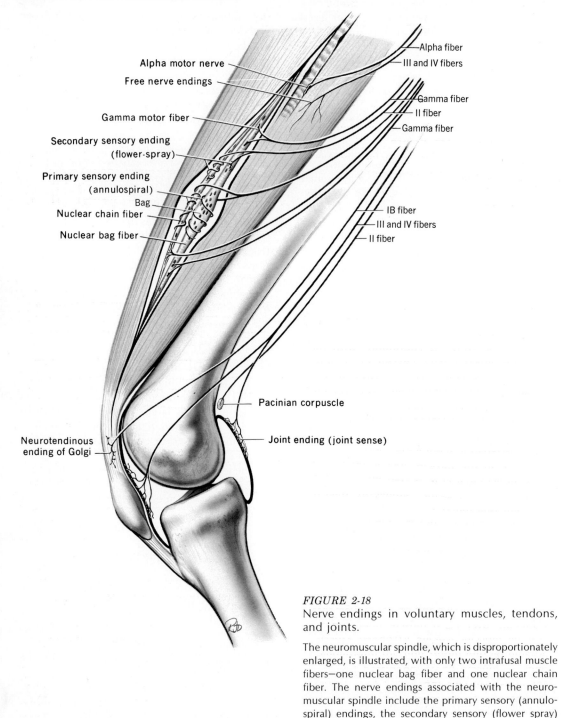

Alpha fiber

III and IV fibers

Gamma fiber

II fiber

Gamma fiber

Alpha motor nerve

Free nerve endings

Gamma motor fiber

Secondary sensory ending
(flower-spray)

Primary sensory ending
(annulospiral)

Bag

Nuclear chain fiber

Nuclear bag fiber

IB fiber

III and IV fibers

II fiber

Pacinian corpuscle

Joint ending (joint sense)

Neurotendinous
ending of Golgi

FIGURE 2-18

Nerve endings in voluntary muscles, tendons, and joints.

The neuromuscular spindle, which is disproportionately enlarged, is illustrated, with only two intrafusal muscle fibers—one nuclear bag fiber and one nuclear chain fiber. The nerve endings associated with the neuromuscular spindle include the primary sensory (annulospiral) endings, the secondary sensory (flower spray) endings, and motor end plates.

endings) are the terminals of group IA nerve fibers; the "secondary sensory endings" (flower spray endings) are the terminals of group II nerve fibers; neurotendinous endings of Golgi are the terminals of group IB nerve fibers; and cutaneous endings are the terminals of groups III and IV.

EFFERENT (MOTOR) ENDINGS (Fig. 2-3)

The *motor end plates* are the specialized efferent endings which terminate on the voluntary (striated) muscles. Each branch terminates as one motor end plate. Practically all muscle fibers are innervated by just one motor end plate. This ending is actually a synapse between a nerve fiber and a muscle fiber. The myelin sheath ends just before the axon reaches the muscle fiber. Distal to the myelin sheath are neurolemma cells (called *teloglia*), which are associated with the axonal branches. The nerve fiber terminates as a flattened plate in a depression, called a *trough, synaptic gutter,* or *primary synaptic cleft,* which indents the surface of the muscle fiber. The primary synaptic cleft is about 200 to 500 Å wide. Within the synaptic cleft is an amorphous material which is continuous with the basement lamina of the muscle cell on the outer surface of the sarcolemma. The axon tip just proximal to the presynaptic membrane contains many mitochondria and synaptic vesicles. These agranular vesicles, of 400 to 500 Å in diameter, contain acetylcholine.

The postsynaptic membrane (postjunctional membrane) on the muscle fiber is thickened, and its surface area is increased by secondary foldings (*secondary clefts, "subneural apparatus,"* or *junction folds*). Close to the secondary foldings in the muscle fiber are many nuclei and mitochondria. The muscle portion of the end plate is called the *sole plate.* A motor unit to the muscle of the eye, with its delicate and dexterous movements, includes three to six muscle fibers. A motor unit to the gastrocnemius muscle, with its massive and cruder movements, may include over 2,000 muscle fibers (motor units of leg muscles average 250 fibers). Muscles innervated by one motor unit are intermingled among the muscle fibers innervated by other motor units. Muscles innervated by relatively more motor units are capable of exerting fine gradations of tension.

The motor endings of the autonomic nervous system terminate as free nerve endings, often in the form of beads and varicosities. These are the endings that innervate muscles (smooth involuntary muscle), glands, and cardiac muscle.

Degeneration and regeneration

An injured neuron reacts to insult, whether it is a transection, a crush, a toxic substance, or a deprivation of blood supply. The entire neuron responds, for the trauma acts as a potent stimulus, through a series of events, which may result in the repair of the neuron.

DEGENERATION

Some of the changes which occur following the simple transection of an axon will be outlined. The reactions, known as the axon reaction, following a transection may be divided into changes in *1* the cell body (chromatolysis), *2* the nerve fiber on the side of the cell body proximal to the trauma (primary degeneration), and *3* the nerve fiber distal to the trauma (secondary, or Wallerian, degeneration).

The cell body imbibes water, triples in volume, and becomes turgid. The Nissl bodies undergo "dissolution" or chromatolysis. The cell swelling precedes the *chromatolysis*. The nucleus may be displaced to the side of the cell body; it assumes an excentric location. The Golgi apparatus is disrupted and dispersed. The chromatolysis is actually accompanied by an increase in ribonucleoproteins, which now stain less intensely. Following the axotomy, there is an increase in ribonucleic acid synthesis in the nucleus, in ribonucleic acid content in the nucleolus, and in the rate of passage of newly synthesized ribonucleic acids from the nucleus to the cytoplasm. The increase in the cytoplasmic ribonucleic acid is followed by an increase in the protein and enzyme content of the cell body. Many of these newly synthesized substances are conveyed by axoplasmic transport and flow down the axon. These are manifestations of metabolic activities which can ultimately lead to the regeneration of the severed process. The chromatolysis is indicative of the enhanced protein synthesis in the cell body. The nerve fiber proximal to the cut usually shows only a few degenerative changes, including the breakdown of the myelin sheath and the axis cylinders in several internodes bordering the injury.

The nerve distal to the cut undergoes several changes (Fig. 2-19). The axis cylinders swell and, after the first week, fragment. The myelin sheath breaks up after a few days into elongated segments and during the next few weeks into smaller spherical and oval fragments. Macrophages phagocytize these breakdown products and remove them from the nerve. Some myelin-sheath fragmentation products may persist for many months after the initial trauma.

REGENERATION (Terminal regeneration)

It is not possible to segregate the degenerative processes from the regenerative processes, for, in a real sense, all the activities of the neural tissue are primarily directed to reconstitution of the nerve. Regeneration is essentially a process of reorganization and growth (Fig. 2-19).

The neurolemma cells in the segment near the trauma and those throughout the entire distal segment undergo mitotic activity. The proliferating neurolemma cells form continuous cords or "tubes" of cells that maintain the orderly longitudinal pattern of the nerve. These cells also migrate into the gap between the distal and proximal stumps and may form a bridge between the two stumps. The cell body synthesizes proteins and other metabolites that flow distally into the injured nerve process. The severed axon tip or terminal forms a new cell membrane, and within a few days several axonal branches or sprouts extend from each original nerve process. Because regeneration of a new axon commences at the severed tip of a terminal, this type of regeneration has been called *terminal regeneration.* When conditions are favorable, many of these growing tips will enter the distal stump. Each of these regenerating processes will contact a neurolemmal cord. This cord will act as a guide, for the regenerating axon will grow along the cord to a nerve ending

at the optimal rate of 4 mm per day. Many processes will enter the distal stump and follow the neurolemmal cords to the nerve endings. If the gap between the two stumps is too long, the regenerating axons may not be able to bridge it. Hence, approximating the cut ends is desirable. Later the neurolemma cells surround the regenerating nerve fibers. Some regenerating fibers become myelinated within 10 days. In time the axon diameters and the myelin sheaths thicken. Each regenerated nerve fiber tends to have an internodal length, a diameter, and a conduction velocity of about 80 percent of those of the original fiber.

The functional effectiveness of peripheral nerve regeneration is related to some other factors. Each regenerating axon of the proximal stump may divide many times, to form as many as 50 branches. Each neurolemmal cord in the distal stump may act as a guiding scaffold for many regenerating axons. If regeneration is successful, there may be more nerve fibers in the distal stump than in the proximal stump several months later. By a year later, many of these fibers will have degenerated. The survivors are those axons that terminate in the proper nerve endings and form functional endings. In effect, the numerous regenerating branches from one axon are a means by which the parent axon increases the possibilities of reaching a proper nerve ending. The capacity of each neurolemma cord to guide many axons is the means of increasing the possibility of the nerve ending's being innervated by a proper nerve fiber. Motor fibers will eventually degenerate if they are located in a neurolemma cord that terminates in a sensory ending.

Transected nerve fibers in the adult mammalian central nervous system attempt to regenerate. Some axons form *sprouts* and growing tips. Many are apparently incapable of mobilizing the metabolic responses which sustain extensive axonal regeneration. The most widely accepted explanation for the failure of fibers to regenerate for any distance is that the regenerating axon tip is unable to penetrate through the glial scar formed at the site of injury.

COLLATERAL NERVE REGENERATION

Collateral branches from an axon may sprout from an intact undamaged nerve and enter into an adjacent denervated neurolemma cord (Fig.

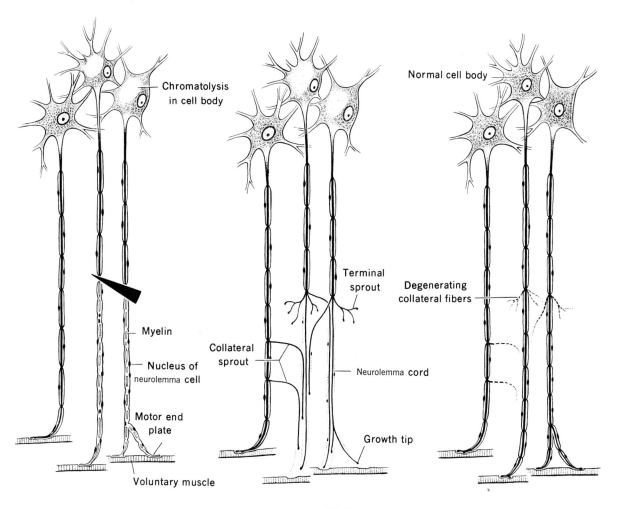

Chromatolysis
in cell body

Normal cell body

Terminal
sprout

Degenerating
collateral fibers

Myelin

Collateral
sprout

Nucleus of
neurolemma cell

Neurolemma cord

Motor end
plate

Growth tip

Voluntary muscle

FIGURE 2-19
Degeneration and regeneration of peripheral somatic motor nerve fibers.

A Several days after transection (at the wedge). Note the chromatolysis and eccentric nuclei, increase in number of neurolemma cells, and fragmentation of myelin sheaths.
B Several weeks later the neurolemma cord receives regenerating axis cylinders from the transected fibers and collateral branches from the adjacent normal fiber.
C Several months later collateral branches of axis cylinders that failed to innervate motor end plates degenerate. The regenerated portions of the fibers contain more internodes than before; hence they conduct nerve impulses more slowly.

2-19). This is known as *collateral nerve regeneration* or *preterminal axonal sprouting.* This collateral sprouting may occur at any node of Ranvier along the axon in the vicinity of the degenerating fibers.

According to one concept, the nearby degenerating nerve fibers exert a stimulus to which the normal nearby fibers respond by forming collateral branches that are, in turn, attracted to the axonless neurolemma cord. This stimulus is presumed to be elicited by chemical substances released by the degenerating nerve fibers, interstitial cells, or denervated structures.

According to another concept, the primary stimulus for activating nerve fibers to sprout collateral branches is provided by tissues of the target organ which is being innervated. In a sense these substances activate each nerve to express its inherent potentiality to generate more collateral branches. In this view, the expression of the potentiality to sprout is inhibited by chemical substances "secreted" by adjacent nerve fibers. Each normal nerve fiber releases such substances, which tend to inhibit adjacent nerve fibers from sprouting. Experimental evidence indicates that these chemical substances are transported from the cell body with the help of the microtubules by fast axoplasmatic flow.

These concepts provide the theoretical bases of understanding why axons utilize their potential to form new collateral branches and to reinnervate the denervated peripheral nerve endings. They offer an explanation for the fact that many muscle fibers denervated in poliomyelitis, for example, may be reinnervated by a branch of an adjacent normal fiber, so that the initial paralytic symptoms are ameliorated. The anesthetic area in the skin following a nerve injury may gradually shrink as a result of collateral sprouting.

Collateral nerve regeneration occurs in both the peripheral and the central nervous systems. Functional synaptic connections may occur after collateral regeneration in both systems.

FUNCTIONAL CONSIDERATIONS OF NERVE REGENERATION

Return of function after regeneration of severed nerves may be excellent. Sensory, motor, and autonomic functional activity may closely resemble that of the original state. However, functional recovery may be poor, especially if the injury is very traumatic and the cut nerve stumps are not properly approximated.

Cross unions of the proximal part of one nerve with the distal segment of another nerve (*crossed-nerve anastomoses*) are followed by successful regeneration of the nerve fibers; e.g., anastomosis of the proximal portion of the hypoglossal nerve (to the tongue) to the distal portion of the facial nerve (responsible for facial expression). The muscles of facial expression,

when reinnervated, will regain their lost muscle tonus and can then be contracted voluntarily. However, the integrated complex functional activity will be modified. The movement of facial muscles can occur only when the patient attempts to move the tongue. The mammalian nervous system is limited in its ability to readapt the function of its disarranged nerves.

Bibliography

Bloom, W., and D. W. Fawcett: *A Textbook of Histology.* W. B. Saunders Company, Philadelphia, 1968.

Bodian, D.: The generalized vertebrate neuron. Science, 137:323–326, 1962.

Bourne, G. H. (ed.): *The Structure and Function of Nerve Tissue* (6 vols.). Academic Press, Inc., New York, 1968, 1969, 1972.

Bunge, R. P.: Glial cells and the central myelin sheath. Physiol. Rev., 48:197–251, 1968.

Clemente, C. D.: Regeneration in the central nervous system. Int. Rev. Neurobiol., 6:257–301, 1964.

Copenhaver, W. M., R. P. Bunge, and M. B. Bunge: *Bailey's Textbook of Histology.* The Williams & Wilkins Company, Baltimore, 1971.

Gray, E. G., and R. W. Guillery: Synaptic morphology in the normal and degenerating nervous system. Int. Rev. Cytol., 19:111–182, 1966.

Greep, R. O., and L. Weiss: *Histology,* 3d ed. McGraw-Hill Book Company, New York, 1973.

Guth, L.: Regeneration in the mammalian peripheral nervous system. Physiol. Rev., 36:441–478, 1956.

Hydén, H. (ed.): *The Neuron.* American Elsevier Company, New York, 1968.

Minckler, J. (ed.): *Pathology of the Nervous System,* vol. 1. McGraw-Hill Book Company, New York, 1968.

Nakai, J.: *Morphology of Neuroglia.* Charles C Thomas, Publisher, Springfield, Ill., 1963.

Nauta, W. J. H., and S. O. E. Ebbesson: *Contemporary Research Methods in Neuroanatomy.* Springer-Verlag, Berlin and New York, 1970.

Peters, A., S. L. Palay, and H. deF. Webster: *The Fine Structure of the Nervous System: The Cells and Their Processes.* Harper & Row, Publishers, Incorporated, New York, 1970.

Winkelmann, R. K.: *Nerve Endings in Normal and Pathological Skin: Contributions to the Anatomy of Sensations.* Charles C Thomas, Publisher, Springfield, Ill., 1960.

CHAPTER 3
BASIC NEUROPHYSIOLOGY

The ability to react to a stimulus is a fundamental property of all living organisms. Glands secrete, muscles contract, cilia sweep, and certain cells ingest foreign organisms. Two systems are specialized to enable the organism to coordinate and to mobilize its resources in responding to the internal and external environments. These are the nervous system and the endocrine system. In fact, the two systems are interrelated and integrated (Chap. 11). The *endocrine system* is a coordinator, utilizing *chemical messengers* (*humoral agents or hormones*) that are transmitted through the bloodstream from their source in an endocrine gland to their site of action in a target organ. The reactivity of this system is slow but sustained. The *nervous system* is also a coordinator utilizing *chemical messengers* (*neurotransmitter agents*); an agent is secreted by a nerve cell into a narrow synaptic cleft where it acts to influence another nerve cell, a muscle cell, or a glandular cell. The reactivity of the nervous system is rapid but less sustained. All neurons have essentially the same biophysical properties; this applies not only to neurons in different regions of the same brain but also to neurons in all kinds of animal brains.

Resting neuron and resting potential

The *resting neuron* is a charged cell that is not conducting a nerve impulse. The difference in electric (bioelectric) potential between the interstitial fluid outside the neuron and the intracellular fluid (neuroplasm) inside the neuron is of critical significance to the maintenance of this dynamic equilibrium of the resting neuron, and to the generation and propagation of the nerve impulse. It is important to realize that the inter-

stitial compartment and the intracellular compartment are each electrically neutral. The resting potential is a result of the difference in the electric potential between the two compartments.

The *cell membrane* of the neuron acts as a thin boundary (50 to 100 Å thick) between the two fluids. Sodium (Na^+) and chloride (Cl^-) ions are in higher concentration in the interstitial fluid (which is similar to sea water); potassium (K^+) and protein (organic) ions are in higher concentration in the intracellular fluid (Fig. 3-1). Because ions tend to diffuse away from regions of high concentration, sodium ions tend to diffuse across the plasma membrane into the neuron and potassium ions tend to diffuse out of the neuron into the interstitial fluid. However, this diffusion gradient is modified by the plasma membrane of the resting axon; the resting membrane has a higher selective permeability for potassium ions than for sodium ions. As a result, potassium ions tend to leak out of the axon rapidly. The potassium leakage continues until an equilibrium is attained when the inside of the axon reaches an electrically negative potential relative to the interstitial fluid. This equilibrium is the resting potential measured in millivolts (thousandths of a volt). As a result, the interstitial fluid has a positive charge in relation to the net negative charge of the intracellular fluid. The *resting membrane potential* across the plasma membrane of the resting neuron is about $\frac{1}{10}$ volt (from 70 to 100 millivolts). The potential difference of this biologic battery across a membrane that is one-millionth of a centimeter thick is actually high, for it is equivalent to a field of 100,000 volts across a membrane 1 cm thick.

These differential concentrations of sodium ions and potassium ions are thought to be pro-

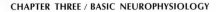
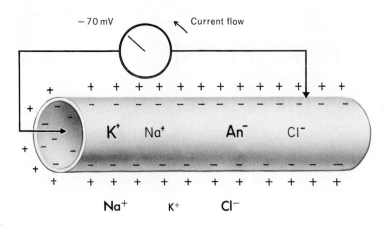

FIGURE 3-1
Resting (steady) potential.

The intracellular neuroplasm potential of the normal nerve fiber "at rest" is negative to the extracellular potential. Sodium (Na^+) and chloride (Cl^-) ions are in high concentration in the extracellular fluid, and the potassium (K^+) ions and protein (An^-) are in high concentrations in the neuroplasm. The potential across the plasma membrane is about -70 to -90 millivolts.

duced and maintained by the metabolic activity of the neuron, in which sodium is pumped out of the cell and potassium is pumped into the neuron. Biologic pumping, which is characteristic of many cells, is known as *active transport*. The energy for the pumping is derived ultimately from energy-rich phosphate bonds (adenosine triphosphate, creatine phosphate). In short, the interstitial fluid has high concentrations of sodium ions (10 times higher on the outside) and chloride ions (14 times higher on the outside) than in the intracellular fluid of the neuron which has high concentrations of potassium ions (30 times higher inside in some neurons) and large organic protein ions. The inorganic ions (Na^+, K^+, and Cl^-) can pass across the cell membrane with relative ease, but are prevented by metabolic activity. The potassium ions are held in the neuron by the strong electrostatic attraction of the organic ions which are too large to leak across the plasma membrane. The resting potential is built up by the ionic concentration differences across this selectively permeable membrane, for this plasma membrane has *capacitance* (ability to store charge).

Calcium ions are essential for the structural and functional integrity of the plasma membrane. They act as a "cement" and have a role in membrane excitability. When calcium levels are low, sodium tends to leak into the neuron, the resting potential is lowered, and the cell may fire spontaneously. The muscle tetany in a hy-

poparathyroid patient with low serum calcium concentration is a consequence of the increased electrical excitability of the plasma membrane of both axons and muscle cells. When calcium ion levels are high, the neurons have less excitability; they are harder to fire.

Nerve impulse (Action potential, nondecremental conduction)

GENERATION OF ACTION POTENTIAL

The nerve impulse is an electrochemical phenomenon. If a stimulus applied to an axon lowers the membrane potential to a critical level called the *threshold level value* (in some cases 30 to 50 millivolts), an explosive-like action results and the brief electrical phenomenon or *action potential* (*spike or nerve impulse*) is produced. This nerve impulse is propagated along the axon without *decrement* (*regenerative process*) to all parts of the cell membrane of the axon as a continuous spread (Figs. 3-2, 3-3). The axon possesses the energy for the action potential, and the stimulus merely lowers the membrane potential sufficiently to trigger the axon into action. If a stimulus greater than the threshold is applied, the response from a single axon is exactly the same as the response to a threshold stimulus. The axon gives an *all-or-none (all-or-nothing) response*. The axon, after stimulation,

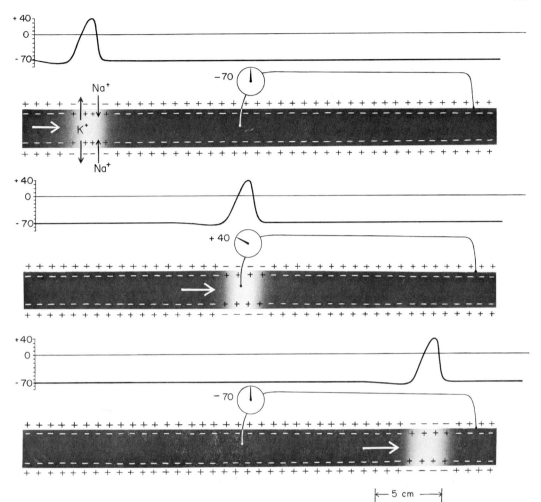

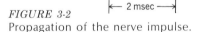

FIGURE 3-2
Propagation of the nerve impulse.

Arrow indicates direction in which nerve impulse is propagated. In the fore of the impulse, sodium rushes into the axon, resulting in a locally positive neuroplasm. In the wake of the impulse, sodium is prevented from passing into the axon, but potassium rushes out of the axon into the extracellular fluid. The normal resting potential is now restored. At the site of the action potential (light region), the potential across the cell membrane is reversed (depolarized) until it approximates +40 millivolts (registered on galvanometer). The length of the depolarized region on the nerve may extend over several centimeters. This type of impulse propagation is found in the squid axon and mammalian unmyelinated nerve fibers.

no longer behaves like a passive conduit but produces its own self-sustaining pulse. If the stimulus does not lower the membrane potential to the critical level, then the resultant *local response* fades and dies (*cable property*) within a few millimeters from the stimulus site. The normal resting potential returns immediately. The local response of a nerve propagates with decrement. The cell membrane of the axon is analogous to a set trap. The potential difference across the cell membrane (resting potential) in the "resting" axon "sets" the axon that is waiting for a stimulus to release the stored energy to spring the trap into action (action potential). The polarization of the resting potential is gen-

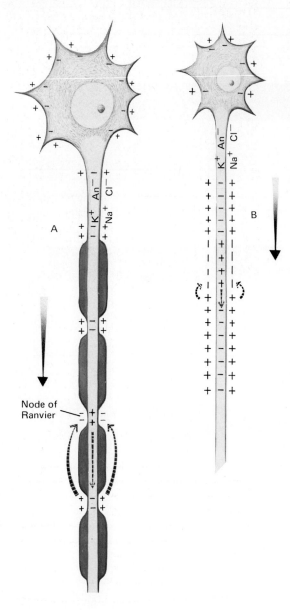

A

Node of
Ranvier

B

FIGURE 3-3
A A neuron with a myelinated axon and *B* a neuron with an unmyelinated axon.

Note the charges on the cell membrane and the location of certain ions in each neuron "at rest" and at active sites (one on each neuron) during conduction of an all-or-none action potential. The minus (−) sign within the neuron signifies negativity with respect to the extracellular fluid outside the neuron. The solid arrows outside the neurons indicate the direction in which the nerve impulses are propagated. The interrupted arrows indicate the direction of flow of the current. Sodium, Na⁺; potassium, K⁺; chloride, Cl⁻; and protein anions, An⁻ ions.

erated by the neuron itself. Gland cells and muscle cells are similar in this respect. The resting potential in muscle cells is about −70 to −90 millivolts, with the minus sign signifying intracellular negativity with respect to the extracellular potential.

PROPAGATION OF ACTION POTENTIAL

With the application of a stimulus to an axon, the local response (local circuit current) may reduce the charge (depolarization) on the plasma membrane from −90 millivolts to the critical threshold (critical point) of −30 to −50 millivolts. The basic mechanisms producing the action potential are unknown. The origin of the action potential is keyed to the loss of permeability of the plasma membrane. The two phases of depolarization are the inrush of sodium ions followed almost immediately by the outrush of potassium ions. These two phases last for less than 1 millisecond. During the sodium inrush phase the plasma membrane becomes selectively permeable to sodium; sodium rushes through the plasma membrane into the axon and produces a positive intracellular charge at the stimulated site. The open "doors" permitting this sodium inrush suddenly close, and the "doors" permitting potassium outrush suddenly open. During the potassium outrush phase the plasma membrane becomes selectively permeable to potassium; potassium rushes out of the axon through the plasma membrane until the resting potential is reconstituted. The critical threshold is that unstable point at which the inrush of sodium ions and the outrush of potassium ions are in balance.

During the interval prior to the critical point, sodium ion permeability (inrush) is dominant, while during the interval following the critical point, potassium permeability (outrush) is dominant. Once this critical threshold is reached, the depolarization continues until the intracellular fluid adjacent to the cell membrane is negative to the interstitial fluid. A reversal in the polarity occurs from that of the resting potential (-90 millivolts) to that of the action potential ($+30$ millivolts). Thus an action potential is triggered when the depolarization reaches a critical point. At the excited locus, the flow of current is inward into the neuron; at the adjacent nonexcited membrane, the flow of current is outward into the interstitial fluid point. The action potential is a sequence of point-to-point flow down the axon with each point acting as a site of sodium inrush into the axon, followed by potassium outrush. This is an electrical signal of the action potential which travels along the cell membrane as a chain reaction and regenerates itself from point to point along the axon (continuous conduction) without loss of amplitude and at a constant speed for that axon (Fig. 3-2). The nerve fiber gains sodium and loses potassium during the passage of the action potential. Later the small amount of sodium which entered the cell is metabolically pumped out.

The amounts of potassium, sodium, and chloride involved in maintaining the potentials are slight as compared with the amount of the ionic stores. Even without the sodium pump working, an axon can be stimulated to produce over 100,000 action potentials before its ionic stores are exhausted. Hence such systems as the sodium pump have plenty of time to redistribute and replenish the ionic stores. In its effect, the pump is electrically neutral, because the pumping of sodium ions out of the neuron is accompanied by an inflow of an equal amount of potassium ions. In an axon the local response is a depolarization that precedes the action potential. It is significant that the nerve impulse is not an electric current, such as one that passes through an electrical wire, but is rather a sequence of ionic exchanges in which the electrical charges are indicative of an action potential. Actually nerve fibers are very poor conductors of electricity. Within a millisecond or so after the action potential has passed by, the cell membrane is restored to its resting potential, in which state the interstitial fluid is positive to the intracellular fluid. This smooth progressive movement of the action potential is the presumed method of conduction in unmyelinated nerves.

SALTATORY CONDUCTION

The action potential in a myelinated nerve is propagated by *discontinuous spread, or saltatory (hop or jump) conduction* (Figs. 3-3, 3-4), in which the nerve impulse hops along the nerve fiber from node of Ranvier to node of Ranvier. The current apparently spreads electronically from active to inactive node. This, along with increasing fiber diameter, is nature's way of obtaining higher speeds of conduction; the greater the distance between nodes of Ranvier in a nerve fiber, the faster its speed of conduction. The myelin sheath acts as an insulator with considerable electric resistance, which constrains ionic flow.

The *node of Ranvier* is the site where ionic interchange readily occurs between the interstitial fluid and the intracellular fluid. This discontinuous ionic movement at the node is effi-

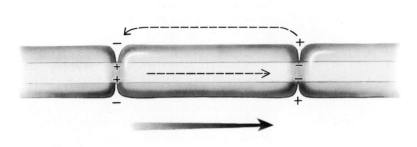

FIGURE 3-4
Saltatory conduction.

The conduction of the nerve impulse in a myelinated nerve fiber probably occurs as a local circuit "leaps" from one node of Ranvier to the next node of Ranvier. Arrow below figure indicates direction in which nerve impulse is propagated.

cient from the energy point of view. The local bioelectrical circuits generated at the node where the impulse is passing can reach out for a considerable distance in advance of the action potential. Eddy currents are produced by the movements of potassium and sodium cations from two or three resting nodes of Ranvier ahead. Each node is a site of self-regeneration. In saltatory conduction, the nerve impulse hops because only small patches of plasma membrane of nerve at the nodes can be depolarized to propagate the impulse. The nodes with low thresholds are linked together by myelinated internodes (segmented insulating jackets) that act as passive conductors. Saltatory conduction may be enhanced by the restraint of extracellular fluid within the periaxonal space of the internode (Fig. 2-12).

The myelinated fibers are analogous to a transoceanic cable; the nodes of Ranvier are repeater relay stations, which, at intervals, boost weakened electric pulses. The distance from node to node (internodal distance) varies from 200 to over 1,000 μm. The ratio of the internodal distance to the diameter of the nerve fiber is approximately 100:1. The more a fiber is myelinated, the longer is its internodal distance, and the faster it conducts an action potential. The myelin improves the signaling efficiency of the nerve fiber.

The astroglia of the central nervous system and the neurolemma cells of the peripheral nervous system may play roles in nerve impulse propagation. Because astroglia contain large amounts of sodium and chloride ions, these cells have been implicated in the bioelectric activity associated with the conduction of the nerve impulse in the central nervous system.

Because of the electric fields created by actively conducting axons, interaction across parallel axons could conceivably occur. The cross talk does take place but the interference is negligible: the talk is analogous to the faint crosstalk conversation occasionally heard on the telephone. However, the efficiency of the nervous system negates an interference.

REFRACTORY PERIODS

Each point on the nerve fiber is not reexcitable for a millisecond after the peak of the action potential has passed it, no matter how intense the stimulus. This millisecond interval is known as the *absolute refractory period.* During this falling phase of the action potential, the sodium channels within the plasma membrane are closed, so that sodium ions cannot enter the neuron at that site. This implies that a nerve fiber cannot transmit more than 1,000 impulses per second (some nerve fibers are thought to have an absolute refractory period of $\frac{1}{2}$ millisecond and hence may transmit up to 2,000 impulses per second). Thus, for example, a fiber of the auditory nerve cannot transmit a sound of 10,000 cycles per second in the form of 10,000 impulses per second.

Immediately following the absolute refractory period is the *relative refractory period,* during which the nerve fiber may propagate an action potential only with stimuli higher than threshold. During this interval when it is difficult to drive the neuron to the equilibrium potential, the potassium channels within the plasma membrane are open. The entire refractory period is over in a few milliseconds.

DECREMENTAL CONDUCTION AND THE RECEPTOR MEMBRANE

The *all-or-none nerve impulse* (*digital spike or pulse*) is characteristic of the axon, which is specialized for conducting long distances. The remainder of the neuron, cell body, and dendrites of a typical neuron may not respond in an all-or-none manner but propagates a response with decrement. Unlike the response of the axon, the local response is not necessarily followed by an action potential. Stimulation of receptor sites on the cell body and dendrites of a motor neuron evokes a *graded response* (*slow potential, local response*) which spreads with decrement (cable property) and fades out in a short distance. The graded response generated at one synapse does not generally reach the initial segment of the axon because, except for the few synapses near an initial segment, most synapses are too far from the initial segment. The initial segment on the axon is the critical site at which an action potential is initiated, and generated in the axon. If the decremental spreading activity of the neuron reaches the initial segment, an action potential may result. The dendrites and the cell body are adapted not for long-distance transmission but rather for integrating synaptic activity.

The terminal segment of a sensory nerve ending may also exhibit decremental conduction without all-or-none activity. The terminal segments, or telodendria, are the unmyelinated portions of the nerve process. Stimulation of the terminal segment results in decremental conduction. Should the activity reach the node of Ranvier (initial segment) in the myelinated portion, an all-or-none action potential is generated in the nerve fiber and is conducted to the central nervous system. The critical site for the initiation of the action potential in many nerve fibers is the first node of Ranvier. The portion of the neuron exhibiting decremental conduction may be called the *receptor membrane* (Fig. 3-11), because it is influenced by synaptic activity of other neurons (dendrites and cell body)

and environmental stimuli (terminal segment of peripheral nerve ending). The precise location of the "initial segment" in an unmyelinated nerve is not known.

STRENGTH-DURATION CURVES AND CHRONAXIE
(Excitation time)

A relationship exists between the strength of a stimulus, whether it is of electric, thermal, mechanical, or chemical origin, and the duration of time the stimulus is applied. The resulting plot is a strength-duration curve (Fig. 3-5). An electric stimulus is most generally used in neurophysiologic experimentation. The weakest current flowing indefinitely but just sufficient to stimulate a nerve to generate an action potential is called the *rheobase*. A current weaker than rheobase cannot stimulate a nerve even if applied indefinitely. The fiber does not fire because ions are not being drained away fast enough from the surface of the plasma membrane; the restorative processes are able to replace the charge as fast as charge is removed.

The time it takes to stimulate a nerve with twice the rheobase strength is called *chronaxie* or *excitation time*. Currents with high frequencies may act over such short intervals that they may never stimulate a nerve, even at high intensities, because each stimulus is of too short a duration. The chronaxie for a nerve is constant. The chronaxie time for a normal nerve fiber is always less than 1 millisecond. In an injured nerve, the chronaxie may reach over 100 times that of the normal. The strength-duration curves of injured nerves and of nerves in other clinical states are also altered. Hence chronaxie and strength-duration curves are useful to a physician.

Classification of nerve fibers

The peripheral nerves and their spinal roots are a composite of populations of different types of fibers. On the basis of several criteria, the nerve fibers of the peripheral nervous system are classified by three different systems. In the *general classification* the fiber types are designated by

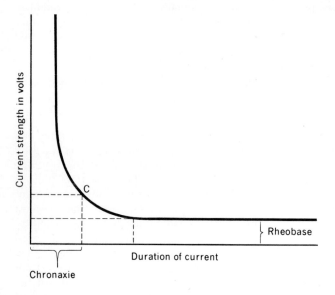

FIGURE 3-5
Strength-duration curve.

The relationship between current strength (strength of stimulus) and the duration of time that stimulus is applied. Rheobase is the least strength of current flowing for an indefinite length of time sufficient to stimulate nerve. Chronaxie (excitation time) is the time interval during which a current twice the rheobase must flow in order to excite the nerve.

capital letters (A, B, and C). In the *dorsal root afferent fiber classification,* the fibers are designated by Roman numerals (I, II, III, and IV). In the *ventral root efferent fiber classification* the fibers are designated by Greek letters (α, β, and γ). All systems are used.

GENERAL CLASSIFICATION

The range of fiber size and velocity are the criteria upon which this system is based. Conduction velocities are directly related to the diameter of the fiber and to the length of the internode; the larger these dimensions are, the greater the speed of conduction. In the medium to large fibers, the *speed of conduction* in meters per second is roughly equal to the diameter of the fiber in micrometers (including myelin sheath) times the conversion factor 6. The conversion factor for fine fibers is 4. Thus a fiber with a diameter of 22 μm should conduct at speeds of 132 meters per second. These highest velocities are at about 200 miles per hour, or a little less than one-third the speed of sound.

The *A fibers* are the myelinated somatic afferent and somatic efferent nerve fibers. This group includes those fibers which transmit im-

pulses from such afferent endings as Meissner's corpuscles, Pacinian corpuscles, neuromuscular spindles, and Golgi neurotendinous endings and impulses to the efferent motor end plates.

The *A group* is further divided into four subgroups: alpha (α), beta (β), gamma (γ), and delta (δ) neurons. These range from the alpha neurons, which have the most heavily myelinated axons with the highest conduction velocities, to the delta neurons, which have lightly myelinated fibers with the slowest conduction velocities of the A group.

The *B fibers* are myelinated efferent preganglionic fibers of the autonomic nervous system. These fibers are up to 3 μm in diameter and conduct at speeds of from 3 to 15 meters per second.

The *C fibers* are unmyelinated fibers including *1* the postganglionic sympathetic axons of the autonomic nervous system, and *2* the unmyelinated afferent fibers of the peripheral nerves and dorsal roots. These fibers are probably associated with the entire spectrum of sensory modalities, as are the A fibers. The postganglionic sympathetic C fibers range from 0.3 to 1.3 μm in diameter and have conduction speeds of from 0.7 to 2.3 meters per second. The afferent C fibers range from 0.4 to 1.2 µm in diameter and have conduction speeds of from 0.6 to 2.0 meters per second. The afferent C fibers commence as free nerve endings.

DORSAL ROOT CLASSIFICATION

All sensory input to the spinal cord enters via nerve fibers of the dorsal roots. These afferent fibers have been classified into groups I, II, III, and IV. As compared to the general classification, groups I and II correspond to A group, alpha subgroup; group III corresponds to A group, delta subgroup; and group IV corresponds to C group.

Group Ia fibers arborize peripherally as the primary sensory endings (annulospinal endings) on the intrafusal fibers of the neuromuscular spindles. *Group Ib fibers* terminate peripherally as the Golgi tendon organs (GTO). Group I fibers range approximately from 12 to 20 (average 16) µm in diameter, with conduction velocities of 70 to 120 meters per second.

Group II fibers are associated with such peripheral nerve endings as the secondary sensory endings (flower spray endings) of the neuromuscular spindle, and with encapsulated receptors such as the cutaneous touch-pressure receptors (Merkel's and Meissner's corpuscles), skin and joint receptors (Pacinian corpuscles), dermal receptors (Krause's and Ruffini's corpuscles), and some joint receptors (laminated paciniform corpuscle). The group II fibers range from approximately 5 to 14 (average 8) µm in diameter, with conduction velocities of from 30 to 70 meters per second.

The *groups III and IV fibers* terminate as nonencapsulated (free) nerve endings; these include the hair receptor endings in the integument and the touch, pressure, and pain-free nerve endings in the skin and blood vessels. The group III fibers range from approximately 2 to 7 µm in diameter, with conduction velocities of 12 to 30 meters per second. The group IV fibers range from approximately 0.5- to 1-µm diameter, with velocities of 0.5 to 2 meters per second.

The terms I, II, III, and IV are usually used in the anatomic sense. The designations Ia, Ib, and secondary spindle group II are used in the physiologic sense. Group I are thickly myelinated, group II are medium myelinated, group III are finely myelinated, and group IV are unmyelinated fibers.

VENTRAL ROOT CLASSIFICATION

Three types of efferent (motor) fibers emerge from the spinal cord and brainstem. The *thickly myelinated α (alpha) fibers* from the alpha motor neurons of somatic motor nuclei terminate as the motor end plates of the extrafusal muscles. The fibers range from 10 to 20 µm in diameter and have conduction velocities of from 15 to 120 meters per second. The *finely myelinated γ (gamma) fibers* from the gamma motor neurons of the spinal cord and brainstem are of two types; one type terminates as discrete motor end plates, and the other type terminates as a fine network ("trail" endings) on the intrafusal muscle fibers of the neuromuscular spindles. These gamma fibers range from 2 to 10 µm in diameter, with conduction velocities of from 10 to 45 meters per second. The *preganglionic autonomic myelinated fibers (group B fibers)* are less than 3 µm in diameter with velocities of 3 to 15 meters per second. The *β (beta) fibers* are few in number; these fibers innervate both extrafusal and intrafusal fibers.

Physiology of the chemical synapse

Of prime significance in the integrative activities of the nervous system is the synapse. Although each nerve fiber may transmit an impulse in either direction within the neuron (toward or away from the cell body), conduction in a sequence of neurons is transmitted in only one direction (unidirectional conduction). In effect, the synapse is rectifying in that it allows the current to flow in one direction only. This one-way transmission occurs because the chemical transmitter, released only by the presynaptic neuron, triggers the postsynaptic neuron to respond in some manner. The synapse acts as a one-way valve, permitting the action potential of an axon to exert its influence across the synaptic cleft on a dendrite (axodendritic synapse) or on a cell body (axosomatic synapse). *Uni-*

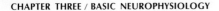

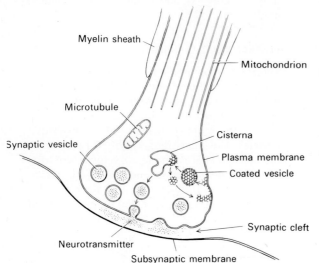

Myelin sheath

Mitochondrion

Microtubule

Synaptic vesicle

Cisterna

Plasma membrane

Coated vesicle

Synaptic cleft

Neurotransmitter

Subsynaptic membrane

FIGURE 3-6
Recycling of synaptic vesicles.

Neurotransmitters are synthesized in a neuron, stored and packaged in vesicles, and released by exocytosis. The transmitters and vesicles are recycled (Fig. 6-5). Following exocytosis, the vesicle membrane fuses with the plasma membrane. New vesicle membranes are reformed by pinocytosis (endocytosis) and form the plasma membrane and its intermediary structures–called cisternae. The coat of the newly formed vesicle is also recycled. (*After Heuser and Reese.*)

directional conduction across the synapse from the presynaptic neuron to the postsynaptic neuron results in the functional or dynamic polarity of any sequence of neurons. The dendrites and cell body of a neuron do not directly affect other neurons but can only influence the axon of the same neuron to generate an action potential which, in turn, synapses with other neurons.

With the arrival of the action potential, neurotransmitters (transmitters) are released from each bouton in packets or quanta rather than in a continuous stream (Fig. 3-6). Each packet is a *biologic "quantum"* in the sense that it is the minimal unit of release. These quanta are released from the synaptic vesicles within the bouton into the synaptic cleft by exocytosis (Chap. 2). The *putative transmitters* include acetylcholine, norepinephrine, dopamine, 5-hydroxytryptamine (serotonin), gamma-aminobutyric acid (GABA), glycine, and others. According to *Dale's law*, each neuron elaborates and releases the same transmitter from all its synaptic terminals. This does not imply that the effects of this neurotransmitter are the same on all postsynaptic cells innervated by each neuron, because the effects are largely determined by the postsynaptic cell. (Refer to "Receptors of the Postsynaptic Membrane," further on.)

The conduction of an impulse along an axon of a neuron in the usual direction toward the axonic synapses is known as *orthodromic conduction*. The conduction of a nerve impulse in the same axon in the opposite direction away from the axonic synapses is known as *antidromic conduction*. For example, when an axon is stimulated an impulse can travel orthodromically toward its telodendria or antidromically toward its cell body.

Transmission of neurotransmitters across the chemical synapse usually requires from 0.3 to 1.0 millisecond (synaptic delay or synaptic latency). Synaptic delays of several milliseconds may occur in the autonomic ganglia. The synapse has a lower safety factor than the axon, for, unlike the axon, which is essentially not fatigable, the synapse is fatigable. During anoxia resulting from an insufficient blood supply or from general anesthesia, synaptic transmission succumbs much sooner than does axonal conduction. This is in line with the fact that the synaptic physiology is altered by many pharmaceutical agents. The fatigability of the synapse is probably the consequence of the depletion of the stores of neurotransmitter chemicals.

Transmission across an electrical synapse is quicker because the current passes directly between two adjacent cells.

Receptor sites are present in the postsynaptic membranes of neurons, muscles, and glands. Putative neurotransmitters have effects on specific receptor sites, which are macromolecules of protein. These receptors on the postsynaptic membrane are chemically reactive but may not be responsive to electric stimuli. The interaction of a transmitter with the postsynaptic membrane may evoke an excitatory response or an inhibitory response. The *excitatory response* is expressed by a *depolarization (graded local response)*, with a sodium ion inrush and a potassium ion outrush of the postsynaptic membrane (Fig. 3-7). The *inhibitory response* is expressed by a *hyperpolarization,* with a chloride ion inrush and a potassium ion outrush across the postsynaptic membrane (Fig. 3-7). The basic difference between the two is that there is a positively charged sodium inrush at the excitatory synapse and a negatively charged chloride ion inrush at the inhibitory synapse. The shift in the chloride ion is significant. By usage, a decrease in the electrical potential is called depolarization, whereas an increase in the electrical potential is called hyperpolarization. The stress is not on absolute potentials but on the potential differences between that on the intraneuronal side of the plasma membrane and that on the extraneuronal side of the membrane. Thus a decrease in the potential difference is called depolarization. The normal dendritic or somal potential of -70 millivolts decreases to -60 millivolts or less and approaches the critical firing level. An increase in the potential difference is hyperpolarization; in the resting neuron hyperpolarization results in a potential shift away from critical firing potential. In hyperpolarization the normal resting dendritic or somal potential of -70 millivolts increases to a value as great as -80 millivolts.

The manner in which a receptor site responds to a specific chemical transmitter must be determined individually. The neurotransmitter may stimulate, but the receptor responds in its own (probably predetermined) way. The neurotransmitter-receptor linkage tells only the chemical combination; it does not indicate the action. *Only the receptor site seems to know the action.* In brief, the postsynaptic effects of a neurotransmitter are determined by the nature of the receptors. Each postsynaptic membrane probably contains hundreds and thousands of receptor sites; each receptor site is a macromolecular protein. These sites are specialized decoders. For example, the combination of the transmitter norepinephrine and receptor sites differs in the response evoked at different synaptic sites. This transmitter facilitates depolarization (excitation) of the cardiac pacemaker cells and of the smooth muscles of the vas deferens. On the other hand, it hyperpolarizes the smooth muscles of the gastrointestinal tract (inhibition) and the secretory cells of the sublingual gland. Acetylcholine can have excitatory or inhibitory effects, depending upon the identity of the postsynaptic cell; acetylcholine is an excitatory agent at the motor end plate (contraction of voluntary muscle) and is an inhibitory agent at the vagus nerve–heart synapse (decrease in heart rate).

ACETYLCHOLINE RECEPTORS

The acetylcholine receptors are classified as nicotinic receptors and muscarinic receptors. The nicotinic receptors are located predominantly at the neuromuscular junctions of voluntary muscles (motor end plates) and in the autonomic ganglia. These receptors are subject to stimulation by nicotine and to blockade by curare. Muscarinic receptors are located predominantly at effector cells (smooth muscle, cardiac muscle, and glands). They are subject to stimulation by muscarine and to blockage by atropine. In both types of receptors, acetylcholine is effective. The differences are thought to reside in the receptor sites; different parts of the acetylcholine molecule are involved at the different receptor sites. Stated otherwise, the differential action of muscarine and nicotine is explained by the concept that each of these chemicals reacts with a different kind of the many receptor proteins on the postsynaptic membrane.

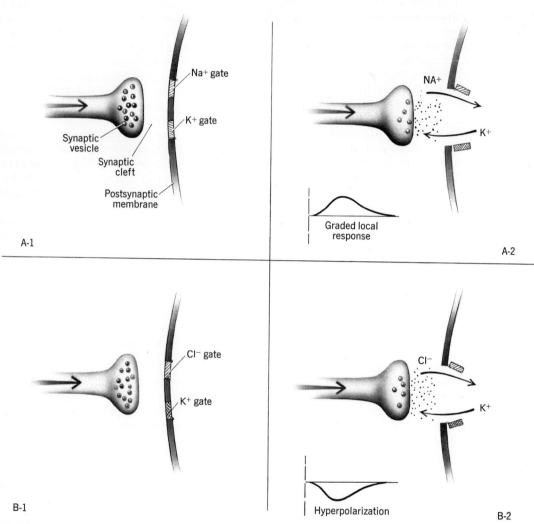

Na⁺ gate

K⁺ gate

Synaptic
vesicle

Synaptic
cleft

Postsynaptic
membrane

A-1

NA⁺

K⁺

Graded local
response

A-2

Cl⁻ gate

K⁺ gate

B-1

Cl⁻

K⁺

Hyperpolarization

B-2

FIGURE 3-7
Excitatory synapses *A* and inhibitory synapses *B*.

A-1 and *B*-1 Synapses prior to release of neurotransmitter.
A-2 Excitatory postsynaptic response following release of neurotransmitter with Na ion inrush through Na gate and K ion outrush through K gate.
B-2 Inhibitory postsynaptic response following release of neurotransmitter with Cl ion inrush through Cl gate and K ion outrush through K gate.

ADRENERGIC RECEPTORS (Adrenoceptive sites)

On the basis of pharmacologic criteria, the adrenergic receptors, those responsive to norepinephrine, have been classified as alpha (α) and beta (β) receptors. The *alpha receptors* have an affinity for norepinephrine and epinephrine; the *beta receptors* have a greater affinity for epinephrine. Some pharmacologic differences between these receptors are as follows: the alpha receptors are directly stimulated by phenylephedrine and blocked by phenoxy-benzamine, and the beta receptors are directly stimulated by isoproterenol and blocked by propanolol. Although the alpha and beta receptors have an affinity for both norepinephrine and isoproterenol, the alpha receptors have a high affinity for norepinephrine, whereas the beta receptors have a high affinity for isoproterenol.

Several factors determine the response of an organ or organ system to sympathetic nerve stimulation. Among these are *1* the distribution of the nerve terminals within the organ, and *2* the relative number and distribution of alpha and beta receptors stimulated by the released neurotransmitter.

In a general way, *alpha receptor stimulation* results in an excitatory response—such as contraction of smooth muscles. *Beta receptor stimulation* usually produces an inhibitory response—such as the dilatation of arterioles to the inhibitory influences upon the smooth muscles. Blood pressure can dilate arterioles when the intrinsic muscles are relaxed. There are two major exceptions to this formulation. These involve the heart and the gastrointestinal tract. The *stimulation of the beta receptors of the heart* produces excitatory effects, comprising increase in heart rate, increase in force of contraction, and increased excitability and automaticity. The *stimulation of the alpha and/or beta receptors* of the gastrointestinal tract results in an inhibitory response; the responses are additive. Gastric motility is decreased.

The so-called gamma receptors are stimulated by acetylcholine and yield an inhibitory response (cholinergic inhibitory). Some blood vessels have gamma receptors; vasodilatation is the response to stimulation. Such blood vessels are located in skeletal muscles, brain, and pia mater.

POSTSYNAPTIC POTENTIALS (PSP)

Excitation may be defined as the response of the postsynaptic membrane to the neurotransmitters which partially depolarizes the membrane, forming an *excitatory postsynaptic potential* (*EPSP*). The postsynaptic membrane becomes momentarily sievelike in character and is more permeable to sodium and potassium cations. The resulting small depolarizing potential is a graded decremental potential which lasts briefly for only milliseconds or tens of milliseconds (Fig. 3-8). Most EPSPs are so small that they are hardly detectable; by themselves they do not generate action potentials because these potentials do not reach the critical firing level.

The EPSPs generated at the postjunctional membrane of the motor end plate of a voluntary muscle are so large that they can generate a muscle action potential. Neurotransmitters capable of evoking EPSPs include acetylcholine and norepinephrine. All EPSPs are summational (Fig. 3-8). The first impulse arriving at the synapse produces an EPSP. If a second impulse arrives at the synapse before the first EPSP has decayed, it positively adds (summates) to whatever remains of the first. In turn a third EPSP adds to what remains of the other two. The addition of successive EPSPs at the same synapse is called *temporal summation*. The addition of EPSPs at different synapses on the same neuron is called *spatial summation*. If the summation of EPSPs can reach the critical level at a nodal point such as the initial segment, an action potential is generated (Fig. 3-8).

Whereas excitation is the act of bringing a cell to a state in which it is more likely to fire, inhibition is the act of preventing a cell from firing. Inhibition may be explained as the response of the postsynaptic membrane to a putative neurotransmitter substance (Fig. 3-8) which raises its membrane potential (i.e., hyperpolarization, or increasing the difference in the potential between the cell and the extracellular fluid) or prevents the release of excitatory chemical substances. In either situation an *inhibitory postsynaptic potential* (*IPSP*) is formed. An IPSP opposes an EPSP. A neurotransmitter acting at some inhibitory synapses is γ-aminobutyric acid (GABA). A neuron may have many excitatory postsynaptic membrane sites and many inhibitory postsynaptic membrane sites. Both excitatory and inhibitory synapses share the ability to alter the ionic permeability of the postsynaptic membrane. On the basis of morphologic criteria, excitatory synapses cannot be distinguished from inhibitory synapses.

The postsynaptic membrane of the dendrites and cell body is presumed to have different properties from the presynaptic membrane of

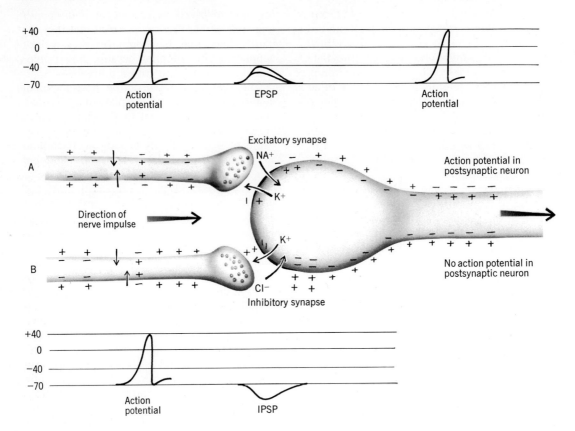

FIGURE 3-8
Sequences in *A* excitatory and *B* inhibitory transmission from presynaptic neurons (left) across synapses to postsynaptic neuron (right).

A The action potential conducted along the presynaptic axon to an excitatory synapse produces an EPSP, which, in turn, can contribute to the generation of an action potential in the postsynaptic neuron.
B The action potential conducted along the presynaptic axon to an inhibitory synapse produces an IPSP, which, in turn, suppresses the generation of an action potential in the postsynaptic neuron.

the axon. These differences are significant in the integrative activity of the neuron. The action potential of an axon is a traveling potential, is not graded (i.e., has an all-or-none response), and exhibits refractoriness immediately following a stimulation. In contrast, the postsynaptic potential is a standing potential (i.e., it does not travel), is graded, and lacks refractoriness immediately following a stimulation. These properties are most significant, for they mean that a second postsynaptic potential can be added to the first potential (temporally, summated subliminal stimuli). The graded responses provide a greater flexibility and plasticity of reaction to the neuron and to the nervous system than the rigidity of the stereotyped all-or-none pulse.

PRESYNAPTIC INHIBITION

Inhibition may be expressed upon a neuron as either postsynaptic or presynaptic. Postsynaptic inhibition operates through axosomatic or axodendritic synapses; it exerts its effect on the receptive segment of the neuron (see "A Structural and Functional Concept of the Neuron," further on in this chapter). On the other hand, presynaptic inhibition operates through axoaxonic synapses located on an axon just proximal to an excitatory (axosomatic or axodendritic) synapse (Fig. 2-5). In presynaptic inhibition the presynaptic neuron, acting through an axoaxonic synapse, releases "excitatory" neurotransmitters which depolarize the excitatory (axosomatic or axodendritic) synapse. In effect the postsynaptic membrane of the axoaxonic synapse is adjacent or close to the presynaptic membrane of the excitatory (axodendritic or axosomatic) synapse. The action of the presynaptic inhibitory synapse is to excite, through a neurochemical transmitter, the excitatory synapse, which now becomes less excitable for a brief period. During this short interval (milliseconds in duration), the effectiveness of the action potentials reaching the excitatory synapse is diminished and the release of excitatory transmitter chemicals is reduced. In effect, the ultimate effect of presynaptic inhibition is expressed through dampening and reducing the release of neurotransmitters at an excitatory synapse (see Chap. 13 for significance of presynaptic inhibition).

NEUROMUSCULAR SYNAPSE

Voluntary muscle The *motor end plate* is a synapse between a nerve and a voluntary muscle fiber; it is called a *neuromuscular synapse or junction*. When the action potential of the motor nerve reaches this junction, a large amount of acetylcholine is released into the synaptic cleft. This triggers the postjunctional membrane (postsynaptic membrane, end plate) of the muscle fiber to generate a muscle action potential, which is conducted along the plasma membrane. This action potential sets off a series of reactions resulting in the contraction of the muscle fiber (Fig. 3-9). The action potential of the alpha motor neuron always evokes an *obligatory response* (viz., the muscle fiber contracts) because more than enough neurotransmitter is always liberated to get a muscle action potential and a contraction.

The sequence of events within a lower motor neuron, motor end plate, and voluntary muscle illustrates some basic phenomena of activities of the nervous system. The motor end plate is actually a neuromuscular synapse between a nerve and a muscle. Acetylcholine is synthesized within the lower motor neuron (or any cholinergic neuron) by the combination of choline and acetyl-coenzyme A (CoA). The reaction is catalyzed by choline acetyltransferase (choline acetylase). Choline is largely transported into the neuron, whereas acetyl-CoA is a product of mitochondrial oxidative activity of the neuron. The choline acetyltransferase originates in the cell body and, either by active transport or axoplasmic flow, flows down to the nerve terminals, where it is present within the cytoplasm and not in the synaptic vesicles (Fig. 6-5).

After being synthesized, the acetylcholine is bound to a protein and stored in the storage granules (synaptic vesicles) of about 400-Å diameter. These roughly spherical vesicles have clear centers (they are called *vesicles with clear centers*). Vesicles may possibly be formed, in part, from neurotubules. Some acetylcholine is continuously liberated from the synaptic vesicles into cytoplasm, from which it crosses the presynaptic membrane into the synaptic cleft (gutter). Each quantum consists of about 10,000 acetylcholine ions. This small amount of acetylcholine stimulates the postjunctional membrane (end plate) of the muscle fiber to produce random generator potentials (nonpropagated depolarization), which are called *miniature end plate potentials* (*MEPPs*). Each MEPP is graded, shows rapid decrement, and lasts only a few milliseconds; an MEPP does not result in muscle contraction. The acetylcholine is released into the synaptic cleft in quanta. Each quantum produces one MEPP. These small transient MEPP are a normal feature of the "resting" postsynaptic membrane. At least 40 to 50 quanta of acetylcholine are required to initiate the synaptic activity which results in the contraction of a muscle fiber. Each nerve impulse activates the release of from 100 to 250 quanta of acetylcholine within a millisecond; this liberated amount is known as *quantal content*. Thus there is a substantial safety margin in neuromuscular transmission; hence an obligatory response.

Calcium ions must be present in the extracellular environment. They are important in the maintenance of the excitability of the

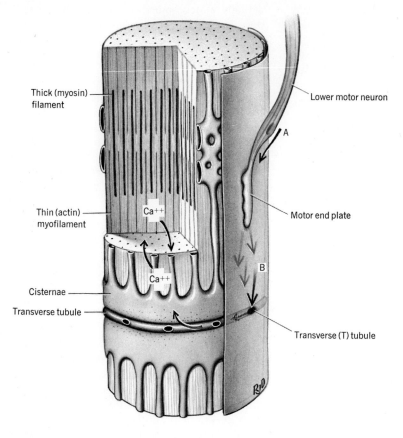

Thick (myosin) filament

Thin (actin) myofilament

Ca++

Ca++

Cisternae

Transverse tubule

Lower motor neuron

A

Motor end plate

B

Transverse (T) tubule

FIGURE 3-9
Neuromuscular linkage.

Sequence of events from the action potential of a motor nerve *A*, to motor end plate, to action potential of muscle cell membrane *B*, to T tubule and to sarcoplasmic cisternae. The release and uptake of calcium ions are involved with excitation-contraction (E-C) coupling.

plasma membrane (transmission) and in the storage and release of neurotransmitters at synaptic junctions. The event initiating neurotransmitter release is probably the influx of extracellular *calcium ions* across the presynaptic membrane in response to depolarization. When no calcium ions are present, there is no release of acetylcholine from the depolarization of the nerve terminals. *Magnesium ions* inhibit the release of neurotransmitters but do not block transmission. The magnesium ions act antagonistically to calcium ions; with an increase in magnesium ions there is a decrease in the release of acetylcholine. *Botulinus toxin*, a most potent poison, prevents the release of acetylcholine from nerve terminals whereas the black widow spider venom induces a rapid release of

acetylcholine, with a resulting depletion of the transmitters.

The acetylcholine released in the synaptic cleft of the motor end plate has several fates. Some molecules diffuse across the cleft and combine with specific cholinergic receptors (protein macromolecules) on the postsynaptic membrane on the muscle fiber. Depolarization of the muscle cell membrane is thus initiated. The rest of the acetylcholine may diffuse away from the synaptic cleft into tissue spaces, be adsorbed upon inert tissue, or be hydrolyzed into choline and acetate by the enzyme acetylcholine esterase. The choline may be restored to the neuron. Acetylcholine, unlike norepinephrine (see below), is not taken up into the nerve terminal.

The events linking the excitation of the muscle membrane (sarcolemma) to actual contraction of the muscle fibers are known as *excitation–contraction coupling (E–C coupling)*. Nerve stimulation results in the synchronous release of many quanta of acetylcholine which act on the postsynaptic membrane by causing a change in the ionic conductance (i.e., conductance of sodium, potassium, and calcium) of the muscle membrane (Fig. 3-9). The result is depolarization of the postsynaptic membrane, known as *normal end plate potential,* which can evoke a muscle action potential. This muscle action potential is similar to a nerve action potential; nerves and muscles are alike in that both can generate impulses.

A voluntary muscle fiber (cell) has a plasma membrane (*sarcolemma*) on its surface; this plasma membrane is continuous with the membrane lining the *transverse tubules (called T tubules)* of the muscle (Fig. 3-9). The cavity of each T tubule is actually an extracellular space which is continuous through its lumen with the connective tissue space surrounding the muscle fiber. In mammalian muscle, two T tubules are associated with each sarcomere (each T tubule is located at the A-I junction; A is the anisotropic and I is the isotropic band of the sarcomere). The surface area of a muscle cell is increased tenfold by the T tubules. The T tubules are the morphologic means by which the electrical signals are rapidly conveyed from the surface to the interior of the muscle fiber to initiate excitation and ensure the synchronous contraction of a fiber as a unit. Within the muscle fiber is a continuous system of membrane-limited tubular network called the sarcoplasmic reticulum (Fig. 3-9). This organelle is a specialized form of endoplasmic reticulum. The channels of the sarcoplasmic reticulum tend to be oriented longitudinally (parallel to the plane of the contractile myofibrils) and continuous with the terminal cisterna. The T tubule is flanked on each side by two terminal cisternae. The T tubule and the two terminal cisternae form the so-called *triads of voluntary muscle.* These triads are important functional units; the T tubules and sarcoplasmic reticulum are anatomically and physiologically linked. Calcium ion stores are located within the sarcoplasmic reticulum. For the details of muscle structure, refer to a textbook of microscopic anatomy.

Contraction of muscles The action potential is conducted rapidly along the muscle cell membrane, and the excitation signal penetrates immediately into the interior of the fiber along the T tubules. The final steps leading to contraction include *1* activity in the T tubules effecting the release of calcium ion stores from the sarcoplasmic reticulum compartment into the myofilament space. *2* The calcium ions are the activators of the contractile mechanism; these ions activate by releasing the inhibitory influences acting on adenosine triphosphatase (ATPase). Thus adenosine triphosphate (ATP) is converted to adenosine diphosphate (ADP), with the release of energy required for contraction of the myofibrils. In brief, the E-C coupling is the means of supplying calcium ions so that energy from ATP can be released for the contraction phase via the sliding filament principle of Huxley. After the action potential passes by a particular region of the muscle fiber, the uptake of calcium ions occurs; a calcium pump in the sarcoplasmic reticulum moves the calcium out of the myofilament space by active transport to the sarcoplasmic reticulum compartment. The reduction in the calcium ion concentration in the environment of the myofibrils prevents further contraction and thereby brings about relaxation of the muscle fibers.

Stated otherwise, following the stimulus from the T tubules the highly organized sarcoplasmic reticulum releases calcium upon excitation; in turn the released calcium triggers contraction, the calcium pump reaccumulates the calcium from the myofibril compartment into the sarcoplasmic reticulum compartment. This results in relaxation of the muscle fiber.

Involuntary (smooth) muscles Smooth muscles are spindle-shaped cells which are in such close apposition with one another as to form gap junctions (nexi, Fig. 6-1). These electrical junctions permit the spread of excitatory waves (contractions) from one muscle cell to another throughout the entire muscle mass. Smooth muscles can be stimulated to contract by postganglionic autonomic neurons (Chap. 6), by certain hormones, and by local changes within the muscle itself. Local contraction may be initiated in

94

CHAPTER THREE / BASIC NEUROPHYSIOLOGY

response to stretching of the muscle fibers. These muscles are capable of slow, sustained contractions; they are efficient because their contraction can be sustained with a minimal expenditure of energy. Smooth muscles maintain an "intrinsic tone" which is the basal tension upon which the other contractions are added.

The basic principles of excitation-contraction coupling and contraction by the sliding-filament principle expressed by voluntary muscles apply to smooth muscles. Excitation at the nerve-muscle junctions produces a membrane depolarization, which is followed by the release (contraction) and uptake (relaxation) of calcium ions so critical to muscle contraction and relaxation. The differences between the voluntary and involuntary muscle contractions—such as force, speed, and holding economy—are probably caused by the less regular arrangement of the myofilaments and the lesser number of contractile linkages in the involuntary muscle filaments.

On the basis of functional criteria, the smooth muscles have been classified as either *unitary muscles* or *multiunit muscles.* Unitary muscles are so called because contraction waves spread throughout the muscle mass as if the muscles were a single unit. These muscles are characterized by spontaneous activity, apparently initiated in pacemakers within the muscle, and by contractile responses to rapid stretch. Neural influences do not initiate contraction in these muscles, but rather, act to coordinate and regulate their contractile activity. Unitary musculature is found in the gastrointestinal tract, ureter, and uterus. *Multiunit muscles* are so called because each muscle mass, which is dependent upon its innervation for activation, is normally stimulated by a multiple number of motor nerves to several regions within the muscle mass. These muscles do not exhibit spontaneous contractile activity, nor do they respond to stretch by contracting. Multiunit muscles are found in the vas deferens, ciliary muscles, iris, and larger blood vessels, and they are associated with hair (pilomotor muscles). The musculature of the urinary bladder is intermediate in that it exhibits properties of both types (Chap. 6).

NEURON AS AN INTEGRATOR

Each neuron is a complex receptor and processor of a mosaic of numerous inputs. After integrating the stimuli from these inputs, the neurons may relay this information, which, in turn, is part of the input to other neurons, muscle fibers, or glandular cells. The synaptic receptor sites for the stimuli from other neurons are primarily located on the dendrites and cell body of a neuron. Quantitatively the dendrites generally contain more synapses than the cell body. In the motor neurons of the spinal cord in the cat, the surface area of dendrites is about 14 times that of the soma. About one-fifth of the thousands of synapses of each motor neuron are located on the soma and proximal 100 μm of the dendrites; about three-tenths are located on the dendrites between 100 to 300 μm from the soma; and the remaining one-half are associated with the dendrites more than 300 μm distal from the soma. The density of synapses on the axon hillock (close to the initial segment) is the same as on the soma (Aiken and Bridger).

In both the developing and mature neuron, the cell membrane is not static but rather is a dynamic trilaminar membrane. The dynamism at its molecular level is presumed to be critical to the variety of physiologic activities expressed by this membrane of each neuron. These expressions include those bioelectrical properties associated with chemical synapses, electrical synapses, excitation and inhibition, decremental nonpropagated potentials, and nondecremental propagated potentials. Molecular recognition of plasma-bound molecules is considered to have a significant role in the development of the precise, complex, and intricate neuronal circuitry of the central nervous system and peripheral nervous system during the prenatal and postnatal life. Similar, cell-to-cell molecular interactions between regenerating neuronal processes and neurolemma cells occur during terminal and collateral nerve regeneration. Molecular-level activity associated with the plasma membrane has been presumed to be involved in some way with memory and learning processes.

Some of the receptor sites on the postsynaptic membrane of the dendrites and cell body are excitatory and some are inhibitory. In *excitatory depolarizing activity* the membrane channels at the receptor sites favor the transmembrane movements of sodium and potassium cations. In *inhibitory hyperpolarizing activity* the membrane channels at the receptor sites presumably favor the transmembrane movements of potassium cations and chloride anions. Interneurons which synapse with excitatory receptor sites are often called *excitatory interneurons;* those which synapse with inhibitory receptor sites are called *inhibitory interneurons.* The nondecremental action potential of either an excitatory or an inhibitory interneuron is "changed" at the synapse to the local decremental event. The dendritic activity is often called a *dendritic potential.*

Stated otherwise, each neuron may be influenced by hundreds or thousands of stimuli on its excitatory and inhibitory receptive sites. The complex interplay of the subliminal excitatory postsynaptic potentials (EPSP) and subliminal inhibitory postsynaptic potentials (IPSP) on each neuron endows the neuron with a variety of inputs; this provides the basis for the great plasticity of activity. Neurons are under continual "synaptic bombardment." In this battleground of activity, the neuron reacts and responds. If the algebraic summation of the polarizing EPSPs and hyperpolarizing IPSPs results in a depolarizing event at the low-resistance, low-threshold axon hillock, an action potential is generated and conducted along the axon. On the other hand, if the algebraic summation of the graded subliminal potentials is not sufficient to stimulate the initial segment sufficiently, an action potential is not generated in the axon. Two EPSPs (or IPSPs) of equal size may not be equally effective. One may be more effective than the other, because it is located closer to the initial segment. Those EPSPs (or IPSPs) generated on the dendrites are less effective in exciting (or inhibiting) the neuron than those generated on the cell body or axon. Those graded postsynaptic potentials on the dendrites cannot reach the initial segment except by summating with other postsynaptic potentials (refer to spatial and temporal summation later on in chapter). In many neurons, synapses producing IPSPs are located on the axon hillock or on the initial segment; these synapses can be effective in throttling or blocking the generation of an action potential because they are located at a critical site.

In summary, each neuron is a miniature "integration" center where the confluences and algebraic summation of all the decremental spreads of EPSPs and IPSPs take place on the dendrites and cell body in relation to their geometric distribution and locations on the neuron. "We are dealing, in these central nervous system cells, with a brain in miniature" (Kuffler and Nicholls). The resulting action potential is, in effect, a code message conveying information about graded events in the dendrites and cell body of one neuron to a distant location where a graded event can be initiated on another neuron. Because the action potential evokes a graded response, the action potential in the central nervous system is said to be *optional;* it is not obligatory. In contrast, the action potential of a motor neuron on the voluntary muscle is *obligatory.*

In addition, a nerve cell fires periodically (ticks like a clock). The basis for this continued background activity is unknown; in effect, this firing is probably determined by some intrinsic mechanism within the neuron. Pacemaker loci may have a role in triggering these spontaneous rhythms.

PHYSIOLOGY OF PERIPHERAL RECEPTORS

The afferent (sensory) neurons conveying information from the internal and external environment to the central nervous system are the unipolar and bipolar cells associated with the cranial and spinal nerves. The short peripheral segments of theses nerves are associated with nerve endings, or peripheral receptors. According to one system, there are three anatomic forms of peripheral receptor. *1* Some nerve fibers actually end at the body surface and are in direct contact with the external environment. The olfactory nerves are the one example in man; these nerve terminals of the olfactory nerve are surrounded only by glandular secretions of the olfactory mucosal surface. *2* The actual nerve endings are in the tissues either as naked nerve endings or as encapsulated endings. *3* The nerve endings may have synaptic contact with a specialized neuroepithelial cell. The hair cells of the vestibular and cochlear system, the rods and cones of the eye, and the "taste cells" of the tongue are neuroepithelial cells.

All receptors are biologic transducers which utilize the stimulus of one form of energy to initiate the "electric" energy of the nerve impulse. Mechanoreceptors utilize mechanical forms of energy that result in sonic sensations in man, in ultrasonic sensations in dogs and bats, in muscle tension, in sensing movement and body position, in touch and pain, and in information on the blood pressure (pressoreceptors or baroreceptors). Chemoreceptors utilize chemical energy that results in taste, in smell, and in evaluating the carbon dioxide content of the blood (chemoreceptors of the carotid body). Light receptors utilize light energy that results in sight. There is some infrared light sensitivity in receptor endings of the rattlesnake. Thermal receptors utilize the temperature gradients that produce the sensations of cold and warmth. The external energies applied to these receptors act only as a trigger to release the energy stored across the plasma membrane. Sensory receptors can be stimulated by more than one form of energy. However, each receptor is especially sensitive to a particular form of energy (as the ear is sensitive to sound waves); this form of energy—actually the lowest intensity stimulus to which a receptor will respond—is known as the *adequate stimulus.*

The result of an effective transduction by the adequate stimulus is the production of a receptor potential (generator potential, generator current) in the nerve terminal. It is called the *generator potential* because it may generate an action potential. This generator potential is actually an EPSP because it is a standing potential, is graded, lacks refractoriness, can be summated as the postsynaptic membrane, and spreads passively with decrement for 1 or 2 mm. A short distance from the nerve ending the fiber is ensheathed by a neurolemma cell and in some cases by a myelin sheath. The generator current may spread along the receptor to a site on the nerve with a low threshold for generating an all-or-none action potential. In the case of a myelinated fiber, this site might be located at the first node of Ranvier (Fig. 3-12). The resulting digital impulse propagates along the nerve fiber to the central nervous system. The neurons through their telodendria have several receptors (a receptor field), each capable of producing a generator potential.

The Pacinian corpuscle serves to illustrate some basic principles of receptor activity (Fig. 3-12). Within the lamellar capsule are an unmyelinated segment and a myelinated segment of the nerve ending. In the "resting" state the afferent neuron, including the unmyelinated segment, has a potential of 70 millivolts, the resting potential. Displacement and movement, not pressure, on the Pacinian corpuscle provide the stimulus which produces changes in the molecular structure of the plasma membrane. This is followed by local changes in the permeability of the unmyelinated portion. The extracellular sodium ions are mainly responsible for the depolarization. The resulting buildup of positive charge on the intracellular side of the plasma membrane is followed by an intracellular flow of current carried by potassium ions toward the first node of Ranvier. This local circuit is closed by the extracellular space at this node of Ranvier. This *local, graded depolarizing potential* is the generator potential. When the depolarization reaches the critical threshold value, the action potential is probably initiated at the first node of Ranvier. When the stimulus at the receptor is weak, no action potential develops; when stimulus is strong but brief, several action potentials develop; and when stimulus is strong and sustained, a train of many impulses follows. The digital pulses of the action potentials are the means by which the coded data from the receptors are transmitted to the central nervous system. In another context the code resides in the chemical events of the sodium and potassium ions. This axonal transmission is analogous to a system utilizing only dots, not both dots and dashes. The frequency of the digital pulses transmitted varies. The greater the stimulus, the greater the frequency of the nerve impulses. In this analogy the afferent neurons utilize frequency modulation (FM), not amplitude modulation (AM).

Adaptation The receptors exhibit a phenomenon known as *adaptation.* This principle is an expression of decreased receptor sensitivity in response to a steady, continuous stimulus. If a stimulus is applied and maintained with an unchanging constant quality, the receptor will discharge initially at a high rate that will progressively be reduced to a lower rate of frequency. The response of the nerve is not maintained; rather, it declines with time.

Slowly adapting receptors are those that are able to maintain the lower rate of discharge for minutes and even hours. Slow adaptors include some touch receptors, neuromuscular spindles, temperature receptors, pain receptors, position sense receptors, and receptors in the carotid sinus and lung. The spindles, the recorders of limb position, adapt slowly if at all. Thus there is no loss of information concerning body position. Temperature and pain receptors are slow adaptors and therefore are efficient sensors for protecting the organism against noxious stimuli. The blood pressure receptors in the carotid sinus and the stretch receptors in the lung are monitors for the vital function of respiration.

Fast-adapting receptors are those whose burst of impulses terminate in less than a second following the initiation of the stimulus. Touch and pressure receptors are rapidly adapting organs. This explains why we are usually unaware of the contact of our clothes. Fast adaptation in the sense of touch permits the receptor to erase its activity and be ready to receive a new stimulus. The mechanism to explain adaptation is unknown. Adaptation may occur at the receptor level. A continuous stimulus applied to the receptor will be followed in time by a decline in the number of action potentials within the nerve. Adaptation may also take place at the synaptic level within the central nervous system; this has been demonstrated to occur in the visual pathways. It is not fatigue of the receptors, for following a shift in the intensity of the stimulus, the receptor fires again until it readapts.

Adaptation may have a significant biologic role. It seems probable that changes per se in the stimulus strength may be more important than the stimulus itself. The neurons respond to the change more effectively than to steady, continuous stimulation.

A structural and functional concept of the neuron

The neuron may be thought of as a cell with *1* a receptive segment, *2* an initial segment, *3* a conductile segment, *4* a terminal transmissive synaptic segment, and *5* a trophic segment (Figs. 3-10, 3-11). The receptive segment is specialized for the reception of stimuli and for the propagation of decrementally propagated responses. In a sense, the receptive segment monitors and integrates neural information. The initial segment is the junctional or trigger zone between the receptive segment and the conductile segment. It is the site at which the initiation of all-or-none action potential in any neuron is triggered. The conductile segment is specialized for the conduction of information for long distances from the receptive segment to the terminal transmissive synaptic segment. To perform this function, the conductile segment conducts the nondecremental all-or-none action potentials. The synaptic terminal segment is incorporated in a synapse. The trophic center is the cell body, which is the metabolic center essential to the maintenance of the viability of the neuron. Note that the trophic segment may be located within the receptive segment or within the conductile segment.

In a peripheral sensory myelinated unipolar neuron the receptive portion is the telodendria, the initial segment is the first node of Ranvier between the telodendria and the myelinated fiber, and the conductile segment includes the remaining cell processes, the axon and dendrite (Figs. 3-11, 3-12). The trophic segment is located within the conductile segment in the spinal ganglion.

In the typical somatic motor neuron (Figs. 3-10, 3-11) the receptive segment includes the dendrites and the cell body; the junctional zone is the initial segment of the axon just distal to the cell body; the conductile segment is the axon; and the synaptic segment is incorporated into the motor end plate. In this motor neuron the trophic segment is within the receptive segment. The location of the trigger point (or trigger points) in the neurons of the central nervous

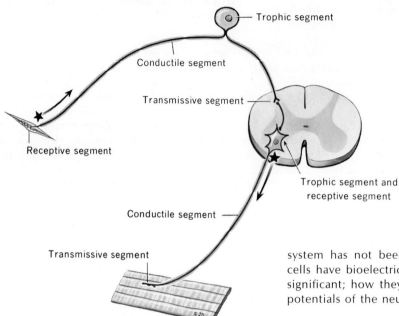

Trophic segment

Conductile segment

Transmissive segment

Receptive segment

Trophic segment and receptive segment

Conductile segment

Transmissive segment

FIGURE 3-10
A structural and functional schema of a neuron.

A neuron may be parceled into segments other than the classical dendrite, cell body, axon, and nerve endings. The sensory neuron may be parceled as follows: The receptive segment, which conducts with decrement, is the nerve ending; the initial segment (star) is the nodal site where the decremental conduction becomes the nondecremental (all-or-none) conduction of the conductile segment; the conductile segment, which conducts without decrement (all-or-none), extends from the initial segment to the synaptic endings within the spinal cord; the terminal (transmissive) segment includes the synaptic endings. In this neuron, the cell body is located within the conductile segment. The motor neuron may be subdivided as follows: the receptive segment includes the dendrites and cell body; the initial segment (star) is located just distal to the cell body; the conductile segment extends from the initial segment to the motor end plates; and the terminal segment is located within the motor end plates. In this neuron the cell body is located within the receptive segment.

system has not been demonstrated. The glial cells have bioelectric potentials which may be significant; how they influence the bioelectric potentials of the neurons is unknown.

General principles of interneuronal activity

The neurons of the nervous system interact in a matrix of organized complexity, which is far from being completely unraveled. Several basic principles of the structure and function operative in the nervous system will be described.

NEURONAL CIRCUITS

The neurons of the nervous system are organized in sequences of cells called *neuron circuits*. Several are shown in Figs. 3-13 and 3-14. Although the examples used below are found in the spinal cord (Chap. 5), these circuits are found in all levels of the central nervous system.

1 The simplest circuit, the two-neuron (monosynaptic) chain, as found in the stretch extensor reflex, consists of an afferent neuron, an intermediary synapse, and an efferent neuron.

2 The three-neuron (disynaptic) open circuit is formed by the intercalation of an interneuron between an afferent neuron and an efferent

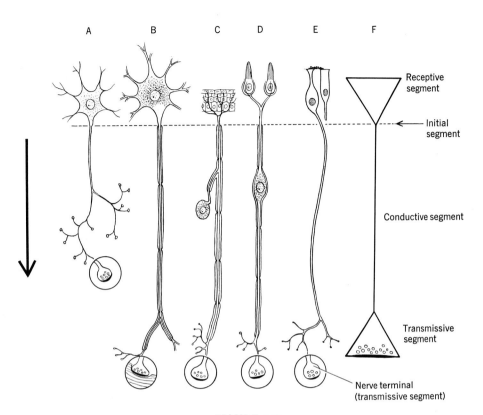

A   B   C   D   E   F

Receptive
segment

Initial
segment

Conductive segment

Transmissive
segment

Nerve terminal
(transmissive segment)

FIGURE 3-11
Structural and functional organization of representative neurons.

Most neurons are composed of a receptive segment,
an initial segment, a conductile segment, and a transmission segment. The transmission segment of each
neuron is encircled. Arrow indicates normal direction
of conduction of nerve impulse. *A* Interneuron; *B*
lower motor neuron; *C* sensory neuron with cell body
in spinal ganglion; *D* neuron of vestibulocochlear
nerve; *E* neuron of olfactory nerve; *F* functional organization of a neuron. Note that the cell body may be
located within the receptive segment (*A*, *B*, and *E*) or
within the conductile segment (*C* and *D*). The neuron
of the vestibulocochlear nerve is associated with a hair
cell in the upper part of figure. (*Adapted from D.
Bodian and H. Grundfest.*)

neuron. An example of this open circuit is the
withdrawal flexor reflex. An open circuit is a
chain of neurons connected with other neurons,
none of which connects (either directly or indirectly) through an axon with a prior neuron
in the chain.

3 The simple closed circuit is formed by the
intercalation of an interneuron between the
recurrent axon collateral branch of an efferent
neuron and the original efferent neuron. A
closed circuit contains an interneuron that connects (feeds back) to a prior neuron in the chain
(Fig. 3-13). This is a simple feedback circuit
whereby the efferent neuron may influence itself. (No neuron has an axon collateral branch
that synapses directly with itself.) An example
of the closed feedback circuit is found in the
anterior horn of the spinal cord in the circuit
of the (alpha) motor neuron and the interneuron neuron (Renshaw cell, Chap. 5).

4 The open multiple-chain circuit is formed by
many interneurons, all linked through collateral
branches and arranged in parallel chains. The
synaptic delays and the variability of conduction

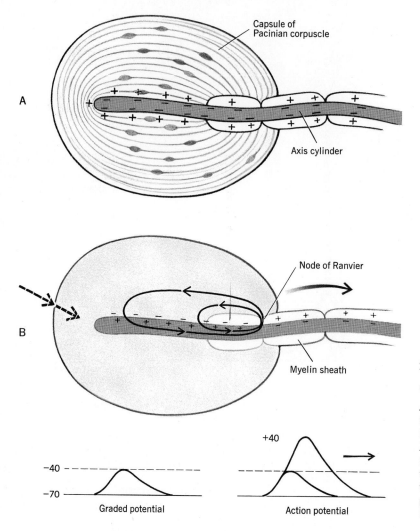

FIGURE 3-12
The Pacinian corpuscle as a receptive segment.

A The Pacinian corpuscle prior to stimulation has an axis cylinder with a resting potential. *B* The stimulated corpuscle (arrows) evokes a graded potential, which, in turn, triggers the generation of an action potential at the first node of Ranvier.

times in the links of these chains are features of this circuit system. A functional consequence of such a chain is that the neurons at the end of these circuits can be subjected to prolonged and variable stimulation.

5 The closed multiple-chain circuit is formed by many interneurons intercalated between the recurrent axon collateral branch of an efferent neuron and the original efferent neuron. These closed multisynaptic chains form feedback cir-

cuits that apparently permit the reverberation of impulses which can thereby raise or lower the excitability of various neurons in the chain.

PRINCIPLE OF DIVERGENCE

Each neuron synapses with many other neurons. An afferent nerve cell that is stimulated by peripheral receptors terminates in the central nervous system by arborizing into many

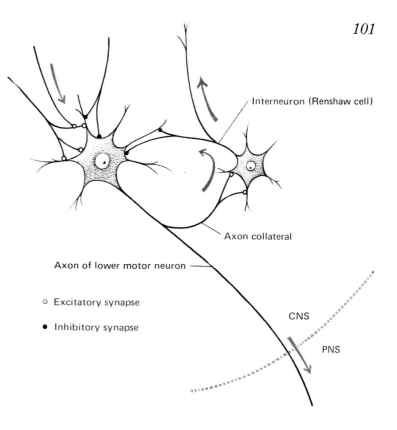

Interneuron (Renshaw cell)

Axon collateral

Axon of lower motor neuron

○ Excitatory synapse

● Inhibitory synapse

CNS

PNS

FIGURE 3-13
The neuron as an integrator.

Arrows indicate the direction in which nerve impulses are progagated. Neurons from many sources in the brain, spinal cord, and body convey influences to each lower motor neuron (Chap. 5), which in turn innervates some voluntary muscle fibers.

branches (telodendria), each branch having synaptic contact with the receptive portion of many other neurons (Fig. 3-14*A*). The axons of some neurons of the central nervous system are estimated to branch sufficiently to synapse with up to 25,000 or more other neurons. The opportunity of a neuron to excite (or to inhibit) numerous other neurons by the divergence of its axonal terminal branches is a fundamental principle underlying the activity of the central nervous system.

PRINCIPLE OF CONVERGENCE

Each neuron of the central nervous system is excited and inhibited by the synaptic activity of many other neurons on its dendrites and cell body (Fig. 3-14*B*). This receptive portion of the neuron is the focus for the convergence of the activity of, in many cases, literally thousands of other neurons. The integrated reactivity of the excitatory and inhibitory synapses on the recep-

tor portion of the neuron may result in the generation of an action potential in the axon of the neuron.

PRINCIPLE OF AFTERDISCHARGE

A stimulus such as a pinprick on a finger will evoke a response, the reflex withdrawal of the finger. Theoretically the time interval from stimulus to response in this three-neuron flexor reflex arc is equal to the time of conduction through the three neurons plus the synaptic delays. However, the muscle may continue to contract for many milliseconds after the withdrawal of the stimulus (i.e., the contraction outlasts the stimulus). This is because of "afterdischarge," which results from the activity of other circuits in addition to the three-neuron reflex arc. The multiple open- and closed-chain circuits provide a succession of discharges which arrive to excite the motor neuron after a slight delay. The neural activity transmitted

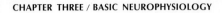
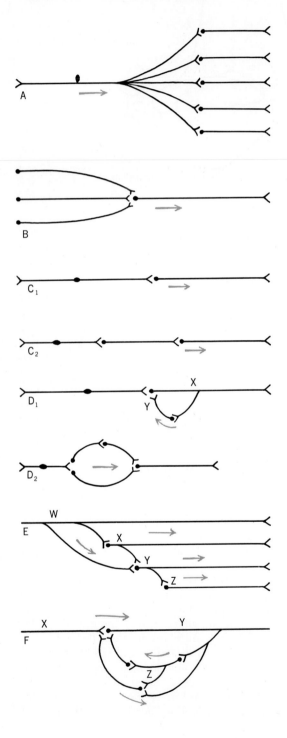

through the longer multineuronal circuits arrives at the motor neurons later than that transmitted through the short pathway circuits. These multi-synaptic systems "recirculate" the neural activity through interneurons, and this results in the sustained excitation of the motor neurons. The (after) discharge, which occurs after the stimulus is off, prolongs the reflex response.

FACILITATION

Facilitation (literally, "making easy") is the phenomenon wherein a normally subliminal (subthreshold) stimulus from a presynaptic neuron "primes" a postsynaptic neuron so that another subliminal stimulus can evoke a discharge of the postsynaptic neuron. In brief, the first stimulus has facilitated the postsynaptic neuron. The start of a sprint race offers an analogy. The starter's

FIGURE 3-14
Schematic representation of some circuits of neurons. Arrows indicate direction in which nerve impulses are propagated.

A Principle of divergence. One presynaptic neuron branches and synapses with several postsynaptic neurons.
B Principle of convergence. Several presynaptic neurons synapse with one postsynaptic neuron.
C Simple open-type circuits. (*C-1*) Two-neuron sequence of afferent neuron synapsing with efferent neuron, found in a two-neuron reflex. (*C-2*) Three-neuron sequence of afferent neuron, interneuron, and efferent neuron, found in a three-neuron reflex.
D Simple closed-type circuits. (*D-1*) Simple feedback circuit, in which the axon collateral branch of neuron X synapses with interneuron Y, which, in turn, synapses with neuron X. Refer to Fig. 3-13. (*D-2*) Simple feedforward circuit, basic to recruitment and afterdischarge, as discussed in text.
E Open multiple-neuronal chain circuit. In this circuit, neuron W through a collateral branch, may influence neuron X and, through another collateral branch, may influence neuron Y. In turn neuron X, through a collateral branch, may influence neuron Y, and, in turn, neuron Y, through a collateral branch, may influence neuron Z. In essence the stimulation of neuron W may influence the activity of three other neurons. This is a form of divergence.
F Closed multiple-neuronal chain circuit (feedback circuit). In this circuit neuron Y, through a collateral branch, may influence a complex of neurons Z, which in turn may influence (feedback) neurons X and Y.

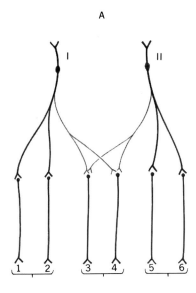

A

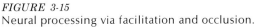

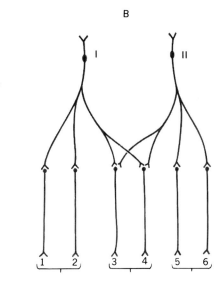

B

FIGURE 3-15
Neural processing via facilitation and occlusion.

A Facilitation. Presynaptic neurons I and II may independently stimulate two postsynaptic neurons to discharge. However, if I and II simultaneously fire, six postsynaptic neurons may discharge. The reason is that 3 and 4, although subliminally stimulated by I or II, are adequately stimulated by I and II firing together. The subliminal effects are facilitated by summation.
B Occlusion. Presynaptic neurons I and II may independently stimulate four postsynaptic neurons to fire. But if I and II discharge simultaneously, only six postsynaptic neurons are stimulated to fire. The reason is that neurons 3 and 4 already receive liminal stimulation from either I or II; the excess stimulation received when both I and II fire has no effect.

instruction of "Get set" is the stimulus that "facilitates" the sprinters for the final stimulus of "Go."

Facilitation has a role in the following expression. The total response to several simultaneously applied stimuli may be greater than the sum of the responses to stimuli separately applied (i.e., the sum seems to be greater than the parts). For example, the simultaneous discharge of two presynaptic neurons into a neuron pool may stimulate six postsynaptic neurons above threshold to fire (Fig. 3-15*A*). However, the discharge of each of the two presynaptic neurons alone stimulates only two postsynaptic neurons to fire liminally (or a total of four postsynaptic neurons). The two remaining postsynaptic neurons are subliminally stimulated by each of the two presynaptic neurons. One presynaptic neuron facilitates and the other stimulates the two postsynaptic neurons to fire.

Many interactions of the central nervous system involve facilitation.

DISINHIBITION

Facilitation may be produced in one of two ways: by the direct activity of excitatory synapses, or by preventing inhibitory synapses from

acting. The latter is known as "disinhibition." Disinhibition is functionally expressed in such a circuit as the sequence of a collateral branch of a motor neuron, to a chain of several interneurons, terminating on a motor neuron. In such a circuit, the collateral branch of a motor neuron (neuron 1) synapses and may excite an interneuron (neuron 2) with inhibitory synaptic endings; these endings stimulate an interneuron (neuron 3) with inhibitory synaptic endings, which, in turn, synapse with the postsynaptic membrane of a motor neuron (neuron 4). When neuron 3 is inhibited from firing by neuron 2, motor neuron 4 is actively inhibited. When this circuit is active, the motor neuron (neuron 4) may be temporarily released from this inhibitory stimulation; this release is an expression of disinhibition. This sequence commences with the facilitatory activity of the recurrent collateral branch of neuron 1 and terminates with active inhibition of the inhibitory interneuron (neuron 3). This recurrent facilitatory activity results in disinhibition (a release phenomenon, Chap. 9) of the motor neuron (neuron 4). Recurrent facilitation (disinhibition) and recurrent inhibition (active inhibition of postsynaptic membrane) are important to the organized circuitry of the nervous system.

The inhibition of an inhibitory pool (or an inhibitory pathway) is also called disinhibition.

OCCLUSION

The total response of several simultaneously applied stimuli may be less than the sum of the responses to the stimuli separately applied (i.e., the response seems to be less than the sum of the parts). For example, the simultaneous discharge of two presynaptic neurons may provide above-threshold stimulation to six postsynaptic neurons (Fig. 3-15B), while discharge of each of the presynaptic neurons alone would stimulate four postsynaptic neurons to fire. The explanation is that two of the postsynaptic neurons are "shared" by axons from the presynaptic neurons. Nerve impulses from either presynaptic neuron are sufficient to cause both postsynaptic neurons to fire. When both presynaptic neurons fire simultaneously, there is thus an excess stimulation which has no effect. This is occlusion. Occlusion has nothing to do with inhibition.

SPATIAL SUMMATION

Summation is an expression of the cumulative effects of a number of stimuli upon a neuron. Spatial summation is the summation (integration) of many EPSPs received almost simultaneously at different sites on the receptive por-

tion of the neuron from several other neurons. This summation may (or may not) produce an action potential. Facilitation depends on spatial summation. The presynaptic neuron activity lowers the threshold of excitation of the postsynaptic neurons (EPSP), thereby facilitating or aiding the stimuli of other neurons to fire the postsynaptic neuron. Spatial summation of the postsynaptic potentials is the rule in the central nervous system.

TEMPORAL SUMMATION

Temporal summation is a form of summation whereby the cumulative effects of repetitive subliminal EPSPs from a single presynaptic neuron on the receptive membrane of a postsynaptic neuron may summate in time to excite the neuron. Because of the short excitable period of the synapse, temporal summation is not considered to be as important as spatial summation.

RECRUITMENT

Recruitment (the recruiting of neurons) is a neurophysiologic phenomenon in which a response (action potential) is obtained only after a rapid succession of afferent stimuli is delivered (Fig. 3-14D). The complex of multiple chains intercalated between the stimulated sites (afferent neurons) and the responsive sites (efferent neurons) is critical to the phenomenon of recruitment. Recruitment is a form of facilitation primarily utilizing closed multineuronal circuits. The following is a simplified explanation of this complex activity. The impulses resulting from the first afferent volleys travel via short circuits (an open loop) to the motor pool. These initial volleys are subliminal and thus not sufficient by themselves to elicit action potentials in the motor neurons of the motor pool. These initial volleys also activate closed multiple-chain circuits, but the resulting impulses arrive at the motor pool too late to summate with those traveling over the short circuits. However, these initial volleys transmitted through the closed multiple circuits arrive at the same time as the subsequent volleys transmitted with the short circuits. The resulting summation facilitates a response from the motor neurons in the motor pool. Recruitment is a form of facilitation obtained by repetitive stimulation. The complexities of the circuits capable of eliciting recruitment stagger the imagination.

SPONTANEOUS ACTIVITY IN THE CENTRAL NERVOUS SYSTEM

The nervous system always shows evidence of activity. It is never quiescent. The continuous input from the peripheral receptors and their afferent nerve contributes to this activity. The intrinsic mechanism that keeps the units of the nervous system activated is unknown. It is theorized that without such an intrinsic mechanism (or mechanisms) the central nervous system could not sustain its activity.

One source might be active pacemaker sites. These sites might resemble the *pacemaker cells of the heart.* The pacemakers of the sinoatrial (SA) node, specialized atrial cells, atrioventricular (AV) node, bundle of His, and peripheral Purkinje fibers are automatic in that they can spontaneously excite themselves regularly. These pacemaker cells cycle. They cannot maintain their resting potential. After reaching the resting potential, the potential drifts toward the critical threshold that generates a return to the resting potential. At this point the cycle repeats. In the heart the SA node cycles about 70 to 90 times per minute, the AV node and bundle of His about 40 to 60 cycles per minute, and the Purkinje fibers about 25 to 30 cycles per minute. The SA node is *the* pacemaker because it has the faster cycles, and through these cycles, the SA node synchronizes the cycles of the other pacemaker cells.

The background of continuous and rhythmic spike discharge of neurons in the absence of known stimulation may be accounted for by similar activity. In a *neuronal pacemaker cycle,* the locally produced generator potential constantly drifts to the critical potential at a critical site of the neuron. At this moment, the neuron fires and the new generator potential repeats. These sites might resemble the pacemaker of the heart. The cells of a pacemaker form locally produced generator potentials that drift slowly toward the critical threshold that initiates and results in an action potential. This is followed immediately by a return to the resting or generator potential, which again commences to drift toward the critical threshold. This may account

for the background of continuous spike discharge in the absence of known stimulation, or, in part, for rhythmic discharge (Chap. 13).

Automatic control systems and feedback

An understanding of the automatic control systems (servomechanisms) used by mathematicians and engineers is useful for gaining some conceptual insight into the operation of certain activities of the nervous system.

Biologic analogues exist both with the open-loop and with the closed-loop control systems. These systems are designed to maintain some predetermined constant state, such as temperature, position, or speed. The open-loop control systems do not utilize feedback in their operation, whereas the closed-loop control systems do. Feedback is the return of a portion of the output of a system to the system proper for the purpose of influencing and automatically regulating the further operation of the system.

OPEN-LOOP CONTROL SYSTEM

An example of this type of automatic system is the operation of a dam in the watershed of water supply. The dam in the reservoir is an automatic control which acts to prevent the water from rising above a certain predetermined level. However, the height of the dam is not regulated automatically by the amount of water drained out of the reservoir. Also when rainfall is low, the water level in the reservoir fluctuates below the dam level. The pertinent features of this system for this discussion are *1* the fact that the system does not utilize its output to effect its operation (the level of the dam), and *2* the degree of inherent instability (fluctuating water level).

A biologic open-loop system is the body temperature control of cold-blooded (poikilothermic) animals. These animals apparently possess no feedback mechanism for the fine regulation of heat production and conservation. As a result their body temperature fluctuates widely. The environmental heat which influences the animal's body temperature is analogous to the watershed, and the ability of the animal to lose heat is analogous to the floodgate of the dam. When the environmental heat increases (or decreases) the temperature of the animal rises (or drops). The analogue is the rise (or fall) of the water in the reservoir.

CLOSED-LOOP CONTROL SYSTEM

The closed-loop (cycle) systems utilize feedback, in which a fraction of the output of the system is *1* fed back into the system and *2* utilized in the further performance of the system. In brief, output can control or regulate input. The closed-loop system may utilize negative (degenerative) or positive (regenerative) feedback.

CONTROL SYSTEM UTILIZING NEGATIVE FEEDBACK

This servomechanism utilizes negative feedback to maintain a predetermined performance (or goal) of the control system. This performance is obtained by making a series of self-correcting adjustments which are based on the feedback of the immediately prior performance (output) of the system to a control box (comparator). The feedback is called negative when the correction is in the opposite (negative) direction of the positive divergence from the predetermined performance. For example, the thermostat (control box) of a heating system (closed-loop control system) directs the maintenance of a constant temperature in a room by utilizing some of the heat (i.e., a feedback of a fraction of the output or controlled quality) to activate the thermostat, which, in turn, attempts to maintain the preset temperature by regulating the heat output of the furnace. In practice, the actual temperature fluctuates about the preset temperature of the thermostat. The system is goal-seeking in its attempt to match the predetermined reference. Information of the actual temperature is fed into the thermostat and compared to the preset temperature control. The sequence of feedback of the actual temperature

(output of furnace), comparison of preset temperature (in thermostat), and adjustment (instructions relayed to furnace) is a continuous repetitive sequence. The feedback is negative because an increase in the room temperature is followed by a reduced activity in the furnace with a subsequent decrease in heat production, while a decrease in the room temperature results in a subsequent increase of heat production. In effect, the negative feedback operates to maintain a relatively constant room temperature.

Control systems that utilize negative feedback act to compensate for the difference between the actual and the predetermined quality. They are self-correcting, error-correcting systems operating to maintain a goal. These systems ensure *stability* and *regulation*. Unless specified, feedback systems generally utilize negative feedback. Negative feedback subtracts from the input to the control center box. Biologic control systems are largely of this type.

The biologic implications of closed-loop control systems utilizing negative feedback are significant and widespread. Actually the control system concept is embodied in a phrase of Claude Bernard's, "constancy of the internal milieu" (internal environment), and in Walter B. Cannon's principle of homeostasis. Homeostasis represents the preset norm; when the homeostatic condition is upset, the organism utilizes its resources to restore the equilibrium (Chap. 6). Homeostasis is crucial to an animal's freedom of action, permitting the animal to function regardless of changes in the external environment. Because of homeostasis the organism is less dependent on the vagaries of the environment.

Examples of activities with negative feedback include the regulation of *1* visceral activities, *2* somatic activities, and *3* learning processes.

1 Maintenance of a relatively constant body temperature with narrow fluctuations is an expression of homeostasis utilizing the nervous system (Chap. 11). Regulation of the water balance in the body and that of the general hormonal levels are expressions of homeostasis which utilize both the nervous system (feedback through nerve cells) and the endocrine system (feedback through circulatory system) (Chap. 11).

2 Coordination and smooth integration among voluntary muscles are effected through complex feedback control systems in the spinal cord (see "Gamma Reflex Loop," in Chap. 5) and the cerebellum (Chap. 9).

3 In the higher neural processes of learning, negative feedback is used, as, for example, in maze learning. The initial trials in this form of learning are relatively random attempts with numerous oscillations from the preset goal. In subsequent trials, the randomness is reduced and the oscillations are less marked.

Many diseases in man involve interferences, malfunction, and change in the efficiency of the feedback regulatory systems.

CONTROL SYSTEM UTILIZING POSITIVE FEEDBACK

A servomechanism which utilizes positive feedback returns part of the output to the control box to increase the output. This is a regenerative (or vicious) cycle system. It is unstable. It tends to explode or "run away." In a positive-feedback heating system, an increase in temperature results in a continuous spiraling increase in heat production until the furnace operates at full capacity, breaks down, or explodes.

The initial stages in the generation of an all-or-none action potential utilize the principle of positive feedback. The decrease in the resting potential (receptor potential or postsynaptic excitatory potential, EPSP) may be followed by the sequence of increased sodium conductance, some depolarization, further increase in sodium conductance, etc., until the threshold is reached. The positive feedback results in regeneration until the explosion of the all-or-none action potential. Positive feedback adds to the input to the control center box.

Integration center and modulation center

Portions of the nervous system operate in feedback systems either as integration centers or as modulators. In a biologic feedback system the integration center is the crucial control center, for it regulates the goal-seeking performance of the system. It is the equivalent of the thermostat in a temperature control system. Without the integrative center the feedback system is essentially uncontrolled.

The hypothalamus acts as the integration center for the regulation of temperature (the controlled quality). When this temperature-regulating region of the hypothalamus is impaired or damaged, temperature control can be so altered that death may result. This feedback system utilizes the temperature of the blood to stimulate the temperature integrative center in the hypothalamus. This activates the nervous system and the organism to set in motion those processes that return the temperature to normal (Chap. 11).

A modulation center or higher control center is a region that may influence the integration center. It is not essential to the operation of the feedback cycle. For example, a timer that changes the setting on a thermostat is a modulator. The timer may raise the setting early in the morning, so that the room may be warm during the day, and lower the setting later in the day, so that the room is cool at night. The essential relation of the thermostat to the furnace is unchanged.

The hypothalamus acts as a modulator of the blood pressure *integration centers* in the lower medulla. Hypothalamic activity can affect the medullary cardiovascular center, causing it to raise (sympathetic effect) or lower (parasympathetic effect) the blood pressure (Chap. 8). It does not have a direct role in the vital feedback mechanism of blood pressure control.

Bibliography

Eccles, J. C.: *The Physiology of Synapses.* Academic Press, Inc., New York, 1964.

Florey, E.: *An Introduction to General and Comparative Animal Physiology.* W. B. Saunders Company, Philadelphia, 1966.

Guyton, A. C.: *Structure and Function of the Nervous System.* W. B. Saunders Company, Philadelphia, 1972.

Hoar, W. S.: *General and Comparative Physiology.* Prentice-Hall, Inc., Englewood Cliffs, N.J., 1966.

Kandel, E. R., and W. A. Spencer: Cellular neurophysiological approaches in the study of learning. Physiol. Rev., 48:65–134, 1968.

CHAPTER THREE / BASIC NEUROPHYSIOLOGY

Katz, B.: *Nerve, Muscle and Synapse.* McGraw-Hill Book Company, New York, 1966.

Kuffler, S. W., and J. C. Nicholls: The physiology of neuroglial cells. Ergeb. Physiol., 57:1–90, 1966.

Loewenstein, W. R. (ed.): Principles of receptor physiology, in *Handbook of Sensory Physiology*, vol. 1, pp. 1–600. Springer-Verlag, Berlin and New York, 1971.

McLennan, H.: *Synaptic Transmission.* W. B. Saunders Company, Philadelphia, 1970.

Mountcastle, V. B.: *Medical Physiology*, The C. V. Mosby Company, St. Louis, 1968.

Quarton, G. C., T. Melnechuk, and F. O. Schmitt: *The Neurosciences.* Rockefeller University Press, New York, 1967.

Ruch, T. C., H. D. Patton, J. W. Woodbury, and A. L. Towe: *Neurophysiology.* W. B. Saunders Company, Philadelphia, 1965.

Schmitt, F. O. (ed.): *The Neurosciences—Third Study Program.* The M.I.T. Press, Cambridge, Mass., 1974.

———, G. C. Quarton, T. Melnechuk, and G. Adelman (eds.): *The Neurosciences—Second Study Program.* Rockefeller University Press, New York, 1970.

——— et al. (eds.): *Neurosciences Research Program.* The M.I.T. Press, Cambridge, Mass., 1966 to date.

Tamar, H.: *Principles of Sensory Physiology.* Charles C Thomas, Publisher, Springfield, Ill., 1972.

CHAPTER 4
DEVELOPMENT AND GROWTH
OF THE NERVOUS SYSTEM

The cardiovascular system and the nervous system are the first organ systems to function during embryonic life. In man, the heart commences to beat late in the third week after fertilization. During the second month, an avoidance reflex in the human embryo evokes withdrawal of the head by contraction of the neck muscles when stimuli are applied to the upper lip. A mother may feel life as early as the twelfth prenatal week.

Differentiation and cell multiplication characterize development during early prenatal life, whereas growth (increase in size) is more prominent during late fetal and postnatal life. The formation of new neurons by mitosis normally ceases during late prenatal life and probably does not occur after birth in man. To generate a human brain of more than 100 billion neurons requires the production and differentiation of an average of about 200,000 neurons per minute throughout the entire length of prenatal life. There are roughly 10 billion neurons in the cerebral cortex and up to 100 billion neurons in the cerebellar cortex. Growth of the nervous tissues continues postnatally, especially during the first 3 years after birth, by the increase in size of neurons and glia, and by myelination.

First prenatal month

When the human embryo is but 1.5 mm long (18 days old), the ectoderm, or the outer germ layer, differentiates and thickens along the future midline of the back to form the neural plate (Fig. 4-1). This neural plate is exposed to the surface and to the amniotic fluid; it is continuous later-

ally with the future skin. Certain portions of the ectoderm differentiate and thicken in the head region to form the placodes (thickened ectodermal anlagen) of organs of special sense such as the eyes (optic placode), ears (auditory placode), and nose (nasal placode). In fact, the neural plate is a giant placode. The neural plate elongates, and its lateral edges are raised to form the neural folds (Fig. 4-1). The anterior end of the neural plate enlarges and will develop into the brain. The lateral edges, or lips, continue to rise and grow medially until they meet and unite in the midline to form the neural tube. This midline union commences in the cervical region and progresses both cephalically and caudally until the entire plate is converted into the neural tube (in 25 days). The tube becomes detached from the skin and sinks beneath the surface (Fig. 4-2). The cavity of the neural tube persists in the adult as the ventricular system of the brain and the central canal of the spinal cord.

The cephalic end of the neural tube differentiates and enlarges into three dilatations called the "primary brain vesicles." Rostrally to caudally, the three divisions are the prosencephalon or forebrain, the mesencephalon or midbrain, and the rhombencephalon or hindbrain (Table 4-1). A bilateral column of cells differentiates from the neural ectoderm at the original junction of the skin ectoderm and the rolled edges of the neural plate. These two columns of cells become the neural crests.

The three-vesicle stage of the brain, the remainder of the neural tube (which will develop into the spinal cord), several placodes, and neural crests constitute the embryonic nervous system at the stage attained by the end of the first month after fertilization in man. Thus, basically

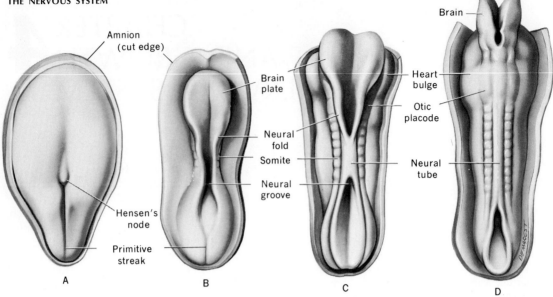

FIGURE 4-1
Dorsal aspect of human embryo.

A Primitive-streak stage of 16-day presomite embryo.
B Two-somite stage of approximately 20-day embryo.
Note first somites, neural fold, and neural groove. *C*
Seven-somite stage of approximately 22-day embryo. *D*
Ten-somite stage of approximately 23-day embryo.
(*Adapted from Scammon, 1953.*)

the nervous system originates as a surface structure and then sinks beneath the body surface.

The neural tube, placodes, and neural crests are derived from ectoderm. The neural tube is the primordial structure for the central nervous system (brain and spinal cord), including all neurons in the central nervous system, oligodendroglia, and astroglia. The neural crests are the primordial structures giving rise to the neurons of the sensory ganglia, some neurons of the peripheral autonomic ganglia, satellite cells of the peripheral ganglia, neurolemma cells of the peripheral nerves, and the piarachnoid meningeal layers (Fig. 4-3).

Several mesodermally derived elements are associated with the nervous system. Those that secondarily invade the central nervous system include the blood vessels and microglial cells.

Surrounding the central nervous system is the dura mater. The extraneural mesodermal elements of the peripheral nervous system include the outer satellite cells of the peripheral ganglia, the epineurium, perineurium, and endoneurium of the peripheral nerves, and the capsules of some peripheral sensory endings.

Embryonic central nervous system

The maturing cells of the embryonic central nervous system are conceived as developing according to one of two general concepts: *classic* and *recent.*

CLASSIC CONCEPT

The neural tube differentiates into three roughly concentric laminae extending through the length of the future central nervous system (Fig. 4-3). The *matrix* (*ependymal*) *layer* is the pseudostratified columnar epithelial layer lining the central canal. This direct descendant of the single-layered neural plate is the germinal layer

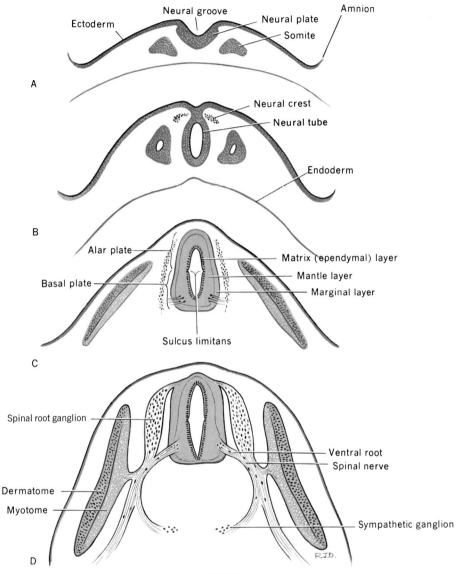

A

B

C

D

FIGURE 4-2
Development of the spinal cord, neural crest, somite, and spinal nerve (transverse sections) in human embryo of the following ages: *A* approximately 19 days; *B* approximately 20 days; *C* approximately 26 days; *D* after 1 month of age.

from which the other laminae are derived. The matrix (germinal) cells of this layer proliferate by mitotic activity to form neuroblast cells and glioblast (spongioblast) cells, which migrate into the two other laminae, viz., the mantle and marginal layers (Fig. 4-3). The *neuroblasts* differentiate into neurons, and the *glioblasts* into the macroglia: oligodendroglia and astroglia. Ac-

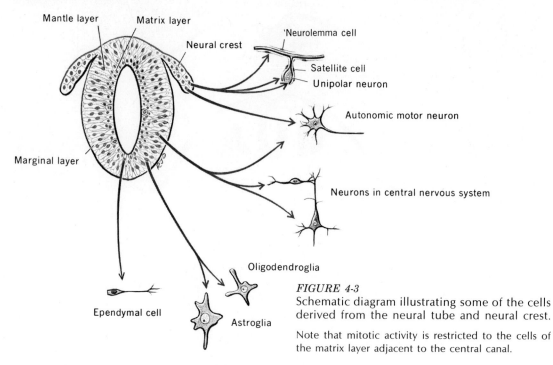

Mantle layer

Matrix layer

Neural crest

Neurolemma cell

Satellite cell

Unipolar neuron

Autonomic motor neuron

Neurons in central nervous system

Marginal layer

Oligodendroglia

Ependymal cell

Astroglia

FIGURE 4-3
Schematic diagram illustrating some of the cells
derived from the neural tube and neural crest.

Note that mitotic activity is restricted to the cells of
the matrix layer adjacent to the central canal.

TABLE 4-1
The derivatives of the neural tube

	Primary vesicles	*Subdivisions*	*Derivatives*	*Lumina or cavities*
Brain	Prosencephalon (forebrain)	Telencephalon (endbrain)	Cerebral cortex Corpora striata Rhinencephalon Rostral hypothalamus	Lateral ventricles Rostral part of third ventricle
		Diencephalon (twixt-brain; between brain)	Epithalamus Thalamus Hypothalamus Ventral thalamus	Most of third ventricle
	Mesencephalon (midbrain)	Mesencephalon (midbrain)	Corpora quadrigemina Tegmentum Crura cerebri	Cerebral aqueduct of Sylvius (iter)
	Rhombencephalon (hindbrain)	Metencephalon (afterbrain)	Cerebellum Pons	
		Myelencephalon (spinal brain)	Medulla oblongata	Fourth ventricle
Spinal cord		Spinal cord	Spinal cord	Central canal

cording to this concept, the germinal cells divide within the matrix layer of the central nervous system and generate postmitotic neuroblasts; these neuroblasts migrate outward through the intercellular spaces of a mass of glioblasts to form the cell-rich mantle layer and the cell-poor marginal layer. The *mantle layer* is composed of maturing postmitotic neuroblasts and glioblasts, while the *marginal layer* is composed of spongioblasts and the axons of the developing neurons. In the fully differentiated central nervous system the matrix layer persists as the mitotically inactive ependymal layer, the mantle layer as the gray matter other than cortex, and the marginal layer as the white matter. The cortical laminae (cerebral cortex, cerebellar cortex, and colliculi of the midbrain) are formed by the peripheral migration of neuroblasts and glioblasts through the mantle and marginal layers to become the outermost lamina in each of these structures.

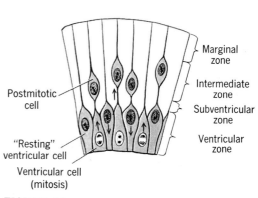

FIGURE 4-4
The four zones of the embryonic central nervous system.

The arrows within the ventricular cells indicate the direction in which their nuclei migrate during a mitotic cycle. The arrow outside the cells indicates the direction in which the postmitotic neuroblasts migrate.

RECENT CONCEPT

The embryonic central nervous system comprises four concentric zones: ventricular, subventricular, intermediate (mantle), and marginal (Fig. 4-4). The adult nervous system is derived from these basic zones, but none of the four corresponds directly to any adult component.

The *ventricular zone* comprises one type of cell—the ventricular cell. Recent studies indicate that the apparent differences among the cells of this lamina are actually differences in the stages of the mitotic cycle of each cell of the pseudostratified columnar epithelial ventricular zone. The nucleus of each ventricular cell migrates to the base of the cell (adjacent to the central canal), rounds up, and undergoes a mitotic division; after dividing, the nuclei of the daughter cells migrate to the apical portions of their respective cells, where the replication of its deoxyribonucleoproteins occurs. Thus the ventricular zone is known as the lamina of the *to-and-fro nuclear movement*. The mitotic and nuclear migration cycle lasts from 5 to 24 hr. Ventricular cells are the progenitors of all neurons and macroglia of the central nervous system. This zone will attenuate and eventually disappear after all its cells differentiate.

The *subventricular zone* is located adjacent to the ventricular zone. The subventricular cells are small cells which proliferate by mitosis. They do not exhibit the to-and-fro nuclear movements during their mitotic cycles. The subventricular zone persists from only a few days in the spinal cord to many months or even years in the cerebral hemisphere. This zone generates certain classes of neurons and all macroglia of the central nervous system. In the spinal cord, the ventricular layer gives rise to the neurons, while the subventricular layer generates all spinal macroglia. Those progenitor cells (neuroblasts) destined to form neurons migrate from the ventricular and subventricular zones during development before those subventricular cells destined to form macroglia. Once neuroblasts move out of the generator zones, they are postmitotic cells. With the possible exception of some microneurons, which differentiate in the subventricular zones of the brain (rhombic lip and ganglionic eminence, see below), in man all neurons appear during prenatal life, whereas macroglia are generated during prenatal and postnatal life. In fact, glia cells may proliferate at a low rate throughout life. Once neuroblasts migrate from the ventricular zone, they lose their capacity to divide—they are postmitotic cells. Neuroblasts migrating out of the subventricular zone may be either postmitotic cells or mitotically capable cells. Those subventricular cells invading cortex may continue to divide.

There are two important specialized areas composed of subventricular cells: the rhombic lip and the ganglionic eminence. The *rhombic lips*, located at the lateral margins of the fourth ventricle, give rise to many cells of the cerebellum (granule, stellate, and basket cells) and the brainstem (neurons of the inferior olivary, reticularis pontine and pontine nuclei, Fig. 4-6). The *ganglionic eminence*, located in the floor of the lateral ventricle near the future caudate nucleus, is the site of origin of cells of the basal ganglia and pulvinar, and possibly of some cells of the association cortical areas. This eminence and primordial nests of cells in the hippocampal region may be the source, in man, for the differentiation of microneurons postnatally in the adult. Recall that some authorities claim that new neurons do not differentiate postnatally in man.

The *intermediate (mantle) zone* is the lamina immediately external to the subventricular zone. The postmitotic neurons migrate to this zone, aggregate into cell groups, and differentiate their cell processes. Macroglial cells also occupy this zone. In general the intermediate zone seems to evolve into the gray matter of the central nervous system with its complex neural organizations. In the potential cerebral and cerebellar areas, other neurons migrate and collect to form the *cortical plate;* these neurons form efferent axons that course inward (these are the future cortical neurons) to and through the intermediate layer. Later other neurons and macroglia migrate in the cortical plate from the subventricular zone (Fig. 4-5). Considerations of the development of the cerebral and cerebellar cortex will be outlined below.

The *marginal zone* is the cell-sparse layer with no primary cells of its own. In the early stages the ventricular cells have processes which extend to the outer margin of the zone. Eventually the marginal layer forms much of the white matter as it is replaced by ingrowing axons, dendrites, synaptic terminals, and macroglia.

Sulcus limitans

A longitudinal groove, called the *sulcus limitans*, is present on either side of the inner surface of the neural tube (Fig. 4-2). The portion of the tube posterior to the sulcus is the *dorsal* or *alar plate;* the portion on the anterior side is the *ventral* or *basal plate.* In the spinal cord, as well as in the brainstem, (1) the sensory (afferent) nuclei associated with the input from the peripheral, spinal, and cranial nerves become differentiated in the gray matter of the alar plate, and (2) the motor (efferent) nuclei of the cranial and spinal nerves differentiate in the basal plate.

Cell migration

During development, neuroblasts migrate from their sites of origin to the locales where the mature cells reside. The mode of the migration of these cells is not fully understood. One possibility is by the "guidance" of cytoplasmic processes of the young neurons; many neuroblasts have branching processes which extend to and are anchored to the pia on the outer surface of the central nervous system. Some neurons may migrate by the shortening of those processes attached to the pia surface. The possibility of migration through guidance by genetically predetermined chemical codes or by contact with preformed submicroscopic guidelines has been proposed.

Spinal cord

Up to about the third fetal month, the spinal cord extends throughout the entire length of the developing vertebral column. At this time the dorsal (sensory) roots and the ventral (motor) roots of the spinal nerves extend laterally at right angles from the spinal cord. The roots unite in the intervertebral foramina to form the spinal nerves. The roots and spinal nerves are products of outgrowths from the spinal cord and neural crests (Fig. 4-4). Because the spinal cord elongates at a slower rate than the bony vertebral column, the cord becomes relatively shorter than the vertebral column after the third fetal month. At birth the caudal end of the spinal cord is located at the level of the L3 vertebra, and at adolescence, as in the adult, this caudal end is located at the level approximately between the L1 and L2 vertebrae. During the long period of the differential growth of the spinal cord and vertebral column, the root filaments between the spinal cord and the intervertebral foramina elongate. As a result of this disparity in growth, the lumbar, sacral, and coccygeal roots become directed caudally at an acute angle to the spinal cord. The subarachnoid space below the first lumbar vertebra in the adult is occupied by dorsal and ventral roots of spinal nerves (cauda equina) and the filum terminale, not by spinal cord (Fig. 5-1).

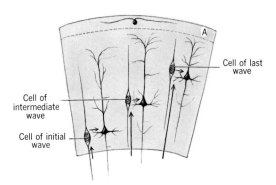

Cell of last wave

Cell of intermediate wave

Cell of initial wave

FIGURE 4-5
The "inside-out" migration of cells forming the cerebral cortex.

The cells migrate (arrows) into the cortical plate to form the cortical laminae sequentially from the deepest (lamina VI) to the most superficial lamina. Lamina I (A) may be a derivative of the marginal zone.

Patterned differentiation of the cerebral cortex and cerebellar cortex

The various regions of the central nervous system evolve during development in an orderly patterned program—probably genetically determined. The general sequences of the states of neuronal migration and maturation in the formation of the cerebral cortex and the cerebellar cortex will be outlined to illustrate the general features of neurogenetic events. The neuronal organization of the adult cerebral cortex and that of the cerebellar cortex are described in Chaps. 16 and 9.

CEREBRAL CORTEX

The neurons of the six-layered neocortex are derived from the ventricular and subventricular zones of the telencephalon. The cells migrate from these zones through the intermediate zone to the cortical plate in an *"inside-out" migration* of successive waves of cells which form the deeper layers before those of more superficial layers (Fig. 4-5). The initial waves of cell migration proceed as far as the cells can go to a location between the marginal layer and the white matter; these cells form the deepest layers of the adult neocortex. Other waves migrate among and past the cells of the initial migration and come to lie in the middle third of the ma-

ture cortex. Other waves of cells migrate among and past the cells of the previous waves and come to lie in the superficial layers of the mature cortex. These migratory patterns of developing neurons passing other developing neurons permit connectivity among neurons which is consistent with the radial columnar organization of the cortex (Chap. 16).

The presumed sequence of differentiation of the major cortical neurons is roughly as follows: pyramidal cells (efferent neurons of cortex), specific thalamic afferent fibers (primary afferent neuron to the cortex), stellate cells (intrinsic interneurons of the major neuronal circuits), horizontal cells and pyramidal axon collaterals (lateral interactions by intrinsic interneurons), and the callosal and association neurons (secondary extrinsic afferent neurons).

The temporal order of development of a pyramidal cell comprises in order: apical dendrite, basilar dendrites, axodendritic synapses, axosomatic synapses, and axodendritic synapses on spines. In man, the apical dendritic system develops primarily during late prenatal life, while the basilar dendritic system develops during the first year postnatally. Even in their earliest developmental stages, the pyramidal cells are radially oriented neurons, which presages

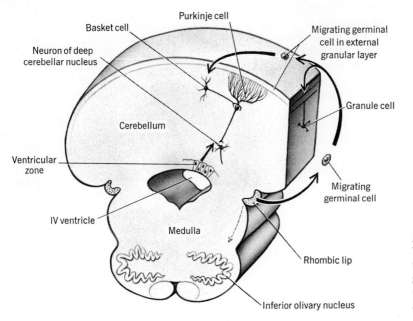

FIGURE 4-6
The routes (arrows) of migration of cells during the histogenesis of the cerebellum. (*Adapted from Sidman and Rakic.*)

the functional columns of the adult (Chap. 16). The radial axis of apical dendrite and cell body of each pyramidal cell is formed before the laterally directed basilar dendrites.

CEREBELLAR CORTEX

The histogenesis of the cerebellum, especially the cortex, is a dramatic example of the migration of germinal cells from two sources in two directions to mesh finally into the functionally integrated unit (Fig. 4-6). Only the most general outlines of a precisely timed and integrated sequence of events will be presented. The two sources are *1* The ventricular and subventricular zones, and *2* the rhombic lip. The two directions are *1* the direct migration of germinal cells from the zones to the cerebellar plate (rudiment of the cerebellum), and *2* the migration of germinal cells from the rhombic lip (subventricular derivative) along the outer surface of the cerebellar plate (external granular layer) and then deep into the cerebellar plate to mesh with the neurons of the direct migration. After differentiating, neuroblasts migrate from the ventric-

ular and subventricular zones into the mantle layer of the cerebellar plate. The mantle layer evolves into two strata: the young neurons of the deep stratum differentiate into the neurons of the deep cerebellar nuclei (fastigii, globose, emboliform, and dentate nuclei), while the young neurons of the more superficial stratum differentiate into the Purkinje cells and the Golgi type II cells. Germinal cells from the rhombic lip migrate over the surface of the cortical plate to form another germinal zone, called the external granular layer. This layer gives rise to the granule cells of the adult granular layer and the stellate and basket cells of the adult molecular layer. Glial cells of the cerebellum are derived from the same sources as the neurons.

The following complex events are thought to be causally related; this comprises the meshing of the zone derivatives (Purkinje cells, Golgi type II cells, and some glial cells) with those of the external granular layer. The Purkinje cells form their dendritic trees within the molecular layer. At the same time the granule cells migrate down from the external granular layer through the molecular layer to the granular layer (deep

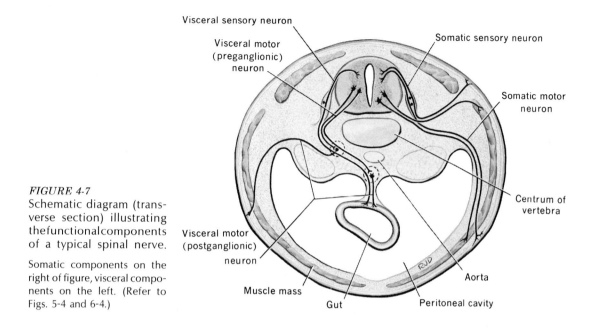

Visceral sensory neuron

Visceral motor (preganglionic) neuron

Somatic sensory neuron

Somatic motor neuron

Centrum of vertebra

Visceral motor (postganglionic) neuron

Muscle mass

Gut

Aorta

Peritoneal cavity

FIGURE 4-7
Schematic diagram (transverse section) illustrating the functional components of a typical spinal nerve.

Somatic components on the right of figure, visceral components on the left. (Refer to Figs. 5-4 and 6-4.)

to cell bodies of Purkinje cells) along the preexisting processes of glial cells (Bergmann glial cells). These processes of Bergmann cells apparently are the guidelines for the migrating granule cells (Rakic). Interactions between the Purkinje cells and the migrating granule cells are presumed to take place within the molecular layer; this results in the formation of the parallel fibers of the granule cells, the complete differentiation of the dendritic trees of the Purkinje cells, and the specific synaptic connections between these two neuron cell types. The development of the cerebellum is further integrated into sequences involving the differentiation and growth of the Golgi type II cells, stellate cells, basket cells, climbing fibers, and mossy fibers.

Peripheral nervous system

Adjacent to the neural tube are 31 pairs of somites. These are the structures that differentiate into muscles, skeleton (including the vertebral column), and connective tissues (Figs. 4-2, 4-7). The somites are segmental (metameric) structures arranged in sequence from the first cervical level through the coccygeal levels (Fig. 4-7).

They form the basis for the segmental innervation pattern of the spinal nerves, in that a pair of nerves is developed in association with each pair of somites (see "Spinal Cord," earlier in this chapter). The apparent segmentation of the spinal cord is dependent on the development of paired segmental nerves. The continuous bilateral neural crest becomes segmented into paired units, one pair for each future sensory ganglion of the spinal and cranial nerves (Fig. 4-5).

The peripheral nervous system develops from the following primordial sources (Figs. 4-2, 4-3):

1 Neuroblasts of the neural crest differentiate into the sensory ganglionic (dorsal root) neurons and their processes.

2 Neuroblasts of the basal plate differentiate into the lower motor neurons. Their axons emerge from the neural tube to the ventral root and innervate the muscles and many glands.

3 Neuroblasts of the neural crest and of the basal plate migrate peripherally to form the ganglia of the autonomic nervous system.

4 Cells of the neural crest differentiate into the satellite cells of the ganglia and the neurolemma cells of the peripheral nerves.

5 Mesodermal cells differentiate into the connective tissue elements such as the endoneurium, perineurium, epineurium, and blood vessels.

An axon has its full complement of neurolemma cells by the time it innervates an end organ (either sensory or motor). Myelination commences when the axon reaches 1 to 2 μm in diameter. During the subsequent growth in length, the internode elongates. Those axons which have the largest diameters when mature are those which commence to myelinate first. Within the same general region of the nervous system, the motor nerves tend to develop before the sensory neurons. Within the ascending sensory pathways (e.g., somatosensory, auditory, and optic), the neurons tend to mature in an ascending order, commencing with those closest to the peripheral receptors and ending with those neurons of the highest order at the most rostral levels of the neuraxis.

The precise mechanisms by which the peripheral nervous system is organized into complex patterns that are basically similar in different individuals are not really understood. Some observations are instructive. The outgrowths from the neural crest and the basal plate occur early in development and invade the adjacent somites. As the somites differentiate and their subdivisions migrate to their respective locations in the body, they maintain their connections with nerve fibers. In effect the elongating nerve processes are "towed" along to the periphery by developing nonneural tissues such as muscle cells. Subsequent outgrowths of other nerve fibers follow their predecessors and form nerve fascicles and future nerves. Neurolemma cells accompany the processes, and subsequently myelination occurs.

The number of nodes of Ranvier is fixed at an early stage of development. As a result, the length of the internodal segments increases as the nerve elongates. All internodal segments are initially of the same length (300 μm). An example of the consequence of the towing of nerve fibers by the primordial muscle cells is found in the innervation of the diaphragm, a voluntary respiratory muscle forming a septum between the thorax and the abdomen. The diphragmatic muscles are derived from somites of the third, fourth, and fifth cervical segments. After these somites are innervated, the primordial muscle cells that will form the diaphragm migrate and tow their innervation with them to the site of the future diaphragm in the lower thoracic region. Other portions of these same somites remain in the vicinity of the midcervical regions. Hence, some fibers of the third, fourth, and fifth cervical nerves innervate the diaphragm via the long phrenic nerve, and other fibers innervate neck muscles by shorter cervical nerves.

A reciprocal relation exists between the peripheral nerves and the peripheral tissues. An uninnervated muscle cell is receptive to becoming innervated, but once innervated it will usually reject further innervation. (This is similar to the fertilization of an egg; immediately after an egg is fertilized by a sperm, no other sperm can penetrate the fertilized egg.) In the terminology of communication engineers, the peripheral nerves are programmed by peripheral structures. This mechanism may help to ensure that all muscle fibers become innervated.

Nerve fibers possess the capacity to branch. Hence several uninnervated muscle cells may become innervated by a single axon. This is another mechanism to ensure the innervation of all voluntary muscle cells. This potential of a nerve fiber to branch is retained throughout life, as is the potential of a nerve process to grow in length. Later in life this is expressed in nerve regeneration and in collateral nerve regeneration (Chap. 2). The inability of neurons to multiply by mitosis after birth may be a liability, but the nervous system compensates for this by having the nerve cells retain the capacity to grow and branch. These capacities are, in effect, the retention of an embryonic potential.

Critical periods: effects of genetic and environmental factors on the development of the nervous system

Although the entire nervous system develops as an integrated organ system, its various parts and subparts mature at different rates and tempos. During its ontogeny, each structure passes through one or more critical or sensitive periods, during which it is sensitive to various influences. These periods are generally times of rapid biochemical differentiation. At such a period, the proper influences have a significant role in advancing normal development. Subsequent normal development is often impaired when these influences are wanting or when abnormal influences are exerted at these critical times. When the impaired development results in anatomic abnormalities which are present at birth, they are called congenital malformations. These abnormalities are usually caused by *genetic factors*—chromosomal abnormalities or mutant genes, and *environmental factors*.

GENETIC FACTORS

Many cases of congenital mental deficiency and retardation are the result of trisomy of autosomes (three chromosomes instead of the usual pair). *Down's syndrome (mongolism)* is a genetic condition in which there are three of the No. 21 chromosome.

Another genetic disease, *phenylketonuria (PKU)*, is a clinical syndrome of marked mental retardation associated with irritability and abnormal EEG patterns. This condition is due to an inherited inborn error of phenylalanine metabolism (transmitted by an autosomal recessive gene) that results in an excessive accumulation of the amino acid phenylalanine and its metabolites. The basic defect is a deficiency of the enzyme phenylalanine hydroxylase in the liver; it is essential for the conversion of phenylalanine to tyrosine. Treatment consists of placing PKU patients on a low-phenylalanine diet commencing in the first year of life; this must be done at this time because the brain damage caused by this condition is due to the accumulation of excess phenylalanine, which reaches its peak between the second and third years of life.

ENVIRONMENTAL FACTORS

Environmental factors have a significant role in the normal ontogeny of the nervous system during prenatal life and infancy. Among these factors, which will be discussed briefly, are nutrition, hormones, external stimulation, and oxygen levels in the circulation. Other causal

factors associated with anomalies, mental retardation, and functional disabilities include: infections such as German measles (rubella) and syphilis; excessive irradiation of the developing organism; birth trauma and injuries; and various chemical substances.

Nutrition Malnutrition during the early rapid period of development and growth of the nervous system can result in permanent damage. In man, this critical period extends from the second trimester of pregnancy through most of the first year after birth. During this interval many neurons and macroglia are being replicated and much of the brain growth is taking place. The evidence indicates that under severe protein malnutrition, the rates of proliferation of new neurons and glial cells are reduced. This reduction occurs during fetal life because even the fetus is *not* protected from maternal malnutrition. The developing brain is vulnerable during the remainder of this critical period of postnatal life; the formation of glial cells is impaired, and myelination is inefficient. Malnutrition during this period in human infants is known as *marasmus.* If the child is fed a nutritionally adequate diet after this period, the damage is not completely repaired, even though normal appearance may be achieved in some subjects. Those who appear to be healthy have brains which are irrevocably damaged by the protein deficiency. The functional abnormalities in children reared on nutritionally inadequate diets may consist of transient apathy, lethargy, or hyperirritability, together with a lesser intellectual development as measured by a decrease of some 10 to 20 percent of mental capacity. The brain fails to become normal because of its inability to replicate new neurons during the postcritical period. Thus undernutrition during fetal and early postnatal life may leave the individual deficient in numbers of neurons and glial cells in the brain, including the cerebral cortex.

Prolonged protein deficiency in children from 1 to 2 years of age may result in *kwashiorkor.* In this condition, the number of neurons is not reduced, because the deficiency occurs after the full complement of neurons is formed; however, the complete differentiation and connectivity of these cortical cells may be impaired. If after being subjected to prolonged, severe malnutrition, such children with kwashiorkor are fed a normal diet, their IQ tests still score below those of other children in the same population, even siblings, who were not subjected to severe malnutrition.

The timing of nutritional deprivation is a critical factor in determining whether or not subsequent recovery from the effects of such deficiencies is possible. In contrast to brains of fetuses and young children, the adolescent and adult brain is most resistant to permanent effects of malnutrition. The young and mature adult victims of starvation during World War II did not show any loss of intelligence after their nutritional rehabilitation.

Although the most serious effects of subnormal physical and mental development result from the prolonged intake of diets deficient in proteins with the essential amino acids, mental and neurologic maturation may be slowed down by deficiencies in vitamins, minerals, and calories during prenatal and circumnatal life.

The effects of malnutrition assume gigantic proportions in the world today. Roughly 60 percent of the world's preschool population—over 300 million children—is exposed to varying degrees of undernutrition. These children live primarily in underdeveloped lands on diets low in proteins and calories. Malnutrition is contributory to the early death of many of them. Survivors grow up in poverty and become adults with physical and mental handicaps. Thus these poverty (nongenetic) conditions are perpetuated through their children—to be passed on from one generation to the next.

Hormones At a critical stage in the growth of mammals, either before birth or during the circumnatal period, the developing brain is especially sensitive to steroid hormones. The androgen hormones are apparently necessary to activate the neural substrates underlying male sexual behavior. The influences of these hormones at this stage effect some permanent change in the brain, which is eventually expressed months and years later in juvenile and adult behavior. These behavior patterns include the typical aggressive rough-house tactics, accompanied by threatening facial gestures, of juvenile male monkeys and the characteristic feminine displays and postures exhibited by female monkeys. For example, androgens injected into female (or male) animals at the critical maturational stage activate those substrates which produce female (or male) animals capable of displaying, in later life, male types of behavioral pattern. Estrogens do not appear to play an active role in imposing a female organization on the developing nervous system. Female development depends more on the absence of androgen at the critical period than on the presence of estrogen. Presumably the brain of a female (or male) animal exposed to androgens at the critical stage is in later life sensitive to androgens and relatively insensitive to estrogens; such a female (or male) animal does not exhibit typical behavior during later life in response to estrogens. Male (or female) animals deprived of androgen stimulation at the critical stage have brains which are sensitive to estrogens and insensitive to androgens. These animals exhibit typical female behavior during later life in response to estrogens; they do not exhibit typical male behavioral patterns in response to androgens.

Masculinizing androgenic effects may occur in human genetic females whose mothers were administered excessive quantities of androgens during their pregnancy. These prenatally androgenized girls typically identify themselves and behaviorally express themselves as tomboys. This indicates that in the human being, androgen can sensitize parts of the developing brain (presumably the hypothalamus and limbic system).

The mental retardation associated with *cretinism* in man is due to a thyroid hormone deficiency at a critical period during the late stages of in utero development (estimated to begin at the seventh fetal month). The cerebral cortex of cretinoid individuals is poorly developed. There is a reduction in number and size of the cell bodies of the neurons, as well as hypoplasia of both their axons and dendrites. Axodendritic synaptic connections are reduced in number. The electrical activity of the cortex is altered, and protein and nucleic acid metabolism in the neurons is impaired. In contrast to the drastic effects from hypothyroidism in the prenatal human fetus, hypothyroidism in children, juveniles, and adults does not seem to produce any adverse effects on the brain or the capacity for learning. Mental retardation of the cretinoid human being can be prevented or effectively remedied if adequate doses of thyroid hormones are given during the first year of life.

External stimulation during ontogeny of the visual system The development of each pathway system in its full anatomic, physiologic, and functional complexities is the expression of the organism's genetic potential supplemented and reinforced by environmental stimuli placed upon the system during ontogeny. In a sensory pathway such as the visual system, the stimuli are a variety of visual experiences. In the motor sphere responses to stimuli are expressed by varied motor activities. The absence or a minimal amount of stimulation at critical periods hampers or even prevents the normal development of a system. The exact age at which a critical period occurs and the precise duration of each critical period are not known in man. Some aspects of the concept of critical periods will be outlined in relation to the visual system.

The differentiation, growth, and precise synaptic connectivity of the visual pathways are primarily predetermined genetically. It appears that the neurons of the visual pathways from both retinas to the visual cortices are instructed and programmed genetically to construct this binocular, topographically organized system. This complex neural connectivity is established before the eyes have received any photic stimulation. Except for a few slight neurophysiologic differences, all types of visual responses of neurons in the optic pathways of visually inexperienced kittens are strikingly similar to those of the adult cat. This indicates that complex neural connections do develop without the benefit of visual experiences.

Drastic reduction and complete deprivation of light stimulation result in morphologic, neurophysiologic, and behavioral deficits in the visual system. The degree to which the visual system is altered is related to the age of the animal and to the length of time the animal is subjected to visual deprivation. If the deprivation occurs only before the critical period, the visual system re-

mains normal. If the deprivation occurs after the critical period, the visual system also remains normal. If the deprivation occurs for a long stretch of the critical period, abnormalities in the visual system occur (e.g., alterations in pattern discrimination, difficulty in fixating objects). The longer the animal has been visually deprived during this critical period, the more severe the effects to the visual system. In the kitten, the critical period is estimated to last from the fourth to the tenth or twelfth week postnatally. The following experiment is illustrative. During the critical period, the right eye of a kitten is exposed to seeing only vertical lines and the left eye of the same kitten is exposed to only horizontal lines; later in life the right eye responds to vertical lines and is indifferent to horizontal lines, while the left eye responds to horizontal lines and is indifferent to vertical lines. This can be demonstrated by behavioral responses of the cat.

Amblyopia, or lazy-eye, in man is presumed to be caused by inadequate stimulation by formed objects of the macula of one eye during the critical stages of postnatal life before 5 years of age. The slightly cross-eyed child favors one eye over the other (to avoid seeing double), with the result that the visual pathway from the macula of one eye is not adequately stimulated and hence fails to maintain normal connections.

This concept of the critical period during childhood is the basis of the suggestion that young children should be exposed to rich visual experiences, even more than they can handle intelligently. This should help to ensure the optimal maturation of the child's visual pathways.

The person who is congenitally blind (from *cataracts*) and whose capacity to receive environmental visual stimuli is surgically restored after several years will never see "normally" because the inadequately developed optic system cannot compensate effectively. Upon reacquiring sight such a person first obtains impressions of brightness and color. Gross differences in the perception of depth eventually develop into the ability to estimate depth. The idea of shape, determined visually, is secondarily acquired, after shape has been consciously interpreted. The functional return is generally limited to crude discriminations, gross depth perceptions, and identifications of large objects. Recognition of large letters is possible, but that of small letters is unlikely. Again, the absence of adequate visual stimulation during the critical period did not permit a normal visual pathway to sustain itself.

Oxygen levels and perinatal brain damage The brain is so dependent upon continuous supplies of oxygen and glucose that the deprivation of either for even a few minutes may result in irreversible brain damage. Depending upon degree and duration, hypoxia during the perinatal period (i.e., the last half of pregnancy and the first month after birth) may lead to pathologic changes, cerebral palsy, and certain types of mental retardation. This *hypoxia* of the fetal circulation to the developing brain may be due to impairment of placental functional activity or to an oxygen deficiency in the maternal blood associated with toxemia, anemia, or cardiac disorders. Experimental studies indicate that several episodes of prolonged partial asphyxia of full-term monkey fetuses lead to cerebral hemispheric damage—including various degrees of cortical atrophy, sclerosis of the white matter, and pathologic changes in the basal ganglia (Myers). This damage is similar to that described in the brains of human beings with perinatal injury, cerebral palsy, or mental retardation. In contrast, a single episode of acute total asphyxia, when of sufficient length, leads to damage restricted to the brainstem; this has little resemblance to the more common pattern noticed in perinatal injury in human infants (Myers).

Prenatal motor activity The early ontogenesis of the neuronal circuits involved with the motor innervation of the somatic musculature has an essential role in the regulation of the muscular contractions which are common during prenatal life. These somatic movements of the fetus are more than the expression of casual contractions. They are activities which are essential to the development of normal musculature. Experi-

mental evidence indicates that in the absence of such movements muscles are small and poorly developed.

Brain

PRENATAL DEVELOPMENT

Early in the second fetal month, the "three-vesicle brain" differentiates into the "five-vesicle brain" (Fig. 4-8). The prosencephalic vesicle is subdivided into the telencephalon, or endbrain, and the diencephalon, or between-(twixt) brain. The mesencephalic vesicle remains as the midbrain; the rhombencephalic vesicle is subdivided into the metencephalon, or afterbrain, and the myelencephalon, or spinal brain. The derivatives of the neural tube and its vesicles are outlined in Table 4-1.

The development of the "contorted" brain from the tubelike structure is the result of the complex integration of several processes: *1* three bends known as flexures, *2* differential enlargements of the different regions, *3* growth of portions of the cerebral hemispheres over the diencephalon, midbrain, and cerebellum, and *4* the formation of sulci and gyri in the cerebral and cerebellar cortices (Fig. 4-9). The flexures are the mesencephalic (midbrain) flexure (forming an acute angle on the anterior surface of the brain), the pontine flexure (forming an acute angle on the posterior surface), and the cervical flexure at the lower medulla (forming an acute angle on the anterior surface). The posterolateral margin of the rhombencephalon is the rhombic lip, which develops into the cerebellum. The differential enlargement is most pronounced in the cerebral and cerebellar hemispheres. The telencephalon during development surrounds most of the diencephalon; there is an intussusception of the diencephalon into the telencephalon. As the result of a partial intussusception of the upper midbrain into the diencephalon, the substantia nigra, nucleus ruber, and surrounding tegmentum protrude rostrally into the diencephalon.

The main outlines of the form of the brain are recognizable by the end of the third fetal month (Figs. 4-9, 4-10). The lateral cerebral sulcus

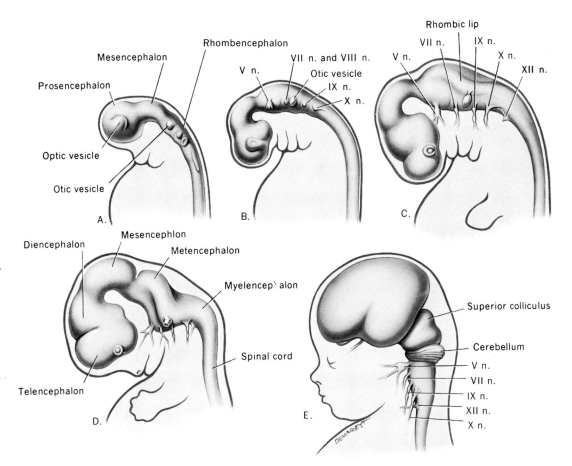

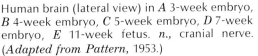

FIGURE 4-8
Human brain (lateral view) in *A* 3-week embryo, *B* 4-week embryo, *C* 5-week embryo, *D* 7-week embryo, *E* 11-week fetus. *n.*, cranial nerve. (*Adapted from Pattern*, 1953.)

appears in the third fetal month. The central sulcus, calcarine sulcus, and parieto-occipital sulcus are indicated by the fifth fetal month; all the main gyri and sulci of the cerebral cortex are present by the seventh fetal month. The external structure of the cerebral hemisphere of the 8-month fetus is characterized by the prominence of the precentral and postcentral gyri, by a wide-open lateral sulcus exposing the insula, and by the presence of all primary and secondary sulci and a few tertiary sulci. The occipital lobe overrides the cerebellum. During the last month of fetal life the frontal and temporal lobes are stubby, the insula is still exposed to the surface, and the occipital poles are blunt. The cortical gyri are broad and plump, and the fissures are shallow. The patterns of the primary and secondary sulci are simple and present a diagrammatic appearance.

The cerebrum of the full-term neonate is more fully developed in the regions posterior to the central sulcus than in the anterior regions. The frontal pole and the temporal pole are relatively short, and the insula is almost completely covered by the adjacent lobes. The number of tertiary sulci is still small. The leptomeninges are not completely adherent to the brain, and they

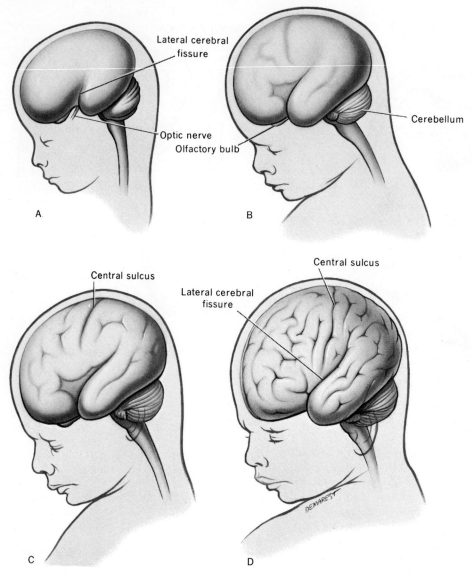

FIGURE 4-9
Human brain (lateral view) in *A* 4-month fetus,
B 6-month fetus, *C* 8-month fetus, *D* newborn
infant. (*Adapted from Patten,* 1953.)

do not dip into all the sulci. The superficial
blood vessels are straight. The brain has a gelatinous consistency because except for some somatic afferent tracts (general somatic, auditory,
and visual systems), the subcortical white matter
is unmyelinated. As a result, the cortex is poorly
demarcated from the white matter. By the end
of infancy, at 2 years of age, the relative size and

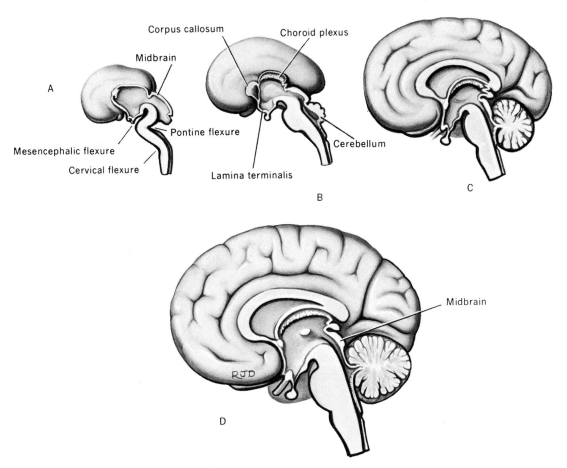

Corpus callosum

Choroid plexus

Midbrain

Mesencephalic flexure

Cervical flexure

Pontine flexure

Lamina terminalis

Cerebellum

Midbrain

RJD

A

B

C

D

proportions of the brain and its subdivisions are essentially similar to those of the adult brain. The brain is firmer. The gray cortex is demarcated from the subcortical white matter, which is now myelinated. The superficial cortical blood vessels are predominately tucked into the fissures and sulci. After the end of the second year the tertiary sulci dominate the topographic pattern of the cerebral surface. These sulci are variable from brain to brain and thereby put the stamp of individuality on each brain. Tertiary sulcation may continue throughout life.

POSTNATAL GROWTH

The large brain in the newborn infant exceeds 10 percent of the entire body weight; in the adult the brain constitutes only approximately

FIGURE 4-10

Human brain (midsagittal view) in *A* 3-month fetus, *B* 4-month fetus, *C* 8-month fetus, *D* newborn infant. (*Adapted from Patten*, 1953.)

2 percent of the total body weight. The postnatal growth of the brain is rapid, especially during the first 2 years after birth (Fig. 4-11). The brain weighs about 350 Gm in the full-term infant and about 1,000 Gm at the end of the first year. The rate of growth slows down after this, and by puberty the brain weighs about 1,250 Gm in girls and 1,375 Gm in boys. It appears that the brain of a girl grows more rapidly than that of a boy up to the third year, but the brains of boys grow more rapidly after that. This brain size is

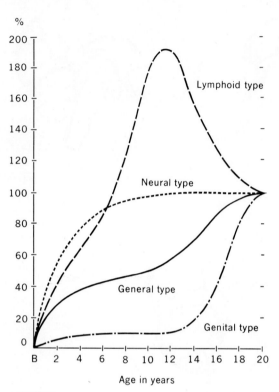

%

FIGURE 4-11
Graph illustrating the postnatal growth of the
major organ systems and general body size.

Note that relative to the other organ systems and general body growth, the nervous system grows most rapidly during the first years after birth. In this graph, the
end of each curve in the upper right represents the
weight of each organ system at 20 years of age, expressed as 100 percent. Other points in the curves
represent weight of each organ system at different ages
as the percentage of the weight at 20 years of age.
(*After Scammon.*)

reflected in the growth of the cranial skeleton.
In contrast to the adult, the young child has a
large cranium in relation to the face. Head circumference is a measure of the growth of the
brain. The head circumference is 34 cm at birth,
46 cm at the end of the first year, 48 cm at the
end of the second year, 52 cm at 10 years, and

only slightly larger at puberty and in the adult.

Man is unusual among mammals in at least
two ways. *1* Of all the large-brained mammals,
man has the largest brain relative to his total
body weight. He does not have the largest
brain—several large-brained mammals, such as
elephants and whales, have brains which are
larger than man's but smaller relative to their
total body weight. There are several monkeys,
all small, with brains which are larger, relative
to their body weights, than man's. *2* The major
increase in the absolute size of the human brain
occurs during postnatal life. The two and one-
half to threefold increase in man's brain during
the first year after birth is unique among mammals (Fig. 4-11). Man might not have survived
as a species but for the evolution of a brain that
grows considerably during postnatal life. A
newborn infant with a brain the size of that of
a year-old infant could not have been delivered
naturally through the human female pelvis.

Aging of the nervous system

Each neuron is as old as the individual, for all
neurons are differentiated before birth. Few, if
any, new neurons are formed after birth in man.
The number of neurons tends to decrease with
age, for as neurons die they are not replaced.
The consequences of a slight loss of neurons are
not noticeable because other neurons may compensate for the decreased number of neurons.
For an estimated loss of one-tenth of our cerebral cortical neurons in the 50 years from 20 to
70 years of age, an average loss of 50,000 neurons
daily is indicated. Neurons undergo senescence.
Aging of the neurons is evidenced by change
in size (either decrease or increase), by the accumulation of pigment, or by the decrease in
amount of Nissl substance. In man, for example,
the quantity of ribonucleoproteins in the alpha
motor neurons of the spinal cord increases significantly from birth to 40 years of age, plateaus
from 40 to 60 years, and decreases from 60 years
on. In elderly people, decrease in the weight of
the brain, increase in the size of the ventricles,
and calcification in the meninges are all signs of
an aging nervous system. Involutory changes

in the surface structure of the cerebral hemisphere occur in old age. Atrophic changes are found in the following cerebral cortical regions, roughly in the following temporal sequence: *1* limbic lobe structures such as the uncus and cingulate gyrus, *2* the insula, and *3* the orbital gyri of the frontal lobe. These regions appear reduced in surface area and width in the elderly as compared with the young. The last to show such gross objective signs of aging are the gyri of the frontal and parietal lobes, since they may appear normal even in persons in their nineties.

An indication of the degree of the aging process after the prime of life is obtained by comparing several parameters in the 30-year-old age group with those in the 75-year-old age group. In the older group, the reduction in brain weight is about 10 percent; in the blood flow to the brain, about 20 percent; in the number of nerve fibers in large nerves, about one-third; in the number of taste buds, about two-thirds; and in the velocity of nerve conduction, about 10 percent.

Development of functional activity of the nervous system

A basic "unit" of neural activity is the simple reflex arc. Stimulation of a receptor and production of a response from an effector indicate the presence of a functional reflex arc. Each component of an arc expresses its functional activity at different times. The sequence for the initiation of activity in the several components is as follows:

1 A muscle cell exhibits intrinsic contractility prior to being innervated.

2 A motor neuron is capable of conducting an action potential and, through the motor end plate, of stimulating muscle cell to contract. The functional unity of the motor neuron, motor end plate, and muscle cell is thus established.

3 The afferent neuron can be stimulated to conduct an action potential to the central nervous system, but the reflex arc is not active.

4 The reflex arc does not become functional until the interneurons form the final synaptic interconnections between the afferent and efferent neurons.

Observation of early functional activity has resulted in two concepts: that of initial mass patterned activity, and that of initial simple reflex patterned activity. Both concepts are valid, and they are not mutually exclusive. Recent studies indicate that both are important during the development of the organism.

According to the *concept of initial mass patterned activity,* the initial movements elicited from sensory stimulation are always integrated mass movements, not simple reflex movements. Two examples of evidence include the observation that the initial movements in an animal such as a salamander are wriggling movements involving many muscle masses of the body, and the observation that the first movement to be elicited in the human embryo is the withdrawal of the head by contraction of the neck musculature in response to a stimulation of the upper lip. The latter activity is a complex avoidance reflex from a noxious stimulus apparently for the protection of the organism. This involves the fifth cranial nerve (sensory nerve), central nervous system integration, and the eleventh cranial nerve and cervical nerves (motor nerves). Two implications from this concept are *1* that complex interneuronal and synaptic interrelationships are functionally integrated before the afferent neurons can exert their effects on the lower motor neurons, and *2* that the simple reflex movements are secondarily individuated out of the mass patterns.

According to the *concept of initial simple reflex activity,* the initial activities are basically simple movements and the complex movements are the result of the progressive integration of the more elementary reflexes into the functional whole. The proponents of this theory claim that the earliest activity is actually not observed in mammals because observations are not made in utero, the natural environment for the embryo.

The development of skilled movements may be considered as a sequence progressing from mass patterns to more individuated patterns, in which inhibition assumes a more significant role. Dexterity, in one sense, involves the deemphasis of nonessential movements and the emphasis of essential ones. In learning to write, for example, the child progresses from stages of making excessive movements to those of pre-serving favorable movements by eliminating unnecessary accessary movements. Develop-ment may be regarded as the evolution of the proper integration of inhibition.

In certain injuries to the nervous system, the intensity of the symptoms and the degree of recovery from the injury are related to the age of the organism. This age factor may be signifi-cant in the interpretation of ablation experi-ments. For example, the bilateral removal of the motor cortex in infant monkeys does not pro-duce as severe symptoms as it does in adult monkeys. In addition, the infant monkeys make more complete recoveries. Stated otherwise, localized ablations of the cerebral cortex, inter-nal capsule, or many other regions in infancy frequently result in less severe functional def-icits than lesions in similar locations in the juvenile or adult mammal, including man. Two factors may explain these observations: other areas of the cortex may assume some of the roles of the ablated area during subsequent develop-ment; and other regions of the nervous system adapt more effectively in the young animal.

Prenatal and postnatal activity in man

MOTOR ACTIVITY

The initial reflex activity in response to external stimuli, as noted above, is the withdrawal of the head from an irritation of the upper lip during the seventh week after fertilization. The area of sensitivity expands until by the fourteenth week tactile stimulation of the face will evoke re-sponses that include rotation of the head, con-traction of the contralateral trunk musculature, extension of the trunk, extension of the upper extremities at the shoulder, and rotation of the pelvis to the opposite side. Reactions of the early fetus to tactile stimulation of the lips in-clude swallowing movements ($10\frac{1}{2}$ weeks), pro-trusion and pursing of both lips (22 weeks), and audible sucking (twenty-ninth week). In the realm of respiratory activities, the chest muscu-lature contractions can be evoked at the thir-teenth week, contractions of the diaphragm have been noted at the twenty-second week, and continuous respiratory movements have been observed at the twenty-seventh week, long before the date of normal delivery. The fetal respiratory movements result in the aspiration of amnionic fluid. Local trunk reflexes and local reflexes of the extremities have been evoked in the third fetal month.

The newborn infant retains many of the fetal flexor attitudes, such as flexed limbs, closed hands, and adducted thumbs. The reaction to a sudden noise is characterized by intense sim-ple and stereotyped motions. The primitive re-flexes involve the overall response of the entire body and limbs. Many visceral activities, al-though well developed, are not fully differen-tiated. Respiration is irregular, the body temper-ature fluctuates, and swallowing and peristaltic activities are not fully coordinated. The reflexes that are easily evoked include hiccups, urina-tion, and sweating. The newborn infant's activi-ties are not dependent on the cerebral cortex, since similar reactions are exhibited by the anencephalic monster, i.e., one with essentially no forebrain. For all intents, the newborn infant is a reflex animal with all motor activity operat-ing through subcortical influences.

The typical neonatal infant's mass move-ments are gradually modified in the early months of life. By the third month, isolated movements and conscious motor activity are in evidence. Mastery of the volitional motor move-ments is expressed first in the proximal joints of the limb, and later by the movements of the more distal joints. The movements of the head, spine, and legs are perfected before a child as-sumes the upright posture and ambulates. The coordinated movements of the shoulders, the flexor-extensor activities of the elbow and wrists, the primitive palm graspings, all precede the coordinated movements of the fingers. In-dividuation of the skilled movements out of the previous generalized movements is indicated.

Progress in motor coordination during the child's first year is expressed, in general, as fol-lows: first month, smiles in response to an adult; second month, vocalizes with such sounds as "ah" and "uh"; third month, head control in-dicated when infant is raised by his hands from supine to sitting position, the head coming forward with the body instead of lagging; fourth month, hand control, indicated by grasping for object held within sight and reach; fifth month, rolls body from supine to prone; sixth month, sits without support for several seconds; seventh month, crawls voluntarily by pushing with legs, rolling, and hitching; eighth month, picks up small objects by opposing the thumb and index finger; ninth month, pulls self up to standing position; tenth month, walks without support but by holding on to adult's hand or stable object; eleventh month, stands alone and without support for several seconds; and twelfth month, walks alone without support for several seconds.

SENSORY ACTIVITY

The newborn infant's initial impressions of the external world come through the touch receptors. Touch is apparently highly evolved. Contact with mother, nipple, and clothes is a primary source of information. The protopathic senses of pain, temperature, touch, kinesthetic sense, and visceral senses are all present at birth but are poorly localized. The tolerance of pain, especially if the child's attention is diverted by sucking a nipple, suggests that the sensitivity to pain is less than in an older child.

The development of visual perception progresses from birth through the first decade of life. During the first few weeks of life, the infant distinguishes light from dark but probably perceives only vague visual images. The baby's eyes move without fixing upon specific objects. A bright light causes the pupil to contract and the eyelids to close. From 1 month after birth, the eye can fix on a bright object and follow the object for a few seconds. During the third and fourth months, the infant commences to fix upon and recognize his mother and such objects as his bottle, and he is able to follow objects well. The child is normally farsighted. By the sixth month, recognition of familiar faces and objects is well developed. Strange objects may evoke crying spells. The eyes and the visual system continue to develop until 7 to 8 years of age. Objects should be large when a child is learning from visual cues.

The newborn infant is actually deaf at birth, mainly because of the absence of air in the eustachian tube and the presence of embryonic tissue in the middle ear. Several days after birth, hearing becomes acute, especially to a high-pitched voice. At 1 month the infant can respond by turning in the direction of a sound, especially an unusual one.

The senses of smell and taste are present at birth. They are well developed by the second and third months.

Genetic code and plasticity of the nervous system

The genetic code, acting through its biochemical control system, is instrumental in establishing the complex structural functional matrix of the nervous system as expressed in the patterning of the nuclei, pathways, circuits, and synaptic connections. The precise modus operandi of these genetic and hereditary influences is unknown. An older version of this modern genetic-biochemical theory as applied to the nervous system employed such general terms as *chemotropism, chemotaxis,* and *neurotropism.* In brief, these concepts imply that biochemical specificity is crucial in determining the differentiation and growth pattern leading to the final detailed organization of the nervous system. For example, the optic pathways are destined to be involved specifically and irrevocably with visual perception and a number of associated correlates. In this interpretation, the biochemical control system is essential in determining the organization not only of the neurons and their processes but also of the extraneuronal elements associated with the neurons and their processes.

Another concept emphasizes the role of mechanical factors in the establishment of the fiber tracts. This "contact guidance" of the growth of nerve fibers into precise patterns stresses the role of extraneuronal elements and their organization as essential in guiding the growing nerve processes to their destinations. Thus these elements are partly responsible for the structuring of the nervous system. The nerve fibers are thus considered to have selective affinities for their own pathways. These affinities of the axons for their location within the nervous system depend on *1* mechanical guidance, *2* biochemical guides (cytochemical codes) stationed along the course to their synaptic termination, and *3* biochemical properties within each neuron.

The postnatal mammalian nervous system that develops under the influence of the specific and selective biochemical regulators becomes a relatively nonplastic nervous system. That is, the functional specificity within the nervous system is probably set down during early development, and any functional readaptation during postnatal life is restricted and confined to relatively narrow limits.

The formation of a relatively nonplastic nervous system in the postnatal mammal is suggested by many experiments, of which two are noted. *1* If the sensory nerves to the right leg of a rat are interchanged with the sensory nerves of the left leg, the animals will associate a stimulus to the right leg as coming from the left leg. For example, the animal with an irritating lesion on the right leg will favor the left leg, not the right leg, because he associates the irritation as coming from the left leg. No amount of experience will change this behavior to that favoring the right leg. *2* If the nerve supply to the flexor muscles of the arm is interchanged with the nerve supply to the extensor muscles in the monkey (after the nerves have regenerated and functional connections are established), the animal will flex when he intends to extend, and vice versa. He never *learns* to flex when he intends to extend. In practice, the monkey learns to restrict his movements on the interchanged side.

Congenital defects and abnormal development

Of all the malformations and congenital defects in man, ranging from minor observable variations from the norm to lethal abnormalities, as many as one-half are estimated to involve the nervous system. Slight decrease in intelligence due to a defect in development is hard to establish. Striking abnormalities definitely attributable to ontogenetic defects include the absence of a brain (anencephalus), extremely small brain (microcephalus), excessive enlargement of the ventricular cavities (hydrocephalus), and the absence of a head (acrania).

Theoretically most of the anomalies of the nervous system arise in one of two ways. *1* Ballooning defects. Pressure develops in the ventricular system. In turn, a ballooning may occur in a specific "weak" part of the nervous system, or a generalized increase in pressure may result in excessive enlargement of the ventricles, producing hydrocephalus (water in the brain). In the latter, the brain is compressed between the high ventricular pressure and the unexpandable skull, with the result that severe brain damage occurs unless the pressure is relieved. *2* Lip defects in the neural folds. The lips of the neural folds exhibit developmental flaws that result in variable defects, the most extreme being the nonfusion of the lips leading to the formation of an abnormal open neural tube. These two ways by which anomalies are formed are not causal but mechanistic. The causes of anomalies are not fully known. They have genetic and environmental bases. The environmental causes include the lack of an important metabolite (e.g., oxygen) at a critical stage or the presence of a noxious substance (e.g., a poison) which might inhibit a vital metabolic action at a critical time.

Spina bifida is one of the more common examples of defects; the term is used to cover a wide range of closure defects, usually located in the lower lumbar region (Fig. 4-12). The most extreme version occurs when the neural plate in the lumbar region remains as a plate exposed to the outside. An infant with this defect has bladder and bowel incontinence, sensory loss, and motor paralysis of the lower extremities. In less severe cases the meninges or the meninges along with the spinal cord, though displaced backward, are still covered by the skin. In a minor form, only the bony vertebral arches may be defective. The persistence of an attachment of the caudal end of the spinal cord in a minor form of spina bifida results in the stretching of

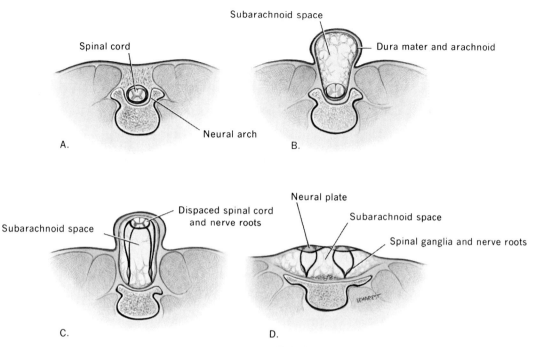

A.

Spinal cord

Neural arch

B.

Subarachnoid space

Dura mater and arachnoid

C.

Subarachnoid space

Dispaced spinal cord and nerve roots

D.

Neural plate

Subarachnoid space

Spinal ganglia and nerve roots

FIGURE 4-12
Some anomalies which may occur in the lumbo-sacral region.

A Spina bifida occulta results from the failure of the neural arches of the vertebrae to fuse dorsally. *B* Spina bifida with meningocele is a defect with a subarachnoid fluid-filled meningeal cyst bulging through unfused neural arches. Cyst is covered with skin. *C* Spina bifida with myelomeningocele is a defect with meningeal cyst containing spinal cord and nerve roots. *D* Spina bifida with myeloschisis is a defect in which neural plate (having failed to close) is exposed to surface. (*Adapted from Patten.*)

the spinal cord as far caudal as the fifth lumbar vertebra. The degenerative changes associated with this *tethering of the spinal cord* are accompanied by some motor deficits. Severing the attachment by surgery will relieve the stretch and can arrest any further degenerative changes.

Bibliography

Altman, J.: Autoradiographic and histological studies of postnatal neurogenesis. J. Comp. Neurol., 128:431–474, 1966.

Angevine, J. B., Jr., et al.: Embryonic vertebrate central nervous system: revised terminology. Anat. Rec., 166:257–261, 1970.

Caley, D. W., and D. S. Maxwell: Development of the blood vessels and extracellular spaces during postnatal maturation of rat cerebral cortex. J. Comp. Neurol., 138:31–48, 1970.

Edds, M. V., Jr., et al.: Development of the nervous system, in F. O. Schmitt (ed.), *The Neurosciences.* Rockefeller University Press, New York, 1970.

Grenell, R. G., and R. E. Scammon: An iconometrographic representation of the growth of the central nervous system in man. J. Comp. Neurol., 79:329–354, 1943.

Hamilton, W. J., and H. W. Mossman: *Human Embryology.* W. Heffer & Sons, Ltd., Cambridge, England, 1972.

Hess, A.: The experimental embryology of the foetal nervous system. Biol. Rev., 32:231–260, 1957.

Jacobson, M.: *Developmental Neurobiology.* Holt, Rinehart and Winston, Inc., New York, 1970.

CHAPTER FOUR / DEVELOPMENT AND GROWTH OF
THE NERVOUS SYSTEM

Kalter, H.: *Teratology of the Central Nervous System.* University of Chicago Press, Chicago, 1968.

Langman, J.: *Medical Embryology. Human Development, Normal and Abnormal.* The Williams & Wilkins Company, Baltimore, 1969.

Moore, K. L.: *The Developing Human.* W. B. Saunders Company, Philadelphia, 1973.

Morest, D. K.: The growth of synaptic endings in the mammalian brain: A study of the calyces of the trapezoid body. Z. Anat. Entwicklungsgesch., 127:201-220, 1968.

Myers, R. E.: Two patterns of perinatal brain damage and their conditions of occurrence. Am. J. Obstet. Gynecol., 112:246-276, 1972.

O'Rahilly, R., and E. Gardner: The timing and sequence of events in the development of the human nervous system during the embryonic period proper. Z. Anat. Entwicklungsgesch., 134:1-12, 1971.

Patten, B. M.: *Human Embryology,* 3d ed. McGraw-Hill Book Company, New York, 1968.

Rakic, P.: Kinetics of proliferation and latency between final cell division and onset of differentiation of cerebellar stellate and basket neurons. J. Comp. Neurol., 147:523-546, 1973.

Rockstein, M. (ed.): *Development and Aging in the Nervous System.* Academic Press, Inc., New York, 1973.

Snell, R. S.: *Clinical Embryology for Medical Students.* Little, Brown and Company, Boston, 1972.

Timiras, P. S.: *Developmental Physiology and Aging.* The Macmillan Company, New York, 1972.

Winick, M.: Fetal malnutrition. Clin. Obstet. Gynecol., 13:526-541, 1970.

CHAPTER **5**
THE SPINAL CORD

Gross anatomy

The *spinal cord* is that portion of the central nervous system which is surrounded and protected by the vertebral column. The flexible *vertebral column* consists of a series of bony vertebrae, including seven cervical vertebrae, twelve thoracic vertebrae, five lumbar vertebrae, five fused sacral vertebrae (sacrum), and the coccyx. On the sides of the column are located paired openings called *intervertebral foramina*; one pair of foramina is typically located between two successive vertebrae.

The spinal cord, which is continuous with the medulla, is a cylinder that is slightly flattened posterolaterally (i.e., it is wider than it is deep) surrounded by the three meninges: pia mater, arachnoid, and dura mater (Fig. 5-1). It lies within the upper two-thirds of the vertebral canal (the cavity within the vertebral column) and terminates caudally as the cone-shaped *conus medullaris*, at the level between the first and second lumbar vertebrae (the upper small of the back). The pia mater continues caudally from the tip of the conus as a nonneural thread, the *filum terminale*, to the end of the bony vertebral column where it is anchored into the ligament on the posterior side of the coccyx. The piarachnoid and the dura mater continue as tubular sheaths to the level of the second sacral vertebra, where they fuse with the filum terminale. Note that the subarachnoid space with its cerebrospinal fluid extends below the level of the spinal cord to the second sacral vertebral level.

The spinal cord is suspended from the dura mater by a series of 20 to 22 pairs of *denticulate ligaments*, which are flanges of epipial tissue extending laterally from the pia mater to the dura mater. These collagenous ligaments of pial tissue are attached medially to a continuous line on either side of the entire spinal cord from the medulla to the conus medullaris midway between the dorsal and ventral roots. The lateral, free edges of the denticulate ligaments are scalloped (Fig. 5-2). Each ligament extends laterally to a pointed process, which passes through the arachnoid, and then it attaches to the dura mater; this point of attachment is located between sites of the emergence of two successive spinal nerve roots. In general, denticulate ligament is found above the first cervical roots and between all successive roots through the first lumbar; at the latter site the ligament is continuous with the filum terminale.

Spinal nerves

An almost continuous series of *nerve rootlets* emerges from the posterolateral sulcus on the dorsolateral aspect, and another series emerges from the sulcus on the anterolateral aspect of the spinal cord (Figs. 5-1 and 5-2). These rootlets collect laterally as *spinal roots* and finally form the 31 pairs of spinal nerves (Figs. 5-2, 5-3). A typical spinal nerve passes through an intervertebral foramen and is then distributed to a segment of the body. (The first cervical nerve, an exception, passes between occipital bone and the first cervical vertebra.) There are eight pairs of cervical, twelve pairs of thoracic, five pairs of lumbar, five pairs of sacral, and one pair of coccygeal spinal nerves. Each of the first seven cervical nerves is named from the bony vertebra immediately below its exit through the intervertebral foramen (e.g., the third cervical nerve passes through the intervertebral foramen located between the second and the third cervical vertebrae). The eighth cervical nerve passes

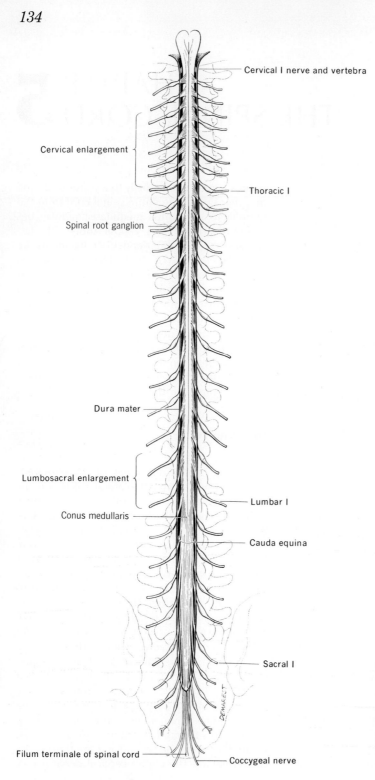

Cervical I nerve and vertebra

Cervical enlargement

Thoracic I

Spinal root ganglion

Dura mater

Lumbosacral enlargement

Lumbar I

Conus medullaris

Cauda equina

Sacral I

Filum terminale of spinal cord

Coccygeal nerve

FIGURE 5-1

The spinal cord and its relation to the vertebral column (as viewed from behind).

The first cervical dorsal root and spinal ganglion are absent. Each spinal ganglion is located in the region of an intervertebral foramen. The length and caudally directed slant of the spinal roots increase progressively from cervical to coccygeal levels.

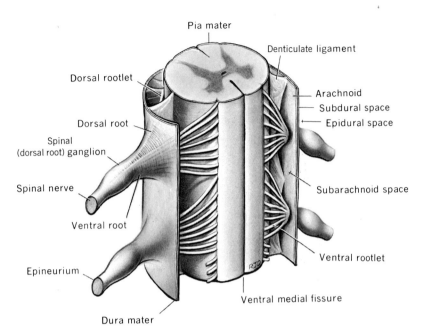

Pia mater

Denticulate ligament

Dorsal rootlet

Arachnoid

Subdural space

Epidural space

Dorsal root

Spinal
(dorsal root) ganglion

Spinal nerve

Subarachnoid space

Ventral root

Epineurium

Ventral rootlet

Ventral medial fissure

Dura mater

FIGURE 5-2
Two segments of the spinal cord and its meningeal coverings.

Note that *1* several rootlets merge to form one spinal
nerve, *2* the dura mater and arachnoid, as the dural
sleeve, are continuous with the epineurium of each
spinal nerve, *3* the pia mater is continuous with the
denticulate ligament, and *4* the subarachnoid space
extends with the dural sleeve into the region of the
spinal ganglion.

through the intervertebral foramen between the
seventh cervical and the first thoracic vertebrae.
Each of the other spinal nerves is named after
the vertebra above its exit from the vertebral
column. In this conventional system, the nerve
is named in relation to the level of its exit from
the bony vertebral column. Because the spinal
cord is shorter than the vertebral column, the
level for the exit of a specific spinal nerve from
the cord is usually different from the level of
its exit from the vertebral column (Fig. 5-1 and
Table 5-1). For example, the rootlets of the first
cervical nerve exit from the spinal cord at the
level of the first cervical vertebra, the rootlets
of the first thoracic nerve exit at the level of the
seventh cervical vertebra, the rootlets of the first
lumbar spinal nerve emerge at the level of the
twelfth thoracic vertebra, and the rootlets of all
sacral nerves exit at the level of the first lumbar
vertebra.

The spinal cord is actually a nonsegmented
structure; this is indicated by the presence of
a continuous series of emerging rootlets and the
gradual changes in the internal structure of the
spinal cord. Its apparent segmentation into 31

spinal segments (Fig. 5-3) is an expression of 31
pairs of spinal nerves, which develop embryologically in relation to the segmented somites.
On the posterior aspect of the cord are three
longitudinal shallow grooves—the *posterior median sulcus, posterior intermediate sulcus,* and
posterolateral sulcus; on the anterior aspect are
two longitudinal grooves—the *anterior median
fissure and anterolateral sulcus.* Except for the
posterior intermediate sulcus, which extends
through the cervical and upper half of the thoracic spinal levels, all these grooves extend
throughout the entire length of the spinal cord.
The posterior medial sulcus and anterior median
fissure are located in the midsagittal plane. The

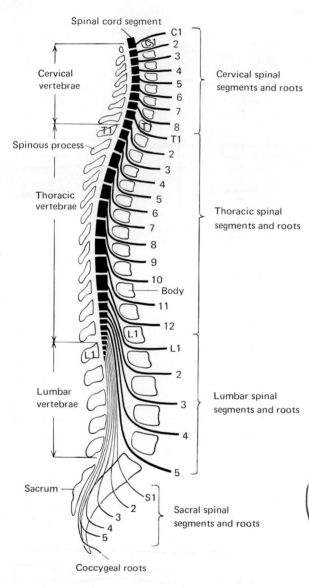

Spinal cord segment

Cervical vertebrae

Spinous process

Thoracic vertebrae

Lumbar vertebrae

Sacrum

Coccygeal roots

Cervical spinal segments and roots

Thoracic spinal segments and roots

Lumbar spinal segments and roots

Sacral spinal segments and roots

Body

FIGURE 5-3
The topographic relations of the spinal cord segments, spinous processes, and bodies of the vertebrae, intervertebral foramina, and spinal nerves.

Refer to Table 5.1. Each spinal cord segment (except upper cervical segments) is located at a higher vertebral level than the spinal nerve emerging through its intervertebral foramen. (*Adapted from Haymaker, Bing's Local Diagnosis in Neurological Diseases, The C. V. Mosby Company, St. Louis.*)

posterolateral sulci and anterolateral sulci are paired grooves located at the emergence of the posterior and anterior spinal rootlets, respectively. The posterior intermediate sulci are paired grooves located between the posterior median sulcus and the posterolateral sulci.

All rootlets pass through the subarachnoid space and the cerebrospinal fluid surrounding the spinal cord before joining the arachnoid and dural meningeal layers which form the *dural sleeve* around the emerging roots before they unite to form the spinal nerves (Fig. 5-2). The dural sleeve is continuous distally with the epineurium of the peripheral nerves. The piarach-

TABLE 5-1

137

Levels of spinal cord segments

Spinous process of vertebra	Interspace between vertebral bodies*	Spinal cord segment
C1		C1–2
C6	C6	T1
T10	T10	L1
T12	T12	S1
	T12–L1	All sacral and coccygeal levels
	S2 or S3	Caudal termination of subarachnoid space
	Coccyx	Termination of filum terminale

*Named from centrum of vertebra above interspace.

noid is said to be continuous with the perineural epithelial sheath of the peripheral nerve. The subarachnoid space caudal to the conus medullaris contains cerebrospinal fluid and the cauda equina (horse's tail). The cauda equina is composed of the roots of the lower lumbar, sacral, and coccygeal nerves. The lower lumbar approach of inserting a hypodermic needle between the neural arches of the third and fourth lumbar vertebrae into the subarachnoid space (*spinal puncture or tap*) is used to obtain samples of cerebrospinal fluid. In this procedure, the spinal cord cannot be injured and the occasional nicking of a root by the needle in the cauda equina is of minor consequence. Between the dura and the vertebrae is the epidural space, which is filled with blood vessels and fat. The anesthetic that produces caudal (sacral) anesthesia (as for painless childbirth) is introduced into the epidural space below the second sacral vertebral level, so that it reaches the sacral nerves and avoids the subarachnoid space with its circulating cerebrospinal fluid.

Spinal nerve—its components

Each *spinal nerve* has a dorsal root and a ventral root (Figs. 5-2 and 5-4). The *dorsal, or sensory, root* consists of the sensory or afferent fibers

that transmit impulses (input) from sensory receptors in the body to the spinal cord. This root contains a *spinal (sensory dorsal root) ganglion* that is located within the intervertebral foramen. This ganglion contains the cell bodies of the sensory neurons. The *ventral, or motor, root* consists of the motor or efferent nerve fibers whose cell bodies are located within the gray matter of the spinal cord. The motor fibers transmit impulses (output) from the spinal cord via motor roots and spinal nerves to the muscles and glands of the body. Distal to its emergence through the vertebral column, a spinal nerve divides into four rami (Fig. 5-4). The large *dorsal ramus (division)* branches into the nerves that innervate the general region and intrinsic muscles of the back. The large *ventral ramus (division)* branches into the nerves and plexuses (in combination with branches of other ventral divisions) that innervate *1* the region and muscles of the body wall (neck, chest, and abdominal wall), *2* the limbs, and *3* the "perineal" region. The small rami communicantes are connected to the sympathetic trunk. The small recurrent meningeal branches innervate the meningeal membranes and blood vessels of the spinal cord.

The ventral rami of the spinal nerves form *plexuses,* which are located just distal to the sites where the nerves emerge from the intervertebral foramina. These plexuses give rise to peripheral nerves. By convention, C indicates cervical; T, thoracic; L, lumbar; S, sacral; and Co, coccygeal spinal levels or nerves. The *cervical plexus* is derived from the anterior rami of spinal nerves C1 through C4; these innervate the neck and back of the head. The *brachial plexus,* derived from spinal nerves C5 through T1 or T2, gives rise to the nerves innervating the upper extremity. Except for the contribution of T1 and T2 to the brachial plexus and of T12 to the lumbar plexus, the thoracic nerves (T3 through T11) are simple in their course and distribution; they do not form plexuses. The *lumbar plexus* is derived from spinal levels T12 through L4, the *sacral plexus* from L4 through S4, and the *coccygeal plexus* from spinal nerves S4 through Co. T12 does not always join the lumbar plexus. L4 and S4 contribute branches to both the lumbar

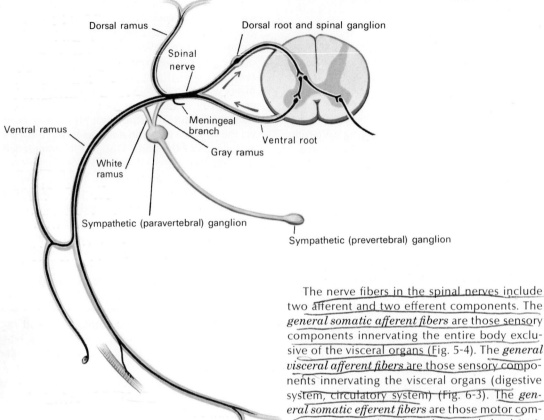

FIGURE 5-4
Diagram of a typical thoracic spinal nerve.

The union of the dorsal and ventral roots forms a spinal nerve. The nerve divides into a posterior primary ramus, an anterior primary ramus, a meningeal ramus, and white and gray rami communicantes.

and sacral plexuses. The nerves innervating the lower extremity are derived primarily from L2 through S3 of the lumbar and sacral plexuses. Nerves from the upper lumbar levels of the lumbar plexuses innervate the lower trunk above the level of the lower extremity, while nerves from the lower sacral levels of the sacral plexus and from the coccygeal plexus innervate the perineum.

The nerve fibers in the spinal nerves include two afferent and two efferent components. The *general somatic afferent fibers* are those sensory components innervating the entire body exclusive of the visceral organs (Fig. 5-4). The *general visceral afferent fibers* are those sensory components innervating the visceral organs (digestive system, circulatory system) (Fig. 6-3). The *general somatic efferent fibers* are those motor components innervating the voluntary skeletal (striated) muscles. The *general visceral efferent fibers* are those motor components innervating the involuntary smooth (nonstriated) muscles, cardiac muscle, and glands (Chap. 6, Fig. 6-4). All spinal nerve components are in the general categories because they are widely distributed throughout the body.

Each spinal nerve is distributed to a specific segment or region of the body. The dorsal root of each spinal nerve supplies the sensory innervation to a body segment known as a *dermatome* (Figs. 5-5, 5-6). Theoretically there are 31 pairs of dermatomes, one pair for each spinal nerve. Actually there are 30 dermatomes, for the first cervical nerve has either no dorsal root, or a tiny one; it does not directly innervate a dermatome. The minute dorsal root of the coccygeal nerve joins the fifth sacral nerve. The second dermatome is located in the back of the head behind the ears and upper part of the neck, the third and fourth dermatomes are in the neck, the fifth through eighth cervical and first thoracic dermatomes are in the upper extremity, the second through twelfth thoracic and the first lumbar dermatomes are in the thoracic and abdominal walls, and the other dermatomes are located in the lower extremity and the gluteal and coccygeal regions (Table 5-2).

The ventral root of each spinal nerve is composed of nerve fibers from one spinal segment. These fibers supply the somatic motor innervation to several voluntary muscles. The following is a list of representative muscles and the spinal segments involved with their innervation:

1 biceps brachii muscle (flexes elbow and supinates forearm), by segments C5 and C6

2 triceps muscle (extends elbow), by C6 through C8

3 brachialis muscle (flexes elbow), by C6 and C7

4 intrinsic muscles of the hand, by C8 and T1

5 thoracic musculature, by T1 through T8

6 abdominal musculature, by T6 through T12

7 quadriceps femoris muscle (knee jerk), by L2 through L4

8 gastrocnemius muscle (ankle jerk for extension of foot), by L5 through S2 (Table 5-3).

The spinal cord has two enlargements (Figs. 5-1, 5-7): the cervical enlargement includes the fifth cervical through the first thoracic cord levels; and the lumbosacral enlargement includes the L2 or L3 through the S3 spinal cord levels. The cervical enlargement contributes the innervation to the upper extremities; the lumbosacral enlargement contributes the innervation to the lower extremities.

The dermatomes are not exactly distinct and separate segments. There is considerable overlapping between any two adjacent dermatomes. A dermatome will often overlap with about one-half of the dermatome more rostrally located and with about one-half of the dermatome more caudally located. As a consequence, if one spinal nerve were completely nonfunctional, no area of complete anesthesia on the skin would be found, for the nerve fibers from the two adjacent dermatomes would pick up the

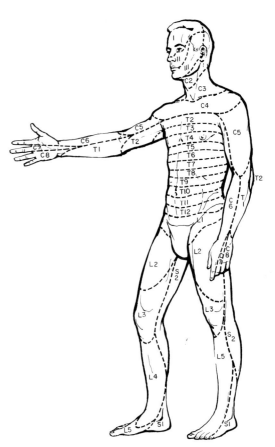

FIGURE 5-5
Segmental innervation of the skin (dermatome).

Each dorsal (sensory) spinal root innervates one dermatome. The first cervical nerve usually has no cutaneous distribution. The trigeminal nerve supplies most of the general somatic sensory innervation to the anterior aspect of the head (ophthalmic division I, maxillary division II, and mandibular division III).

sensory stimuli. On the other hand if a dorsal root of one spinal nerve is irritated, as in herpes zoster (shingles, a viral infection of a spinal ganglion), the noxious stimuli would be felt subjectively from the entire dermatome, including the overlap. The dermatomal area associated with pain and thermal sense is larger than that associated with the tactile sensations.

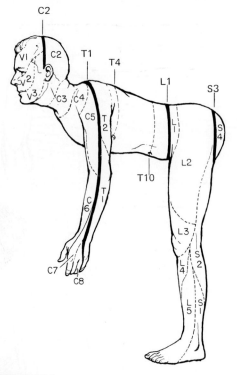

FIGURE 5-6
Dermatomes of the skin. (Refer to Table 5-2.)

The trigeminal nerve is represented by the ophthalmic division (V1), maxillary division (V2), and mandibular division (V3). (*Adapted from Haymaker, Bing's Local Diagnosis in Neurological Diseases, The C. V. Mosby Company, St. Louis.*)

Simple reflex arc

The circuit known as a *simple reflex arc* includes (Fig. 2-2) *1* a sensory receptor (e.g., a neuromuscular spindle or a Meissner's corpuscle), *2* a sensory or afferent neuron (a unipolar neuron with cell body in the spinal ganglion) which enters the posterior gray column of the spinal cord, *3* interneurons (association, intercalated, or internuncial neurons) that lie wholly within the gray matter of the spinal cord, *4* a motor or efferent neuron in the anterior (ventral) horn of the gray matter, and *5* an effector (muscle

TABLE 5-2
Innervation of dermatomes by dorsal spinal roots

Dorsal spinal root	Body region innervated*
C2	Occiput
C4	Neck and upper shoulder
T1	Upper thorax and inner side of arm
T4	Nipple zone
T10	Umbilical girdle zone
L1	Inguinal region
L4	Great toe, lateral thigh, and medial leg
S3	Medial thigh
S5	Perianal region

*Dermatome and region to which radicular pain is referred.

cell). This three-neuron reflex arc (comprises an afferent neuron, interneuron, and efferent neuron) is typical of a flexor reflex such as the elbow flexing. The simple spinal reflex arcs are actually "abstractions" out of the complex neural circuitry.

Reflexes can be named by the number of neurons in the sequence from receptor to effector. *Monosynaptic reflexes* comprise the sequence of afferent neuron and efferent neuron. *Disynaptic reflexes* comprise the sequence of afferent neuron, interneuron, and efferent neuron. *Polysynaptic reflexes* include the sequence

TABLE 5-3
Innervation of voluntary muscles by ventral spinal roots

Ventral spinal root	Muscles innervated
C5–6	Biceps brachii (flexes elbow)
C6–8	Triceps brachii (extends elbow)
T1–8	Thoracic musculature
T6–12	Abdominal musculature
L2–4	Quadriceps femoris (knee jerk, patellar tendon reflex)
L5–S1–2	Gastrocnemius [Achilles tendon reflex (ankle jerk)]

of afferent neuron, several interneurons, and efferent neurons. The afferent limbs of these reflexes include afferent fibers IA, IB, II, and III from muscle receptors and afferent fibers II, III, and IV from cutaneous receptors.

Sensory unit and motor unit

One sensory neuron, its processes, and its sensory receptors form a *sensory unit.* One sensory unit may terminate peripherally as one process, as the neuron associated with one Pacinian corpuscle. Another unit may terminate in many branches over an area as great as a square millimeter. In functional terms, the spatial region or area from which stimuli can influence the firing of the one neuron is known as the *receptive field* of that neuron. These stimuli should be of adequate intensity and proper quality. The receptive area of a "light-touch neuron" is that area of the skin the touching of which provokes an action potential in that neuron. In brief, some receptive fields may be diffuse and others located precisely in a limited area. Extensive overlapping among receptive fields occurs.

One motor neuron and the muscle fibers it innervates form a *motor unit.* This comprises the *anterior horn neuron* (sometimes called the *motoneuron, alpha motor neuron,* or *lower motor neuron),* its axon, and all terminal branches, motor end plates, innervating muscle fibers. In man, a motor unit is composed of from 10 to 25 to over 2,000 muscle fibers. Muscles under delicate control have small motor units; in such muscles the number of muscle fibers in each motor unit is stated to be 13 for the opponens pollicis, 23 for the extraocular superior rectus, and 25 for the platysma muscles. The sartorius, rectus femoris, and first dorsal interosseous muscles have motor units, each composed of about 300 muscle fibers. The powerful gastrocnemius has motor units of just over 2,000 muscle fibers. The average motor unit may be taken to consist of about 200 muscle fibers. In general, each muscle fiber of man is innervated by one or occasionally by two motor end plates. Multiple innervations of some muscle fibers have been reported. The motor end plate is most often located in the middle of a muscle fiber. When the motor neuron is stimulated, all the

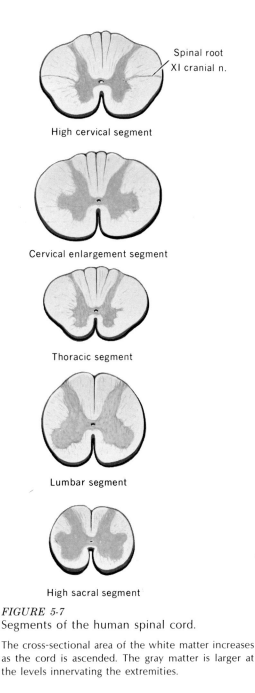

High cervical segment

Cervical enlargement segment

Thoracic segment

Lumbar segment

High sacral segment

FIGURE 5-7
Segments of the human spinal cord.

The cross-sectional area of the white matter increases as the cord is ascended. The gray matter is larger at the levels innervating the extremities.

muscle cells of the motor unit contract. The nerve impulse of a motor fiber results in excitatory activity in the synapse at the motor end plate—hence an *obligatory contraction* is elicited from the stimulation of its innervating nerve fiber. The muscle fibers in each motor unit are not necessarily adjacent but are usually interspersed among muscle fibers of other motor units.

Under certain conditions some motor units may innervate up to 10 times more muscle fibers than normally. These so-called *macromotor units* are formed by the addition of more muscle fibers to the normal motor unit through collateral regeneration (Chap. 2). In some cases of poliomyelitis, for example, many, but not all, the motor nerve fibers to a skeletal muscle may degenerate and form neurolemma bands (Chap. 2). In turn, an axon of a normal motor unit regenerates preterminal sprouts, which invade the neurolemma bands of adjacent degenerated axons. These sprouts elongate within the cords until they reinnervate the denervated muscle fibers. With these macromotor units, the muscle regains much lost function. The degree of control over that muscle is less than that over the normally innervated muscle.

Organization of gray matter and white matter of spinal cord

The spinal cord is organized as white matter surrounding the butterfly-shaped (in cross section) gray matter. The white matter consists of both lightly myelinated and unmyelinated fibers oriented parallel to the long axis of the spinal cord; cell bodies are absent. The gray matter consists of cell bodies and many unmyelinated and some lightly myelinated fibers oriented at right angles to the long axis of the spinal cord. A *nucleus* is an anatomically defined group or column of cell bodies within the central nervous system; each has a more or less specific function. A *lamina* is an anatomically defined group or column of cell bodies; 10 laminae are recognized (Fig. 5-10). A *neuron pool* is a physio-

logically defined group of functionally similar cell bodies; each cell body tends to function together with the others when stimulated. Glial cells and blood vessels are found throughout the entire spinal cord. The rich vascularity and the unmyelinated fibers produce the color of the gray matter, whereas the white myelinated fibers produce the color of the white matter.

The *white matter* in each half of the spinal cord is arranged into three *funiculi* (*columns*): the *posterior funiculus*, located between the posterior median septum and posterior horn; the *lateral funiculus*, located between the posterior and anterior horns; and the *anterior funiculus*, located between the anterior horn and the anterior median fissure (Fig. 5-8). The funiculi are subdivided into bundles of fibers called tracts or fasciculi, which will be analyzed further on with the pathways. The *gray matter* is subdivided into the posterior horn, the intermediate zone with a lateral horn, and the anterior horn (Fig. 5-7).

Regional differences are present at various levels of the spinal cord (Fig. 5-7). The amount of gray matter at any spinal level is largely related to the richness of the peripheral innervation. Hence the gray matter is largest in the spinal segments of the cervical and lumbosacral enlargements innervating the upper and lower extremities; such large structures require a massive innervation. The thoracic and upper lumbar levels have relatively small amounts of gray matter because they innervate the thoracic and abdominal regions.

The absolute number of nerve fibers in the white matter increases at each successive higher spinal segment. Stated otherwise, the white matter of a spinal level caudal to another level contains fewer fibers. This difference results because *1* additional fibers of the ascending sensory pathways join the white matter at each higher spinal level, and *2* fibers of the descending pathways from the brain leave the white matter before terminating in the gray matter at each successive spinal level.

The cell bodies in the gray matter are grouped into clusters of *nuclei* or *laminae*, which extend through the long axis of the spinal cord (Figs. 5-9, 5-10). These nuclei and laminae are characterized by microscopic criteria. On the basis of the course of their axons, two types of neurons are recognized: *root neurons* (*cells*) and

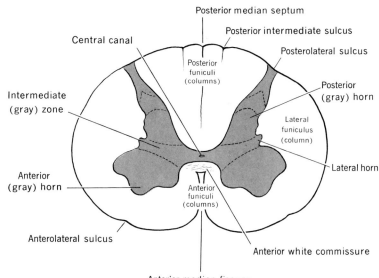

FIGURE 5-8
Section through a cervical level of the spinal cord to illustrate some subdivisions of the gray matter and white matter.

The white matter is composed of three funiculi (columns). The gray matter is divided into two horns and an intermediate zone. The posterior gray commissure and anterior gray commissure are located on either side of the central canal.

FIGURE 5-9
Composite diagram of a spinal cord segment illustrating the nuclei in the gray matter.

The nuclei in the posterior horn and intermediate gray matter are labeled. The intermediolateral nucleus contains visceral efferent neurons (Chap. 6). A neuron pool composed of interneurons is located in the intermediate gray matter. The motor nuclei of alpha and gamma efferent neurons include *1* dorsomedial, *2* ventromedial, *3* anterior, *4* central, *5* ventrolateral, *6* dorsolateral, and *7* retrodorsolateral nuclei. On left of main figure and in the lower diagrams are illustrated the general topographic locations of the muscle groups innervated in the upper extremity (C_5 to T_1), the lower extremity (L_2 to S_5), and the thoracoabdominal region (T_2 to L_1). The nucleus pericornualis anterior is located in the cervical and lumbar segments.

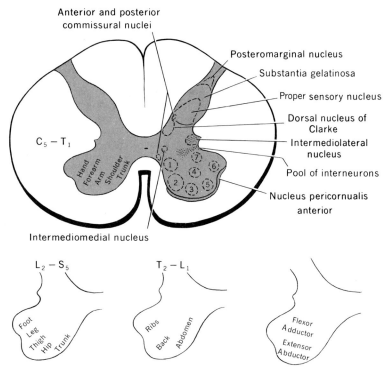

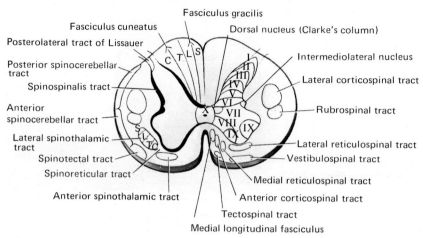

FIGURE 5-10
Composite diagram of Rexed's laminae and the tracts of the spinal cord.

The ascending tracts are represented on the left, and the descending tracts on the right. The lamination of the posterior columns and the lateral spinothalamic tract is indicated: C., cervical; T., thoracic; L., lumbar; S., sacral.

column neurons (cells). The cell bodies of the root neurons give rise to the axons which emerge from the spinal cord through the ventral roots; these are neurons with cell bodies in the central nervous system and axons terminating in the periphery outside the central nervous system. They include the alpha and gamma motor neurons of the somatic nervous system and preganglionic neurons of the autonomic nervous system.

The *column neurons* have axons which terminate within the central nervous system, both in the spinal cord and in the brain. These include *1 intrasegmental neurons*—those with axons which arborize and terminate within the gray matter of the spinal segment in which the cell body is located; *2 intersegmental neurons*—those with axons which bifurcate into branches which ascend or descend in the white matter before arborizing and terminating in the gray matter of many spinal segments; *3 commissural neurons*—those with axons which cross

over (decussate) from one side of the spinal cord to the other side before bifurcating, arborizing, and terminating in the gray matter of the same and other spinal segments on the opposite side from the location of the cell bodies; and *4 suprasegmental neurons*—those with axons which ascend on the same side (ipsilaterally) or decussate and ascend on the opposite side (contralaterally) before terminating in the brain (Fig. 5-11).

According to the *schema of nuclei*, the gray matter comprises a number of nuclei (Fig. 5-9). The more important include the posteromarginal nucleus, substantia gelatinosa, and proper sensory nucleus (nucleus proprius) of the posterior horn, the dorsal (thoracic) nucleus of Clarke, the intermediomedial nucleus and intermediolateral nucleus of the zona intermedia, and the medial nuclear column and lateral nuclear column of the anterior horn.

According to Rexed's *schema of laminae*, the gray matter comprises 10 laminae (Fig. 5-10). Laminae I through VI are located in the posterior horn. Lamina VII is coextensive with the zona intermedia, although it may extend into the anterior horn. Laminae VIII and IX are located in the anterior horn, while lamina X is present in the gray matter surrounding the central canal. The laminae and the corresponding nuclei are outlined in Table 5-4.

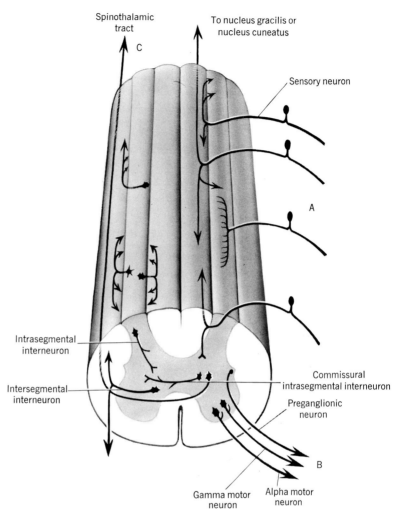

Spinothalamic tract

To nucleus gracilis or nucleus cuneatus

C

Sensory neuron

A

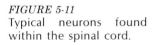

Intrasegmental interneuron

Intersegmental interneuron

Commissural intrasegmental interneuron

Preganglionic neuron

B

Gamma motor neuron

Alpha motor neuron

FIGURE 5-11
Typical neurons found within the spinal cord.

The axons of the sensory neurons (*A* on right) enter the posterior horn. The collateral branches may terminate there in the gray matter or may ascend or descend in the white matter (fasciculi proprii or posterolateral fasciculus) and terminate at other spinal levels. The axons of the three types of motor neurons pass via the ventral spinal roots (*B* on lower right). The intrinsic spinal interneurons (mainly on left side of figure) have main branches and collaterals which *1* terminate at once within the gray matter or *2* ascend and descend for many spinal levels before terminating in the gray matter of other spinal levels. Some main axons ascend to the brain (*C*).

The *posteromarginal nucleus, substantia gelatinosa,* and *proper sensory nucleus* are found in all levels of the spinal cord. These nuclear columns receive input from the general somatic afferent fibers of the spinal nerves and from some descending fibers from the brain. Just lateral to the posterior horn within the white matter of cervical levels 1 and 2 is a nucleus called the *lateral cervical nucleus.* The *dorsal (thoracic) nucleus of Clarke* is present at all levels from segments T1 through L2 or L3; it is largest in the lower thoracic and lumbar levels. This is the nucleus of origin of the posterior spinocere-

bellar tract. The *intermediomedial nucleus* probably receives the main input from the general visceral afferent fibers of the spinal nerves. The *intermediolateral nucleus* is located from T1 through L2 or L3 in the lateral horn. It is the nucleus of origin of most preganglionic sympathetic fibers; some fibers may arise from cell bodies located in the zona intermedia. Cells in the lateral aspect of lamina VII of spinal levels S2 through S4 form the so-called sacral autonomic nuclei. These are the cell bodies of the preganglionic parasympathetic neurons; their axons pass through the ventral roots of the sacral nerves and join the "pelvic nerves." The nuclear columns of the anterior horn contain the cell bodies of the lower motor neurons (alpha and gamma motor neurons) of the general somatic efferent system. The *medial nuclear column* (ventromedial and dorsomedial nuclei) contains the cell bodies of neurons innervating the neck, back, intercostal, and abdominal musculature. Some of the intercostal and abdominal musculature may be innervated by neurons located in the lateral nuclear column. The medial column is found at all spinal levels. The *lateral nuclear column* (ventrolateral, dorsolateral, and retrodorsal nuclei) contains the cell bodies of neurons innervating the musculature of the extremities. Hence this lateral column is prominent in the *cervical enlargement* (C5 through T1), which innervates the upper extremity, and in the *lumbosacral enlargement* (L2 through S3), which innervates the lower extremity. The nucleus of origin of the neurons innervating the diaphragm via the phrenic nerve is located in the lateral aspect of lamina IX in the midcervical segments, especially C4. The cells of origin of the fibers of the *spinal accessory cranial nu-*

TABLE 5-4
Laminae and corresponding nuclei

Lamina	Corresponding nucleus
I	Posteromarginal nucleus
II	Substantia gelatinosa
III and IV	Proper sensory nucleus (nucleus proprius)
V	Zone anterior to lamina IV
VI	Zone at base of posterior horn
VII	Zona intermedia (includes intermediomedial nucleus, dorsal nucleus of Clarke, and sacral autonomic nuclei
VIII	Zone in anterior horn (restricted to medial aspect in cervical and lumbosacral enlargements)
IX	Medial nuclear column and lateral nuclear column

cleus are located in the lateral aspect of lamina IX in spinal levels C1 through C6.

Except for lamina VI, which is absent from levels T4 through L2, all laminae are located at all spinal cord levels. Laminae V and VI are often divided into medial and lateral regions. Lamina VI is well developed in the cervical and lumbosacral enlargements. Lamina VIII is located on the medial aspect of the anterior horn in the cervical and lumbosacral enlargements; in the other levels this lamina extends laterally across the anterior horn ventral to lamina VII.

General aspects of afferent input and efferent output

CLASSIFICATIONS OF AFFERENT (SENSORY) INPUT (Table 5-5)

The streams of impulses conveyed by the peripheral nerves from both the external and internal environments are the sources of the information fed into the central nervous system. The number of senses exceeds the proverbial five sensations of touch, sight, sound, smell, and taste. The several classifications outlined below point up various aspects of afferent, or sensory, input. None is wholly satisfactory.

Subjectively, afferent stimuli may produce either unconscious or conscious sensations. The unconscious "sensations" are ultimately expressed in such varied activities as breathing, muscle coordination, and digestion. The conscious sensations encompass a wide spectrum such as pain, sight, and well-being.

The distribution of the sensors is the basis of a widely used classification. The general afferent receptors have a widespread distribution over the body and include receptors that result in such sensations as pain, touch, visceral sense, and thermal appreciation, and in unconscious responses such as the reflexes. The special afferent receptors are associated with highly specialized senses and are concentrated in small areas of the body. They include the receptors for such sensations as smell, sight, hearing, and taste. In man, they are located in the head and are conveyed only by cranial nerves.

The location of the sensors is used as the basis of the classification of afferent input: The *exteroceptive* (cutaneous or superficial) *modalities* are sensed by those receptors which are located in the skin or its derivatives and which respond mainly to external agents and changes in the external environment. Exteroceptive sensations include the classical four cutaneous sensations of pain, warmth, cold, and light touch (tactile sense). Modalities associated with the position and movements of the body and sensed by receptors located deep in the body tissues are called *proprioceptive* by anatomists and physiologists, *kinesthetic* by experimental psychologists, or *deep sensibilities* (all are synonyms). They include such conscious senses as the appreciation of movement or of position of the body and limbs, the judging of weight, shape, and form, and the feeling of vibratory sense (as ascertained by a tuning fork applied to a joint), deep pain, and pressure. The kinesthetic sense is generally limited to the appreciation of movement and position of the body and limbs. The *interoceptive or visceral senses* have a role in the visceral activities of digestion, circulation, and others, including such sensations as fullness of the stomach or bladder, pain from excessive distention, and cramps from muscle spasms. These visceral senses are poorly localized and diffuse. Nerve fibers associated with the exteroceptive and proprioceptive senses are known as general somatic afferent fibers; those associated with the interoceptive senses are known as general visceral afferent fibers. "Somatic" refers to the body wall and limbs; "visceral" refers to the "vital" organ systems, including the circulatory, digestive, respiratory, and excretory systems.

The terms *protopathic sensations* and *epicritic sensations* have special usages. The protopathic sensations are the poorly localized modalities such as crude touch, crude temperature, and awareness of pain; they are considered to be phylogenetically old. The epicritic sensations are the precise modalities, such as fine temperature and touch discrimination, and are considered to be phylogenetically new.

ROLE OF PERIPHERAL SENSORY RECEPTORS

Our contact with the world—both the internal and external environments—is through our receptors. The role of the receptors to the subjective senses is controversial. The wide range of subjective expressions includes the sensations of pain, touch, warmth, cold, itching, wetness, tickling, malaise, well-being, and position ap-

TABLE 5-5
Classification of sensory receptors (probable functional roles)

I. Receptors of general sensibility
   A. Endings in epidermis
     1. Free nerve endings (tactile, pain, thermal sense)
     2. Terminal disks of Merkel (tactile)
     3. Nerve (peritrichial) ending in hair follicle (tactile)
   B. Endings in connective tissue (skin and connective tissue throughout body)
     1. Free nerve endings (pain, thermal sense)
     2. Encapsulated nerve endings
       a. End bulbs of Ruffini [thermal sense, warmth (?), touch-pressure]
       b. End bulbs of Krause [thermal sense, cold (?), touch-pressure]
       c. Genital corpuscles (thermal sense, touch-pressure)
       d. Corpuscles of Meissner (tactile)
       e. Corpuscles of Pacini (vibratory sense, touch-pressure)
       f. Corpuscles of Golgi-Mazzoni (touch-pressure)
   C. Endings in muscles, tendons, and joints
     1. Neuromuscular spindles (stretch receptors)
     2. Golgi tendon organs, neurotendinous endings (tension receptors)
     3. End bulbs of Ruffini in joint capsule (touch-pressure, position sense)
     4. Corpuscles of Pacini (touch-pressure, vibratory sense)
     5. Free nerve endings (pain, thermal sense)
II. Receptors of special senses
   A. Bipolar neurons of olfactory mucosa (olfaction)
   B. Taste buds (gustatory sense)
   C. Rods and cones in retina (vision)
   D. Hair cells in spiral organ of Corti (audition)
   E. Hair cells in semicircular canals, saccule, and utricle (equilibrium, vestibular sense)
III. Special receptors in viscera
   A. Pressoreceptors in carotid sinus and aortic arch (monitors arterial pressure)
   B. Chemoreceptors in carotid and aortic bodies and in or on surface of medulla (monitors arterial oxygen and carbon dioxide levels)
   C. Chemoreceptors probably located in supraoptic nucleus of hypothalamus (monitors osmolarity of blood)
   D. Free nerve endings in viscera (pain, fullness)
   E. Receptors in lungs (respiratory and cough reflexes)

preciation. Each of these sensations has many variations, e.g., sharp pain, burning pain, and dull pain. Even the primary sensory modalities of pain, warmth, cold, and touch are actually defined in abstract philosophical terms.

The law or doctrine of specific nerve energies (law of specific energy of senses) implies that the primary modalities are subserved by morphologically specific nerve endings: pain by free nerve endings, light touch by Meissner's corpuscles, cold by Krause's end bulbs, warmth by Ruffini's corpuscles, and deep sensibility and pressure sense by Pacinian corpuscles. The law states that each sensation is dependent on 1 the nature of the stimulus, and 2 the nerve endings stimulated. Each receptor may be characterized by its adequate stimulus, which is that form of energy to which the receptor is most sensitive.

Evidence is available that such a simplified correlation between structure and function is unlikely. The concept of a specific nerve fiber for each sense has been supplanted by the pattern theory of sensation, which implies that groups of nerve endings, each associated with different nerve fibers, form a complex or "spot." Such a group of endings constitutes a cold spot, a warm spot, or a touch spot. A specific stimulus evokes a stream of nerve impulses which are dispersed spatially and temporally and which are conveyed by the various fibers innervating the spot. It is theoretically possible for such sensations as pain, itch, and tingle to arise from the same complex of endings stimulated in different ways and combinations. The peripheral spots are primarily initiators of a train of impulses that may reach and activate these brain centers. The interplay of various combinations of impulses is basic to the intricacy of the input to the central nervous system. Actually conscious sensations are primarily an expression of the complex interactions in the centers of the brain.

AFFERENT (SENSORY) INPUT

The dorsal roots are composed of sensory neurons conveying input to the spinal cord. Each of these neurons is a pseudounipolar neuron with its cell body in the spinal (dorsal root) ganglion. Before entering the spinal cord, the fibers of the dorsal roots segregate into a medial bundle and a lateral bundle. The medial bundle is composed of relatively thick myelinated fibers from such receptors as Golgi tendon organs, neuromuscular spindles, Meissner's corpuscles, and Pacinian corpuscles. The myelinated fibers pass through the posterior funiculus adjacent to the gray matter and medial portions of laminae II, III, and IV of the posterior horn. The main fibers branch into collaterals which 1 may extend to, and terminate in, the gray matter at the spinal level of entrance, 2 may ascend or descend within the posterior columns and terminate in the gray matter of other spinal segments, and 3 may ascend to terminate in some nuclei of the medulla (Figs. 5-11, 5-12). Many fibers recurve in lamina IV and extend back into laminae II, III, and IV. Many fibers terminate in the medial and central regions of laminae V, VI, and VII, especially in the dorsal nucleus of Clarke and the intermediomedial nucleus. Other branches terminate 1 in lamina VIII and medial lamina IX, and 2 in lateral lamina IX, respectively.

The lateral bundle, composed of finely myelinated and unmyelinated fibers, passes into the posterolateral tract of Lissauer, where each fiber bifurcates into an ascending branch, which extends rostrally for from one to three spinal segments, and a descending branch, which extends caudally for a segment or so. Collaterals from these branches terminate largely in lamina I and to a lesser degree in laminae II and III. In general, the terminal fibers are distributed primarily to the laminae at the segmental level of entrance and to the same laminae, but in lesser numbers, in the segmental levels just above and below the level of entrance (Fig. 5-12). The intermediomedial nucleus receives direct input from dorsal root fibers; this nucleus may be the terminal nucleus for visceral afferent fibers. On the other hand, the intermediolateral nucleus does not receive any direct input from dorsal root fibers; this is the nucleus of origin of preganglionic sympathetic neurons (Chap. 6).

EFFERENT (MOTOR) OUTPUT

The integrated activity of the central nervous system can be expressed ultimately only in terms

FIGURE 5-12 149

Schema illustrating *1* the course and termination of dorsal root fibers within the spinal cord (right half of figure), and *2* the major ascending tracts of the spinal cord (left half of figure).

The lateral bundle (L) of lightly myelinated fibers passes into the posterolateral tract of Lissauer (DTL), and into laminae I, II, and III. The medial bundle (M) of heavily myelinated fibers passes into the posterior column and to many laminae including the anterior horn. The bifurcation of fibers into ascending and descending branches forms the posterolateral tract and posterior column. The ascending tracts include the fasciculus gracilis (FG), fasciculus cuneatus (FC), posterior spinocerebellar tract (PSCT), anterior spinocerebellar tract (ASCT), anterior spinothalamic tract (ASTT), lateral spinothalamic tract (LSTT), spinotectal tract (ST), and spinoreticular tract (SRT). (*From Noback and Harting, Spinal Cord, S. Karger, Publisher, Basel*, 1971.)

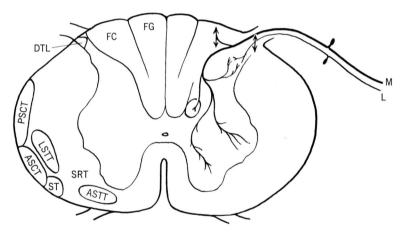

of the contraction of muscle fibers and the secretion of glands. Through these effectors, the organism responds to internal stimuli and to influences from the external environment. The voluntary (striated) muscles are innervated by the general somatic efferent neurons. These neurons have their cell bodies in the anterior horn of the spinal cord (Fig. 5-9). The large alpha efferent neurons (lower motor neurons) innervate the muscle fibers proper; the small gamma efferent neurons innervate the small muscle fibers of the neuromuscular spindle sensory endings. The involuntary (smooth) muscles, cardiac muscle, and glands are innervated by the general visceral efferent neurons of the autonomic nervous system (Chap. 6).

Ascending pathways

Information from the peripheral sensors is conveyed through the nervous system by sequences of neurons organized into ascending pathway systems. The major ascending systems are composed of a sequence of three neurons (each neuron has a long axon). These are *1* neuron of the first order (cell body in a spinal ganglion or a sensory ganglion of a cranial nerve), *2* neuron of the second order (cell body in the central nervous system), and *3* neuron of the third order (cell body in the thalamus). Interneurons with short axons interact with these neurons (Chap. 13). In general, these major sensory systems and their pathways to the cerebral cortex are somatotopically organized. In addition, they project to both primary and secondary cortical areas (Chap. 16).

GENERAL ASPECTS OF THE ASCENDING PATHWAYS FROM THE SPINAL CORD TO THE BRAIN

Environmental energies from both inside and outside the body stimulate sensory receptors, which are located throughout the organism. Following the transduction of these energies at the receptors, coded information is transmitted as nerve impulse patterns (action potentials) via fibers in the spinal nerves to nuclei within the central nervous system for neural processing. Some of this input may be integrated into spinal reflex loops or arcs. Other inputs may be relayed via ascending sensory pathways consisting of groups of nerve fibers (*tracts*) linking *processing centers (nuclei)* until information eventually reaches the higher centers in the brain (e.g., the cerebral cortex or cerebellar cortex). These inputs may reach the conscious sphere and may be utilized at the unconscious levels. The processing within the nuclei and cortices involves neural interactions among the terminal endings of the ascending fibers, small interneurons within the nuclei, and descending fibers from higher centers.

Basic pathways In a general way, the ascending pathway systems of the spinal cord which terminate in the cerebral cortex or cerebellar cortex may be subdivided into *three basic tract systems: anterolateral system, posterior column–medial lemniscal system,* and *spinocerebellar system*. The *anterolateral system,* so called because its components ascend through the anterolateral part of the spinal cord, comprises several tracts: *1* lateral spinothalamic tract, *2* anterior spinothalamic tract, *3* indirect spinoreticulothalamic pathway, and *4* the spinotectal tract. The *posterior column–medial lemniscal system* includes the posterior column–medial lemniscal pathway and, in addition, the spinocervicothalamic (spinocervicolemniscal) pathway. The *spino-*

cerebellar system includes the anterior and posterior spinocerebellar tracts, the cuneocerebellar tract, and the rostral spinocerebellar tract. The first two systems ascend to the cerebral cortex while the third ascends to the cerebellar cortex.

Basic organization The pathways from the periphery to the cerebral cortex of which the spinothalamic tracts and posterior column–medial lemniscus are components are basically composed of sequences of three neurons and three processing centers. These neurons, each with a long axon, are called neuron of the first order, neuron of the second order, and neuron of the third order. The long nerve process (axon) of the neuron of the second order generally crosses (decussates) from one side (ipsilateral side) to the other side (contralateral side). The other two neurons have axons which do not decussate. Within each processing center are many interneurons. In these pathways, the *neuron of the first order,* with its cell body in a spinal ganglion, conveys information from a sensory receptor to a nucleus within the spinal cord or lower medulla. In turn, the *neuron of the second order,* with its cell body located in the above-noted nucleus, conveys information via an axon which decussates to the contralateral side, and ascends in a tract (spinothalamic tracts or medial lemniscus) to a nucleus of the thalamus. The *neuron of the third order,* with its cell body in the thalamus, has an axon which terminates in the sensory area of the cerebral cortex. This organization is illustrated in Figs. 5-14 and 5-17. The somatic sensory areas to which these pathways project are (1) the postcentral gyrus of the parietal lobe, also called the primary somesthetic cortex, areas 3, 1, and 2, or somatic sensory area I; and (2) the opercular part of the upper bank of the lateral (Sylvian) sulcus, also called somatic sensory area II (Chap. 13).

In clinical usage, the appreciation of pain and of extremes in warmth and cold is called *"protopathic,"* and these modalities are *protopathic sensations.* The appreciation of small temperature differences, light touch, and other discriminatory general senses (e.g., two-point discrimination) is called *"epicritic,"* and these modalities are *epicritic sensations.*

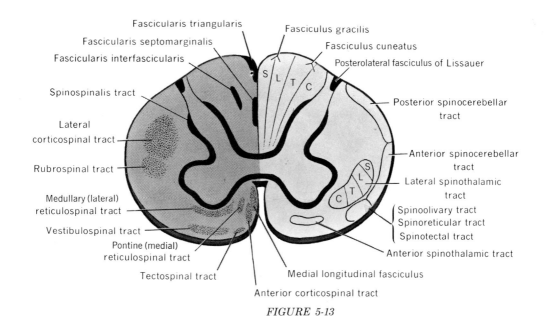

Fascicularis triangularis
Fascicularis septomarginalis
Fascicularis interfascicularis
Spinospinalis tract
Lateral corticospinal tract
Rubrospinal tract
Medullary (lateral) reticulospinal tract
Vestibulospinal tract
Pontine (medial) reticulospinal tract
Tectospinal tract
Anterior corticospinal tract

Fasciculus gracilis
Fasciculus cuneatus
Posterolateral fasciculus of Lissauer
Posterior spinocerebellar tract
Anterior spinocerebellar tract
Lateral spinothalamic tract
Spinoolivary tract
Spinoreticular tract
Spinotectal tract
Anterior spinothalamic tract
Medial longitudinal fasciculus

FIGURE 5-13
The spinal cord tracts.

The ascending tracts are represented as plain outlines on the right, the descending tracts as stippled outlines on the left, and the intrinsic spinal tracts (composed of descending and/or ascending fibers) as solid outlines. The representation of the tracts is arbitrarily drawn. The lamination of the posterior columns and lateral spinothalamic tracts is indicated (C, cervical; T, thoracic; L, lumbar; S, sacral).

PAIN AND TEMPERATURE PATHWAY

Modalities of pain and temperature The pathways concerned with the modalities of pain and thermal senses take parallel courses through the nervous system. Pain is a warning signal to the organism. It is inherently a subjective experience with unpleasant qualities, psychologically determined. Emotional and cultural attitudes color its intensity. The Indian fakir and the professional boxer cultivate an emotional detachment which enables them to disregard pain, while a slightly injured child heightens the feeling. On the one hand, pain has an essential role in our survival, but, on the other hand, it can be, when intractable or accompanied by fear, our enemy.

Pain can be initiated in several ways—by mechanical, thermal, electrical, and chemical stimuli. Three types of pain include the fast-conducted, sharp, prickling pain; the slowly conducted, burning pain; and the deep, aching pain (in joints, tendons, and viscera). Some tissues are more likely to exhibit pain than others. A needle inserted into the skin evokes intense pain, while one probed into a muscle produces little pain. An arterial puncture is painful; a venous puncture (venopuncture) is almost pain-

less. The distention of the ureters by a kidney stone produces what is probably the most excruciating pain. Distention of hollow viscera and muscle spasms (cramps) are painful, yet burning or cutting the intestines evokes scarcely any painful sensation. The tenderness of an inflammation is related to the turgor of the tissues. Slight mechanical traction on the abdominal mesenteries evokes intense pain.

Pain perception may be subdivided into two phases: initial sensation and reaction following that sensation. Soldiers with potentially painful wounds inflicted during intense battle conditions usually experienced minimal pain. To them, the wounds meant the war was over. On the other hand, civilians with much less trauma may complain of severe pain, amelioration of which requires narcotics. This suggests that the suffering may be a consequence of the reaction or processing phase. The reactivity to pain is subjective and difficult to evaluate. No sensations are evoked when the exposed human brain is cut or cauterized; this is because the brain proper has no sensory receptors.

Cold spots and warm spots cover the body, with the cold spots being more numerous. For example, the lips have both warm and cold spots, while the tongue is only slightly sensitive to warmth. The rationale of placing a cool wet towel on the forehead on a hot day is valid, because the forehead is more sensitive to cold than to warmth.

Direct spinothalamic pathway (Neospinothalamic pathway, lateral pain system, or spinal lemniscus; Figs. 5-14, 5-15)   Fine naked free nerve endings are probably the pain receptors. They are the only endings in such pain-producing sites as the pulp cavity of a tooth and the cornea of the eye. Corpuscles of Ruffini and of Krause are said to be associated with the reception of warmth and cold, respectively.

It is thought that the *thermal senses are conveyed by one pathway system and that pain is conveyed by two pathway systems.* The thermal pathway and one of the pain pathways form the *direct or lateral spinothalamic* (spinal cord to thalamus) *tract*, which consists of a sequence of at least three neurons with long axonal processes. The other pain pathway is the *indirect spinoreticular thalamic pathway,* which consists of a sequence of many neurons.

In the *direct spinothalamic pathway* (*classical or neospinothalamic pathway*), the neurons of the first order of both fine myelinated A fibers and unmyelinated C fibers pass through the dorsal root of a spinal nerve into the posterolateral fasciculus of Lissauer of the spinal cord to terminate and to synapse in the posterior horn. Small interneurons within the posterior horn and intermediate zone are intercalated between the neurons of the first order and the neurons of the second order. From cell bodies

located in the posterior horn and intermediate zone (most of them in laminae V, VI, and VII), axons of the neurons of the second order decussate transversely or in an upward oblique course through the anterior white commissure to the anterolateral aspect of the spinal cord on the opposite side. In its oblique course, each fiber traverses the equivalent of one spinal segment. At this site the axons bend and project rostrally through the lateral funiculus and brainstem tegmentum (hence called the lateral pain system or spinal lemniscus) to terminate primarily in the ventral posterolateral nucleus of the thalamus and also in the posterior thalamic region (magnocellular portion of the medial geniculate body) and in some intralaminar nuclei of the thalamus (parafascicular and central lateral nuclei). Some uncrossed fibers terminate in the posterior thalamic region and intralaminar nuclei; these nuclei are said to receive bilateral input. The posterior thalamic region receives various types of input (polysensory), including noxious stimuli. Within these nuclei are small interneurons. From cell bodies within these nuclei, axons course through the posterior limb of the internal capsule and corona radiata to the postcentral gyrus and somatic sensory area II. The precise significance of the cortex in pain perception is not known. Lesions of the postcentral gyrus may be accompanied by hypalgesia, rarely by analgesia, and possibly by a minor loss of pain sensibility in the appropriate body part on the contralateral side. Stimulation of the postcentral gyrus may produce the sensations of numbness and tingling but rarely that of pain. Anesthesia of any region may be produced by a lesion of the cerebral cortex. The thalamus and the somatic sensory area II may contain the critical substrates underlying conscious pain appreciation.

The first-order neuron has its cell body in a spinal ganglion. Its arborization in the spinal cord exhibits the principle of divergence as its short ascending and descending terminal branches in the posterolateral tract of Lissauer extend up (or down) one or two spinal segments before terminating in the posterior horn. Small interneurons, located between the first-order and the second-order neurons, process the input before relaying influences to the anterior horn for reflex activities or to the higher centers of the brain (Fig. 5-14). The second-order neuron

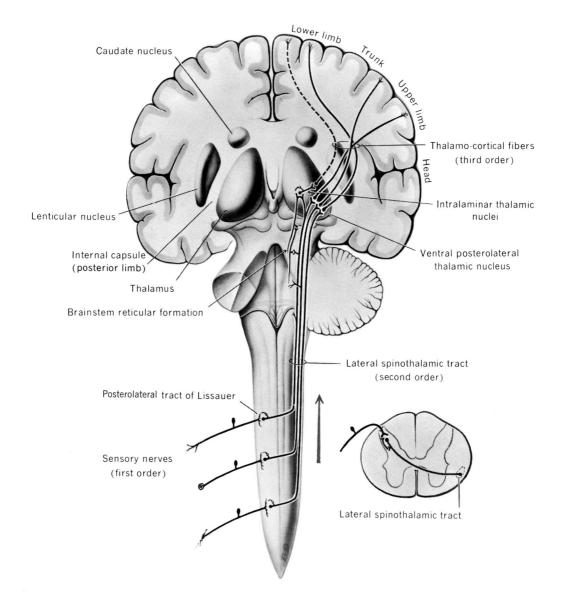

FIGURE 5-14
The spinothalamic pathways.

The direct spinothalamic pathway comprises *1* neurons of the first order with cell bodies in the spinal ganglia, *2* neurons of the second order with cell bodies in the posterior horns and with axons that decussate and ascend as the lateral spinothalamic tract to the thalamus, and *3* neurons of the third order with cell bodies in the thalamus and with axons that project to the cerebral cortex.

The indirect spinothalamic pathway is composed of *1* neurons of the first order, *2* sequence of several neurons of the second order that project through the brainstem reticular formation to the intralaminar thalamic nuclei, and *3* neurons of the third order with cell bodies in the thalamus and with axons that project to the cerebral cortex (the latter is represented in broken line because course is not precisely known). Note interneurons in the relay nuclei (see Fig. 13-2).

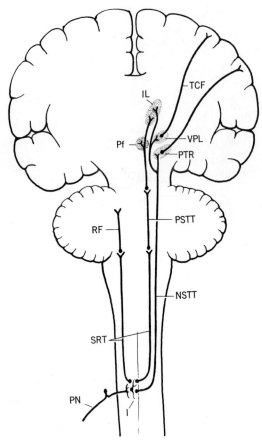

FIGURE 5-15
The spinothalamic pathways.

The ascending tracts of the spinothalamic system consist of *1* the lateral spinothalamic tract (neospinothalamic tract, NSTT), *2* the spinoreticulothalamic pathway (paleospinothalamic tract, PSTT), and *3* the anterior spinothalamic tract. Interneurons (I) stand between central terminations of the peripheral nerves
(PN) and the ascending tracts, including the spinoreticular tract. (SRT) and lateral spinothalamic tract. [The
paleospinothalamic tract includes interneurons located
in the brainstem reticular formation (RF).] The thalamic
nuclei, integrated within the spinothalamic pathways,
include the intralaminar nuclei (IL), parafascicular
nucleus (Pf), posterior thalamic region (PTR), and ventral
posterior lateral nucleus (VPL). Influences from the
thalamus are projected by thalamocortical fibers (TCF).
(*From Noback and Harting, Spinal Cord, S. Karger,
Publisher, Basel.*)

has collateral branches which extend from its
ascending axon to the matter of the spinal cord
at higher levels, into the brainstem reticular
formation, and into the periventricular gray
matter and superior colliculi of the midbrain. In
fact, some of the fibers of the tract terminate
as spinoreticular fibers in the brainstem reticular
formation. Probably only about one-third of the
2,000 or so fibers of the lateral spinothalamic
tract actually reach the thalamus. Within the
brainstem the lateral spinothalamic tract is
called the spinothalamic tract. This phylogenetically new pathway in mammals, called the neospinothalamic tract, conveys sensory influences
perceived as sharp, localized pain sensations.
The lateral spinothalamic tract exhibits both
anatomic and physiologic lamination. Fibers
from the lower segments of the spinal cord tend
to be located posterolateral to those that are
added to the tract at higher levels (Fig. 5-12).
This anatomic somatotopic lamination results
because the fibers decussating through the anterior white commissure are added from each
successive higher level on the medial aspect of
the tract. Within the brainstem this tract is less
precisely somatotopically organized. Claims are
made that the fibers conveying pain impulses
tend to be located laterally in the tract and that
those conveying thermal impulses tend to be
located medially in the tract.

Indirect spinothalamic pathway (Spinoreticulothalamic pathway, paleospinothalamic pathway,
or medial pain system; visceral sensory pathway,
Fig. 5-14) The spinoreticulothalamic pathway is
a multineuronal, multisynaptic pathway that
courses from the spinal cord through the brainstem reticular formation before terminating in
the parafascicular and other intralaminar nuclei
of the thalamus. From cell bodies in the posterior horn and intermediate zone, fine axons ascend as both crossed and uncrossed fibers in the
white matter of the anterolateral regions of the
spinal cord; some of these fibers are interspersed among the fibers of the lateral spinothalamic tract. These fibers course through the
reticular formation of the medulla posterior to
the inferior olivary nuclear complex and anteromedial to the descending trigeminal tract. These
fibers (sometimes called spinoreticular or spinobulbar fibers) terminate in nuclei of the medial
reticular formation of the medulla, pons, and
midbrain. This pathway, composed of sequences

of neurons within the brainstem reticular formation, terminates in thalamic intralaminar nuclei, the posterior thalamic region, and in the hypothalamus. Influences are probably projected to general somatic area II. This fine-fibered medially located pain pathway is the phylogenetically old system concerned with the disagreeable, diffuse, and burning aspects of pain; it is likely that visceral sensations are conveyed by this system.

The pathway to the hypothalamus and the limbic system (Chaps. 11 and 15) presumably conveys some pain influences which may evoke responses associated with the autonomic nervous system activity (e.g., gastrointestinal activity) and with aggressive and aversive behavioral patterns (e.g., facial grimaces).

An *anterolateral chorodotomy* (cutting of the spinal cord) is a neurosurgical procedure designed for the relief of intractable pain in the body. *Intractable pain* is an obstinate form of pain which persists for weeks or months and renders the patient unable to sleep normally or carry out his usual daily duties. In the operation, each of the two anterior quadrants of the spinal cord is cut (anterior to the denticulate ligament, corticospinal tract, and rubrospinal tract) at a spinal level. Pain and temperature sensations are lost below the transected level because the fibers of the lateral spinothalamic tract and spinoreticulothalamic pathway have been severed. After an elapse of some time, some pain and temperature sense may return in some patients. Two explanations have been suggested: *1* some persisting spinoreticular fibers may reconstitute a functional pathway, and *2* a new functional pain pathway may develop through the posterolateral tract of Lissauer and bridge the sectioned region. A unilateral section through the spinal cord does not abolish visceral pain, because such influences are projected rostrally in both crossed and uncrossed ascending fibers.

Strong analgesic drugs have no effect on the peripheral receptors. They act by modifying either the perception of pain or the emotional reaction to pain.

NEURAL MECHANISMS ASSOCIATED WITH PAIN

What is pain? The answer depends on the respondent. With some reservations, pain is viewed by psychologists as a basic sensory modality; by neurophysiologists, neurologists, and neurosurgeons as a pattern of neurophysiologic activity in certain neural centers; by biologists as an activity of significance to survival; by psychiatrists as affect or emotion; by the psychoanalyst as the product of internal psychic conflict. Objectively, pain is an expression of the interpretation by some centers in the brain of the input to these centers.

Several clinical conditions indicate that the influences conveyed from the free nerve endings via the A fibers and the C fibers have different critical roles in the appreciation of pain. Some persons are congenitally insensitive to pain. In certain such subjects, with markedly elevated pain thresholds, the small-diameter C fibers are absent, whereas the A fibers are relatively intact (Swanson et al.). In contrast, patients afflicted with *herpes zoster*—a skin eruption due to a virus infection—experience excruciating pain when the involved skin area is exposed to normally innocuous stimuli such as light touch. In this condition there is a reduction in the number of A fibers relative to C fibers in the peripheral nerve (Noordenbos). This abnormal sensitivity to pain may be a consequence, in part, of the inability of the fewer lightly myelinated A fibers to exert suppressor effects on the fine-fiber activity. As explained below, the intense delayed pain may be a response to repetitive stimulation of C fibers.

The A and C fibers terminate in the substantia gelatinosa (lamina II), which is a processing center. One concept of the role of this region of the posterior gray matter is the gate-control theory (Melzack and Wall, 1965). The A and C fibers may synapse directly with and excite neurons called T (central transmission) cells within the gray matter. These T cells are presumably involved in some way with the anterolateral tracts, which convey pain impulses to the brain. Collateral branches from the A and C fibers enter the substantia gelatinosa and interact with a complex of short-axon neurons which excite or inhibit substantia gelatinosa interneurons (SG interneurons) with axons which may inhibit the A and C fibers (presumably by presynaptic inhibition) before they synapse with the T cells (Fig. 5-16). Within this complex the gate-control system operates. These SG interneurons are, in

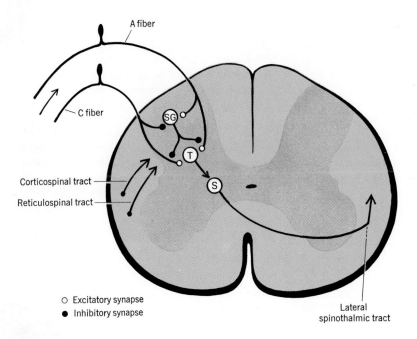

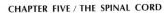

FIGURE 5-16
Gate-control theory of pain.

The A and C fibers are presumed to synapse with interneurons in the substantia gelatinosa (SG cells) and transmission neurons (T cells). The latter neurons synapse with the neurons of the lateral spinothalamic tract (S). The descending fibers of the corticospinal and reticulospinal tracts may exert influences upon sensory input.

a sense, the "guardians of the gates" over the pain traffic. The balance of the input activity of the A and C fibers upon the SG interneurons regulates the input to the T cells. Discharges by A fibers tend to close the gates because they excite the SG interneurons to exert their presynaptic inhibitory influences (Fig. 5-16). This is consistent with the concept, noted previously, that the subjects with A fibers but with few C fibers have elevated pain thresholds; their A fibers tend *"to close the gates."* On the other hand, the activity of the C fibers tends *"to open the gates,"* because they inhibit SG interneurons from exerting their presynaptic inhibitory influences. The differential input conveyed by the A and C fibers is important in the operation of the gate. The cells of the gate may be continuously regulated by central mechanisms through feedback circuits and may be under prime control of descending influences from the brain. These supraspinal influences, which can modify the effect associated with pain, may be conveyed from the cerebral cortex and other subcortical centers to the gate-control system in the poste-

rior horn. These descending pathways include the corticospinal tract (especially from the parietal lobe) and other descending fibers to the brainstem reticular nuclei within the reticulospinal tracts. Many of our subjective experiences of pain are modified through higher centers in the brain. Anxiety and depression may magnify the intensity of pain; hypnosis and intense emotional involvement or cognitive activity can suppress it. After prefrontal lobotomy (Chap. 16), the affective component of intractable pain may be markedly reduced, with the retention of the discriminative component.

SPINORETICULAR TRACT

The *spinoreticular (spinobulbar) tract* is composed of fibers originating from cells in the posterior horn and intermediate zone of all levels of the spinal cord. The fibers ascend in the anterior and anterolateral funiculi and brainstem reticular formation; they terminate in the medial two-thirds of the medullary and pontine reticular formation. The spinoreticular tract is not somatotopically organized. The fibers of this tract which terminate in the nucleus reticularis gigantocellularis and lateral reticular nucleus are primarily uncrossed axons, whereas those which terminate in the nucleus reticularis pontis oralis and caudalis are both crossed and uncrossed axons. These pathways are integrated into the "ascending reticular system" and the spinoreticulothalamic pain pathway, and, in addition, probably convey visceral sensory impulses from the thoracic, abdominal, and pelvic viscera.

SPINOTECTAL TRACT

This *spinotectal tract* is composed of fibers which originate in the intermediate gray zone, decussate in the anterior white commissure, and ascend as a small bundle located adjacent to the spinothalamic tract. Its fibers terminate in the deep layers of the superior colliculus and in the central gray substance. This pathway of unknown significance may have a role in the transmission of tactile, thermal, pain, and other noxious stimuli. In a sense, the spinotectal fibers may be considered as one expression of the spinoreticular and spinoreticulothalamic pathways.

TOUCH AND DEEP-SENSIBILITY PATHWAYS

The nerve endings associated with the conscious pathways for touch and deep sensibility include Merkel's disks, Meissner's corpuscles, terminals surrounding the hair follicles (peritrichial arborization), and Pacinian corpuscles. These modalities are conveyed by two pathways: light (tickle or crude) touch (stroking without deforming skin or moving hair) via the *anterior spinothalamic tract* (Fig. 5-15); and tactile discrimination, stereognosis, pressure (deep touch), and associated discrimination senses via the *posterior column (spinal cord)–medial lemniscal (brainstem) pathway* (Figs. 5-15, 5-17, and 5-18).

Anterior spinothalamic pathway (Figs. 5-15, 5-18) The first-order neuron of this system consists of myelinated fibers that pass through the dorsal root into the posterolateral tract of Lissauer and terminate in the posterior horn. The short ascending and descending collateral branches in the posterolateral tract of Lissauer

extend up and down through about three spinal segments. The second-order neuron projects its axon obliquely from a cell body located in the gray matter (several spinal levels) through the anterior white commissure to the anterior funiculus of the spinal cord, where it bends and projects rostrally through the spinal cord and brainstem to terminate in the ventral posterolateral nucleus of the thalamus. In the brainstem the fibers of the tract join either with the lateral spinothalamic tract to form the spinothalamic tract or with the medial lemniscus. The third-order neuron in the thalamus projects its axon through the posterior limb of the internal capsule to the postcentral gyrus of the cerebral cortex. Because the lateral and anterior spinothalamic tracts overlap, the two and the spinotectal tract are often considered as one, called the *anterolateral system.*

POSTERIOR COLUMN–MEDIAL LEMNISCAL PATHWAY (Figs. 5-17, 5-18)

Modalities This major system conveys information from mechanoreceptors in the skin, muscles tendons, and joints. Their activity is subjectively perceived in basically three forms of sensibility: touch-pressure, kinesthesia, and vibratory sense (in flutter-vibration). Touch-pressure is the sense resulting from the deformation of the skin; kinesthesia includes the sense of position and movement of joints (angle-movement detectors). Vibrations sensed from skin are called flutter-vibrations, while that from deep structures such as joints and bone is called the vibratory sense. Vibratory sense is actually a sensing of rapid successive stimuli of tactile sense. In general, the fibers of first order of this posterior column–lemniscal system are modality specific. In turn, this modality specificity is preserved throughout this system, including the processing nuclei (nuclei gracilis and cuneatus and ventral posterolateral nucleus of the thalamus), second- and third-order neurons, and in the neurons of the postcentral gyrus (primary somesthetic cortex).

Touch-pressure and the flutter component of flutter-vibration are monitored by the fast-

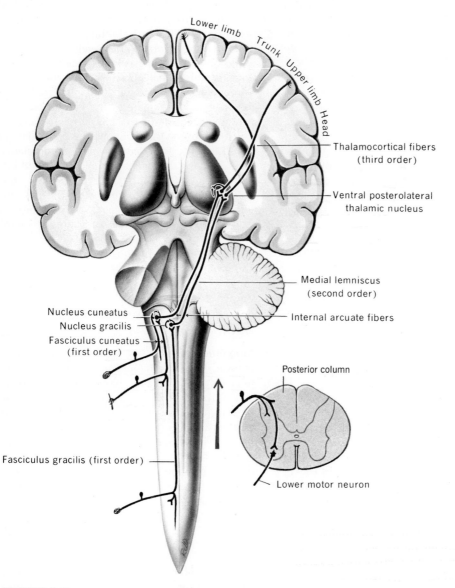

Lower limb · Trunk · Upper limb · Head

Thalamocortical fibers
(third order)

Ventral posterolateral
thalamic nucleus

Medial lemniscus
(second order)

Internal arcuate fibers

Nucleus cuneatus
Nucleus gracilis
Fasciculus cuneatus
(first order)

Posterior column

Fasciculus gracilis (first order)

Lower motor neuron

FIGURE 5-17
Posterior column–medial lemniscal pathway.

This pathway is composed of: *1* neurons of the first order with cell bodies in the spinal ganglia and with axons that ascend in the posterior column to the nuclei gracilis and cuneatus; *2* neurons of the second order with cell bodies in the nuclei gracilis and cuneatus and with axons that decussate as the internal arcuate fibers in the lower medulla and ascend in the medial lemnis- cus to the thalamus; and *3* neurons of the third order with cell bodies in the thalamus and with axons that project to the cerebral cortex (postcentral gyrus). Col- lateral branches of the neuron of the first order pass to the posterior horn, the anterior horn (Fig. 5-12), and the posterior column; the last are descending associa- tion fibers.

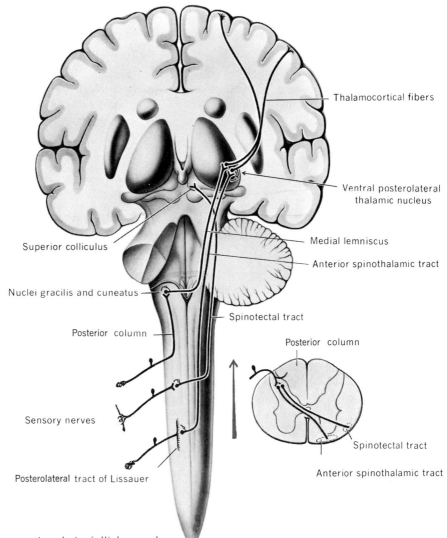

Thalamocortical fibers

Ventral posterolateral thalamic nucleus

Medial lemniscus

Anterior spinothalamic tract

Superior colliculus

Nuclei gracilis and cuneatus

Spinotectal tract

Posterior column

Posterior column

Sensory nerves

Spinotectal tract

Posterolateral tract of Lissauer

Anterior spinothalamic tract

adapting fibers innervating hair follicles and Meissner's corpuscles (movement detectors) in the skin. Touch-pressure is also sensed by slowly adapting fibers innervating Merkel disks in the epidermis and Ruffini-like endings in the dermis of the skin, fascia, and periosteum. Vibratory sensibility (high-frequency sense) is picked up by Pacinian corpuscles of the dermis and deep tissues, while kinesthesia is sensed by receptors in the joint capsules and joint ligaments. The receptors in the joint "know" where the limb is (angle of joint). This information, signaling positive active movement and resistance to

FIGURE 5-18
Touch pathways and spinotectal tract.

The touch pathways include *1* the posterior column–medial lemniscus–thalamocortical pathway, and *2* the anterior spinothalamic tract–thalamocortical pathway. The spinotectal pathway is composed of *1* neurons of the first order with cell bodies in the spinal ganglia, and *2* neurons of the second order with cell bodies in the posterior horn and with axons that decussate and ascend as the spinotectal tract to the superior colliculus.

160

movement to the nervous system, is essential for the regulation of normal movements.

Pathway The first-order neurons of this system with their cell bodies located in the spinal ganglia consist generally of heavily myelinated fibers which pass the spinal cord through the medial bundle of the dorsal root. Upon entering the cord of the medial aspect of the posterior horn, the fibers divide into ascending and descending branches which are located within the *posterior column (fasciculi gracilis and cuneatus*) on the same side of the spinal cord. About one-fourth of the ascending fibers extend rostrally and terminate in the nuclei gracilis and cuneatus, which are located in the lower medulla. Collateral fibers branch off the main axon within the segment of entrance and also from the ascending and descending branches into other segments; these collaterals terminate in the spinal gray matter. Approximately one-fifth of the ascending fibers terminate in the immediate gray matter within two or three spinal segments above their segment of entry. Many of these intraspinal collaterals are involved with intersegmental spinal reflexes. The ascending fibers are somatotopically organized within the posterior columns. Those conveying input from the lower body caudal to T6 (including the lower extremity) are located more medially, in the *fasciculus gracilis*, and those from the upper body rostral to T6 (including the upper extremity) are located more laterally, in the *fasciculus cuneatus.* Fibers from each spinal segment are added successively on the lateral aspect of the posterior column; this maintains the somatotopic organization within the posterior columns. Thus at the cervical levels, the lamination from posteromedial to lateral consists, in order, of fibers from the sacral, lumbar, thoracic, and cervical segments of the body (Fig. 5-12). Thus, the fibers from the sacral, lumbar, and lower six thoracic segments form the fasciculus gracilis, and those from the upper six thoracic levels and all cervical levels (including the back of the head) form the fasciculus cuneatus. The longest neurons in the body are those of the fasciculus gracilis; they extend without interruption from

the foot to the nucleus gracilis in the medulla. These neurons in a 7-ft-tall giant are over 6 ft long. Each posterior column fiber terminates after dividing into two or three branches which, through collaterals, synapse directly with several neurons of the second order.

The somatotopic organization is maintained in the nuclei gracilis and cuneatus. Neural processing within these nuclei occurs through synaptic interactions among the nerve terminals of the ascending fibers, intrinsic interneurons, descending (centrifugal) corticonuclear fibers from the cerebral cortex, and the neurons of the second order. The corticonuclear fibers originate in the somatosensory (postcentral gyrus) cortex and course through the corona radiata, internal capsule, and basilar portion of the brainstem (among the fibers of the pyramidal tract) before terminating with the posterior column nuclei. Each descending fiber divides before spreading over wide areas of these nuclei. The interneurons are not intercalated between the first- and second-order neurons, but rather are integrated into recurrent circuits (recurrent collateral fibers from second-order neurons) and are interposed between the corticonuclear fibers and second-order neurons. These neuronal connections with these nuclei are organized into center-surround units (see Chap. 12). Within this organization the discriminative nature of the sensations (e.g., two-point discrimination) maintains individuality within the processing nuclei by the excitatory center and inhibitory-surround organization. The information from each distinct point on the body is preserved and prevented from being dispersed from the center by the inhibitory activity of the surround.

The second-order neurons, with their cell bodies in the nucleus gracilis and nucleus cuneatus, have axons which course transversely in an arc as the decussating *internal arcuate fibers* of the medulla into the contralateral *medial lemniscus* and ascend through the brainstem to the *ventral posterolateral nucleus* of the thalamus. Apparently all fibers of this pathway decussate in the low medulla and terminate in cone-shaped bushy endings in the ventral posterolateral nucleus. In the medulla, the medial lemniscus is located in the anterior portion just posterior to the pyramid between the midline raphe and the inferior olive. In the pontine region, the medial lemniscus shifts laterally along the anterior margin of the tegmentum of the pons. In the midbrain it shifts posterolaterally as a crescent-shaped bundle lateral to the nucleus ruber and medial to the medial geniculate body before terminating in the ventral posterolateral nucleus (Figs. 8-4 through 8-11).

Although the lamination is not precise, the somatotopical organization is maintained within the medial lemniscus. In general, the second-order fibers from the nucleus gracilis ascend in the anterior portion of the medial lemniscus within the medulla and lateral portion of the medial lemniscus within the pons and synapse in the lateral portion of the ventral posterolateral nucleus of the thalamus. Those fibers from the nucleus cuneatus ascend in the posterior portion of the medial lemniscus within the medulla and the medial portion of the lemniscus within the pons and synapse in the medial portion of the ventral posterolateral nucleus.

Axons of neurons of the third order with their cell bodies in the ventral posterolateral nucleus of the thalamus pass through the posterior limb of the internal capsule and corona radiata before terminating in the general somatic area I (primary somatic area, postcentral gyrus) and somatic sensory area II (general somatic area II, secondary somatic area).

In summary, the modalities associated with the posterior column–medial lemniscus system include discriminative touch, two-point discrimination, stereognosis, awareness of shape, size, and texture, awareness of passive movement, position sense, flutter vibration, vibratory sense (as in use of a tuning fork), and weight perception.

Spinocerebellar pathways

GENERAL CHARACTERISTICS (Fig. 5-19)

Receptors in the extremities and body wall, especially those in the muscles and tendons, are continually monitoring the immediate status of muscle contraction and the momentary degree of tension within the tendons. The resulting "unconscious" proprioceptive information from the muscles, tendons, and joints is projected to the cerebellum via four pathways. Some input to the cerebellum comes from exteroceptive receptors in the skin. The *posterior and anterior*

spinocerebellar tracts convey these influences from the lower extremities and the caudal half of the body, while the *cuneocerebellar tract* and the *rostral spinocerebellar tract* (the latter as yet unidentified in man) convey influences from the upper extremities and upper half of the body. In general, the posterior spinocerebellar and cuneocerebellar pathways receive their input from the muscle spindles, tendon organs, touch receptors, and pressure receptors, while the anterior spinocerebellar and rostral cerebellar pathways receive input via neurons with large receptor fields of Golgi tendon organs and flexor reflex afferents. These flexor reflex afferents are those receptors in skin and joints conveying information via neurons of groups II and III; they are involved with the general flexor reflex, with two or more neurons intercalated within the reflex.

POSTERIOR SPINOCEREBELLAR TRACT

The neurons of the first order with cell bodies in the spinal ganglia convey coded information from the stretch receptors directly to the neurons of the second order in the dorsal nucleus of Clarke (Clarke's column) of lamina VII. The neurons of this nucleus receive monosynaptic excitatory influences mainly from group IA and IB fibers with some from group II afferents. Fibers from receptors in other muscles may contribute inhibitory influences. The axons of the dorsal nucleus of Clarke (located at levels T1 through L3) ascend ipsilaterally as the somatotopically organized uncrossed spinocerebellar tract (Fig. 5-19). The fibers of this tract are among the fastest conducting fibers—120 meters per second. Its large fibers ascend successively through the posterolateral aspect of the lateral funiculus of the spinal cord, the inferior cerebellar peduncle, and the white matter of the cerebellum before terminating in the ipsilateral anterior (lobules I to IV) and caudal (pyramis and paramedian lobule) portions of the cerebellar vermis. Within the spinal cord the tract is superficial to the lateral corticospinal tract.

Because the dorsal nucleus of Clarke does not extend caudal to L3, *1* the fibers entering the spinal cord via the dorsal spinal roots of

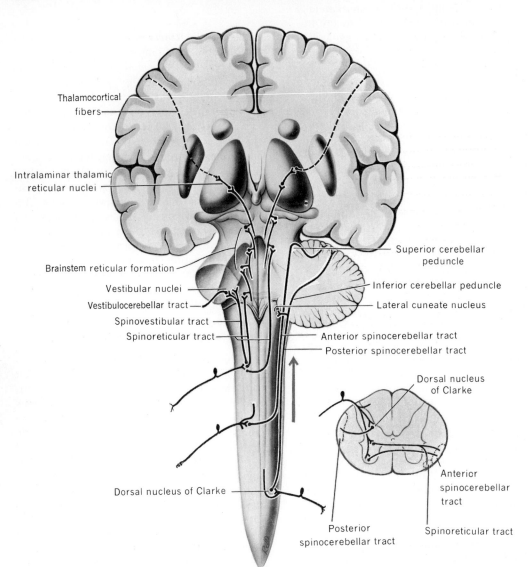

Thalamocortical fibers

Intralaminar thalamic reticular nuclei

Brainstem reticular formation

Vestibular nuclei

Vestibulocerebellar tract

Spinovestibular tract

Spinoreticular tract

Superior cerebellar peduncle

Inferior cerebellar peduncle

Lateral cuneate nucleus

Anterior spinocerebellar tract

Posterior spinocerebellar tract

Dorsal nucleus of Clarke

Dorsal nucleus of Clarke

Anterior spinocerebellar tract

Posterior spinocerebellar tract

Spinoreticular tract

FIGURE 5-19
Spinocerebellar tracts, spinovestibular tract, and spinoreticular tract.

The spinocerebellar tracts include *1* the uncrossed posterior spinocerebellar tract that passes through the inferior cerebellar peduncle and terminates in the paleocerebellum, and *2* the crossed anterior spinocerebellar tract that passes through the superior cerebellar peduncle and terminates in the paleocerebellum. The spinovestibular tract includes fibers that terminate in the vestibular nuclei. The spinoreticular tract is composed of crossed and uncrossed fibers that terminate in some brainstem reticular nuclei.

lumbar and sacral levels ascend in the posterior columns before synapsing with the neurons of the dorsal nucleus of Clarke, and *2* the posterior spinocerebellar tract, as such, is not found within the spinal cord caudal to the L3 level. In summary, the somatotopically organized posterior spinocerebellar tract relays unconscious proprioceptive information from the caudal half of the body and lower extremities to the cerebellar cortex via a two-neuron linkage with synaptic connections in the dorsal nucleus. This pathway has a role in the fine coordination of individual muscles during postural adjustments and movements.

ANTERIOR SPINOCEREBELLAR TRACT

Fibers of neurons of the first order from the Golgi tendon organs and flexor reflex afferent receptors located in the lower extremity and lower half of the body enter the spinal cord via the dorsal roots and terminate with neurons in laminae V, VI, and VII in the lumbosacral levels. Each second-order neuron receives monosynaptic excitatory influences derived primarily from IB afferents of Golgi tendon organs located in widely separated muscle tendons. The flexor reflex afferent fibers include those of groups II and III which evoke flexor reflexes via polysynaptic circuits mediated via two or more interneurons. These neurons also receive inhibitory and excitatory stimuli from the cutaneous afferent fibers. The axons of the neurons of the second order decussate in the anterior white commissure and ascend as the somatotopically organized anterior spinocerebellar tract located in the anterolateral aspect of the lateral funiculus. Some fibers of this tract are uncrossed. The tract can be identified as low as the lower lumbar levels. The tract courses through the lateral brainstem and along the posterior surface of the superior cerebellar peduncle before terminating in the vermis of the anterior lobe (lobules I to IV). This pathway has a role in the general coordination of posture and movement of the entire limb.

CUNEOCEREBELLAR TRACT

Group IA and some cutaneous afferent fibers of first-order neurons innervating the upper extremities and rostral half of the body pass through the dorsal roots, ascend in the ipsilateral fasciculus cuneatus, and terminate in the somatotopically organized accessory cuneate nucleus. The accessory cuneate nucleus, located in the lower medulla just lateral to the cuneate nucleus, is the rostral equivalent to the dorsal nucleus of Clarke. Axons of the accessory cuneate nucleus course via the uncrossed cuneocerebellar tract through the inferior cerebellar peduncle and terminate in the ipsilateral lobule V of the cerebellar cortex. This pathway is the rostral counterpart of the posterior spinocerebellar tract.

ROSTRAL SPINOCEREBELLAR TRACT

This pathway serves the same role for the rostral half of the body and upper extremity as the anterior spinocerebellar tract for the lower extremity. Although its presence has been established so far only in the cat, it is presumed to exist in man. This rostral spinocerebellar pathway relays influences from the group I muscle afferents and flexor reflex afferents (movement patterns of the whole extremity) from the ipsilateral upper extremity via uncrossed fibers. These course through both superior and inferior cerebellar peduncles and terminate in the upper-extremity region of the cerebellar cortex.

SPINOCERVICOTHALAMIC PATHWAY
(Spinocervicolemniscal pathway)

This pathway has an, as yet, unknown role in the transmission of tactile and kinesthetic information from the periphery to the ventral posterolateral thalamic nucleus and cerebral cortex. It differs from the spinothalamic and posterior column–medial lemniscal pathways in that it is composed of both three and four orders of neurons (Fig. 5-20). This pathway has been demonstrated in the rhesus monkey and is thus assumed to be a functioning pathway in man. The influences from the afferent fibers of first-order neurons reach the ipsilateral lateral cervical nucleus (nucleus located in the lower medulla and upper three cervical spinal levels) directly or indirectly; the indirect connections are via two routes: *1* collateral branches of the posterior spinocerebellar fibers and *2* axons of neurons located in the gray matter of the lumbosacral region. Axons of the lateral cervical nucleus decussate in the lower medulla, ascend in or near the medial lemniscus within the brainstem, and terminate in the ventral posterolateral nucleus of the thalamus. The pathway projects from the thalamus to both the primary and secondary somatic areas of the cerebral cortex (somatic sensory area I and area II).

OTHER ASCENDING PATHWAYS

Fibers have been described that project directly to the cerebral cortex (*spinocortical tract*), to

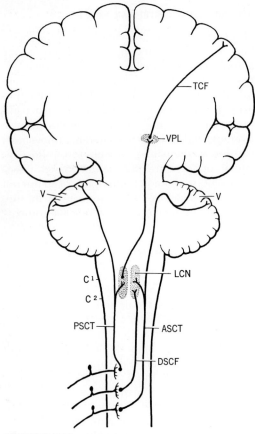

FIGURE 5-20

Spinocervicothalamic pathway.

This tactile and kinesthetic system relays influences via the lateral cervical nucleus (L.C.N.) to the ventral posterolateral (V P L.) nucleus of the thalamus. This pathway projects to both the primary and secondary somatosensory areas of the cortex. ASCT, Anterior spinocerebellar tract; DSCF, Direct spinocervical fibers; PSCT, Posterior spinocerebellar tract; TCF, Thalamocortical fibers; V, Vermis; VPL, Ventral posterolateral nucleus. (*From Noback and Harting, Spinal Cord, S. Karger, Publisher, Basel,* 1971.)

the (inferior) vestibular nuclei (*spinovestibular tract*), and to the pons (*spinopontine tract*). The nuclei of origin of these tracts are in the gray matter. The general visceral afferent influences conveyed to the spinal cord are probably relayed rostrally via the *spinoreticular tract.*

Spinal reflexes

The descending motor pathways from the brain to the spinal cord exert their influences on the intrinsic neural circuits of the spinal cord. These intrinsic neurons are important because they form the basic circuitry that eventually interacts with the lower motor neurons which innervate the voluntary muscles.

The *neuromuscular spindles* are arranged in parallel to the voluntary muscle fibers; they monitor *muscle length (length detectors).* The *Golgi tendon organs* are arranged in series with the voluntary muscles; they are *tension detectors.* When the muscle is stretched (lengthened), the spindle and the bag region of its intrafusal fibers are passively stretched and "loaded." The "loaded" spindle stimulates the IA fibers to increase their firing rate. When the muscle is contracted, the spindle and its bag region are shortened and "unloaded." The "unloaded" spindle fires less actively. The Golgi tendon organs are not activated by passive stretch. Rather they respond to increases in tension during the contraction of a muscle by increasing their rate of discharge. The roles of the spindle and Golgi tendon organs are discussed further on in this chapter under "Monosynaptic Extensor Reflex." These sensory receptors are integral elements of negative feedback or servo loops; the feedback information is utilized by the various reflex circuits.

RED AND WHITE MUSCLE FIBERS

Each gross muscle is composed of red muscle fibers, white muscle fibers, and some intermediate fibers. *Red fibers* are adapted for slow, efficient contractions which are sustained for long durations without fatiguing. *White fibers* are adapted for noncontinuous rapid and powerful contractions, which are not sustained. The relative number of these fiber types in a muscle is related to the nature of the contractions characteristic of specific muscle. The reddish coloration of the red muscles is due to the high concentrations of mitochondria and enzymes associated with oxidative metabolism within the fiber; a dense capillary network surrounds each small dark muscle fiber. The white fibers are large and pale, with an abundant sarcoplasmic reticulum and T-tubule system elements, high levels of glycogen and glycolytic enzymes, and few mitochondria; a poor capillary network surrounds each fiber. Their rapid fatigability is associated with their anaerobic metabolism. Red fibers are referred to as "oxidative" fibers, and white fibers as "glycolytic" fibers.

The red fibers are normally utilized for dexterous movements requiring the graded use of large numbers of small motor units and for postural stance requiring sustained contractions. White fibers are utilized less frequently; their role is to contract in response to sudden and transient demands requiring extra activity. As a rule, red fibers are found in deep muscles and deeper aspects of superficial muscles. White muscle fibers are found in superficial muscles. Muscles with a high proportion of red fibers include such antigravity muscles as the neck musculature and the one-joint brachialis and soleus muscles. Muscles with a high proportion of white fibers include the phasic two-joint biceps brachii, hamstring, and gastrocnemius muscles.

NEURONS OF SPINAL REFLEX ARCS AND THE LOWER MOTOR NEURONS

The neurons that comprise the intrinsic circuits within the spinal cord are classified into three categories (Figs. 5-21 through 5-24):

1 The afferent neurons, those that enter the spinal cord via the dorsal roots and terminate in the gray matter. These neurons commence distally as endings in receptors within muscles, joints, and tendons, and in cutaneous receptors in the skin. The deep receptors include the annulospiral endings and flower spray endings of the neuromuscular spindles, and the Golgi tendon organs (GTO) (associated with groups IA, IB, II, and III fibers, Chap. 3). The cutaneous (superficial) receptors include encapsulated endings (Meissner's corpuscle, Pacinian corpuscle) and free nerve endings of the skin (associated with groups II, III, and IV fibers).

2 The interneurons, those that lie wholly within the spinal cord and interact with other interneurons or with lower motor neurons. These interneurons are classified as *a* intrasegmental interneurons, those located entirely within a spinal cord segment on one side; *b* commis-

sural interneurons, those projecting their axons to the same segment on the opposite side; and *c* intersegmental interneurons, those projecting their axons to other segments of the same side and of the opposite side (see "Intrinsic Spinal Interneurons and Fasciculi Proprii," later on).

3 The lower motor neurons. Each has its cell body in the anterior horn; it projects its axon through a peripheral nerve to a voluntary muscle. The lower motor neurons are of two types, alpha and gamma (Figs. 2-1, 2-3). The alpha motor (skeletomotor) neuron is a heavily myelinated, fast-conducting neuron that terminates in the motor end plate of a voluntary muscle (extrafusal) fiber. The gamma efferent (fusimotor) neuron is a lightly myelinated, slowly conducting neuron that innervates the small muscle (intrafusal) fibers within the neuromuscular spindle receptor. The lower motor neurons have their cell bodies located within the central nervous system (anterior horn of the spinal cord for spinal nerves and motor nuclei of cranial nerves III, IV, V, VI, VII, XII and nucleus ambiguus of the brainstem). They have axons coursing within the peripheral nerves before terminating as motor end plates with extrafusal muscle fibers or intrafusal muscle fibers of the neuromuscular spindles. In summary, lower motor neurons include all alpha and gamma motor neurons associated with the cranial and spinal motor nerves. Movements of the body are produced by the contractions of skeletal muscles; muscle contractions result from the discharge of lower motor neurons. When adequately stimulated, each lower motor neuron conveys excitatory influences which evoke the contraction of all voluntary muscle fibers of the motor unit. This results because all motor end plates are obligatory excitatory synapses. All inhibitory synaptic influences upon the somatic motor circuits occur within the central nervous system.

MONOSYNAPTIC EXTENSOR REFLEX (Fig. 5-22)

The *simple knee jerk* results from the tapping of the tendon of the relaxed quadriceps femoris muscle—the muscle that extends the knee joint. This reflex is also known as the *patellar reflex,*

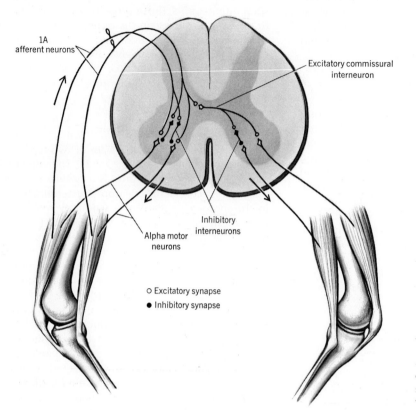

1A
afferent neurons

Excitatory commissural
interneuron

Inhibitory
interneurons

Alpha motor
neurons

○ Excitatory synapse
● Inhibitory synapse

FIGURE 5-21
Reciprocal innervation of the agonist and antagonist muscles in an ipsilateral reflex (left side) and in a contralateral "crossed" reflex (right side).

myotatic reflex, deep tendon reflex, or *stretch extensor reflex.* It may be characterized as two-neuron (i.e., it involves a sequence of a set of afferent neurons and a set of efferent neurons), ipsilateral (it is restricted to the side tapped), and intrasegmental (each receptor stimulates an afferent neuron which excites alpha motor neurons in the same spinal segment). The sudden tap stretches the muscle and the neuromuscular spindles within the muscle. The stretched spindles (bag region) excite the sensitive low-threshold annulospiral endings to set up generator potentials that initiate a volley of impulses in the group IA afferent fibers. The resulting action potentials are conveyed via these fibers through the dorsal roots of the L2 or L3 levels to the ipsilateral alpha motor neurons. In turn, these bombarded alpha neurons convey excita-

tory influences via the axons, which course through the ventral roots, spinal nerves, and peripheral nerves, to excite the motor end plates of muscle fibers of the quadriceps femoris to contract, thereby producing the knee jerk. During contraction, the spindles are passively short-ened. The *brisk knee jerk* is a *phasic motion* (as in kicking a football); it is initiated by the synchronous discharges of many spindles. The *slow knee jerk* (as in contractions during stance) is a *tonic or postural jerk;* it is initiated by the asynchronous discharges from many spindles. The spindle acts as a *strain gauge monitor (length detector)* for these extensor reflexes. It is not a receptor associated with conscious sensations. Because the spindles are oriented "in parallel" to the extrafusal muscle fibers, the contraction of the extrafusal fibers results in the

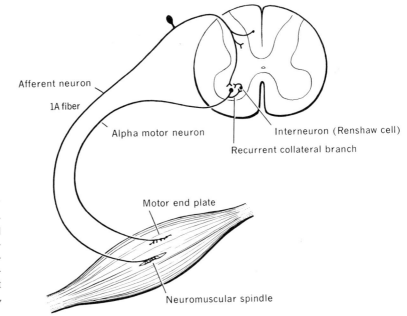

Afferent neuron

1A fiber

Alpha motor neuron

Interneuron (Renshaw cell)

Recurrent collateral branch

Motor end plate

Neuromuscular spindle

FIGURE 5-22
Extensor reflex (knee jerk).

This two-neuron, monosynaptic, ipsilateral, intrasegmental reflex is composed of a "primary secondary ending" (annulospinal ending) of the neuromuscular spindle, afferent neuron, alpha motor neuron, and voluntary muscle.

shortened spindles; this "unloads" the spindle so that it may cease to discharge momentarily (*"silent" period of spindle discharge*). As soon as the muscle relaxes, the spindle is stretched and firing resumes. Thus the spindles are involved in the autogenic excitation of the extrafusal fibers.

This two-neuron reflex, consisting of the afferent neuron innervating the spindle and the alpha motor neuron to a muscle, is known as the alpha (reflex) loop. Actually this monosynaptic reflex does not exist in isolation; collateral branches from the IA afferent fibers (Figs. 5-21, 5-22) are integrated into a polysynaptic flexor reflex (reciprocal innervation).

GAMMA REFLEX LOOP (Fig. 5-23)

As a muscle contracts, the neuromuscular spindles within the muscle become passively shorter; with this shortening there is a concomitant reduction in the rate of spindle firing via the IA afferent neurons to the alpha motor pool. With this rate reduction, the system is not able to maintain the continuous contraction of any

muscle mass. Continuous contraction of a muscle mass results when the muscle fibers are in various degrees of contraction in response to asynchronous volleys of alpha motor neurons (a volley is the firing of a group of neurons). This continuous contraction is dependent upon the gamma reflex loop, which comprises *1 gamma motor neuron, 2 neuromuscular spindle, 3 afferent neuron, 4 alpha motor neuron,* and *5 voluntary muscle.* Note that the gamma loop commences with the gamma efferent neuron.

The *gamma control of spindle sensitivity to stretch* by the contraction of the intrafusal muscle fibers is important because the gamma neurons influence the quality of the sensory input from the spindle to the spinal cord. Gamma activation has a critical role in alpha motor neuron output. This process of sensitization of the spindle through the gamma efferents is known as *"gamma bias";* it modulates the activity of the spindle. When intrafusal fibers contract, the equatorial region (bag) is stretched just as if the main muscle has been extended; the ensuing deformation pulls the coils of the annulospiral part and increases the rate of firing in the IA

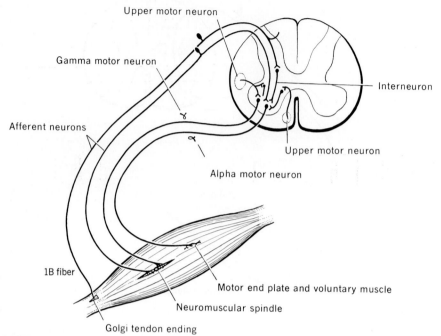

Upper motor neuron

Gamma motor neuron

Interneuron

Afferent neurons

Upper motor neuron

Alpha motor neuron

1B fiber

Motor end plate and voluntary muscle

Neuromuscular spindle

Golgi tendon ending

FIGURE 5-23

Gamma reflex loop and the Golgi tendon endings.

The gamma loop comprises gamma motor neuron, neuromuscular spindle, afferent neuron, alpha motor neuron, and voluntary muscle. The upper motor neurons can facilitate the gamma motor neurons.

The Golgi tendon endings are involved in the loop composed of Golgi tendon endings, afferent neuron, spinal intrasegmental neuron, and alpha motor neuron.

fibers. Through gamma efferent stimulation, the slack in the muscle spindle (a consequence of the shortened muscle) is taken up by the pull on the bag by the intrafusal muscle fibers. This acts to maintain spindle firing, which, through excitatory influences conveyed via IA fibers to the alpha motor neurons, acts to smooth out the muscle contraction. The "biasing mechanism" of the gamma system is readily altered by changes in muscle tension. In general, increasing the load on the muscle will increase the gamma efferent activity. When the slack occurs in the initial phase of the extrafusal muscle contrac-

tion, the spindle bags are unloaded and their firing ceases. This cessation is known as the *silent period.* Thus one role of the gamma efferents is to wipe out the silent period by stimulating the intrafusal fibers to contract; thus the bag assumes its normal tension status and firing rate of its IA fibers is resumed. In effect, this activity sustains the smooth ongoing muscular contraction. To summarize, the gamma motor neurons have two roles: they can change the sensitivity of the spindle—with the gain in the sensitivity of the bag region the firing rate of the IA fibers increases; and they can obliterate the silent period.

The gamma neurons can be stimulated *1* by IA fibers from the muscle spindle, *2* actively from the periphery through cutaneous stimulation by direct connections through interneurons synapsing with the gamma neurons, and *3* actively by upper motor neurons, especially those originating in the brainstem reticular formation. The cutaneous input acts rapidly; the reticular input via the upper motor neurons acts more slowly. Facilitatory and

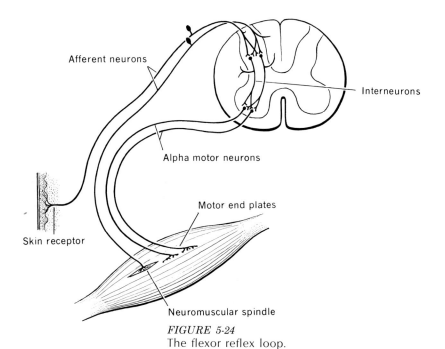

Afferent neurons

Interneurons

Alpha motor neurons

Motor end plates

Skin receptor

Neuromuscular spindle

FIGURE 5-24
The flexor reflex loop.

inhibitory influences from the brainstem reticular formation are conveyed via the medial and lateral reticulospinal tracts to laminae VII and VIII. Other descending tracts also contribute. The upper motor neurons stimulate the gamma motor neurons to excite the infrafusal muscle fibers slightly before stimulating the alpha motor neurons. This prior excitation of the gamma loop slightly before the alpha motor neuron discharge, acts, in a sense, to condition the muscle. In effect, the gamma motor neurons act to load the spindle at the same rate as it is unloaded through the muscle contraction; this results in a smooth, coordinated muscle activity. Stated otherwise, to get a smooth contraction, the tension remains constant when the length shortens. The normal gamma motor neuron activity acts to prevent jerky, clonic movements.

There are two types of gamma motor neurons or systems: *static fusimotor* and *dynamic fusimotor.* The static gamma neurons are involved preferentially with the tonic reflexes (muscle tone). The rigidity associated with the increased tonic stretch reflexes (as in Parkinson's disease, Chap. 14) may be due to the increased activity of

This three-neuron, disynaptic, ipsilateral, intersegmental reflex is composed of a sensory receptor in the skin, afferent neuron, spinal intersegmental neurons, alpha motor neurons, and voluntary muscles. This reflex can be facilitated by the "secondary sensory ending" (flower spray ending) of neuromuscular spindle, afferent neuron, spinal interneurons, alpha motor neurons, and voluntary muscles.

the static fusimotor system. The dynamic gamma neurons are involved with the phasic stretch reflexes (e.g., deep tendon reflexes). The spastic signs expressed in upper motor neuron paralysis (Chap. 5) may be primarily due to increased activity of the dynamic fusimotor system.

ROLE OF GOLGI TENDON ORGAN

The *Golgi tendon organs (GTOs)* have a critical role in the maintenance of muscle tension through an inhibitory three-neuron reflex arc of afferent neuron, interneuron, and alpha motor neuron (Fig. 5-23). In contrast to the spindles, which are muscle length detectors, the GTOs are muscle *tension detectors.* Because the GTOs within the tendons are *in series* with the extrafusal muscle fibers, they respond to an increase in tension within the tendon. They are believed to be continually monitoring tension in these muscles. As the tension within the tendon mounts, these endings are stimulated to increase the rate of discharge in the IB fibers conveying influences from the GTOs to interneurons, which, in turn, increase their rate of discharge of inhibitory stimuli into the alpha motor neuron pool. In this way, the GTOs tend to counteract the excitatory effects of the gamma loop on the alpha motor neurons. The GTOs, through the IB fibers, are thought to provide a steady inhibitory feedback so that the stretch reflex develops consistently less tension than it would in the absence of GTO influences. The exquisite balance of the excitatory effects of the gamma loop and the inhibitory effects of the Golgi tendon arcs are basic to the precise integration and timing of reflex activity. Through reciprocal innervation the GTO in a tendon inhibits the agonist but excites the antagonist. In this arrangement, the antagonists are said to be protected against excessive stretch by the IA on the agonists. The GTOs are not affected by passive stretch. Because the inhibition is generated within the muscle tendon, this activity is an expression of autogenic inhibition. At the present time the GTOs are *not* conceived as receptors with a high threshold for their appropriate stimulus; rather they provide the central nervous system with signals, which are suitable for the role of continuously regulating the strength of the muscular contraction regardless of the tension. Unlike the spindles, the sensitivity of the GTOs cannot be adjusted by the central nervous system. Autogenic inhibition appears to be a principle function of the GTOs.

TONUS

When muscles are completely at rest, some muscle fibers in any muscle are always contracted. This results in a residual tautness known as *muscle tone*. It is due to the continuous asynchronous discharge of a few motor units. Tonus is related primarily to the functional activity of the muscle spindles. Because muscles inserted to bones are in a continuous state of stretch, some of their muscle spindles must also be partially stretched. As a consequence some muscle spindles are always firing asynchronously. This is sufficient to produce the activity essential to maintain muscle tonus.

FLEXOR REFLEX (Fig. 5-24)

The reflex withdrawal of the hand from a noxious stimulus (heat or pinprick) is a protective reflex. It is a *three-neuron, disynaptic, ipsilateral, intersegmental flexor reflex* (*superficial, nociceptive*, or *cutaneous*). Clinically, it is called the superficial reflex. The circuit includes skin receptors, afferent neurons, spinal intersegmental interneurons, and alpha motor neurons to the flexor muscles of the upper extremity. This reflex can be facilitated by another three-neuron reflex arc consisting of the flower spray ending of the neuromuscular spindle, afferent neuron, spinal interneurons, and alpha motor neurons. Unlike the intrasegmental extensor reflex, the flexor reflex is an intersegmental ipsilateral reflex.

PRINCIPLE OF RECIPROCAL INNERVATION
(Fig. 5-21)

In a movement of a joint, the contraction of the agonist (prime mover) muscles is coordinated with the synchronous relaxation of the antagonist muscles. For example, to obtain the smooth flexion movement, the flexor muscle groups (agonist muscles) contract while the extensor muscle groups (antagonist muscles) relax synergistically during the movement. In the reflex circuits, interneurons integrate the excitatory and inhibitory stimuli (*reciprocal inhibition of an antagonist*) upon the lower motor neurons; this ensures the coordinated reciprocal innervation of the agonist and the antagonist. In the monosynaptic extensor reflex (knee jerk), the IA fibers from the stretched neuromuscular spindles of the quadriceps muscles facilitate monosynaptically the alpha motor neurons innervating the extensor quadriceps muscles to contract. In addition, a collateral branch of the IA fibers facilitates the "inhibitory" interneurons which inhibit the alpha motor neurons innervating the antagonistic flexor muscles. The IB afferent fibers may also be integrated into this circuitry. The influences conveyed via the IB fibers from the stimulated Golgi tendon organs *1* may excite the inhibitory interneuron, which, in turn, inhibits the alpha motor neurons innervating the agonist, and *2* may facilitate an excitatory interneuron, which, in turn, excites the alpha motor neuron innervating the antagonist muscles. In *crossed extensor reflexes*, the coordination of the ipsilateral limb with the contralateral limb reflex activity is possible because of a double reciprocal innervation via commissural neurons.

POLYSYNAPTIC EXTENSOR REFLEXES
(Fig. 5-21)

The *crossed extensor reflex* and the *extensor thrust reflex* are two important polysynaptic extensor reflexes.

In the crossed extensor reflex, the stimuli from peripheral receptors that initiate flexion in an extremity are also involved with the extension of the contralateral extremity. This reflex can be elicited in spinal animals (i.e., animals in which the spinal cord has been severed from the brain) by painful stimuli. Noxious stimuli on the foot produce the flexor reflex withdrawal of the stimulated ipsilateral extremity accompanied by the extension of the contralateral extremity. The flexion is based on the principle of reciprocal innervation, in which the afferent influences are relayed via excitatory interneurons to the flexor muscles and via inhibitory interneurons to the extensor muscles. The concurrent extension is based on the *principle of double reciprocal innervation*. At the same time commissural interneurons provide for the facilitation of extensor muscles and the inhibition of flexor muscles on the contralateral extremity. This interplay is utilized in the alternate rhythms of the extremities during walking and running.

With moderate pressure exerted on the sole of the foot, the pressure receptors in the foot project influences which elicit the extension (*extensor thrust reflex*, Fig. 5-21) of the stimulated extremity. This reflex involves the activity of reciprocal innervation through interneurons facilitating the extensor muscles and inhibiting the flexor muscles.

DISYNAPTIC FLEXOR REFLEX (Fig. 5-24)

A *disynaptic flexor reflex (stretch flexor reflex or "mark-time" reflex)* is the flexor reflex involved, for example, in the stepping movements of a spinal animal. Stimuli from flower spray endings of the neuromuscular spindles (sensors with a higher threshold than annulospiral endings) in either the flexor or extensor muscles are responsible for this flexor reflex. In general, one set of interneurons is intercalated between the type II afferent neurons and the alpha motor neurons. Thus it is a three-neuron, disynaptic intersegmental flexor reflex.

The flower spray endings tend to fire following sustained stretch and thus are capable of signaling information about muscle length. These receptors are usually included in the widespread system of *flexor reflex afferents (FRAs)*; they are presumed to excite flexors and to inhibit extensors. Their role is not fully understood; to the contrary, one school claims these secondary sensory endings produce autogenic excitation rather than inhibition.

MONOSYNAPTIC FLEXOR REFLEX

The *jaw jerk* or *pluck reflex* is a powerful antigravity action which results in clenching the teeth. A tap on the jaw evokes a set of synchronous volleys from the annulospiral endings of the spindles in the flexor muscles of mastication. The IA neurons of the trigeminal nerve (cell body in trigeminal ganglion) monosynaptically excite the alpha motor neurons in the motor nucleus of the trigeminal nerve; hence a monosynaptic reflex.

POLYSYNAPTIC FLEXOR REFLEX
(Flexor Twitch)

The reflex withdrawal of the hand from a noxious stimulus (cutaneous pain or heat receptors) is a *primitive protective reflex*. It is a polyneuronal, polysynaptic, ipsilateral, intersegmental flexor reflex (superficial or cutaneous). The circuit includes skin receptors, type II afferent neurons, several spinal intersegmented neurons, and alpha motor neurons to the flexor muscles of an extremity. This reflex can be facilitated by a three-neuron reflex consisting of flower spray endings of the neuromuscular spindle, afferent II neuron, spinal interneurons, and alpha motor neuron.

The scratch reflex in a dog is elicited when an irritation ("tickle" of pressure receptors in the skin) evokes a scratching response by the lower limb. This is considered to be a polysynaptic flexor reflex, which utilizes the intersegmental interneurons that project axons down the spinal cord in the fasciculi proprii of the white matter adjacent to the gray matter. The intrinsic ascending and descending pathways of the spinal cord are known as the *fasciculi proprii* (*spinospinalis tracts or propriospinal tracts*).

INTRINSIC SPINAL INTERNEURONS AND FASCICULI PROPRII (Fig. 5-11)

The spinal interneurons whose axons course and terminate within the spinal cord are organized into complex circuits which have not, as yet, been described in detail. Some spinal interneurons have axons which are distributed ipsilaterally within their own spinal segment on one side. These interneurons are actually intercalated within the circuits of ipsilateral intrasegmental multineuronal reflexes. Other spinal interneurons, called *commissural interneurons*, have axons which cross to the contralateral side and terminate in the same and other spinal segments. Most interneurons have collateral branches which extend up and down for a number of segments. Some of these fibers course within the gray matter. Others pass into the white matter adjacent to the gray matter as intersegmental fibers and ascend or descend for various distances before entering and synapsing within the gray matter. These fibers form the *fasciculi proprii* (*propriospinal or spinospinalis tracts*). These fasciculi are present in all three funiculi (Fig. 5-11).

The *commissural interneurons* and the *intersegmental interneurons* of the fasciculi proprii have significant roles in the more complex reflexes. The *crossed extensor reflex* utilizes commissural neurons to relay neural information across the midline. A painful stimulus on the foot may result in the reflex flexor withdrawal of the ipsilateral extremity and especially the enhancement of extensor musculature contractions of the contralateral limb to enable this contralateral extended limb to support the body when the flexed ipsilateral limb is off the ground. This interplay is utilized in the alternate rhythms of the extremities during walking and running, as one extremity is in active flexion while the contralateral extremity is in active extension.

A reflex utilizing ipsilateral intersegmental interneurons is the scratch reflex in a dog. This reflex is elicited when an irritation of the chest wall evokes a scratching response by the ipsilateral lower limb. This reflex utilizes intersegmental neurons with axons coursing through the ipsilateral fasciculi proprii.

DESCENDING FIBERS IN THE POSTERIOR COLUMNS

Most of the descending branches of the dorsal root fibers within the posterior columns extend caudally only a few segments, although some may project for as many as 10 spinal segments. These descending fibers cluster into small bundles which tend to locate medially and posteriorly to the ascending pathways. In the sacral region, the descending fibers, called the *triangle of Gombault-Philippe*, are located in the dorsal part of the posterior column near the midline. In the lumbar region, the descending fibers, called the *septomarginal fasciculus*, are located deep adjacent to the posterior septum. In the cervical and most thoracic segments, the descending bundle of fibers, called *fasciculus interfascicularis*, is located in the middle of the posterior column, between the fasciculus gracilis and fasciculus cuneatus.

RENSHAW CELL

An interneuron, called the *Renshaw cell*, is intercalated between the recurrent collateral branches of the axon of the alpha motor neuron and the dendrites of the same alpha motor neuron (Fig. 3-13). This negative feedback circuit

(Chap. 3) acts as an autoinhibitor which dampens the alpha motor neuron (Chap. 13). This circuit probably serves to inhibit momentarily (recurrent inhibition) the discharge of the alpha motor neuron. The fiber of the Renshaw cell that synapses with the alpha motor neuron is probably a collateral branch of a neuron with connections with other neurons. The alpha motor neurons originating in the medial anterior horn (lamina IX) do not have recurrent collateral branches; this suggests that the neurons innervating the axial musculature do not require this form of antidromic feedback to the Renshaw and other neurons. The alpha motor neurons originating in the lateral anterior horn (lamina IX) do have recurrent collateral branches, suggesting that the neurons innervating the appendicular musculature require feedback inhibition.

Each alpha motor neuron receives input through its 2,000 to 10,000 excitatory and inhibitory synapses with other neurons. This neuron is the final integrative battleground for excitation (EPSPs), inhibition (IPSPs), spatial summation, temporal summation, occlusion, and other neural processes. The integration of these activities by this neuron can result in the generation of an action potential in the axon capable of stimulating muscle contraction.

CENTRAL CONTROL OF SENSORY INPUT

The central nervous system has a significant role in regulating the sensitivity by which the sensory receptors respond to both external and internal environmental stimuli. Through these centrally derived influences, the sensitivity of receptors may be enhanced or suppressed. This is one means by which the organism selects, biases, or rejects certain environmental stimuli. The details of these phenomena for most receptors are not known.

After an animal is stressed, the sensitivity of the corpuscles of Meissner is enhanced so that these receptors are more responsive to tactile stimulation. Apparently the activity of the sympathetic nervous system is responsible, because the hypersensitivity is due, at least in part, to the increased concentrations of norepinephrine within the receptors. The central control of the responsiveness of the neuromuscular spindle by the gamma efferent neurons is an example of the influences exerted by the central nervous system in biasing the activity of a peripheral receptor. The sensitivity of the hair cells of the spiral organ of Corti is suppressed by the activity of the efferent cochlear bundle (olivocochlear bundle, Chap. 10). The fibers of this bundle arise in the superior olivary complex of the brainstem and terminate by synapsing on the hair cells. Influences conveyed by these fibers are inhibitory, making the hair cells less responsive to auditory stimuli.

Descending pathways from the brain
(Upper Motor Neurons)

The neurons that form the descending motor pathways from the brain to the spinal cord (and from the cerebrum to the brainstem) are known as upper motor neurons (Figs. 5-25 through 5-30). In contrast to the lower motor neurons, which commence in the central nervous system and terminate in the muscles of the body, the upper motor neurons are wholly within the central nervous system. The pathways of these neurons are listed and outlined below according to the locations of their nuclei of origin. Opinions differ concerning many of the detailed features of the pathways. Those descending fibers that terminate in the cervical spinal segments are largely involved with the motor activities of the neck (position of the head) and of the upper extremity, and those that terminate in the lumbosacral spinal segments are largely involved with the motor activities of the lower extremity. All spinal cord segments have a role in axial (trunk) muscle integration.

The upper motor neurons exert their influences primarily upon the spinal reflex loops and circuits by modifying and biasing their activities. Other descending fibers exert influences to the preganglionic fibers of the autonomic nervous system (Chap. 6) and to nuclei of the ascending pathways (Chap. 8). In general, the upper motor neurons synapse with interneurons which, in turn, terminate on either the alpha motor neurons or the gamma motor neurons. Some upper motor neurons terminate directly on alpha and

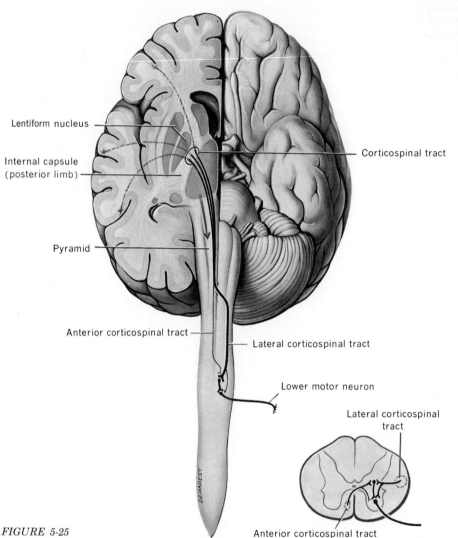

Lentiform nucleus

Internal capsule
(posterior limb)

Corticospinal tract

Pyramid

Anterior corticospinal tract

Lateral corticospinal tract

Lower motor neuron

Lateral corticospinal
tract

Anterior corticospinal tract

FIGURE 5-25
Corticospinal pathways.

These pathways are composed of descending fibers that originate from wide areas of the cerebral cortex, pass through the posterior limb of the internal capsule, crus cerebri, pons, pyramid, and spinal cord. Many of these fibers terminate upon spinal interneurons that, in turn, synapse with the lower motor neurons. Some fibers terminate directly upon lower motor neurons. The lateral corticospinal tract crosses over at the lower medulla as the pyramidal decussation, and the anterior corticospinal tract crosses over in upper spinal cord levels.

gamma motor neurons. Through these connections, the higher centers of the nervous system can control the alpha motor neurons independently of the gamma motor neurons.

CEREBRAL CORTEX

The *corticospinal tracts* (*cerebrospinal tracts, pyramidal tracts*) originate from widespread areas of the cerebral neocortex and descend

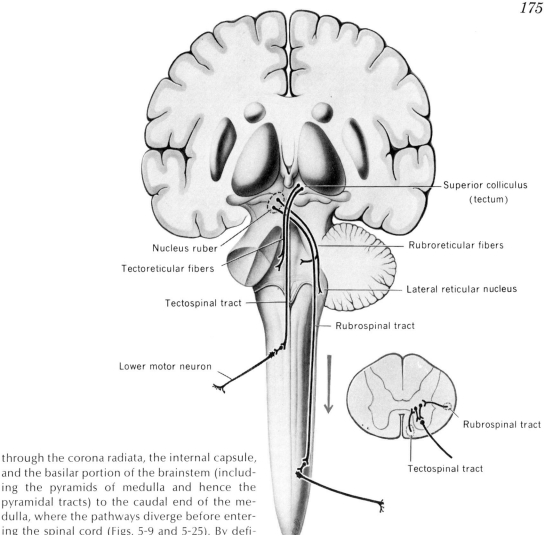

Superior colliculus
(tectum)

Nucleus ruber

Tectoreticular fibers

Tectospinal tract

Lower motor neuron

Rubroreticular fibers

Lateral reticular nucleus

Rubrospinal tract

Rubrospinal tract

Tectospinal tract

through the corona radiata, the internal capsule, and the basilar portion of the brainstem (including the pyramids of medulla and hence the pyramidal tracts) to the caudal end of the medulla, where the pathways diverge before entering the spinal cord (Figs. 5-9 and 5-25). By definition the corticospinal tracts are long pathways found in mammals, originating in the cerebral cortex, passing through the pyramids of the medulla, and terminating in the spinal cord. About 60 percent of the corticospinal fibers originate from areas 4 and 6 of the frontal lobe (Fig. 5-25); the remaining 40 percent arise from areas 3, 1, 2, and 5 of the parietal lobe. Of the pyramidal fibers, about 90 percent are small fibers ranging in diameter from 1 to 4 μm in diameter, fewer than 9 percent range from 5 to 10 μm in diameter, and fewer than 2 percent are large fibers, ranging from 10 to 22 μm in diameter.

Approximately 85 to 90 percent of the 1 mil-

FIGURE 5-26
Rubrospinal tract and tectospinal tract.

The rubrospinal tract originates in the nucleus ruber, decussates as the ventral tegmental decussation in the midbrain, and descends into the spinal cord. The tectospinal tract originates in the superior colliculus, decussates as the anterior tegmental decussation in the midbrain, and descends into the spinal cord. The descending fibers of these tracts terminate largely upon interneurons, which, in turn, synapse with the lower motor neurons. The rubroreticular and tectoreticular (tectobulbar) fibers terminate in the brainstem reticular nuclei, which, in turn, are integrated into other pathways (Chap. 8).

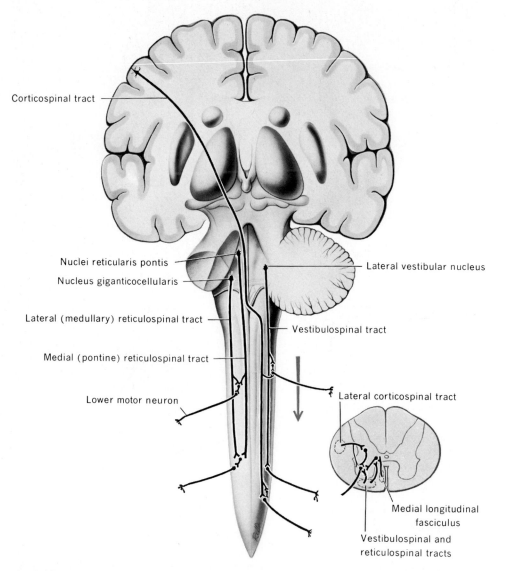

Corticospinal tract

Nuclei reticularis pontis

Nucleus giganticocellularis

Lateral (medullary) reticulospinal tract

Medial (pontine) reticulospinal tract

Lower motor neuron

Lateral vestibular nucleus

Vestibulospinal tract

Lateral corticospinal tract

Medial longitudinal fasciculus

Vestibulospinal and reticulospinal tracts

FIGURE 5-27
Reticulospinal tracts, vestibulospinal tract, and corticospinal tract.

The pontine reticulospinal tract originates in the nuclei reticularis pontis oralis and caudalis of the tegmentum of the pons. The medullary reticulospinal tract originates in the nucleus gigantocellularis of the medulla. The vestibulospinal tract originates in the lateral vestibular nucleus. The medial longitudinal fasciculus is illustrated in Fig. 10-10.

lion or more fibers cross over as the pyramidal decussation to form the lateral corticospinal tract of the spinal cord. Most of the remaining fibers continue as the anterior (ventral) corticospinal tract, as uncrossed fibers. A few uncrossed fibers are present in the lateral corticospinal tract. The lateral corticospinal tract extends throughout the spinal cord, with roughly 50 percent of its fibers terminating in the cervical segments, 20 percent in the thoracic segments, and 30 percent in the lumbosacral segments. The anterior corticospinal tract terminates largely in laminae VII and VIII of the cervical segments. Although its fibers are uncrossed, most of its terminal branches cross over to the opposite side before synapsing in the gray matter. In man, an estimated 90 percent of the corticospinal fibers synapse with interneurons in the base of the posterior horn and the intermediate zone (laminae IV, V, VI, and VII), and the remainder synapse directly with the alpha lower motor neurons (lamina IX, Fig. 5-25).

The corticospinal tract plays a significant role in precise and dexterous voluntary movements, mainly by facilitating flexion in the extremities. When this tract is damaged, there is a marked impairment of volitional activity, especially of the finer movements in the distal segments of the extremities. The movements of the proximal joints and the grosser actions are less severely and less permanently affected, the descending fibers originating from the postcentral gyrus and adjacent parietal cortex (areas 3, 1, 2, and 5 of the "sensory" cortex) terminate within laminae IV, V, and VI of the spinal gray matter; these fibers convey cortical influences to the nuclei of the posterior horn, which process and relay peripheral influences conveyed by the spinothalamic and spinoreticular pathways (pain, temperature, and light touch) to the brain. These tracts are presumed to have a role in precise and dexterous voluntary movements.

MIDBRAIN

Three tracts originate in the midbrain and terminate in the gray matter of the spinal cord: the rubrospinal, tectospinal, and interstitiospinal tracts (Figs. 5-12, 5-26, 5-29).

The *rubrospinal tract* originates in the nucleus ruber of the midbrain tegmentum. Its fibers cross immediately to the opposite side as the ventral tegmental decussation, and many descend through the entire length of the spinal cord. The nucleus ruber receives its major input from the motor cortex (precentral gyrus) of the same side (*corticorubral tract*) and from the emboliform nucleus of the contralateral cerebellar hemisphere (*cerebellorubral fibers*). Within the spinal cord, the fibers of the rubro

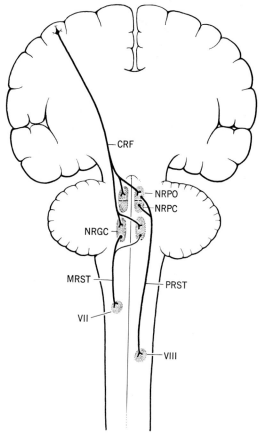

FIGURE 5-28
The reticulospinal tracts and the corticoreticulospinal system.

CRF, corticoreticular fibers; MRST, medullary reticulospinal tract; NRGC, nucleus reticularis gigantocellularis; NRPC, nucleus reticularis pontis caudalis; NRPO, nucleus reticularis pontis oralis; PRST, pontine reticulospinal tract. (*From Noback and Harting, Spinal Cord, S. Karger, Basel,* 1971.)

spinal tract are located anterior to and overlap with the fibers of the lateral corticospinal tract. They terminate upon interneurons in the lateral aspect of laminae V and VI and in the central portions of lamina VII. Most of the fibers which originate in the dorsal and dorsomedial parts of the red nucleus terminate in cervical levels.

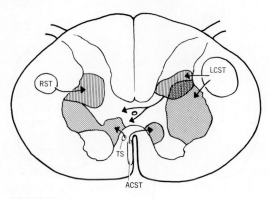

FIGURE 5-29
The location of some major descending (motor) tracts within the white matter and their sites of termination within the gray matter.

ACST, anterior corticospinal tract; LCST, lateral corticospinal tract; RST, rubrospinal tract; and TS, tectospinal tract. (*From Noback and Harting, Spinal Cord, S. Karger, Publisher, Basel, 1971.*)

Fibers which arise from the ventral and ventrolateral parts of the red nucleus terminate in the lumbosacral levels, while those from the intermediate zone between the two parts terminate in the thoracic segments. Because of this arrangement, the rubrospinal tract is said to be somatotopically organized. The rubrospinal tract has a role in the control of tone, especially in flexor muscles; it facilitates flexor activity and inhibits extensor activity.

The *tectospinal tract* originates from cells in the deep layers of the superior colliculus of the midbrain tectum (Figs. 5-26, 5-29). After crossing through the region around the periaqueductal gray of the upper midbrain as the dorsal tegmental decussation, its fibers descend through the brainstem as a bundle located anterior to the medial longitudinal fasciculus (MLF). These fibers join the MLF in the anterior funiculus of the spinal cord. These fibers terminate upon interneurons in laminae VIII, VII, and medial VI of all cervical levels, but mainly those of the upper four cervical segments. Because the superior colliculus is a major subcortical center of the visual system, it is probable that the tecto-

spinal tract mediates visually directed reflex movements of the head through the musculature of the neck.

The small *interstitiospinal tract* originates from the *interstitial nucleus of Cajal* located in the midbrain dorsolateral to the oculomotor nuclei. Its fibers descend without decussating within the MLF and terminate in parts of lamina VIII of all spinal levels.

PONS AND MEDULLA

Two significant pathway complexes originate in the lower brainstem and terminate in the spinal cord: the vestibulospinal and the reticulospinal tracts.

The *vestibulospinal tracts* arise from cells located in the vestibular nuclei of the upper dorsolateral medulla (Figs. 5-12, 5-27, 5-30). The vestibular nuclei receive their input from receptors in the vestibular labyrinth and from the cerebellum. The main input to the lateral vestibular nucleus is from the vestibular labyrinth of the utricle. The (*lateral*) *vestibulospinal tract* originates from the lateral vestibular nucleus and descends as uncrossed fibers within the lateral tegmentum of the medulla and throughout the entire length of the spinal cord within the anterolateral funiculus. The fibers of this somatotopically organized tract originating in the rostroventral lateral vestibular nucleus terminate in the cervical levels; those originating in the dorsocaudal part of the nucleus terminate in the lumbosacral levels; and those originating in the intermediate part terminate in the thoracic levels. The fibers synapse primarily with interneurons of lamina VIII and the medial part of lamina VII, although a few terminate directly on lower motor neurons in lamina IX. The descending influences of this tract act by facilitating spinal reflex activity and extensor muscle tone in the ipsilateral extremities. The amount of inhibitory activity on flexor neurons is insignificant. The role of vestibular influences upon equilibrium and posture is expressed by the numerous fibers which terminate in the cervical levels (musculature of the neck and upper extremities) and in the lumbosacral levels (musculature of the lower extremities).

The *medial vestibular nucleus* gives rise to fibers (sometimes called the *medial vestibulospinal tract*) which descend ipsilaterally within the MLF primarily to cervical levels. These fibers terminate as do those of the vestibulospinal tract, in lamina VIII and adjacent portions of lamina VII. These fibers exert inhibitory influences upon extensor muscle tone. There may be a reciprocal innervation by both vestibulospinal pathways upon the same alpha motor neurons to the neck musculature. In one respect these fibers from the medial vestibular nucleus are unusual; they are the only supraspinal descending fibers known to exert inhibitory effects directly upon alpha motor neurons.

The *reticulospinal pathways* include the descending fibers whose nuclei of origin are tegmental nuclei of the brainstem reticular formation (Figs. 5-12, 5-27, 5-28, 5-30). The *pontine (medial) reticulospinal tract* originates in the medial pontine tegmentum from the *nucleus reticularis pontis oralis* (located in the rostral pons) and the *nucleus reticularis pontis caudalis* (located in the caudal pons). It descends primarily as an uncrossed tract in the vicinity of the MLF in the brainstem and within the anterior funiculus throughout the entire spinal cord. The fibers terminate upon interneurons in lamina VIII and adjacent portions of laminae VII and IX. Some of its fibers decussate in the anterior white commissure. The *medullary (lateral) reticulospinal tract* originates from the *nucleus reticularis gigantocellularis*, located in the medial reticular formation of the rostral medulla. It descends as an uncrossed tract, with some crossed fibers, within the anterior aspect of the lateral funiculus throughout the entire spinal cord. The fibers terminate upon interneurons in lateral lamina VII and adjacent parts of laminae VI and IX.

The input to these pontine and medullary reticular nuclei is largely derived from *1* descending corticoreticular fibers from the pre- and postcentral gyri (motor, premotor, and somesthetic cortex), and *2 spinoreticular fibers* from the spinal cord. The descending fibers are distributed bilaterally, but most of them terminate contralaterally in the lower brainstem tegmentum. These *corticoreticulospinal tracts* are not somatotopically organized; they apparently exert their influences through interneurons upon the gamma motor neurons. The medial reticulospinal fibers terminate in the same neuronal pool as the vestibulospinal fibers, while the lateral reticulospinal fibers terminate in

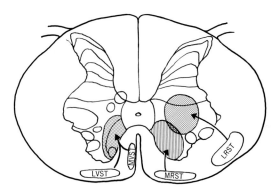

FIGURE 5-30

The location of some major descending (motor) tracts within the white matter and their sites of termination within the gray matter.

MRST, pontine (medial) reticulospinal tract; MVST, "medial" vestibulospinal tract; LRST, medullary (lateral) reticulospinal tract; LVST, "lateral" vestibulospinal tract. (*From Noback and Harting, Spinal Cord, S. Karger, Publisher, Basel,* 1971.)

some of the neuronal pools as the corticospinal and rubrospinal fibers (Figs. 5-29, 5-30).

In general, the reticulospinal tracts convey influences which regulate motor activities related to posture and muscle tone. The medial reticulospinal tract facilitates the extensor myotatic reflex and inhibits the flexor reflex (reciprocal innervation); the lateral reticulospinal tract inhibits the extensor myotatic reflex and facilitates the flexor reflex. Stimulation of the medullary reticular formation generally inhibits myotatic reflexes and muscle tone and movements evoked by cerebral cortical stimulation (*cortically induced movements*). Stimulation of the pontine reticular formation generally produces opposite effects. The reciprocal effects depend primarily upon the organization of the intrinsic circuits within the spinal cord.

MEDIAL LONGITUDINAL FASCICULUS (MLF)

The *medial longitudinal fasciculus* (MLF) is a composite bundle of fibers extending from the upper midbrain (level of the nucleus of the oculomotor nerve) through the spinal cord. It is located in the posteromedial part of the anterior funiculus. The MLF of the lower brainstem and spinal cord is composed of the descending fibers of the tectospinal, interstitiospinal, pontine reticulospinal, and "medial" vestibulospinal fibers.

DESCENDING AUTONOMIC FIBERS

Within the lower brainstem reticular formation are neuronal pools of the autonomic nervous system which receive inputs from the hypothalamus (via the midbrain reticular formation), other levels of the brain, and cranial nerves (Chaps. 6 and 11). From these pontine and medullary pools, influences are relayed via "reticulospinal" fibers to interneurons within the spinal gray matter. These interneurons are in synaptic contact with the preganglionic neurons of the sympathetic system located in levels T1 through L2, and with preganglionic neurons of the parasympathetic system located in levels S2 through S4. The descending spinal autonomic (reticulospinal) fibers are apparently located in the anterior and anterolateral funiculi in close proximity to the spinal gray matter.

DESCENDING SOMATIC INFLUENCES

The descending pathways from the higher centers in the brain probably produce movements *1* by sending "direct" influences to the alpha motor neurons, and *2* by sending "indirect" influences to the gamma motor neurons and thereby acting through a feedback loop from the spindle to produce the desired contraction. Upon stimulation, the central nuclei in the brain have been shown to produce or to inhibit movement; hence the basic generalization that each central nucleus probably is able to excite (or to inhibit) the alpha and gamma motor neurons involved in the same basic contraction in much the same manner. In brief, both alpha and gamma motor nuclei are normally coinfluenced by descending pathways (this is called *"servo-assistance" of movement*). Thus in finger movements and respiratory movements, for example, the essential contraction of a muscle group through the alpha motor neurons

commences just prior to the rise in the spindle firing from gamma stimulation. The latter has facilitated the essential contraction. Stated simply, the descending tracts from the brain convey influences which essentially bias the intrinsic activity of the spinal reflex circuitry.

In general usage, spinal reflexes are basically responses to neural influences conveyed as action potentials from the peripheral receptors. In contrast, voluntary activities are responses to neural influences conveyed as action potentials from the brain to the spinal cord. Voluntary activities need not be initiated by volitional drives. Under natural conditions neurons function in groups; thus a natural stimulus evokes many action potentials, called a volley, which influence the functional activity of a group of physiologically characterized neurons—called a neuronal pool. The inputs to a neuronal pool are expressed as excitatory and inhibitory postsynaptic potentials (EPSPs and IPSPs), whereas the output of reflex and voluntary activity via the lower motor neurons is expressed as obligatory excitatory responses of muscle contractions.

Coactivation The state of contraction of the infrafusal muscles of the neuromuscular spindles and that of the extrafusal muscles are synchronized by the integrated stimulation from the alpha and gamma motor neurons. This coordination is accomplished by the stimultaneous activation of these motor neurons (called *coactivation*) by influences from each of the following: IA fibers from the spindles, IB fibers from the Golgi tendon organs, and some fibers of descending tracts from the brain. The functional role of this alpha-gamma coactivation system in a voluntary movement can be illustrated by the activity initiated by the influences through the corticospinal tract.

In a voluntary movement such as pointing a finger, the impulses in the pyramidal system activate the alpha and gamma motor neuronal complex controlling the finger movements in an approximately synchronous pattern. The alpha motor neurons are stimulated to produce an obligatory contraction of extrafusal muscle fibers. At the same time the gamma motor neurons are stimulated to convey impulses which excite the intrafusal fibers of the spindles to contract. In this way the appropriate gamma loop is activated. The slight time it takes for the influences to travel over the gamma loop means that the resulting alpha motor neuron discharge, generated by the IA fibers from the spindle, occurs just after the extrafusal fibers had commenced to contract following the direct stimulation of the alpha motor neurons by the pyramidal system. Thus the voluntary stimulation of the extrafusal fibers by the corticospinal fibers occurs at the precisely right moment just prior to the onset of the servomechanism control via the gamma loop from the spindle to the extrafusal muscle fibers. In a voluntary movement, therefore, the pyramidal influences excite the initial contraction of the extrafusal fibers just prior to a close follow-up from the excitatory stimulation from the gamma loop. The automatic adjustments at the spinal level associated with voluntary movements are further regulated by influences conveyed from the spindles and Golgi tendon organs via the IA and IB fibers. In turn these fibers can coactivate both the alpha and gamma motor neurons.

Other descending tracts of unknown significance have been described. For example, the inferior olivary nucleus of the medulla may project some fibers to the cervical segments as the olivospinal tract. The descending pathways terminate in different zones in any spinal level: the corticospinal tract and rubrospinal tract to the base of the posterior horn and adjacent intermediate gray; tectospinal tract to the lateral aspect of the anterior horn; and reticulospinal tracts and vestibulospinal tract to the medial aspect of the anterior horn.

The influences of the descending tracts are upon the reflex arcs of the spinal cord. The spinal reflex arcs contain the basic substrates for trunk and extremity movements essential to walking and running. In addition to their function of modifying and coordinating the spinal reflexes, the descending pathways are crucial to the ability to stand; a *"spinal man"* is unable to stand (see "Paraplegia," farther on in this chapter). This is the basis of the statement that a spinal man (or animal) could walk or run, if he could stand unsupported.

Blood supply of the spinal cord

The adult spinal cord derives its arterial supply from a variable number of small spinal arteries

which are branches of larger arteries just outside the vertebral column. These larger arteries include the *vertebral, ascending cervical, deep cervical, intercostal,* and *lumbar* and *sacral arteries.* The small spinal arteries travel along with the spinal nerves, pass through the intervertebral foramina, penetrate through the dura mater, and divide into the *dorsal and ventral radicular arteries,* which accompany the corresponding nerve roots. There is a great deal of variation in the number of large and small radicular arteries. Generally the anterior radicular arteries are larger than the posterior radicular arteries. The number of larger radicular arteries on both sides ranges from 15 to 34 in man (average 24).

These arteries form three main longitudinal channels along the entire spinal cord: an *anterior spinal artery (anterior longitudinal arterial channel)* at the anterior median fissure, and a pair of *posterior spinal arteries (posterior longitudinal arterial channels)* adjacent to the entering dorsal spinal rootlets. An anastomotic network of branches from the anterior and posterior spinal arteries, called the *arterial vasocorona,* is located on the anterior and lateral surface of the spinal cord. Branches from the vertebral arteries supply most of the cervical spinal segments; these include the anterior spinal, posterior spinal, and inferior cerebellar arteries (Chap. 1). The *ascending and deep cervical arteries* give rise to the radicular arteries to spinal segments C7 to T2. The spinal cord levels caudal to T2 derive their blood supply from branches of the *aorta* and *internal iliac arteries.* The *anterior and posterior spinal arteries* arise from the intracranial portion of the vertebral arteries. These arteries supply part of the lower medulla and upper cervical spinal segments. The posterior spinal arteries descend and join the posterior longitudinal arterial channels. The anterior spinal arteries join on the anterior median surface of the medulla (Fig. 5-31) to form the unpaired spinal artery, which descends to join the anterior longitudinal arterial channel of the spinal cord.

Each segment of the spinal cord is supplied by the *anterior spinal artery* (and its branches, the sulcocommissural arteries), the paired *pos-*

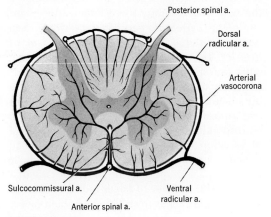

FIGURE 5-31
The arterial supply of the spinal cord.

terior spinal arteries, and surface branches of these arteries, comprising the *arterial vasocorona.* The *sulcocommissural branches* supply the anterior two-thirds of the cord, except for the peripheral portions of the anterior and lateral funiculi, which are supplied by the arterial vasocorona. The posterior spinal arteries supply the rest of the spinal cord—the posterior funiculi and most of the anterior horn. Because anastomoses among arteries within the spinal cord do not occur, except at the capillary level, the arteries in the gray matter are end arteries. The interconnections among the arterial beds of the arterial vasocorona and the anterior and posterior spinal arteries are relatively weak, and blood may not be readily shunted from one bed to the other. Thus in some spinal levels, the arterial vasocorona may not act as efficient safety valves against a reduced blood flow in either of the other true vascular beds.

Certain levels of the spinal cord, especially those in a zone between two regions deriving their blood supply from different major arteries, have sparse collateral circulatory anastomoses. These levels are vulnerable to vascular injury, i.e., *ischemic necrosis,* which may result in a transection of the cord. C2 to C3, T1 to T4, and L1 are considered to be such vulnerable levels (Fig. 5-32).

The distribution of the veins of the spinal cord is similar to that of the spinal arteries. They course along with the arteries and drain outward via the dorsal and ventral roots into the massive *internal vertebral venous plexus (spinovertebral venous plexus, epidural venous plexus)* located between the dura mater and the periosteum of the vertebral column. There are about 6 to 11 large anterior radicular veins and roughly an equal number of posterior radicular veins. This valve-free venous plexus has rich and ample connections with the azygous vein and other veins of the thoracic, abdominal, and pelvic cavities.

Functional and applied considerations

Some functional aspects of the spinal cord are emphasized in the following illustrations (Fig. 5-33).

AFFERENT CORRELATIONS

Dorsal roots and posterior columns The irritation of the fibers of one *dorsal root (radix)* by mechanical compression (by a slipped disk or extramedullary tumor) or a local inflammation may produce pain with a *radicular distribution* over the entire *dermatome* (Fig. 5-33). In herpes zoster (shingles) there is either a spontaneous severe, intense pain, or a pain readily evoked by touch or pressure on one or more dermatomes. This pain is a consequence of the varicella zoster virus, which primarily affects one or more spinal ganglia. Because adjacent dermatomes overlap, the destruction of but one dorsal root (e.g., by transection, called rhizotomy) results in a diminution of all sensations (hypesthesia) in that part of the dermatome innervated by the dorsal root. Destruction of several consecutive dorsal roots results in the complete absence of all sensations (anesthesia) in all but the rostral and caudal dermatomes of the roots sectioned. Irritation to the dorsal root fibers may result in paresthesia (abnormal spontaneous sensations such as numbness and prickling) or hyperesthesia (excessive sensibility to sensory stimuli in pain). The stimulation of a dorsal root may result in a dermatomal vasodilatation (due to the reflex arc involving the autonomic nervous system).

If a limb is completely deafferented, it is generally not used. For example, if all the dorsal roots innervating the upper extremity are sectioned (C5 through T1), the upper extremity is completely anesthetic (i.e., there is a complete absence of all forms of sensibility because of the lack of input). Because the afferent limbs of the reflex arcs are interrupted, reflex activity is absent (areflexia) and the muscles lack tone (i.e., they are hypotonic or atonic). Although the limb muscles are not paralyzed (lower motor neurons are intact), motor activity is impaired. The deafferented limb hangs by the side and is generally not used. The loss of muscle tone illustrates the significance to motor activity of peripheral sensory input from the neuromuscular spindles and Golgi tendon endings. Contraction of muscle is obtained when the volleys from the brain conveyed via upper motor neurons are sufficient to stimulate alpha motor neurons. On the other hand, a limb with only one dorsal root intact may be useful, as, for example, if dorsal root C8 is present but dorsal roots C5 to 6 and 7 and T1 are interrupted. Cervical 8 innervates the skin of the hand and palm. This indicates the importance of the skin sensations from this sensitive region in influencing movements.

A monkey with a completely deafferented limb does not use the limb; in the free situation no purposive movements occur. If the normal limb is restrained, the deafferented limb will make crude movements (e.g., grasp food). A monkey with both upper limbs completely deafferented will use both limbs for climbing the sides of the cage or one limb to grasp food. These actions are due to motivation, attention to body parts, and reinforcement.

Lesions and irritation of the dorsal roots or posterior horn result in segmental (dermatomal) sensory disturbances. In dorsal root lesions all general senses are involved, whereas in posterior horn lesions a *dissociated sensory loss* may occur in the dermatome, with pain and temperature sensibilities lost or reduced, but with touch and other associated general senses intact and normal. Dissociated sensory loss (loss of one sensation and preservation of others) of pain and temperature also occurs with lesions in the vicinity of the central canal (see "Syringomyelia," farther on in this chapter).

The degeneration of the dorsal column neu-

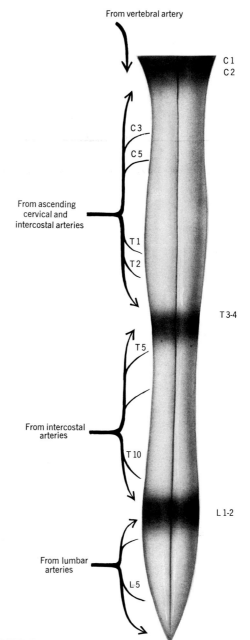

From vertebral artery

C 1
C 2

C 3

C 5

From ascending cervical and intercostal arteries

T 1

T 2

T 3-4

T 5

From intercostal arteries

T 10

L 1-2

From lumbar arteries

L 5

FIGURE 5-32
The sources of the arterial supply of the spinal cord.

The upper cervical, upper thoracic, and upper lumbar spinal segments are zones located between two regions deriving their blood supply from different major arteries.

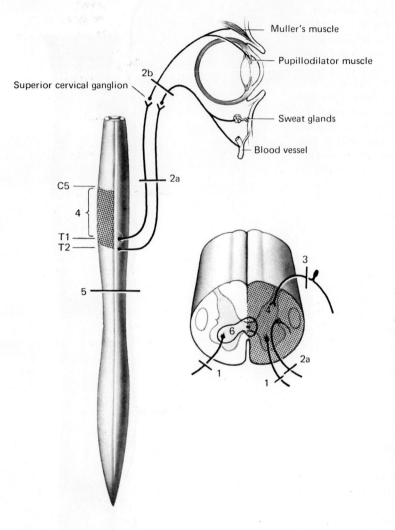

FIGURE 5-33
Some lesions of the spinal nerves and spinal cord.

Lesions discussed are at *1* ventral roots of spinal nerves; *2a* preganglionic sympathetic fibers from T1 and T2 levels; *2b* postganglionic sympathetic fibers from the superior cervical ganglion; *3* posterior roots of spinal nerves; *4* hemisection of the spinal cord (Brown-Séquard syndrome) extending through the cervical enlargement; *5* transection of the spinal cord at a midthoracic level; and *6* region surrounding central canal throughout the cervical enlargement and extending into the anterior horn at the C8 and T1 level on one side. C5 to T1 is the cervical enlargement.

rons of the lumbosacral nerves in the disease *tabes dorsalis* impairs the proprioceptive and discriminative touch pathways. Tabes dorsalis is a consequence of a syphilitic infection of the dorsal roots with secondary degeneration of the posterior columns. General tactile sensibility is retained, but two-point tactile discrimination is lost. A stumbling, staggering gait known as *locomotor ataxia* is characteristic. The motor impairment is a result of a deficiency in proprioceptive input, not in the motor pathways per se. The patient is not fully aware of the location

of his lower extremities; consequently he feels as though he is walking on a floor of soft, downy pillows. His feet slap sharply on the ground with each step. The use of visual cues by looking at his feet helps to compensate for the proprioceptive deficit.

Referred pain Pain of visceral origin is usually vaguely localized on the body surface. The pain may be interpreted as being located on the surface of the body somewhat removed from the primary source. This phenomenon, when visceral pain is subjectively felt in a somatic area, is known as "referred pain." The pain of coronary heart disease (angina pectoris) is referred to the left axilla, where the pain is subjectively felt. Irritation of the gallbladder may actually be felt under the shoulder blade. A stone in the ureter (duct from the kidney) results in an intense pain in the loin and groin.

Several explanations have been advanced to account for the subjective misinterpretation of the source of pain. Because the visceral source-location of the pain and the somatic area where the pain is felt are innervated by neurons utilizing a common dorsal root, the visceral sensory fibers and the somatic sensory fibers are presumed to discharge into a small common pool of neurons in some region of the central nervous system. Discharges from this pool to the cerebrum result in the referral of the pain. The fact that we are normally more continuously aware of somatic sensations than of visceral sensations may be contributory.

Phantom limb An amputee is normally aware of his amputated extremity. This phantom limb moves easily, even through objects or the normal limb. The ring and wristwatch that were formerly worn can be felt on the finger and wrist, respectively. The phantom sensations of pain, pins and needles, aches, and thermal sense are felt by some amputees for many months, even years, following the amputation. Usually the phantom limb seems short, telescoped, embedded in the stump of the limb, or even separated from the stump; the distal segments of the phantom are felt to the exclusion of the proximal segments. The joints are felt more than the interjoint segments. With a limb amputated at the knee, the amputee is more aware of his foot than of his leg; with a limb amputated at the ankle, the amputee is more aware of his toes than of the rest of his foot. The phantom perceptions disappear last in those regions with the largest representation in the cerebral cortex (i.e., the thumb, hand, and foot). Pain may be considerable; the patient often feels that if he could only open his hand, the pain would leave. The neural mechanisms involved in the phantom limb have not been conclusively explained; some of the pain may be psychologically based. By some means, pools of neurons associated with sensory perception of the miss-

ing segments are activated. These pools, perhaps in the thalamus and cortex, are hypersensitive (see "Denervation Hypersensitivity," in Chap. 6) and in an abnormally disturbed state. Irritation of the proximal stump of the peripheral nerve may initiate a series of impulses that trigger these pools of neurons in the central nervous system.

EFFERENT CORRELATIONS

Lower motor neuron paralysis When the lower motor neurons to the voluntary muscles are severed physically or impaired metabolically (poliomyelitis is caused by a neurotropic virus which has a predilection for impairing the function of the lower motor neurons), the voluntary muscles become denervated. A lower motor neuron (flaccid) paralysis results. This paralysis is characterized by muscle weakness and loss of reflexes (areflexia), loss of muscle tone (atony), wasting away of muscle tissues because of the loss of the trophic influences of the nerve (atrophy), lack of resistance to passive movement (movement produced by another source, another person), and prolonged chronaxie. Fasciculations (muscle spasms) are exhibited by the denervated muscles. These spasms are probably due to denervation sensitivity (see Chap. 6) to trace amounts of acetylcholine or some unknown chemical substance. If only a percentage of the muscle fibers of a muscle mass is denervated, the reflexes are weaker (hyporeflexia), the tone is reduced (hypotonia), and the atrophy is less pronounced.

Upper motor neuron paralysis When the descending motor tracts on one side of a segment of the spinal cord are interrupted, a paralysis known as an *upper motor neuron (spastic) paralysis* results in the body segments innervated by spinal segments below the level of the lesion. Many clinicians equate the upper motor neuron with the corticospinal pathway; hence the common conception that the signs exhibited in an upper motor neuron paralysis are due to the lesion of the corticospinal tract. This is not correct, because confirmed lesions limited to the corticospinal tract do not produce all the upper motor neuron signs. Thus the interruption of the fibers of the corticospinal system and portions of other descending systems are necessary to produce the classical upper motor neuron paralysis.

Immediately after the occurrence of the lesion, the deep tendon reflexes are temporarily depressed (*areflexia*) and the paralyzed muscles are flaccid. In time, weeks and months later, the muscles become *spastic*, i.e., *increased muscle tone* (*hypertonus*), *increased deep tendon reflexes* (*hyperreflexia*), and other signs are present. In upper motor neuron paralysis, *spasticity* is associated with hypertonicity of the antigravity muscles. Hence an upper motor neuron paralysis is called a *spastic paralysis*. Hypertonus and muscle weakness are significant features of a spastic paralysis. Such a paralysis of the upper and lower extremities on one side is called a *hemiplegia*.

Several weeks or months after the lesion occurs, an upper motor neuron paralysis is characterized by a *paresis* (the impairment of motor function, partial paralysis with incomplete loss of muscle power) or *paralysis* (loss of motor function), hyperactive deep tendon reflexes (hyperreflexia), increase in muscle tone (hypertonus), clonus, increased resistance to passive movement and clasp-knife (jackknife) response, loss or diminution of cutaneous or superficial reflexes, positive Babinski reflex, and disuse atrophy. The *brisk knee jerk* (*hyperactive myotatic reflexes*) following the tapping of the quadriceps tendon is an example of hyperreflexia. *Hypertonus* is expressed in the firmness and stiffness primarily, but not exclusively, of the flexors in the upper extremity and in the extensors in the lower extremity. Apparently the stronger groups of muscles in each limb predominate. The more powerful muscle groups are the antigravity muscles, because they help the body oppose gravity—the extended lower extremity supports the body during standing, and the flexed upper extremity elevates the limb. The spasticity is primarily due to an increase in gamma motor neuron activity, and the increased sensitivity of the neuromuscular spindles to the stretch of the antigravity muscles. Gravitational forces act as a trigger to sustain hypertonus or spasticity. Apparently the loss of certain inhibitory upper motor neuron influences sets the stage.

Clonus is the rhythmic oscillation of a joint (e.g., ankle or knee) which occurs when a second party suddenly dorsiflexes the foot (pressure on the sole of the foot pushes toes toward the knee) and maintains the dorsiflexion under elastic pressure. The dorsiflexion actually puts the gastrocnemius muscle and its Achilles tendon under moderate stretch. The stretched neuromuscular spindles fire, and the activated myotatic reflex results in contraction of the gastrocnemius and plantar flexion (extension) of the ankle. The plantar flexion produces a stretch of its antagonist, the anterior tibialis muscle; its sensitive neuromuscular spindles activate a myotatic reflex which produces a contraction of the anterior tibialis muscle and dorsiflexion of the ankle. The dorsiflexion of the ankle produced by the contraction of the anterior tibialis muscle and the elastic pressure produced by the second party maintain the cycle of the rhythmic oscillation. Clonus is actually a self-perpetuating rhythmic series of myotatic reflexes. It persists as long as a muscle agonist is kept under a moderate state of stretch. Clonus ceases as soon as the state of stretch ceases.

The *increased resistance to passive movement* and the *"clasp-knife response"* are expressed as follows: When a second party attempts to extend the elbow by applying pressure on the palmar side of the hand, the spastic flexors of the elbow resist stretch. At the beginning of the action the resistance is strong; if the pressure on the hand is maintained, the resistance yields suddenly, in a clasp-knife (jackknife) fashion. When the tension stretches the biceps muscle to a certain point, the Golgi tendon endings suddenly commence to fire; their inhibitory influences act upon the unstable positive-feedback situation, maintaining the spasticity by inhibiting the hyperreflexia; hence the marked sudden shift in the passive resistance of the clasp-knife reflex. This so-called *inverse myotatic reflex* is a consequence of the activity of the Golgi tendon endings triggered by the lengthening of certain muscles involved in the movement (*lengthening reaction, autogenic inhibition*). The characteristic of Golgi tendon endings to fire inhibitory influences into neuronal pools has been regarded as a safety device to prevent a muscle from being damaged by excessive externally applied forces.

The *loss or diminution of the cutaneous reflexes* is difficult to explain on a neuronal basis. Stimulation of the skin of the thorax, abdomen, or extremities evokes weak or no reflex response—these are all disynaptic and multisynaptic reflexes. The *Babinski reflex (sign)* accompanies an upper motor neuron paralysis. When the lateral aspect of the sole of the foot is stroked with a blunt point, the big toe dorsiflexes (hyperextension), the tip of the toe points to the knee, and the other toes spread (fan). This reflex can be elicited in the newborn infant and baby during the first months after birth. Atrophy of these innervated muscles occurs because of disuse, hence it is called *disuse atrophy.* Passive exercise of the muscle is helpful in delaying disuse atrophy.

Several additional explanations have been suggested to account for some of the signs associated with upper motor neuron paralysis. All may be contributory. The spinal cord below the lesions retains its basic intrinsic neural circuits. These circuits have been deprived of many of the excitatory and inhibitory influences from the brain. In one interpretation, the basic intrinsic circuits are released more from the inhibitory influences than from the excitatory influences derived from supraspinal levels. Greater release from inhibition than from excitation may account for the hyperactivity. Denervation sensitivity (Chap. 6) and collateral regeneration (Chap. 2) of more nerve fibers have been proposed as explanations. In fact, the central mechanisms accounting for spasticity are not fully known.

Hemisection of the spinal cord
(Brown-Séquard Syndrome)

A hemisection (unilateral transverse lesion) of the spinal cord damages structures, which results in a number of changes in the body at, and below, the levels caudal to the lesion (Fig. 5-33). For instructional purposes, assume that the lesion is a hemisection extending from spinal levels C5 through T1; the peripheral nerves associated with these spinal levels innervate the upper extremities.

In relating the side of a lesion (right or left) in the nervous system to the side of the body where signs are expressed, one must relate the site of the pathway's crossing over to the location of the lesion. Symptoms occur on the same side (ipsilateral) and below the level of the lesion when the damaged neurons are those which normally convey influences from the same side of the body (ascending sensory tract) or to the same side of the body (descending motor tracts). In the spinal cord, structures involved with ipsilateral functional roles include the posterior columns, dorsal roots, lateral corticospinal tract (and other upper motor neurons), and ventral roots. Symptoms occur on the opposite (contralateral) side below the level of the lesion when the damaged neurons convey information from or to the opposite side of the body. In the spinal cord, this includes the decussated fibers of the lateral and anterior spinothalamic tract. In the brain, this includes the spinothalamic tract, medial lemniscus, and corticospinal tract. The fiber tracts injured and resultant symptoms and signs include:

1 Posterior column (fasciculi gracilis and cuneatus). Loss of position sense, appreciation of passive movement, vibratory sense, and two-point discrimination on the same side at and below the spinal levels of the lesion. The modalities from the neck are unaffected because the fibers conveying them are located wholly above the level of the lesion.

2 Lateral spinothalamic tract. Loss of pain and temperature on the opposite side at and below the spinal levels of the lesion. This includes the contralateral upper extremity, because lateral spinothalamic fibers decussate within one or two levels of the spinal root origin.

3 Anterior spinothalamic tract. Tactile sensibility is probably little affected on the opposite side below the spinal level of the lesion because this modality is also conveyed in the uncrossed fasciculi gracilis and cuneatus.

4 Corticospinal tracts and other descending supraspinal tracts. The spastic syndrome following the interruption of these fibers results in an upper motor neuron paralysis including spasticity, hyperactive deep tendon reflexes (*DTRs, hyperreflexia*), diminution or loss of superficial reflexes, Babinski sign, and muscle clonus below (but not at the level of) the site of lesion on the ipsilateral side. The hyperactive DTRs are illustrated by a brisk knee jerk.

5 At the spinal levels of the transection (C5 through T1), the entering fibers of the dorsal roots and the emerging fibers of the lower motor neurons and preganglionic sympathetic fibers (C8 and T1) are interrupted. The result is the complete absence of all sensations in the upper extremity on the lesion side and loss of pain and temperature on the contralateral upper extremity. Paresthesias and radicular pain may be sensed over the ipsilateral C5 and T1 dermatomes from the irritation of some intact dorsal root fibers; because of dermatome overlap from C4 and T2, the C5 and T1 dermatomes have a hypesthesia. The upper ipsilateral limb is flaccid; it exhibits all the signs of a lower motor neuron paralysis. Horner's syndrome on the ipsilateral side of the face and trophic changes in the ipsilateral upper extremity are due to the interruption of the preganglionic sympathetic neurons.

Amyotrophic lateral sclerosis

Amyotrophic lateral sclerosis is a degenerative motor tract disease with bilateral involvement of the pyramidal tracts and anterior horns; there is degeneration of both upper and lower motor neurons. Most of the affected muscles show evidence of the degeneration of lower motor neurons, including paralysis, atrophy, fasciculations, and weakness; these signs are initially expressed by the muscles of the hands and arms. Some muscles exhibit signs of upper motor neuron paralysis, hyperreflexia, and, at times, Babinski signs. The lower motor neurons of cranial nerves may also exhibit signs of degeneration.

Combined system disease

Combined system disease is a complication of pernicious anemia—lack of intrinsic factor for the absorption of vitamin B_{12}—in which there is a subacute degeneration bilaterally of the fibers of the posterior columns and lateral columns, especially those involved with the lumbosacral cord. The clinical symptoms include *1* loss of position and vibratory senses, numbness and dysesthesias in the lower extremities, and *2* such upper motor neuron signs as spasticity, muscle weakness, hyperactive deep tendon reflexes, and Babinski reflexes.

Transection of sympathetic fibers to the head

Lesion of preganglionic sympathetic fibers in the ventral roots of T1 and T2, the cervical sympathetic trunk, or of the postganglionic sympathetic neurons of the superior cervical ganglion (see Chap. 6) will result in *Horner's syndrome* on the ipsilateral side of the face (Fig. 5-33). The affected pupil is smaller than the pupil of the opposite eye; it does not dilate when the pupil is shaded (pupillodilator muscle unit is not stimulated to contract). The affected eyelid droops a bit (ptosis) because the superior palpebral smooth muscle (Muller's muscle) is denervated. The face is dry (denervated sweat glands), red, and warm (vasodilatation of cutaneous blood vessels). In man, Horner's syndrome regresses because of denervation hypersensitivity (Chap. 6).

Syringomyelia

A syrinx (cavity) may develop in the region of the central canal of the cervical enlargement; from there the gliosis and cavitation may extend to other sites (Fig. 5-33). The initial clinical signs are the loss of pain and temperature sensibility with a bilateral segmental distribution in both upper extremities. This dissociated sensory loss is due to the interruption of the decussating lateral spinothalamic fibers in the anterior white commissure. There is no sensory loss in the body and lower extremities because the spinothalamic tracts and posterior columns are intact. The extension of the degeneration into the anterior horn (lower motor neurons) results in a lower motor neuron paralysis.

Paraplegia

Paraplegia is the condition in which both lower extremities are paralyzed; *quadriplegia (tetraplegia)* is the paralysis of all four extremities. The paralysis of the upper and lower extremity on one side is called *hemiplegia.*

Paraplegia is a direct consequence of a complete transection of the spinal cord. Several aspects of this condition in a man who has had a midthoracic transection are outlined. Immediately after the complete transection of the spinal cord, the body innervated by spinal segments caudal to the lesion site is devoid of detectable neural activity. All voluntary movements and somatic and visceral reflex activities are abolished. During the first month or so following the trauma, several symptoms are noted below the level of the lesion: loss of all sensations, loss of all reflex activities, bilateral flaccid paralysis of the lower extremities, visceral deficits such as loss of thermoregulatory control (dry, cool skin with no sweating), loss of voluntary control of a spastic urinary bladder, and loss in sexual potency. Tidal drainage of the urinary bladder must be maintained to prevent retention of urine. This extremely depressed neural activity, called *spinal shock,* usually lasts about 2 to 3 weeks in man though the period varies from 4 days to 6 weeks. Spinal shock is apparently due to the sudden withdrawal of influences from the descending excitatory supraspinal regions, especially from the corticospinal tracts. Experimentally, spinal shock occurs at the moment of complete transection.

In time, the intrinsic spinal cord circuits become active. The isolated spinal cord and its spinal nerves gradually exhibit autonomous neural activity, which is divided into a sequence of phases of variable lengths: *1* minimal reflex activity, *2* flexor spasm activity (superficial reflexes), *3* alternation between flexor and extensor spasm activities, and *4* predominant extensor spasm activity (deep reflexes). Some symptoms are retained, while others are altered, until a stabilized condition is reached within a year or so. No sensations, no voluntary control of motor activities, and no thermoregulatory mechanisms can ever be elicited below the transection site. The muscular reflex activities are modified with the return of muscle tone and flexor reflex activities. A slight pinprick on the foot, for example, may initiate a mass withdrawal of the entire lower extremity by the *triple reflex*—flexion at the hip, knee, and ankle. This response is considered to be an expression of the protective primitive withdrawal of the limb from noxious stimuli, even though no sensation is felt. Later, extensor activities become more marked, until some spasticity may occur. At times the body weight may be supported in a transitory manner by the extended lower extremity, but the patient cannot stand on his own without support. After a year or two, the paraplegic patient will be in one of several conditions: *1 paraplegia-in-extension,* in which extensor spasms predominate over flexor spasms (observed in about two-thirds of paraplegics); *2 paraplegia-in-flexion,* in which flexor spasms predominate; *3* flaccid paralysis (occurring in fewer than 20 percent). The basic reason why the paraplegic subject cannot stand or walk is that the extensor monosynaptic reflexes are depressed; adequate extensor reflex activity is essential to maintain the upright posture for standing or walking. The excitatory influences from the upper motor neurons are apparently necessary to facilitate the subliminal excitatory influences from the neuromuscular spindles; otherwise our lower extremities cannot support our weight. In theory, the brain projects neural influences which bias and facilitate the basic activity of the intrinsic circuits of the spinal cord.

The urinary bladder may be evacuated by reflex activity (reflex bladder) but is not under voluntary control. The absence of influences from the higher centers of the autonomic nervous system in the brain results in a variety of disturbances in the control of the autonomic activity in the urinary, genital, and anorectal systems. A spinal tap may induce *spinal reflex sweating*—this may be a phenomenon related to denervation sensitivity. Similarly, sweating may be associated with anxiety (e.g., as a consequence of the insertion of a hypodermic needle).

Bibliography

Brodal, A.: *Neurological Anatomy in Relation to Clinical Medicine.* Oxford University Press, New York and London, 1969.

Chambers, W. W., C. N. Liu, G. P. McCouch, and E. D'Aquli: Descending tracts and spinal shock in the cat. Brain, 89:377–390, 1966.

Gilman, S., and L. A. Marco: Effects of medullary pyramidotomy in the monkey. Brain, 94:495–514, 1971.

Ha, H., and C. N. Liu: Organization of the spino-cervico-thalamic system. J. Comp. Neurol., 127:445–470, 1966.

Iggo, A. (ed.): Somatosensory system, in *Handbook of Sensory Physiology,* vol. II, pp. 1–851. Springer-Verlag, Berlin and New York, 1973.

Matthews, P. B. C.: *Mammalian Muscle Receptors and Their Central Actions.* The Williams & Wilkins Company, Baltimore, 1972.

Melzack, R., and P. D. Wall: Pain mechanisms, a new theory. Science, 150:971–979, 1965.

Noordenbos, W.: Some aspects of anatomy and physiology of pain, in R. S. Knighton and P. R. Dumke (eds.), *Pain,* pp. 249–254. Little, Brown and Company, Boston, 1966.

Nyberg-Hansen, R.: Functional organization of descending supraspinal fibre systems to the spinal cord. Ergeb. Anat. Entwicklungsgesch., 39:1–48, 1966.

Oscarsson, O.: Functional organization of spinocerebellar paths, in A. Iggo (ed.), *Handbook of Sensory Physiology,* vol. II, pp. 339–380. Springer-Verlag, Heidelberg, 1973.

Pubols, B. H., and L. M. Pubols: Forelimb, hindlimb and tail dermatomes in the spider monkey (*Ateles*). Brain, Behav. Evol., 2:132–159, 1968.

Ralston, H. J., III: Dorsal root projections to the dorsal horn neurons in the cat spinal cord. J. Comp. Neurol., 132:303–330, 1968.

Rexed, B.: A cytoarchitectonic atlas of the spinal cord in the cat. J. Comp. Neurol., 100:297–380, 1954.

Scheibel, M. E., and A. B. Scheibel: Spinal motoneurons, interneurons and Renshaw cells: A Golgi study. Arch. Ital. Biol., 104:328–353, 1966.

Shriver, J. E., B. M. Stein, and M. B. Carpenter: Central projections of spinal dorsal roots in the monkey. Am. J. Anat., 123:27–74, 1968.

Sinclair, D. C.: *Cutaneous Sensation.* Oxford University Press, London, 1967.

Swanson, A. G., G. C. Buchan, and E. C. Alvord: Anatomic changes in congenital insensitivity to pain. Arch. Neurol., 12:12–18, 1965.

CHAPTER **6**
THE AUTONOMIC
NERVOUS SYSTEM

The regulation of the internal environment

The autonomic nervous system is the regulator, adjuster, and coordinator of vital visceral activities, including digestion, body temperature control, blood pressure, and many expressive facets of emotional behavior. Many of the activities are mediated below the conscious level or are recognized by the mind in a vague way. Synonyms for this system reflect these functional expressions: *involuntary nervous system, vegetative nervous system,* and *general visceral efferent system.*

The primary function of the autonomic nervous system is to help maintain a stable internal environment, or *milieu interne,* in the body against those forces that tend to alter it. The concept expressing the maintenance of the steady state of the internal environment is that of *homeostasis.* It is a form of negative feedback (Chap. 3) and represents the equilibrium level of activity. For example, a relatively constant body temperature is critical for the survival of warm-blooded animals. Compensatory thermostatic mechanisms are constantly operating to adjust and to prevent excessive fluctuations of this temperature. Heat is produced by such metabolic activities as the oxidation of glucose, active muscular movements, and shivering; it is conserved by the constriction of the skin blood vessels (to reduce loss by radiation); and it is dissipated by perspiration and dilatation of skin blood vessels.

Blushing, pallor, palpitations of the heart, clammy hands, and dry mouth are several emotional expressions mediated through the autonomic nervous system.

The concept of the autonomic nervous system

The autonomic nervous system is represented in both the central nervous system and the peripheral nervous system. Classically the autonomic nervous system is defined as the motor (efferent) system innervating visceral organs; hence it is called the "general visceral efferent system." In this traditional view, both the somatic and visceral afferent (sensory) systems act as the input arm of the reflex arcs, utilizing the general visceral efferent system as an output channel.

A more inclusive view broadens the older definition so that the autonomic nervous system includes both the general visceral afferent and the general visceral efferent systems. Both definitions are used and are valid.

The visceral nervous system and the somatic nervous system—
some interactions, differences, and similarities

Although the nervous system is conceptually divided into the visceral nervous system and the somatic nervous system, the two divisions are not mutually exclusive. Many neural activities are the product of interactions between these two divisions. For example, the somatic sensory input from "light," conveyed via the optic pathways, may be expressed via the visceral motor system by the dilation or constriction of the pupil of the eye, and via the somatic motor system by the movements of the eye or of the head and body. The sensory input from visceral

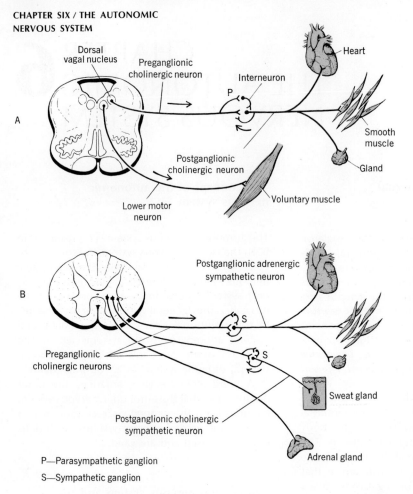

Dorsal
vagal nucleus

Preganglionic
cholinergic neuron

Interneuron

Heart

A

P

Smooth
muscle

Gland

Postganglionic
cholinergic neuron

Lower motor
neuron

Voluntary muscle

B

Postganglionic adrenergic
sympathetic neuron

S

S

Preganglionic
cholinergic neurons

Sweat gland

Postganglionic cholinergic
sympathetic neuron

Adrenal gland

P—Parasympathetic ganglion

S—Sympathetic ganglion

FIGURE 6-1
Motor innervation to the
peripheral effectors.

A The parasympathetic outflow from the medulla innervates the heart, smooth muscle, and glands. The lower
motor neuron innervates a
voluntary muscle.

B Sympathetic outflow from
the spinal cord innervates the
heart, smooth muscle, and
glands. See text for discussion
of the various types of neurons.

receptors within the body may be expressed
1 via the somatic motor system, as the respiratory rhythms of voluntary muscles, and *2* via
the visceral motor system, as adjustments in the
rate and force of the heartbeat. The response
to cold may be reflected by the visceral motor
system, which stimulates the contraction of involuntary skin muscles (goose pimples), and by
the somatic motor system, which stimulates the
activity of voluntary muscles (shivering). In addition, a variety of influences acts upon the
autonomic nervous system, including pain from
both somatic and visceral sources, memory, and
worry; these may be expressed in the form of
blushing, pallor, sweating, and heart palpitations.

Fundamental differences and similarities between the two systems are expressed in the
anatomy (Fig. 6-1) and the physiology of their
peripheral motor neurons (Table 6-1).

Anatomy Each effector cell influenced by the
autonomic nervous system is innervated by a
sequence of two neurons called, respectively,
the *preganglionic neuron* and the *postganglionic neuron* (Figs. 6-1 through 6-4). Each preganglionic neuron has a cell body (and dendrites)
that is located within the central nervous system; it has a lightly myelinated axon that courses
through the peripheral nerves and terminates by
synapsing with postganglionic neurons. Each
postganglionic neuron has a cell body which is

found in a peripherally located ganglion (i.e., outside the central nervous system) and an unmyelinated axon that terminates at or near an effector cell.

The autonomic nervous system innervates three types of effector cells: the involuntary (smooth) muscle cells, cardiac (heart) muscle cells, and glandular (secretory) cells. In contrast, each effector cell influenced by the somatic motor system is innervated by a neuron with a cell body (and dendrites) located within the central nervous system and with an axon that courses through the peripheral nerves and directly synapses at a motor end plate with a voluntary muscle cell. The somatic motor system innervates only one type of effector cell: a voluntary (striated) muscle cell (including the intrafusal muscle of the neuromuscular spindle). The anatomic relationship of the autonomic nerve terminals with the smooth muscles, cardiac muscles, and glandular cells is unresolved; the terminations do not form identifiable end plates on these target cells. Neurotransmitter chemicals are released from the axon terminals and act upon several effector cells.

The spinal nerves of the somatic system form interjoining branches of relatively simple, proximally located *plexuses* (e.g., cervical, brachial, or lumbosacral plexuses). In contrast, the nerves of the autonomic nervous system form peripherally located plexuses, which are complex networks along blood vessels and associated organs. These *terminal plexuses* include among others the cardiac, pulmonary, mesenteric, and pelvic plexuses.

Physiology The autonomic nervous system acts more slowly than the somatic system. The more slowly conducting fine fibers and the synaptic delay in the autonomic nervous system contrast with the faster-conducting, more heavily myelinated fibers (alpha neurons and gamma neurons, Chap. 5) of the somatic motor nerves. The

TABLE 6-1
Comparison of somatic motor system with the autonomic nervous system

Structure or function	Somatic motor system	Autonomic nervous system
1. Morphologic		
a. Structures innervated	Voluntary (skeletal) muscle	Cardiac and smooth (involuntary) muscles and glands
b. Ganglia outside central nervous system	None	Paravertebral (chain), prevertebral (collateral), and terminal ganglia
c. Neurons from central nervous system to effector	One	Two
d. Fibers	Myelinated lower motor neuron	Preganglionic fibers, myelinated; postganglionic fibers, usually unmyelinated
e. Peripheral plexus	None	Numerous (e.g., aortic, hypogastric plexuses)
2. Functional		
a. Role in periphery	Excitatory	Either excitatory or inhibitory
b. Effect of denervation on effectors	Paralysis and atrophy	Remains functional, little change in automaticity
c. General role	Adjustments with external environment	Adjustments with the internal environment (homeostasis)
3. Neurotransmitter	Acetylcholine	Acetylcholine and norepinephrine

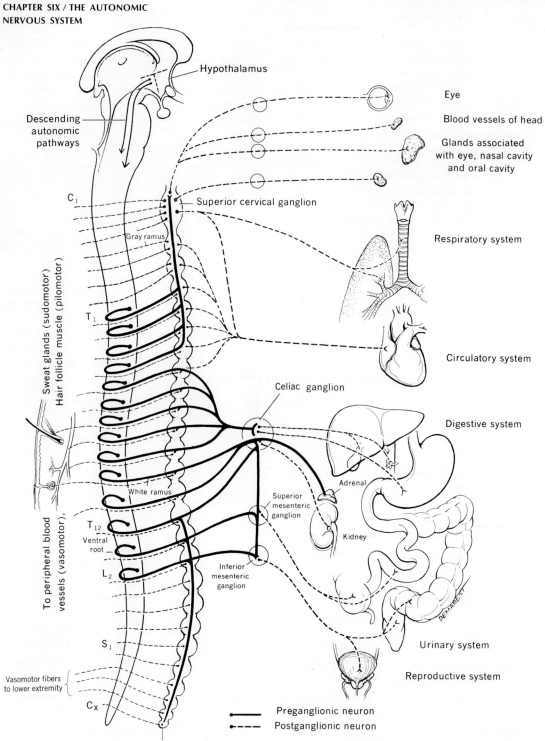

Hypothalamus

Eye

Blood vessels of head

Glands associated
with eye, nasal cavity
and oral cavity

Descending
autonomic
pathways

C_1

Superior cervical ganglion

Gray ramus

Respiratory system

Sweat glands (sudomotor)

Hair follicle muscle (pilomotor)

T_1

Circulatory system

Celiac ganglion

Digestive system

Adrenal

Superior
mesenteric
ganglion

To peripheral blood
vessels (vasomotor),

White ramus

Kidney

T_{12}
Ventral
root

Inferior
mesenteric
ganglion

L_2

Urinary system

S_1

Reproductive system

Vasomotor fibers
to lower extremity

C_x

DEMAREST

——— Preganglionic neuron
–·–·– Postganglionic neuron

Sympathetic trunk

nature of the neurotransmitter substances associated with these two systems is significant. The neurotransmitter substance *acetylcholine* is released at the synaptic junctions between each preganglionic neuron and each postganglionic neuron. *Acetylcholine* is released at each parasympathetic effector junction between a postganglionic neuron and an effector cell, while *norepinephrine* is released at each sympathetic effector junction between a postganglionic neuron and an effector cell (see below). *Acetylcholine* is the chemical mediator released at the myoneural junction (motor end plate) between a somatic motor nerve and a voluntary muscle. A neurotransmitter released by the autonomic nervous system may evoke either an excitatory response or an inhibitory response from an effector (e.g., it may stimulate or inhibit muscle contraction). In the somatic nervous system the neurotransmitter (acetylcholine) always evokes an excitatory response (e.g., obligatory contraction of the muscle).

An effector is not completely dependent on its innervation by the autonomic nervous system. A smooth muscle and a gland express their "functional independence" by not atrophying if deprived of their innervation (see "Denervation Hypersensitivity," at the end of this chapter); they remain functional. In contrast a voluntary muscle is dependent on its somatic motor innervation; in time it atrophies and becomes functionless if deprived of its innervation.

VISCERAL AFFERENT SYSTEM

Influences from the viscera are conveyed via *visceral afferent fibers* to the central nervous system. These fibers are located in the somatic

FIGURE 6-2
The sympathetic (thoracolumbar) division of the autonomic nervous system.

The preganglionic neurons are cholinergic. The postganglionic neurons are adrenergic (see Table 6-3 for cholinergic sympathetic neurons). A preganglionic cholinergic neuron innervates the adrenal medulla. The posterior portion of the hypothalamus is involved with sympathetic activities (Chap. 11). The white rami with their preganglionic fibers are located at spinal levels T1 through L2. The gray rami with their postganglionic fibers are located at all spinal levels.

nerves (e.g., the sciatic nerve) and the visceral plexuses (e.g., cardiac and mesenteric) and nerves (e.g., the vagus and splanchnic). Although some of these afferents are lightly myelinated fibers, most of them are unmyelinated. Those afferent fibers terminating in the spinal cord have their cell bodies in the spinal ganglia, while those coursing in the glossopharyngeal and vagus nerves to the medulla have their cell bodies in the inferior ganglia of these nerves (Chap. 7). One estimate indicates that about four-fifths of the fibers in the vagus nerve are visceral afferent fibers. Influences from the peripheral blood vessels, especially those of voluntary muscles, and from glandular structures in the skin pass via afferent fibers in the somatic nerves.

Apparently these fibers of the afferent limb of a reflex arc of the autonomic nervous system terminate and synapse upon interneurons in the spinal cord. In turn, these interneurons have connections with the preganglionic sympathetic neurons. The visceral afferent fibers do not synapse directly with the preganglionic fibers of the autonomic nervous system.

The visceral afferent fibers are involved with the mediation of *1* visceral sensations, including pain, referred pain, cramps, fullness, and others, *2* vasomotor, respiratory, and viscerosomatic reflexes, and *3* interrelated visceral activities (e.g., digestion and peristalsis). The glossopharyngeal and vagus nerves convey the afferent influences from the chemoreceptors in the carotid and aortic bodies (they monitor O_2 and CO_2 levels of the blood) and the vasopressor receptors in the carotid sinus and the aortic arch (mechanoreceptors) to the medulla. These are involved in the reflex control of heart rate, blood pressure, and respiration.

The sympathetic nervous system and the parasympathetic nervous system

The autonomic nervous system is subdivided into two parts, the sympathetic (orthosympathetic) and the parasympathetic (Figs. 6-2 and 6-3). In general, the *sympathetic system* stimu-

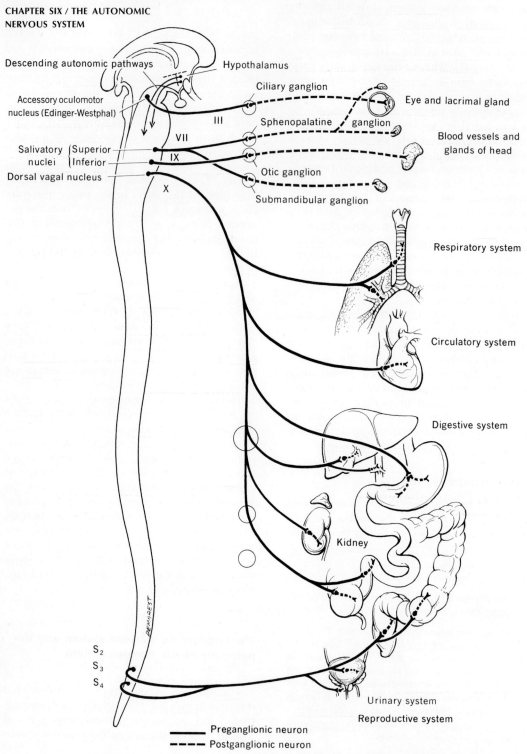

Descending autonomic pathways

Hypothalamus

Ciliary ganglion

Accessory oculomotor
nucleus (Edinger-Westphal)

Eye and lacrimal gland

III

Sphenopalatine ganglion

VII

Blood vessels and
glands of head

Salivatory {Superior
nuclei {Inferior

IX

Dorsal vagal nucleus

Otic ganglion

X

Submandibular ganglion

Respiratory system

Circulatory system

Digestive system

Kidney

S_2
S_3
S_4

Urinary system

Reproductive system

—— Preganglionic neuron
- - - Postganglionic neuron

lates those activities which are most dramatically expressed and *mobilized* during emergency and stress situations—otherwise called the "fight, fright, and flight activities." These reactions are accompanied by the expenditure of energy stores: the acceleration of the rate and force of the heartbeat, increase in the blood pressure, increase in the concentration of blood sugar, and an emphasis on directing the blood flow largely to the voluntary muscles at the expense of flow to the viscera and the skin. Although this system operates at all times in the moment-to-moment adjustments throughout life, it is during stress that it acts with its stops removed.

In contrast, the *parasympathetic system* stimulates those activities that are associated with the conservation and restoration of the energy stores of the organism. The reactions to accomplish these functions are associated with the decrease in the rate and force of the heartbeat, with the decrease in the blood pressure, and with the stimulation of the digestive system to encourage the digestion, movement, and ultimate elimination of ingested food and water.

The two systems integrate their actions and are not antagonistic. In the economy of the body they usually act synergistically, although at times some actions are executed independently. They function in concert to maintain the internal activities of the organism at a level commensurate with the intensity of the stress situation and with the emotional state of the individual (Table 6-2).

SYMPATHETIC (ORTHOSYMPATHETIC) NERVOUS SYSTEM

Anatomy The *sympathetic nervous system* (Fig. 6-1) is also called the *thoracolumbar system* (*thoracolumbar outflow*), because all preganglionic neurons of this system emerge from the spinal cord via the motor roots of all thoracic and the upper two lumbar spinal nerves (T1

FIGURE 6-3
Diagram of the parasympathetic (craniosacral) division of the autonomic nervous system.

The preganglionic and postganglionic neurons are cholinergic. The rostral portion of the hypothalamus is involved with parasympathetic activities (Chap. 11).

through L2). The preganglionic neurons terminate and synapse with postganglionic neurons located either in the paravertebral ganglia (ganglionic chain) or in the prevertebral ganglia. The *paravertebral ganglionic chain* is a series of ganglia located on and along the entire length of the bony vertebral column, extending from the upper cervical to the coccygeal region (Fig. 6-2). Some of the synaptic linkages between the preganglionic neuron and the postganglionic neurons are displaced from the paravertebral ganglion toward the spinal nerve. This displaced linkage is called an intermediate ganglion. When present, these ganglia may escape removal in a paravertebral sympathectomy. They are not reached in a "complete sympathectomy."

The preganglionic neurons projecting from the spinal cord to the paravertebral ganglia pass successively through the ventral roots, spinal nerves, and white rami communicantes (Figs. 6-2 and 6-4). These rami are called white rami because the preganglionic fibers are myelinated. Many fibers ascend or descend through several paravertebral ganglia.

The postganglionic neurons of the paravertebral ganglia reach their effector cells via several routes. Some fibers return to the spinal nerves via the gray rami (gray because the postganglionic fibers are unmyelinated) and are then distributed to smooth muscles (blood vessels, hair follicles) and sweat glands of the skin, extremities, and body wall (Fig. 6-4). Other fibers form small nerves and plexuses around major blood vessels and reach the smaller blood vessels and organs in the head, neck, and thorax (Fig. 6-2).

The preganglionic fibers reach the prevertebral ganglia (located in the abdomen) by passing successively through the ventral root, spinal nerve, white rami, and small nerves terminating in the ganglia (Figs. 6-2 and 6-4). The postganglionic fibers reach their effector cells via perivascular plexuses and are distributed to the blood vessels and organs of the abdomen and pelvis. In general, the sympathetic outflow is distributed as follows: T1 to T4, to the head and neck; T2 to T9, to the upper extremity; T9 to L2, to the lower extremity; C8 and T1 to the eye; T1 to T5, to the heart and lungs; T4 to T9, to the upper abdominal viscera; T10 to T11, to the adrenal gland; and T12 to L2, to the urinary, genital, and lower digestive systems, including the kidney, ovary, testis, and pelvic organs.

Note that the origin and outflow of the preganglionic neurons is restricted to the thoracic and upper two lumbar levels, but that the chain extends the entire length of the vertebral column. The postganglionic neurons projecting from these chain ganglia provide the sympathetic innervation to the visceral muscles and glands of the eye, lungs, heart, and skin and the muscles of the blood vessels of the head, neck, body wall, and extremities.

The *prevertebral (collateral) ganglia* are located in the abdomen in close proximity to the aorta and its major branches, after which the ganglia are named (celiac ganglia, superior mesenteric ganglia, inferior mesenteric ganglion, and others; the celiac ganglia and their associated nerves are known as the solar plexus). These *prevertebral ganglia* receive their innervation from neurons whose cell bodies are located in the lower six thoracic and first two lumbar levels. The postganglionic neurons in these ganglia have axons that terminate distally in association with the smooth muscles and glands of the abdominal and pelvic viscera and their blood vessels, including those of the digestive, urinary, and genital systems. The medulla of the adrenal gland is innervated by preganglionic neurons.

The preganglionic neurons are outnumbered by the postganglionic neurons. Each preganglionic fiber may synapse with as many as 30 or more postganglionic neurons (the postganglionic neurons innervated by one preganglionic neuron may be located in several ganglia—an expression of divergence). In turn, each postganglionic neuron receives synaptic stimulation from many preganglionic neurons—an expression of convergence. The axons of the preganglionic neurons of the sympathetic system are relatively short, while those of the postganglionic neurons are relatively long, with many terminal branches (cf. "Parasympathetic Nervous System," further on).

Sympathetic reflex (Fig. 6-4) The *autonomic visceral reflex arc* comprises a sequence of *1* afferent neuron (general visceral afferent neuron), *2* interneurons within the gray matter, and *3* a sequence of two efferent neurons (a preganglionic general visceral and a postganglionic general visceral neuron). The postganglionic neurons innervate involuntary muscle, cardiac muscle, and glandular cells. The afferent neurons convey influences from visceral structures via somatic and visceral nerves and the dorsal roots to interneurons in the base of the posterior horn. These interneurons interconnect with preganglionic neurons in the intermediolateral nucleus (sympathetic nervous system). The preganglionic neurons course through the ventral root and terminate in sympathetic ganglia with both intraganglionic interneurons and postganglionic neurons. The interneurons are involved with processing within the ganglia.

TABLE 6-2
Biosynthetic pathways of some neurotransmitters

Precursor	Intermediates and enzymes		Neurotransmitter product
L-Tyrosine $\xrightarrow{\text{tyrosine hydroxylase}}$ L-dopa $\xrightarrow{\text{dopa decarboxylase}}$ dopamine $\xrightarrow{\text{dopamine-}\beta\text{ hydroxylase}}$			
	L-norepinephrine $\xrightarrow{\text{phenylethanolamine } N\text{-methyltransferase}}$ epinephrine		
Choline + acetyl CoA $\xrightarrow{\text{choline acetylase}}$ acetylcholine			
L-Tryptophan $\xrightarrow{\text{tryptophan hydroxylase}}$ L-5-hydroxytryptophan $\xrightarrow{\text{5-HTP-decarboxylase}}$ 5-hydroxytryptamine (5-HT, serotonin)			
L-Glutamate $\xrightarrow{\text{glutamate decarboxylase}}$ gamma amino butyric acid (GABA)			

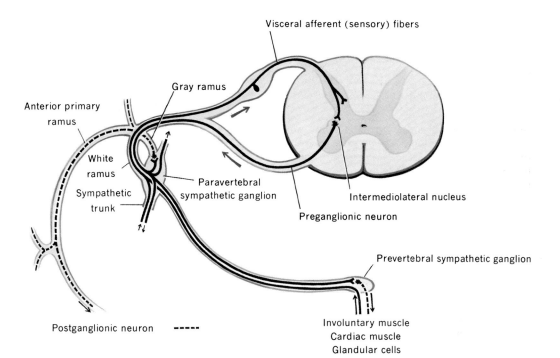

Visceral afferent (sensory) fibers

Gray ramus

Anterior primary ramus

White ramus

Sympathetic trunk

Paravertebral sympathetic ganglion

Intermediolateral nucleus

Preganglionic neuron

Prevertebral sympathetic ganglion

Postganglionic neuron - - - - -

Involuntary muscle
Cardiac muscle
Glandular cells

FIGURE 6-4
A visceral reflex arc of the sympathetic nervous system.

An arc comprises an afferent neuron (general visceral afferent neuron), an interneuron (not illustrated), and a sequence of two efferent neurons (a preganglionic general visceral and a postganglionic general visceral).

Physiology The neurotransmitter mediator at the postganglionic effector junction is norepinephrine (Noradrenaline), one of the catecholamines. Thus the sympathetic system is referred to as an *adrenergic system,* and its postganglionic fibers as *adrenergic fibers,* or *noradrenergic fibers.* Norepinephrine is slowly deactivated in the body. Some postganglionic neurons of the sympathetic nervous system are cholinergic neurons. Postganglionic sympathetic cholinergic fibers innervate *1* some blood vessels in voluntary muscles, and *2* most sweat glands. The sweat glands of the palms are innervated by postganglionic adrenergic fibers.

The sympathetic nervous system is geared to act as a total unit throughout the body for sustained periods of time. Thus the catecholamine effect of the sympathetic nervous system can be widespread and lasting. Anatomic and biochemical factors contribute to this prolonged unit action. Wide distribution and sustained activity result because *1* each preganglionic neuron with a short axon synapses with many postganglionic neurons, each having a long axon with many neuroeffector junctions, and *2* the blood-distributed epinephrine of the adrenal gland [see "Adrenal (Suprarenal) Gland," further on] and the neurotransmitter norepinephrine are largely of adrenergic sympathetic nerve origin and are deactivated slowly.

The sympathetic nervous system is not essential to life, but it is critical for proper reactions to stress and strains. Animals without a sympathetic nervous system or an adrenal medulla can have a "normal" existence if kept in a sheltered environment. Their digestive, cardiovascular, and growth activities are essentially normal. They are sensitive to cold and have a slightly lowered basal metabolic rate. Under stress, such animals do not get excited, cannot adjust their body temperatures properly to heat or cold, and do not raise their blood pressure or their blood sugar levels.

Adrenergic neuron and synapse   Several monamines are regarded as putative neurotransmitters in the nervous system (Table 6-2). Three of these are catecholamines—organic compounds that consist of a catechol nucleus and an amine group. They include dopamine (DA, dihydroxyphenylethylamine), norepinephrine (NE, Noradrenaline), and epinephrine (E, Adrenaline). Another is serotonin, which is an indoleamine called 5-hydroxytryptamine (5-HT). *Dopamine,* a precursor of norepinephrine, is also localized in the substantia nigra, nigrostriatal fibers, and striatum (Chap. 14). *Norepinephrine* is the catecholamine in the postganglionic sympathetic neurons of the autonomic nervous system; it is also found in the noradrenergic neurons of the brain (Chap. 8) and in the adrenal medulla (Chap. 6). *Epinephrine* is present in the adrenal medulla (absent in postganglionic sympathetic neurons). After its release into the circulation, epinephrine acts as a hormone. *Serotonin* is associated with the raphe nuclei of the brainstem (Chap. 8). Because these amines are synthesized in vivo, they are called biogenic amines.

Life cycle of the catecholamines (Table 6-2) Each neurotransmitter has a metabolic cycle which comprises synthesis, storage, combination with receptor sites, and, finally, degradation. The *metabolic cycle of NE,* as demonstrated in the postganglionic sympathetic neurons, is probably similar in the adrenergic neurons of the central nervous system. Each postganglionic sympathetic neuron has axons which terminate by arborizing into many branches with numerous varicosities; there may be as many as 25,000 varicosities per neuron (Figs. 2-5 and 6-5).

The catecholamines are synthesized from the amino acid tyrosine in the following steps: tyrosine → dopa (dihydroxyphenylalanine) →

dopamine → NE. Different enzymes are involved in each of these steps (Table 6-2). The synthesis of NE takes place within the postganglionic sympathetic neurons, in some neurons of the central nervous system (Chap. 8, Fig. 8-17) and in the cells of the adrenal medulla. The epinephrine of the adrenal medulla is formed by the *methylation of NE.* The metabolic cycle of the catecholamines in the cells of the central nervous system is thought to be similar to that described as occurring in postganglionic sympathetic neurons. All enzyme proteins involved in the biosynthesis of the neurotransmitter are formed by the action of the ribosomes of the endoplasmic reticulum in the cell bodies (not in the axons) of the neurons. The rate-limiting step in this biosynthesis is the conversion of tyrosine to dopa by the enzyme tyrosine hydroxylase. A feedback relation exists between NE and tyrosine hydroxylase: when the stores of NE are low, the tyrosine hydroxylase becomes active; when NE stores are high, the reverse occurs. After their formation, the enzymes are transported from the cell body via active transport and axoplasmic flow, or in conjunction with microtubules to the nerve terminals. Tyrosine is taken up from the bloodstream by active transport into the neurons. The synthesis of NE takes place within the cell body and in the varicosities of the axon terminal endings. The dopamine enters the dense-core vesicles, where it is converted to NE. From 90 to 95 percent of the NE is located in the dense-core vesicles (sometimes called storage granules). They are about 500 Å in diameter, with a 280-Å-diameter electron-dense core. These dense-core vesicles may possibly be derived from microtubules. Most vesicles are located in the varicosities. Estimates indicate that there are 1,500 granules per varicosity. The NE is mainly bound with ATP (adenosine triphosphate), in the ratio of 4 NE to 1 ATP. The remaining 5 to 10 percent of NE is located in the axoplasm or on the plasma membrane; some is in a free form unbound to ATP. Some clear vesicles are present in the varicosities.

Some dense-core vesicles may be formed in the soma. Following their synthesis by the ribosomes of the endoplasmic reticulum, the enzymes and other components may be transferred to the Golgi apparatus, where they are enclosed in the membrane-limited vesicles. The NE may be synthesized within the soma or in the axon as the vesicle "flows" somatofugally. Most NE is elaborated in the nerve terminals. These sites of NE formation account for the observation that NE is found in varying amounts throughout the neuron.

Normally small amounts of free NE are released in quantal units into the synaptic cleft. A *quantum* is probably less than the quantity of NE found in one vesicle. The activity of these small amounts on the postsynaptic receptor sites accounts for the miniature graded postsynaptic membrane potentials (equivalent to miniature end plate potentials at the motor end plate of muscles). An action potential at the nerve terminal triggers the influx of some calcium ions into the neuron, which, in turn, triggers, within the nerve ending, the conversion of bound NE to free NE and the release of free NE into the synaptic cleft. The release of NE is dependent on calcium ions. Calcium is essential in the electrosecretory coupling process, i.e., the conversion of the action potential to the "secretion" of the neurotransmitter. One concept states that some synaptic vesicles aggregate near the presynaptic membrane and that, following the action potential, the entire contents of each vesicle is released by exocytosis through a formed opening in plasma membrane into the synaptic cleft. From these events, initiated by the action potential, the many quanta of NE in the synaptic cleft combine with enough receptor sites on the postsynaptic membrane to elicit the formation of an action potential on the postsynaptic neuron (central nervous system) or on the effector.

The released NE within the synaptic cleft has several fates (Fig. 6-5). Some combines with receptor sites on the postsynaptic membrane. Most of the synaptically discharged catecholamines are inactivated by *re-uptake* through active transport into the nerve terminals that had released them. They end up in the synaptic vesicles or in the extragranular pool. Some NE in the cleft diffuses into tissue spaces or is absorbed on inert material.

Two enzymes—*monoamine oxidase (MAO)* and *catechol-O-methyl transferase (COMT)*—are primarily involved in the metabolic degradation of the catecholamines. Monoamine oxidase is considered to be the intraneuronal enzyme, located largely in the outer membrane of the mitochondria or in the axoplasm. It converts catecholamines by deamination to their corre-

sponding aldehydes by acting on the amine group. The MAO probably acts on free NE and dopa and functions to regulate the amount of NE and dopa in the nerve ending; in effect MAO prevents the accumulation or release of an excess amount of NE from the nerve terminal. Catechol-O-methyl transferase is considered to catabolize the NE extracellularly by O-methylation; thus COMT terminates the action of NE liberated into the synaptic cleft. It converts catecholamines by transferring the methyl group from the catechol group. Neither MAO nor COMT is involved in the rapid inactivation of the neurotransmitter.

The catecholamine hypothesis of mood suggests that this group of chemicals has a role in our states of depression, euphoria, and wellbeing. A fall in the catecholamine level in the central nervous system results in a "catecholamine depression." A higher-than-normal central nervous system catecholamine level may result in euphoria. Some antidepressant drugs (e.g., nialamide) are MAO inhibitors which act by inhibiting the degradation of catecholamines. The resulting increase in the amount of catecholamines has an antidepressant role.

Amphetamine (pep pills) has an effect on the NE content in the brain. This drug blocks the re-uptake of NE into the neuron, and, in addition, acts as an MAO inhibitor. This is presumed to be contributory to the euphoria and hallucinations which may follow administration of this drug. Amphetamine abuse from continued use may produce an "amphetamine psychosis," which is virtually indistinguishable from paranoid schizophrenia.

Chlorpromazine has been found to be useful in the treatment of schizophrenia. Chlorpromazine acts by preventing the re-uptake of NE by the nerve ending, and hence by producing more adrenergic activity. Prolonged intake of chlorpromazine may result in Parkinson-like symptoms (Chap. 14).

PARASYMPATHETIC NERVOUS SYSTEM

Anatomy The parasympathetic nervous system (Fig. 6-3) is also called the *craniosacral system (craniosacral outflow)*, because the pregangli-

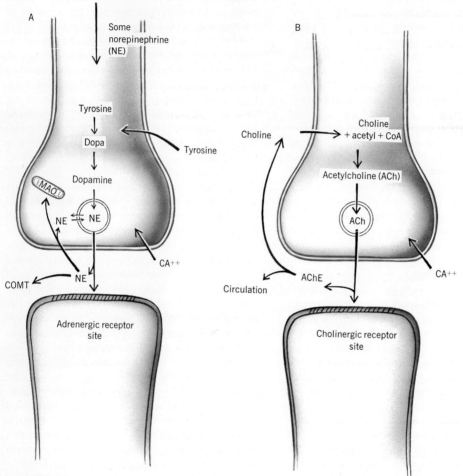

FIGURE 6-5

A The adrenergic synapse, and *B* the cholinergic synapse.

AChE, acetylcholinesterase; CA++, calcium ions; COMT,
catechol-*O*-methyl transferase; MAO, monoamine oxidase. The postsynaptic receptor sites are cross-hatched.

onic neurons of this system leave the brain via
the cranial nerves from the brainstem and leave
the spinal cord via the second through fourth
sacral spinal nerves (S3 through S4). Each preganglionic neuron usually has a long axon that
terminates and synapses with postganglionic
neurons that are close to and located within the
organ to be innervated. Each postganglionic
neuron has a relatively short axon. This is in
contrast to the neurons of the sympathetic
nervous system.

The cranial portion of the parasympathetic
system is associated with *1* four cranial nerves
that supply the parasympathetic innervation to
the head, thoracic viscera, and most of the abdominal viscera, and *2* the sacral spinal cord
that supplies the innervation to the lower abdominal and pelvic viscera (Fig. 6-3).

The third (oculomotor) cranial nerve supplies

the parasympathetic innervation to the eye; this nerve has its preganglionic neurons originating in the accessory oculomotor nucleus (of Edinger-Westphal) in the midbrain, and its postganglionic neurons originating in the ciliary ganglion behind the eye. The seventh (facial) cranial nerve and the ninth (glossopharyngeal) cranial nerve supply the parasympathetic innervation to the glands of the head, including the lacrimal (tear) glands of the eye, glands of the nasal cavities, and the salivary glands of the mouth; these nerves have their preganglionic neurons originating in the salivatory nuclei of the upper medulla and their postganglionic neurons originating in the sphenopalatine ganglion (seventh nerve), the submandibular ganglion (seventh nerve), and the otic ganglion (ninth nerve). The tenth (vagus) cranial nerve supplies the parasympathetic innervation to such organs as the heart, lungs, esophagus, stomach, liver, pancreas, small intestine, upper half of the large intestine, and numerous blood vessels; this nerve has its preganglionic neurons originating in the dorsal vagal nucleus of the medulla and its postganglionic neurons located in or near the visceral organs innervated.

The sacral (pelvic) nerves supply the parasympathetic innervation to the lower half of the large intestine, rectum, urinary system, and genital system, including the uterus and erectile tissues. The preganglionic fibers from the sacral region pass successively through the ventral sacral roots, pelvic spinal nerves, and their plexuses to the effectors (Fig. 6-3). These nerves have their preganglionic neurons originating in the sacral region and their postganglionic neurons located near or within the visceral organs innervated. The blood vessels and other visceral structures of the limbs and the body wall have no direct innervation from the craniosacral outflow.

Physiology The neurotransmitter substance at the parasympathetic postganglionic effector junction is acetylcholine. Thus the parasympathetic system is referred to as a "cholinergic system," and its postganglionic fibers are called "cholinergic fibers" (Fig. 6-5). This chemical mediator is rapidly deactivated by the enzyme cholinesterase in the synaptic area. Hence each parasympathetic discharge has an effect that is of short duration.

The parasympathetic nervous system is geared to act in localized and discrete regions, rather than as a mass response throughout the body. Localized responses of short duration to a specific stimulus result because *1* each preganglionic neuron synapses with a limited number of postganglionic neurons; in turn, each of the latter exerts its effector action on a relatively limited number of neuroeffector (muscle and glandular cell) junctions; and *2* the neurotransmitter acetylcholine is rapidly deactivated by the enzyme cholinesterase. In contrast to the lasting widespread catecholamine effect of the sympathetic nervous system, the acetylcholine effect of the parasympathetic system is discrete. There is no central nervous system mechanism to give a mass discharge of acetylcholine. For example, a drop in the blood pressure is not a response to the generalized action of acetylcholine activity on the cardiovascular system; actually the drop is due to the inhibition of the sympathetic nervous system.

The parasympathetic system is the conserver and the restorer of the energy stores of the body. The parasympathetic system is active when we are at rest and content. At these times there are a deceleration in the rate and force of the heartbeat, decrease in the blood pressure, and increased activity of the digestive system through glandular secretion and peristalsis. The protection of the eye from increased illumination (pupillary constriction) and the stimulation of urinary and bowel excretion are the result of parasympathetic activity. Because of the organs they innervate, the cranial parasympathetic portion is known as the "conserver of bodily resources," and the sacral portion as the "mechanism of emptying."

Massive discharges of the entire parasympathetic system do not usually occur. An excessively intense massive discharge could even be detrimental to the organism; the heart could be decelerated to the point where beating would be reduced excessively.

The sympathetics are the total movers and the parasympathetics are the selective movers. As Cannon expressed it, "The sympathetics are like the loud and the soft pedals, modulating all the notes together, the cranial and sacral innervation like the separate keys."

The autonomic nervous system and the organ systems

A dual innervation of the organs of the body by both the sympathetics and the parasympathetics is general but not universal.

1 The heart has a *true reciprocal (dual) innervation*, with the sympathetics acting to increase and the parasympathetics acting to decrease the force and rate of the heartbeat.

2 The salivary glands are stimulated *synergistically*, with sympathetic activity producing a thick, viscous secretion, and with parasympathetic activity producing a profuse watery secretion.

3 The constriction and dilation of the pupil offer an example of an activity resulting from the stimulation of different muscle groups. The pupil of the eye dilates when the dilator muscles (innervated only by sympathetic fibers) are stimulated by the sympathetics, and it constricts when the constrictor muscles (innervated only by parasympathetic fibers) are stimulated by the parasympathetics.

4 Some structures are innervated by only one system; the hair muscles (goose pimples) and the sweat glands are stimulated only by sympathetic fibers.

Not all the smooth muscle cells of a group or the cardiac muscles need be directly innervated by postganglionic fibers in order to respond to the influences conveyed by these fibers. This is so because smooth muscle cells of a group and the cardiac muscle cells are electrically coupled together by *gap junctions* (see "Nerve Impulse," Chap. 3). The junction between two smooth muscle cells is called a nexus, and that between two cardiac muscle cells is called an *intercalated disk* (Figs. 2-5, 2 8). A group of smooth muscles of the heart behaves like an *electrical syncytium,* because there is electrical continuity between these cells at their gap junctions. This method of propagation is essentially like that of a nerve. In effect, the neural influences sufficient to evoke a muscle action potential in some muscle cells of a group to contract

can, via the gap junctions, stimulate all the muscle cells of the group to contract. The postganglionic autonomic fibers to the heart stimulate the conducting system (nodes, bundle of His, and Purkinje fibers) of the heart, which, in turn, stimulates the cardiac muscle cells through gap junctions.

Eye and lacrimal gland Parasympathetic stimulation results in the constriction (miosis) of the pupil, in the accommodation of the lens to near vision, and in the secretion of tears by the lacrimal gland. Pupillary constriction results from the contraction of the circular (constrictor) muscles of the iris. Accommodation requires a rounder (less flat) lens to effect the focusing on nearby objects.

Sympathetic stimulation results in the dilation of the pupil (mydriasis) by the contraction of the dilator muscles of the iris, slight elevation of the upper eyelid (there is some involuntary muscle in the eyelid), and possibly some accommodation to far vision.

Glands of the nose and mouth, including the salivary glands Parasympathetic stimulation conveyed via secretomotor fibers results in vasodilatation in the glands and in the secretion of a profuse watery secretion. Sympathetic stimulation results in vasoconstriction and in a diminution of blood flow through the glands and in a sparse, thick, viscous, mucinous secretion. The parotid glands lack an adrenergic innervation.

Heart Parasympathetic stimulation results in a slower rate of the heartbeat (bradycardia), decrease in the blood volume expelled with each stroke, and probably the constriction of the coronary arteries (arteries supplying the heart muscle). The automatic rhythmic activity of the heart is basically maintained by the spontaneous depolarization of the automatic, or pacemaker, cells of the heart. In the order of the rate of rhythms (Chap. 3), the automatic cells are located in the sinoatrial node, specialized atrial fibers, atrioventricular node, bundle of His, and Purkinje fibers of the ventricle. Because the sinoatrial node has the fastest rate, it is *the pacemaker.* Acetylcholine slows the rate of depolarization and of the spontaneous depolarization; because the critical level is reached later than normally, the heart rate is slowed down.

Of the automatic cells, acetylcholine acts only upon the sinoatrial node and the specialized atrial fibers.

Sympathetic stimulation results in a higher rate of the beat (tachycardia), increase in the blood volume expelled with each stroke, and dilatation of the coronary arteries. By increasing the rate of depolarization, both NE and epinephrine raise the rate of the heartbeat. All the automatic cells of the heart are activated by both NE and epinephrine.

Lungs Parasympathetic stimulation results in the constriction of the bronchi and bronchioles of the lungs and in an increased secretion of the glandular cells of these tubes.

Sympathetic stimulation results in the dilatation of the bronchi and bronchioles. Respiration, per se, or the inhalation and exhalation of air, is a function of the somatic nervous system, which innervates the respiratory voluntary muscles.

Digestive system Parasympathetic stimulation results in the increase in the contractility, motility, and tone of the digestive tract (peristalsis), in the relaxation of the muscle sphincters (between stomach and intestine, between small and large intestine, and at the anal orifice), and in the increase in the secretion of the digestive glands such as the pancreas. All these activities are directed to the digestion of food and its passage through and out of the digestive tract. The normal mechanical and secretory activities of the digestive tract are not wholly dependent on neural stimulation. Hormonal (humoral) agents are important. For example, contractions of the gallbladder are stimulated by the hormone cholecystokinin.

Sympathetic stimulation results in a decrease in the contractility, motility, and tone of the digestive tract, constriction in the sphincter muscles, inhibition of the secretion of the digestive glands, and an increase in the amount of glucose in the bloodstream. In times of excitement the organism does not readily digest food. Chewing and swallowing of food are essentially functions of the somatic motor system.

Genital system Parasympathetic stimulation results in the engorgement of the erectile tissues of the penis and clitoris and in the active secretion of the accessory glands of the reproductive system (glands of the cervix in the female, and prostate and seminal vesicles in the male).

Sympathetic stimulation results in the ejaculation of the semen by the involuntary muscles of the genital glands and ducts, accompanied by the somatic nervous stimulation of the voluntary muscles. Except for their blood vessels, the ovary, testis, and uterus do not respond to autonomic stimulation.

Urinary system Parasympathetic stimulation results in the increased tone and motility of the ureter and in urination as a consequence of the contraction of the urinary bladder (by the detrusor muscle).

Sympathetic stimulation inhibits urination by stimulating the relaxation of the detrusor muscle. Except for their blood vessels, the kidneys have no autonomic innervation. The voluntary sphincter of the bladder is innervated by the somatic motor system. A more complete discussion is presented below, under "The Pelvic Viscera."

Blood vessels The normal volume of blood is not sufficient to fill all blood vessels should all dilate (vasodilatation) simultaneously. The organism circumvents this consequence normally by dilating some vessels, especially arterioles, while constricting others, thereby maintaining a relatively constant blood vessel volume. In a fight, fright, or flight situation, the vasodilatation in the voluntary muscles is accompanied by vasoconstriction in the abdominal viscera and in the skin. In general, sympathetic stimulation results in dilation of the coronary arteries of the heart and of the arteries of the voluntary muscles, and in the constriction of the blood vessels to the lungs, digestive system, and skin. Parasympathetic stimulation results in the dilation of the blood vessels to the digestive system, as well as to the glands in the head, face (blushing), kidneys, and erectile tissues of the genital system.

The effect of the nervous system is largely over the tone of the arterioles. Vasoconstrictor fibers, by increasing the tone of the smooth muscles, decrease the size of these arterioles. Vasodilator fibers, by inhibiting the contractility of the smooth muscles, decrease the tone of the vessels and thereby allow the blood pressure to increase the diameters of these vessels. Humoral agents may influence the state of contractility of the blood vessels. For example, the cerebral vessels in man react mainly to the circulating metabolic products, rather than to the autonomic nervous system. Carbon dioxide tends to enhance dilatation, and oxygen tends to stimulate constriction of the cerebral vessels.

Sweat glands and pilomotor (hair) muscles of the skin Sympathetic stimulation results in the secretion of sweat glands (actually sympathetic fibers with cholinergic endings) and the contraction of the pilomotor muscles (goose pimples and hair standing on end). The cholinergic fibers to the sweat glands are usually called sympathetic because they are part of the thoracolumbar outflow. The sweat glands of the palms are innervated by sympathetic adrenergic fibers. These are involved in *"adrenergic" palm sweating*, which occurs during emotional stress.

Adrenal (suprarenal) gland The medulla of the adrenal gland secretes both epinephrine and NE into the bloodstream. In this respect, these catecholamines are hormones. The NE is produced by one type of cell. By the methylation of NE, epinephrine is formed in another type of cell. About 80 to 90 percent of the catecholamines secreted by the adrenal gland are epinephrine; the other 10 to 20 percent are NE. These catecholamines are released by *exocytosis* (Fig. 3-6); in this process the vesicles discharge their contents directly through an opening in the plasma membrane into the extracellular space before it diffuses into the bloodstream. The adrenal medulla is controlled by the preganglionic cholinergic fibers of the sympathetic system.

The effect of the secretion of the adrenal medulla is similar to the action of the sympathetic system. This sympathetic activity of the adrenal medulla has a logical basis. The cells of the adrenal medulla, which are actually specialized postganglionic neurons, form the equivalent of a ganglion. These cells are embryologi-

cally derived, just as are many neurons, from neural crest cells (Chap. 4), and they are directly innervated by preganglionic cholinergic fibers (Fig. 6-1). The term *sympathoadrenal system* epitomizes this interrelationship. The widespread and sustained effects of the secretion of the adrenal medulla are the result of the distribution of epinephrine via the bloodstream and its slow deactivation. The adrenal medulla is not essential; its absence can be fully compensated for by the NE produced by the adrenergic fibers of the sympathetic system. Some differences do exist in the pharmacologic properties of NE and epinephrine. One difference, for example, is that epinephrine is more effective than NE in effecting a rapid increase of blood glucose from the glycogen stores in the liver.

The autonomic nervous system and the pelvic viscera

Innervation The peripheral innervation to the urogenital viscera and the rectum is derived from three sets of nerves: *sympathetic nerves* from the lower thoracic and upper lumbar spinal levels, *parasympathetic nerves* from the midsacral spinal levels, and *pudendal nerves* from the second, third, and fourth sacral spinal levels. Within each of these sets are afferent as well as efferent fibers.

The sympathetic outflow passes from the spinal levels via the inferior mesenteric plexus (where synapses between the pre- and postganglionic neurons occur in the inferior mesenteric ganglion), hypogastric plexus (presacral nerve), and pelvic plexus to the pelvic viscera. The parasympathetic outflow passes from the S3, and 4 spinal levels via the pelvic splanchnic nerves (nervi erigentes) and hypogastric plexus to the pelvic viscera. The pudendal nerves convey the somatic motor influences via fibers (lower motor neuron) to the external sphincter of the bladder and external anal sphincter. Afferent fibers conveying the feeling of fullness and pain course via the pelvic splanchnic nerves to the midsacral levels. Other afferent fibers conveying pain may also pass via the hypogastric and inferior mesenteric plexuses to the lower thoracic and upper lumbar levels.

Urinary system Urine formed in the kidney drains into the renal calyces. When the pressure exerted by this urine reaches only 3 to 4 mm Hg, the slightly stretched smooth muscles of the calyces are intrinsically stimulated into spontaneous contraction waves. This low-pressure response propels the urine along the ureter and protects the kidney from back pressure. The urine is forced along to the ureter by peristaltic waves. Higher pressures are necessary within the ureter to stretch the ureteric musculature to initiate local responses, which are again followed by peristaltic waves toward the urinary bladder. Apparently these waves can be influenced but are not under direct central nervous system control. The sensory nerves in the ureter can, when stretched by a stone, evoke a most excruciating pain.

The emptying of the urinary bladder involves the following sequence of events. When the bladder fills (50 to 150 ml), influences from Pacinian receptors in the bladder wall are conveyed via afferent fibers in the pelvic nerves to the sacral cord, and from there pathways ascend to the cerebrum, where the conscious desire to urinate originates.

Voiding of urine is initiated primarily by the stretching of the detrusor muscle of the bladder. This muscle is unusual in that it can be stretched to $2\frac{1}{2}$ times its normal resting length. As the bladder enlarges, the pressure upon the wall is elevated until it reaches the point that induces the external sphincter (voluntary muscle innervated by the pudendal nerve) to relax. This sphincter cannot relax voluntarily; it is actually a passive sphincter. The coordination between the detrusor muscle and the external sphincter is also under reciprocal central control. The stimulation of the spinal cord centers comes from stretch receptors (neuromuscular spindles) in the bladder wall and external sphincter. Strong contractions by the detrusor muscle combined with relaxation of the external sphincter further elevate the pressure and tension. At the same time the detrusor muscle fibers which extend into the bladder neck and proximal urethra contract. These fibers, which are oriented parallel to the long axis of the urethra, will, when they contract, elevate the bladder neck and convert the narrow-mouthed orifice to a wide-mouthed opening, through which the urine passes. There is no distinct internal sphincter of the bladder.

Voluntary voiding can occur in the absence of spontaneous detrusor contractions. The intraabdominal pressure is increased with the contractions of the voluntary muscles of the abdominal wall (somatic fibers of the thoracic and lumbar nerves). The voluntary musculature of the perineum, external urinary sphincter, and pelvic floor relaxes. The involuntary detrusor muscle is induced to contract, with the result that the orifice at the bladder neck is elevated and enlarged as the intravesicular pressure increases; then voiding of urine takes place. Voiding quickly ceases as the voluntary muscles of the pelvic floor and external sphincter contract and the orifice of the bladder closes.

The initiation of voiding can be prevented by strong contractions of both the external urinary sphincter and the pelvic floor musculature.

Rectal system The events during defecation are organized in the following sequence. Afferent influences from the stretch receptors monitoring rectal filling are conveyed via pelvic splanchnic nerves to the midsacral spinal levels and ascending pathways to the cerebrum. The volitional influences descend to the spinal cord and project peripherally via lower motor neurons in the thoracic and lumbar nerves to the voluntary muscles of the abdominal wall (the contraction of this musculature and the resulting increased intraabdominal pressure produce the detrusor action) and in the pudendal nerve to the external voluntary anal sphincter (it relaxes). In a concomitant reflex response, the parasympathetic fibers from the midsacral spinal levels convey influences which result in the contraction of the smooth muscles of the sigmoid colon and rectum and in the relaxation of the involuntary internal sphincter.

Disturbances in function of the bladder and rectum Lesions in various sites result in varying degrees of malfunction of these structures. A complete transection of the spinal cord above the sacral levels (supranuclear) results in an *automatic bladder*—also called a *reflex bladder* because its function depends upon the intact sacral spinal reflex arc. The retention of urine in the weeks immediately following the injury is due to the deranged reflex. Later, automaticity of the bladder occurs; it fills and empties, but never completely. Reflex voiding may be spontaneous or may follow the application of a stimulus to the skin of the perineum, abdomen, or lower, extremity. Fecal retention is a consequence of the loss of the sense of rectal urgency and of voluntary control of the external sphincter.

In lesions of the dorsal roots of sacral nerves or of posterior columns, as in tabes dorsalis, the afferent limb of the arc is interrupted. The result is a stretched and enlarged atonic bladder. The patient is unaware that his bladder is filled. Voluntary voiding is possible but is incomplete and is accompanied with dribbling and incontinence.

Genital system The coordination of the influences of the sacral parasympathetic motor innervation to the urethra and of the sacral somatic motor innervation to the ischiocavernosus and bulbocavernosus muscles activates ejaculation. The sympathetic fibers of the reflex arc from spinal levels T12 to L2 to the detrusor muscle and trigone region of the bladder have a significant role. By inhibiting these bladder muscles from contracting, they prevent the voiding of urine and retrograde flow of semen into the bladder during ejaculation. Following surgical sympathectomy of fibers to the region, patients often experience impotence. In other patients, the semen backs up into the bladder during an ejaculation.

The medulla and the spinal cord contain all the reflex mechanisms and pathways which can initiate all the reflexes and activities essential for coitus. In fact, some *spinal male human subjects* can, following the manipulation of their genitalia, respond by having an erection accompanied by an ejaculation. Spinal females have become pregnant and have carried a child to full term. These activities are possible only with the integrity of the lumbosacral cord.

Representation of the autonomic nervous system in the brain and spinal cord

Structurally and functionally the autonomic nervous system is represented in the central nervous system as an intricate complex of centers and pathways whose details have been only partially unraveled.

The *segmental reflex arcs* are the fundamental anatomic and physiologic units of organization. In general, these arcs resemble the somatic reflex arcs. They are composed of *1* afferent neurons with their cell bodies in the spinal ganglia and in the geniculate ganglion of the facial nerve and inferior ganglia of the glossopharyngeal and vagus nerves, *2* interneurons in the central nervous system, *3* efferent neurons consisting of the sequence of preganglionic and postganglionic neurons, and *4* effector cells (smooth muscle, cardiac muscle, and glandular cell). Some reflex arcs involve other sequences of neurons; e.g., the afferent neurons of the light reflex arc located in the retina, optic nerve, and optic tract (Chap. 12). The afferent neurons do not terminate in the nuclei containing the cell bodies of the preganglionic neurons (dorsal vagal nucleus and intermediolateral nucleus); apparently at least one interneuron is intercalated between the afferent neuron and the preganglionic neuron of either the sympathetic or the parasympathetic system.

These reflex arcs respond to the ever-changing and fluctuating demands of the internal environment. It is through these segmental arcs that the higher centers of the autonomic system in the brain ultimately exert their effects. The "centers" and the descending pathways of the system are identified essentially on the basis of physiologic criteria (e.g., the "respiratory center") and secondarily on the basis of anatomic criteria. Although some centers are relatively discrete morphologically (e.g., the hypothalamus and the dorsal vagal nucleus), many others are not (e.g., the cardiovascular centers in the brainstem tegmentum). The autonomic system in the brain and spinal cord may be thought of as a complexly organized, interacting network of pathways, with the centers as focal or nodal sites physiologically influencing a functional activity. The autonomic nervous system acts not alone but in concert with the somatic nervous system. Fight and flight reactions are expressions of both the somatic and the visceral systems. All autonomic activities are geared to function ultimately to maintain the homeostatic and homeokinetic balance of the organism.

The general visceral afferent input to the central nervous system is conveyed via the spinal nerves and the seventh, ninth, and tenth cranial nerves (Chap. 7). These visceral influences are *1* integrated into segmental visceral reflex arcs, whose motor nerves are the preganglionic and postganglionic neurons, and *2* relayed to higher centers via the spinoreticular tract and ascending tracts associated with the brainstem reticular system (Chap. 8).

Spinal cord   The autonomic centers of the spinal cord are subject to the facilitatory and inhibitory stimuli from the centers in the brain. These stimuli are conveyed via descending pathways located mainly in the white matter in the anterior half of the spinal cord. Presumably the cord centers feed modulating influences back to the centers in the brain via ascending pathways. Ultimately this integrated activity is conveyed *1* via the preganglionic sympathetic neurons through the thoracolumbar outflow, and *2* via the preganglionic parasympathetic neurons in the sacral gray matter through the sacral outflow.

Brainstem and cerebellum   Many vital activities are mediated through the brainstem by "centers" definable largely by physiologic criteria. In the ventromedial tegmentum of the medulla is an inhibitory cardiovascular center; in the lateral tegmentum is an excitatory cardiovascular center. Stimulation of the lateral tegmentum may result in an acceleration of the heartbeat and an elevated blood pressure. Salivation may be a consequence of stimulation of the dorsolateral medullary tegmentum. Respiratory centers are located in the pons and medulla (Chap. 8). These centers and others project their influences via the reticulospinal tracts to the autonomic outflow in the spinal cord and through the reticular formation to the cranial nerve outflow in the brainstem.

The cerebellum may influence autonomic

responses, probably acting through the brainstem reticular formation.

Hypothalamus   The hypothalamus is a complex of visceral centers involved with the elemental visceral activities and behavioral patterns (Chap. 11). The visceromotor expressions of autonomic functions are transmitted from the hypothalamus by multineuronal pathways to visceral neuronal pools in the brainstem and spinal cord before being conveyed via the peripheral autonomic fibers to effectors.

The descending central visceromotor pathways from the hypothalamus to the brainstem and spinal cord are difficult to define precisely because direct descending hypothalamic efferents have not been demonstrated to project to the pons, medulla, or spinal cord. The caudally projecting fibers from the hypothalamus may be divided into two basic groups, both of which terminate in the midbrain.

1 The descending component of the medial forebrain bundle originates from cells in the lateral zone of the hypothalamus and descends *a* as the lateral division to the lateral midbrain tegmentum, and *b* as the medial division to the paramedian midbrain tegmentum.

2 The descending component of the dorsal lateral fasciculus of Schütz originates from the more medial hypothalamus and descends to the anterior half of the periaqueductal gray substance. The nuclei of the paramedian tegmentum receiving input from these fibers include the superior central tegmental nucleus (raphe nucleus of Bechterew), dorsal tegmental nucleus, and ventral tegmental nucleus. This paramedian midbrain tegmentum, also known as the *"limbic midbrain area"* (Nauta), is the origin of ascending fibers which terminate in the hypothalamus (Chap. 13). They course in the dorsolateral fasciculus of Schütz and the mammillary peduncle. This "limbic midbrain area" is the caudal portion of the reciprocally organized hypothalamomesencephalic circuit.

Descending fibers from the midbrain tegmental nuclei terminate in the tegmental nuclei of the pons and medulla, including the nuclei reticularis pontis oralis and caudalis and the nucleus reticularis gigantocellularis. These descending reticulospinal pathways from the rhombencephalic tegmentum project through the white matter in the anterior half of the spinal cord to all spinal levels and terminate in the spinal gray matter. None terminate directly on the cells of the intermediolateral nucleus. Interneurons are the linkages between the fibers originating from the lower brainstem and the preganglionic sympathetic neurons. Interactions within these descending pathways from the hypothalamus occur through the rich interconnections and cross-linkages among the dendritic and axonal arborizations. In summary, the influences from the hypothalamus to the preganglionic neuronal outflow are conveyed via processing nuclear complexes in the midbrain, rhombencephalon, and spinal cord.

On the more elemental level, stimulation of the hypothalamus may result in the increase or decrease of the arterial pressure and the rate of the heartbeat, sweating, dilation of the pupil, increase of the blood glucose concentration, stimulation or inhibition of activity in the gastrointestinal tract, and contraction of the urinary bladder.

On the behavioral level the hypothalamus affects *1* such behavioral patterns as savageness, rage, domestication, and wildness, *2* the sleep-wake mechanisms, *3* patterns of sexual behavior, *4* the overall metabolic activities related to such phenomena as food and water intake, obesity, and emaciation, and *5* the endocrine system through the pituitary gland.

Cerebrum and thalamus The neocortex, limbic lobe cortex, corpus striatum, and thalamus have their effects on autonomic activities. Details of the anatomy and physiology are scant. Cerebral structures are important to the emotional component of the total pattern of behavior. Animals live in a psychologic world with a support that is largely modulated through the autonomic nervous system. These higher centers have a role in such concepts as that excitable individuals are

keyed to the sympathetic system and that placid individuals are keyed to the parasympathetic system. The basal ganglia influence the autonomic nervous system. For example, stimulation of the corpus striatum may produce changes in vascular tonus and in the state of contraction of pupillary, bladder, intestinal, and uterine muscles.

Pharmacology of the peripheral nervous system

Natural chemical mediators of the peripheral nervous system include *1 acetylcholine,* at the cholinergic endings of *a* the preganglionic neurons of the autonomic nervous system, *b* the postganglionic neurons of the parasympathetic nervous system, and *c* the lower (somatic) motor neurons at the motor end plates; *2 norepinephrine,* at the adrenergic endings of the postganglionic neurons of the sympathetic nervous system and secreted by the adrenal medulla; and *3 epinephrine,* secreted by the adrenal medulla. These chemicals are the natural chemical mediators.

PHARMACOLOGIC AGENTS AND THEIR MODE OF ACTION

Many chemical substances have actions that may resemble some of the actions of the natural mediators. Those drugs which mimic the actions of acetylcholine are known as *parasympathomimetic drugs, cholinomimetic agents,* or *cholinergic drugs.* For example, carbachol mimics acetylcholine. Those drugs that mimic the actions of epinephrine and norepinephrine, e.g., ephedrine, are known as *sympathomimetic* or *adrenergic drugs.*

The general principles of neuropharmocology are based mainly on the action of chemical agents on the synaptic membranes of neurons. Some chemical substances modify the neural activity by acting at the synaptic sites to prevent the nerve impulse in the presynaptic neuron from stimulating the postsynaptic neuron (or effector structure). These drugs, known as blocking agents, do not prevent the release of the natural chemical mediators at the nerve endings but act just beyond the ending (probably in the synaptic cleft) to prevent the natural mediator from exerting its normal action.

Some blockers apparently stabilize the receptor site on the postganglionic neuron or effector cell so that the natural mediator cannot depolarize the postganglionic neuron or influence the effector cell. These blocking drugs are called *competitive blocking agents* (e.g., *d*-tubocurarine and tetraethylammonia) because they effectively compete at the synaptic site with the natural mediators.

Other blocking agents prevent the natural mediators from exerting their activity by depolarizing the postganglionic receptive sites, rendering these sites temporarily nonreceptive to further stimulation. These chemical substances are known as *depolarizing blocking agents* (e.g., nicotine). These blocking agents affect the receptor sites proper of the postganglionic cells, not their axons (the axon or the postganglionic neuron can still be directly stimulated to conduct).

The exact mode of action of pharmaceutical agents is not wholly understood. The various agents mimic the natural mediators in a number of ways. These differential activities explain why the search for more agents is continuous. The object is to enhance the specific effects that the physician desires (including ease of administration and duration of the drug action) and to suppress the undesired side effects. The effects of several drugs will be outlined to illustrate some of their pharmacologic properties.

Muscarine, a drug derived from a type of mushroom, is a parasympathomimetic agent that exhibits a cholinergic effect on such effectors as smooth muscles, heart muscle, and glands but has essentially no effect at the ganglionic synapses and at the motor end plates of voluntary muscles. These activities of muscarine are known as the *muscarinic effect*.

Nicotine has a dual effect (i.e., an effect with two phases) on the autonomic ganglia and on the voluntary muscles, but has essentially no effect on smooth muscles, heart muscle, and glands. This agent initially stimulates and subsequently inhibits the excitation of the postsynaptic neuron or muscle. The initial effect of nicotine is to depolarize the postsynaptic membrane (depolarizing phase), which results in stimula-

tion of the postganglionic neuron to fire. The subsequent effect is to maintain the depolarized state or phase so that the postsynaptic membrane cannot be stimulated. This dual action of nicotine is known as the *nicotinic effect*.

CHOLINERGIC AGENTS

The cholinergic endings of the autonomic neurons and of the somatic motor neurons at the motor end plates are the synaptic sites of action of a number of drugs. Carbachol is one such cholinergic drug that acts as a parasympathomimetic drug; its direct effect is similar to that of acetylcholine. Other pharmacologic agents have similar end effects but act by exerting an indirect mimetic action by inhibiting the enzyme cholinesterase; as a result, the concentration of acetylcholine increases in the synaptic clefts. These cholinesterase inhibitors or anticholinesterase agents include physostigmine and diisopropylfluorophosphate (DFP). DFP is a lethal nerve (war) gas. In short, similar cholinergic effects can be obtained either by the acetylcholine-like activity of such drugs as carbachol or by the inhibition of the enzyme cholinesterase (allowing acetylcholine to accumulate) by such drugs as physostigmine.

BLOCKING AGENTS

Some drugs act as *blocking agents* at the synaptic sites. This blockage can be obtained by *1* such depolarizing agents as nicotine (depolarizing phase) and succinylcholine, or *2* such competitive blocking agents as *d*-tubocurarine (derived from curare, the poison placed on arrow tips by certain South American Indians) and tetraethylammonia (TEA). Curare is an efficient blocker at the motor end plate (its paralytic action on the respiratory muscles can be fatal); TEA is a blocker that acts at the ganglionic synapses. Homatropine, a parasympathetic blocker at the postganglionic effector junction, is used by ophthalmologists in eye drops to dilate the pupil of the eye. This drug inhibits the pupillary constrictor muscle fibers from contracting by blocking the cholinergic endings.

Dilation results from the normal sympathetic activity of the unopposed dilator muscles of the pupil. *Atropine* and *homatropine* block the effect of acetylcholine at the neuroeffector receptive sites on the postsynaptic membrane; these agents do not interact chemically with acetylcholine.

ADRENERGIC AGENTS

The *adrenergic mimetic drugs* that simulate some of the actions of epinephrine and norepinephrine include ephedrine and amphetamine. These agents (as constituents of nose drops and nasal decongestants) act to constrict blood vessels and to inhibit mucous secretions.

The effector cells innervated by the autonomic nervous system have two types of *chemically defined adrenoreceptive sites—namely alpha (α) and beta (β) receptors.* The alpha receptors have an affinity for both norepinephrine and epinephrine, while the beta receptors have a selectively stronger affinity for epinephrine.

The *alpha receptors* are generally excitatory, although some may be inhibitory in their response. Stimulation of most alpha receptors results in excitatory activity—contraction of smooth muscles or increased secretory activity of glandular cells. Excitatory responses are evoked in the following: *1* dilator (radial) muscles of the iris, *2* most blood vessels, including the coronary, skeletal muscle, salivary gland, cutaneous, pulmonary, and abdominal visceral vessels, *3* sphincters of the gastrointestinal tract, *4* muscle fibers of the trigone of the urinary bladder and of the vas deferens and uterus of the genital system, *5* sweat glands and pilomotor muscles in the skin, *6* smooth muscle in the capsule of the spleen, and *7* salivary glands (thick and viscous secretion). Inhibitory responses are obtained in some smooth muscle of the digestive system (relax intestine).

The *beta receptors* are generally inhibitory, with two significant exceptions. Inhibitory responses are evoked in the following: *1* ciliary muscles of the eye, *2* some blood vessels, including the coronary, skeletal muscle, pulmonary, and abdominal vessels (dilatation of arterioles), *3* musculature of the gastrointestinal tract (decrease in motility and tone), *4* bronchial muscles of the lung, and *5* detrusor muscle of the urinary bladder and smooth muscles of the uterus.

The two exceptions to the alpha-excitatory and beta-inhibitory responses are expressed by the heart and the gastrointestinal tract. Stimulation of the beta receptors in the sinoatrial node, atria, and ventricles produces excitatory cardiac effects; these include increase in the heart rate, increase in the force of the contraction, and increase in the excitability and automaticity. Stimulation of either the alpha or beta receptors produces inhibitory responses and these responses are additive. Stimulation of both receptors acts to decrease gastrointestinal motility. Sympathetic responses can be eliminated by blocking both alpha and beta receptors. Some adrenergic blocking agents are *alpha receptor blockers* (e.g., dibenamines), while others are *beta receptor blockers* (e.g., dichloroisoproterenol).

Denervation hypersensitivity

When a muscle is deprived of its innervation, it becomes extremely sensitive to chemical mediators (Chap. 4). Smooth muscles are most irritable when deprived of their postganglionic innervation and somewhat less hypersensitive if deprived only of their preganglionic innervation. The rate of beat of a totally denervated heart will increase if the heart is exposed to one part of epinephrine in 1,400 million parts. This hypersensitivity is lost following the regeneration and functional recovery of these nerves. The *paradoxical pupillary reaction* is an example of denervation hypersensitivity to circulating epinephrine. The pupil of the eye without sympathetic innervation remains constricted because of the unopposed intact parasympathetic innervation of the pupillary constrictor muscles. When an individual without this sympathetic innervation is excited, the pupil may dilate. Probably the circulating epinephrine secreted by the adrenal medulla excites the denervated dilator muscles to contract and dilate the pupil.

A denervated skeletal muscle is about 1,000 times more sensitive to acetylcholine than is the normally innervated muscle. At the motor end plate region, the denervated muscle may even be 100,000 times more irritable. The muscle fasciculations associated with lower motor neuron damage probably result from the stimulation (depolarization) of the hypersensitive motor end plate region by the excitatory agents in the bloodstream (Chap. 5).

Denervation hypersensitivity (*supersensitivity*), according to the *law of denervation*, is an expression of the magnified enhancement of the response which can be elicited by minimal concentrations of chemical mediators normally acting and producing an effect at the synaptic junction of a normally innervated structure. This hypersensitivity should be considered as a compensatory mechanism, as an adjustment response utilizing neural junctions which otherwise would be nonfunctional. In the process, the denervated muscle fibers (voluntary and involuntary muscles) apparently retrogress to a more undifferentiated primitive state in which each fiber is spontaneously active to mechanical as well as chemical stimulation.

Trophic effects (Neurotrophism)

The neurons may have other effects, independent of the influences exerted by the neurotransmitter activity, which are essential for the physiologic maintenance of other tissues. These so-called *trophic effects* (*trophic influences*) of neurons are directed to different types of target tissues, including epithelium and nerve endings (e.g., taste buds), muscle cells, and glandular cells. Even the maintenance of the nerve fiber itself may be dependent upon these influences. Chemical substances elaborated in the cell bodies of neurons—called *neurotrophic factors or substances*—are thought to be involved in these *neurotrophic processes*. The precise nature and identity of these factors, or this factor, and the processes involved are not known at present. The concept of neurotrophism has been characterized as the nonimpulse transmitter neural function. It presumably involves some factor(s), which are conveyed by axoplasmic transport along the axon, are released and have a long-term interaction with the innervated tissues. Functionally this factor is essential for the maintenance of these tissues in their normal state. Specifically the trophic effects are "those interactions between nerves and other cells which initiate or control molecular modification in the other cell" (Guth).

The role of the gustatory nerve fibers with respect to the taste buds is illustrative of the effects of these "trophic influences" of the neuron. Not only do the gustatory nerve fibers convey coded "taste" information from the taste buds, but they also have an essential role in maintaining the morphology of the taste bud. Following the transection of the gustatory nerve fibers, the denervated taste buds degenerate. When the nerve regenerates and reinnervates the region, taste buds reappear. If nerve fibers, other than gustatory fibers, reinnervate the region, the taste buds do not reappear. Thus only gustatory nerves are capable of inducing the taste buds to appear. Motor fibers and nontaste fibers are not. The nature of the influences exerted by the nerve on the innervated structure to account for this phenomenon is not known. A plausible explanation is that certain substances—called trophic factors—in the nerves are conveyed via axoplasmic flow to the nerve terminals where they are released to the synaptic cleft. Then these "trophic" substances exert their roles of eliciting the formation of the taste buds and of maintaining their structural integrity.

Motor nerves are also implicated to exert "trophic influences"; these include both somatic motor nerves (neuromuscular trophism) and nerves of the autonomic nervous system (neurovisceral trophism). "Trophic effects" may possibly have a role in some of the anatomic, biochemical, and physiologic differences between slow-red muscles and fast-white muscles. Red muscles are innervated by slowly conducting axons; white muscles are innervated primarily by rapidly conducting axons. Experimentally it is possible to sever the nerves innervating these muscles and have the slowly conducting axons regenerate to reinnervate the white muscles and have the fast conducting axons regenerate to

TABLE 6-3
Some comparisons between the sympathetic and parasympathetic nervous systems

General

	Sympathetic nervous system	*Parasympathetic nervous system*
Outflow from CNS	Thoracolumbar levels	Craniosacral levels
Location of ganglia	Paravertebral and prevertebral ganglia close to CNS	Terminal ganglia near effectors
Ratio of preganglionic to postganglionic neurons	Each preganglionic neuron synapses with many postganglionic neurons	Each preganglionic neuron synapses with a few postganglionic neurons
Distribution in body	Throughout the body	Limited primarily to viscera of head, thorax, abdomen, and pelvis
Metabolism	Energy mobilization during emergency	Conservation and restoration of energy resources
General homeostasis	Central mechanism to obtain mass discharge of system	No central mechanism to obtain mass discharge of system

Specific structures

Structure	*Sympathetic function*	*Parasympathetic function*
Eye		
Radial muscle of iris	Dilates pupil (mydriasis)	
Sphincter muscle of iris		Contraction of pupil (miosis)
Ciliary muscle (accommodation)	Relaxation for far vision	Contraction for near vision
Glands of head		
Lacrimal gland		Stimulates secretion
Salivary glands	Scanty thick, viscous secretion	Profuse, watery secretion
Heart		
Rate	Increases	Decreases
Force of ventricular contraction	Increases	No direct effect
Blood vessels	Generally constricts*	Slight effect
Lungs		
Bronchial tubes	Dilates lumen	Stimulates constriction of lumen
Bronchial glands	Inhibits secretion	Stimulates secretion
Gastrointestinal tract		
Motility and tone	Inhibits	Stimulates
Sphincters	Stimulates	Inhibits (relax)
Secretion	May inhibit	Stimulates
Gallbladder and ducts	Inhibits	Stimulates
Liver	Glycogenolysis increase (blood sugar)	
Spleen (capsule)	Contracts	
Adrenal medulla	Secretion of epinephrine* and norepinephrine	

TABLE 6-3 *(cont.)* *215*

Specific structures

Structure	Sympathetic function	Parasympathetic function
Sex organs	Vasoconstriction, constriction of vas deferens, seminal vesicle, and prostatic musculature (ejaculation)	Vasodilatation and erection
Skin		
Sweat glands	Stimulates*	None
Blood vessels	Constricts	Slight effect
Pilomotor	Contracts	
Urinary tract		
Ureter (motility and tone)	Increases	
Bladder detrusor	Relaxation (usually)	Contraction
Trigone and extension into urethra	Relaxation (see text)	Contraction
Metabolism		
Liver	Glycogenolysis	
Adipose tissue	Free fatty acid release	

Neurochemical basis

	Sympathetic	Parasympathetic
Neurotransmitter at neuroeffector junction	Usually norepinephrine* Adrenergic	Acetylcholine Cholinergic
Inactivation of transmitter	Slow and re-uptake	Rapid
Reinforcement in body	Secretion of norepinephrine and epinephrine by adrenal medulla	

*Exceptions: Some postganglionic neurons of the sympathetic nervous system are cholinergic neurons. Sympathetic neuroeffector transmission mediated by acetylcholine includes (1) some blood vessels in skeletal muscles and (2) most sweat glands. The sweat glands of the palms are innervated by adrenergic fibers. The adrenal medulla is innervated by preganglionic cholinergic sympathetic neurons.

reinnervate the red muscles. In such cross-innervation experiments, there is a conversion of many of the properties that are specific to each muscle type. These changes may be due, in part, to "trophic influences."

Clinically observed trophic changes include alterations that occur after lesions of the fibers of the autonomic nervous system. Among these disturbances are a warm or cool, flushed or cyanotic skin (change in capillary circulation in skin), abnormal brittleness of the fingernails, loss of hair, dryness or ulcerations of the skin and lysis of bones and joints, resulting, at times, in spontaneous fractures.

Bibliography

Albers, R. W., G. J. Siegel, R. Katzman, and B. W. Agranoff: *Basic Neurochemistry*. Little, Brown and Company, Boston, 1972.

Botár, G.: *The Autonomic Nervous System*. Akadémiai Kiado, Budapest, 1966.

Burn, J. H.: *Autonomic Nervous System: For Students of Physiology and Pharmacology*. F. A. Davis Company, Philadelphia, 1971.

Campbell, G.: Autonomic nervous supply to effector tissues, in E. Bülbring, A. F. Brading, A. W. Jones, and T. Tomita (eds.), **Smooth Muscle,** pp. 451–495. E. Arnold, London, 1970.

Code, C. F. (ed.): Section 6: The alimentary canal,

216

Handbook of Physiology, vol. IV. Williams and Wilkins, Baltimore, 1968.

Guth, L.: "Trophic" influences of nerve on muscle. Physiol. Rev., 48:645–687, 1968.

Koelle, G. B.: Neurohumoral transmission and the autonomic nervous system, in L. Goodman and A. Gilman (eds.), *The Pharmacological Basis of Therapeutics*, 4th ed., pp. 402–441. The Macmillan Company, New York, 1970.

Kuntz, A.: *The Autonomic Nervous System.* Lea & Febiger, Philadelphia, 1953.

Mitchell, G. A.: *Anatomy of the Autonomic Nervous System.* Livingstone, Ltd., Edinburgh, 1953.

Neil, E. (ed.): Enterceptors, in *Handbook of Sensory Physiology*, vol. III, sec. 1, pp. 1–233. Springer-Verlag, Berlin and New York, 1972.

Petras, J. M. and J. F. Cummings: Autonomic neurons in the spinal cord of the rhesus monkey. J. Comp. Neurol., 146: 189–218, 1972.

Pick, J.: *Autonomic Nervous System: Morphological, Comparative, Clinical and Surgical Aspects.* J. B. Lippincott Company, Philadelphia, 1970.

White, J. C., R. H. Smithwick, and F. A. Simeone: *The Autonomic Nervous System: Anatomy, Physiology and Surgical Application.* The Macmillan Company, New York, 1952.

CHAPTER **7**
THE CRANIAL NERVES

The cranial nerves are the peripheral nerves of the brain. They transmit input to the brain from the special sensors of smell, sight, hearing, and taste and from the same types of general sensors as do the peripheral spinal nerves. They convey output to the voluntary muscles involved with the movements of the eyes, mouth, face, tongue, pharynx, and larynx. They are the major outlet for the parasympathetic nervous system.

The complexities of the 12 cranial nerves (see Table 7-1) will be outlined as follows:

1 basic theory of the organization of the cranial nerves

2 general structural and functional aspects of the cranial nerves

3 peripheral ganglia associated with the cranial nerves

4 cranial nerve nuclei within the central nervous system

5 the role of the cranial nerves in several activities. Cranial nerves III through XII emerge from the brainstem (Fig. 7-1).

Basic theory of the organization of the cranial nerves

The cranial nerves can be better understood through an analysis of their functional components.

COMPONENTS OF THE CRANIAL NERVES

The cranial nerves comprise the same four components of fibers present in the spinal nerves and three additional components (Fig. 7-2). The four components found both in the spinal

TABLE 7-1
Cranial nerves and location of the cell bodies of their sensory ganglia

Nerve	*Sensory peripheral ganglia*
Olfactory nerve	Bipolar cells in nasal mucosa
Optic nerve	Bipolar cells located within the retina of eye
Trigeminal nerve	Trigeminal (Gasserian, semilunar) ganglion; mesencephalic nucleus of the midbrain
Facial nerve	Geniculate ganglion
Vestibulocochlear nerve	
Vestibular nerve	Vestibular ganglion (Scarpa's ganglion)
Cochlear nerve	Spiral ganglion
Glossopharyngeal nerve	Superior ganglion (somatic afferent)
	Inferior ganglion (visceral afferent)
Vagus nerve and spinal accessory nerve	Superior ganglion (somatic afferent)
	Inferior ganglion (visceral afferent)
Oculomotor nerve, trochlear nerve, abducent nerve, hypoglossal nerve	Cell bodies of proprioceptive neurons probably scattered along nerve, in trigeminal ganglion, or in mesencephalic nucleus of N. V

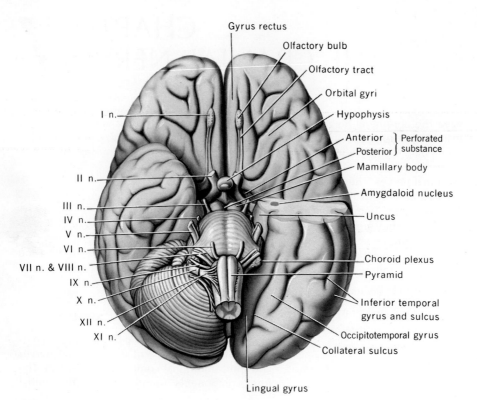

Gyrus rectus
Olfactory bulb
Olfactory tract
Orbital gyri
Hypophysis
Anterior } Perforated
Posterior } substance
Mamillary body
Amygdaloid nucleus
Uncus
Choroid plexus
Pyramid
Inferior temporal gyrus and sulcus
Occipitotemporal gyrus
Collateral sulcus
Lingual gyrus

I n.
II n.
III n.
IV n.
V n.
VI n.
VII n. & VIII n.
IX n.
X n.
XII n.
XI n.

FIGURE 7-1
Basal surface of the brain and roots of the cranial nerves.

Cerebellum and rostral portion of temporal lobe removed on right half of figure.

nerves and in the cranial nerves are the *general somatic afferent fibers* (GSA), the *general visceral afferent fibers* (GVA), the *general somatic efferent fibers* (GSE), and the *general visceral efferent fibers* (GVE). The three additional components found exclusively in the cranial nerves are the *special somatic afferent fibers* (SSA), the *special visceral afferent fibers* (SVA), and the *special visceral efferent fibers* (SVE). The special somatic afferent senses are vision, hearing, and equilibrium; the special visceral afferent senses are smell and taste. The special senses have their receptors located in restricted regions of the body. In contrast, the general senses have their receptors located over extensive regions of the

body. The special visceral efferent fibers are the motor fibers innervating certain voluntary muscles of the head. They are the muscles of the branchial (visceral) arches, which in aquatic vertebrates (fish and amphibia) are the gill arches. Traditionally they are referred to as special visceral efferent musculature (branchiomeric or gill arch musculature). The term *visceral* is applied because these muscles are associated with the jaws, pharynx, and larynx, structures involved with such visceral functions as eating and breathing. No cranial nerve has all seven components.

CATEGORIES OF CRANIAL NERVES BASED ON THEIR FUNCTIONAL COMPONENTS

The cranial nerves are tabulated according to their functional components in Table 7-2. Reference to this table indicates the rationale for the

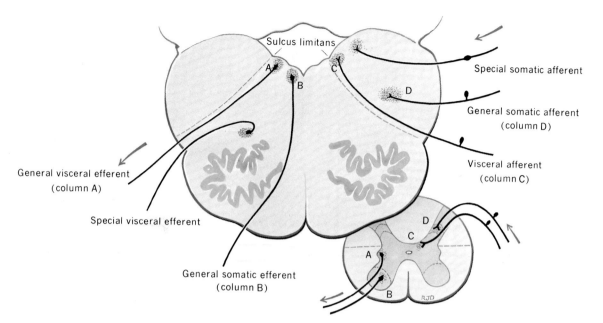

Sulcus limitans

A B C D

Special somatic afferent

General somatic afferent
(column D)

Visceral afferent
(column C)

General visceral efferent
(column A)

Special visceral efferent

General somatic efferent
(column B)

D
C
A
B
RJD

FIGURE 7-2
Functional components of the cranial nerve nuclei in the medulla and the spinal nerve nuclei in the spinal cord.

In both regions, the afferent columns are located dorsal or dorsolateral to the dotted lines (derivatives of the alar plate (Chap. 4), and the efferent columns are located ventral or ventromedial to the dotted lines (derivatives of the basal plate, Chap. 4). In the medulla and the spinal cord, note the comparable locations of the general visceral efferent column (A), general somatic efferent column (B), general visceral afferent column (C), general somatic afferent column (D). Special somatic and special visceral nuclei are present only in the brain. The visceral afferent column in the brainstem is composed of special (such as taste) and general visceral afferent components.

grouping of the cranial nerves into the following three categories.

Special afferent nerves   The nerves primarily conveying special (somatic and visceral) afferent fibers from the special senses include the olfactory nerve (N. I), the optic nerve (N. II), and the vestibulocochlear nerve (N. VIII). The nerves with fibers transmitting the taste modality are located in the three visceral arch nerves noted further on.

General somatic efferent nerves   The nerves conveying general somatic motor fibers to the voluntary muscles of the eye and the tongue include the oculomotor (N. III), trochlear (N. IV), abducent (N. VI), and hypoglossal (N. XII). Each of these nerves has fibers conveying proprioceptive impulses from the muscles to the central nervous system; hence, each possesses general somatic afferent components. The oculomotor nerve has, in addition, general visceral efferent (parasympathetic) fibers to the eye.

Visceral arch nerves (*branchiomeric, branchial, trematic, or gill arch nerves*)   The trigeminal (N. V), facial (N. VII), glossopharyngeal (N. IX),

vagal (N. X), and the cranial root of the spinal accessory (N. XI) are nerves of the branchial arches. Each one of these nerves is associated with a specific gill arch in fish or with its evolutionary successor in higher vertebrates—the trigeminal nerve with the first arch (jaws), the facial nerve with the second arch, the glossopharyngeal nerve with the third arch, and the vagus nerve with the remaining arches. The basic similarities of the facial, glossopharyngeal,

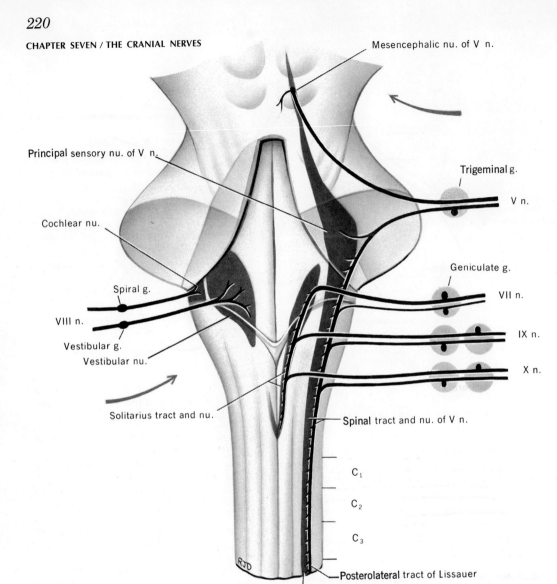

FIGURE 7-3
Location of the afferent (sensory) cranial nerve nuclei within the brainstem.

These nuclei are organized into three nuclear columns. The general somatic afferent column includes the mesencephalic nucleus, the principal sensory nucleus, and the spinal nucleus of the fifth nerve. The general and special visceral afferent column includes the nucleus solitarius. The special somatic afferent column includes the cochlear and the vestibular nuclei. The sensory ganglia of the cranial nerves are indicated. The superior and inferior ganglia of both the ninth and tenth cranial nerves are illustrated but not labeled. G., ganglion.

and vagus nerves are indicated by the fact that all have the same functional components (Table 7-2).

Each of these nerves has one or two sensory ganglia; significantly, these are the counterparts of the spinal ganglia of the spinal nerves (Table 7-1). In addition, parasympathetic ganglia are associated with the general visceral efferent component: the facial nerve is associated with the submandibular and pterygopalatine ganglia;

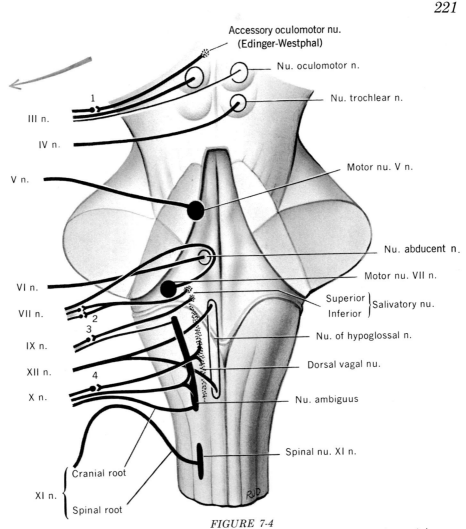

FIGURE 7-4
Location of the efferent (motor) cranial nerve nuclei within the brainstem.

the glossopharyngeal nerve with the otic ganglion; and the vagus nerve with small terminal ganglia within or on the viscera. In these ganglia are located the synapses between the preganglionic neurons and the postganglionic neurons (Chap. 6).

Each gill surrounds a gill slit, or *trema* (a hole from the pharynx to the outside for the passage of water in a fish or tadpole). Typically each of these nerves consists of three divisions: *1* The *pretrematic division,* which passes on the front margin of the trema, is an afferent nerve. *2* The *posttrematic division,* which passes on the hind margin of the trema, is a mixed nerve with afferent and efferent nerve fibers. The efferent fibers

These nuclei are organized into three nuclear columns. The general somatic efferent column includes the nuclei of the third, fourth, sixth, and twelfth cranial nerves (outlined areas). The general visceral efferent (parasympathetic) column includes the accessory oculomotor nucleus (of Edinger-Westphal), salivary nuclei, and dorsal vagal nucleus (dotted areas). The special visceral efferent (gill arch) column includes the motor nucleus of the fifth nerve, facial nucleus, and nucleus ambiguus (solid areas). The numerals indicate the parasympathetic ganglia: *1* ciliary ganglion of the third cranial nerve, *2* pterygopalatine ganglion and submandibular ganglion of the seventh cranial nerve, *3* otic ganglion of the ninth cranial nerve, and *4* terminal parasympathetic ganglia (in the thoracic and abdominal viscera) of the tenth cranial nerve.

TABLE 7-2
Components and functions of cranial nerves

Name	*Components*	*Functions (major)*
I. Olfactory nerve	Special visceral afferent (SVA)	Smell
II. Optic nerve	Special somatic afferent (SSA)	Vision and associated reflexes
III. Oculomotor nerve*	General somatic efferent (GSE)	Movements of eyes
	General visceral efferent (GVE) (parasympathetic)	Pupillary constriction and accommodation
IV. Trochlear nerve*	General somatic efferent (GSE)	Movements of eyes
V. Trigeminal nerve	Special visceral efferent (SVE)	Mastication
		Swallowing
		Movements of soft palate and auditory tube
		Movements of tympanic membrane and ear ossicles
	General somatic afferent (GSA)	General sensations from anterior half of head, including face, nose, mouth, and meninges
VI. Abducent nerve†	General somatic efferent (GSE)	Movements of eyes
VII. Facial nerve	Special visceral efferent (SVE)	Facial expression
		Elevation of hyoid bone
		Movement of stapes
	General visceral efferent (GVE) (parasympathetic)	Lacrimation, salivation, and vasodilatation
	Special visceral afferent (SVA)	Taste
	General visceral afferent (GVA)	Visceral sensation
VIII. Vestibulocochlear nerve	Special somatic afferent (SSA)	Hearing and equilibrium reception
IX. Glossopharyngeal nerve	Special visceral efferent (SVE)	Swallowing movements
		Raises pharynx and larynx
	General visceral efferent (GVE) (parasympathetic)	Salivation and vasodilatation
	Special visceral afferent (SVA)	Taste
	General afferent (GSA, GVA)	General senses in region of posterior third of tongue, tonsils, and upper pharynx
		Receptors of carotid sinus and carotid body
X. Vagus nerve and cranial root of N. XI	Special visceral efferent (SVE)	Swallowing movements and laryngeal control
		Movements of soft palate, pharynx, and larynx
	General visceral efferent (GVE) (parasympathetic)	Parasympathetic to thoracic and abdominal viscera
	Special visceral afferent (SVA)	Taste (epiglottis)
	General visceral afferent (GVA)	Sensory from viscera of neck (larynx, trachea, and esophagus), thorax, and abdomen
XI. Accessory nerve (spinal root)	Special visceral efferent (SVE)	Movements of shoulder and head
XII. Hypoglossal nerve*	General somatic efferent (GSE)	Movements of tongue

*General somatic afferent (GSA)—proprioception from the muscles of the eye and tongue.
†General somatic afferent (GSA)—cutaneous sense from small portion of and just behind external ear and external auditory meatus.

innervate the voluntary musculature of the gill.
3 The *pharyngeal division* is composed of afferent fibers to the pharynx. The relationship of the branchiomeric nerves to a gill slit is retained in a masked form in the land vertebrates, including man. For example, in the trigeminal nerve, the pretrematic division is the maxillary nerve (a sensory nerve), the posttrematic division is composed of the mandibular and lingual nerves (collectively mixed sensory and motor nerves), and the pharyngeal division is the greater palatine nerve (a sensory nerve, Fig. 8-15).

General structural and functional aspects of the cranial nerves

OLFACTORY NERVE (N. I)

The *olfactory, or first cranial, nerve* consists of from 15 to 20 small bundles of unmyelinated axons of neurons whose cell bodies are located in the olfactory mucosa of the nasal cavity. The olfactory neurons are bipolar neurons (SVA) which act as chemoreceptors, transducers of stimuli, and transmitters of nerve impulses to the olfactory bulb. The peripherally directed process of each cell (the "dendrite") commences on the surface of the mucosa. The centrally directed process (the axon) joins one of the bundles, which passes through the cribriform plate of the ethmoid bone and the anterior cranial fossa before terminating in the olfactory bulb (Chap. 15).

These specialized special visceral afferent neurons are unusual among neurons for the following reasons:

1 They are the only sensory neurons in man with cell bodies which are located distally in a peripheral structure (olfactory mucosa).

2 They are both receptors and neurons of the first order.

3 Each dendrite has specialized cilia, which extend into and are bathed in the secretion on the surface of the olfactory mucosa. In man, these are the only nerve processes in direct contact with the external environment. In contrast, gustatory cells in the taste buds are neuroepithelial cells, rather than neurons.

4 The axonal processes of a number of neurons collect into small groups of fibers. Each group is located within a trough ensheathed by neurolemma cells; the axons within each group are not separated from one another by processes of the neurolemma cell (Fig. 2-13).

The total inability to perceive odors is called *anosmia*.

OPTIC NERVE (N. II)

The *optic, or second cranial nerve,* is actually a tract of the central nervous system, not a true peripheral nerve (SSA); it consists of about 1 million fibers of the second order, which are invested by glial rather than neurolemma cells (Chap. 12). The optic nerve comprises the axons of the ganglion cells of the retina. Theoretically the bipolar cells of the retina are the equivalent of the peripheral nerves. These cells are located wholly within the retina and are intercalated between the photoreceptors (rods and cones, which may be considered to be neuroepithelial cells) and the ganglion cells.

The axons of ganglion cells of the retina converge to the optic disk and penetrate through the sclera of the eye (cribriform plate) to form the optic nerve, which is surrounded by all three meninges of the brain. The dura mater is continuous with the sclera of the eye. The subarachnoid and subdural spaces are continuous up to the region of the optic disk. The nerve passes successively through the orbit and the optic canal, including the common tendinous ring which is the origin of the four rectus muscles of the eye. The nerve is continuous with the optic chiasma, which is located in the middle cranial fossa, rostral to the hypophysis. The parasympathetic ciliary ganglion is found within the orbit lateral to the optic nerve. The *central retinal artery* (as well as the vein) enters the optic nerve from below about 10 to 20 mm behind the eye; it supplies the core of the nerve and the entire retina except for the pigment and rod and cone layers. An increase in the intracranial pressure is transmitted to the cerebrospinal fluid of the subarachnoid space surrounding the entire optic nerve, including the region of the optic disk. This increase may result in a condition called *papilledema*. In its early stages, it is characterized by engorgement of the retinal veins, pinkness of the optic disk, and blurring of the margins of the disk. In time, the indentation of the disk is obliterated and elevated.

THE EXTRAOCULAR NERVES—OCULOMOTOR (N. III), TROCHLEAR (N. IV), AND ABDUCENT (N. VI) NERVES (Fig. 7-5)

These three cranial nerves contain the lower motor neurons (GSE) which innervate the six extraocular and levator palpebral muscles. In addition, the oculomotor nerve has preganglionic and parasympathetic fibers (GVE), terminating in the ciliary ganglion with postganglionic neurons which innervate smooth muscles in the eye. Each nerve has proprioceptive fibers (from neuromuscular spindles, GSA), which may have their cell bodies along each nerve, in the trigeminal ganglion or in the mesencephalic nucleus of N. V. The coordinated activities of the extraocular muscles produce the normal conjugate movements of the eyes; the contraction of the levator palpebral muscles elevates the eyelids. The parasympathetic innervation, which is derived from the oculomotor nerve, has a role in accommodation (focusing) and constriction of the pupil. The sympathetic innervation to the eye is derived from postganglionic sympathetic fibers from the internal carotid plexus, which join the third, fourth, and sixth cranial nerves as they pass through the cavernous sinus.

The *nuclear complex of the oculomotor nerve* is located in the anteromedial aspect of the periaqueductal gray at the level of the superior colliculus. The nucleus, which has a triangular shape in cross section, is flanked on its anterolateral sides by the medial longitudinal fasciculus (Fig. 8-10). The root fibers of the oculomotor nerve from this nucleus sweep anteriorly through the medial longitudinal fasciculus, medial tegmentum including the red nucleus and substantia nigra, and enter the interpeduncular fossa as a number of rootlets, which join to form the oculomotor nerve within the interpeduncular cistern. The nerve passes between the posterior cerebral artery and the superior cerebellar artery and then successively through the cavernous sinus, inferior orbital fissure, and

orbit, where it divides into a superior branch (innervating the superior rectus and levator palpebrae muscles) and an inferior branch (innervating the medial rectus, inferior rectus, and inferior oblique muscles).

The oculomotor nuclear complex is subdivided into several longitudinally oriented cell columns and nuclei. The extraocular muscles which are innervated by uncrossed nerve fibers from this complex include the inferior rectus muscle that is innervated by fibers from the posterior cell column, the inferior oblique muscle by the intermediate cell column, and the medial rectus muscle by the anterior cell column. The superior rectus muscle is innervated by crossed fibers from the medial cell column. Each levator palpebral muscle is innervated by both crossed and uncrossed fibers from the caudal central nucleus.

The parasympathetic nuclei (GVE) consists of a pair of narrow columns (accessory oculomotor nucleus of Edinger-Westphal) posterior to the rostral three-fifths of the oculomotor complex; these columns become continuous rostrally with the anterior median nucleus located in the raphe. The accessory oculomotor nucleus and anterior median nuclei give rise to uncrossed preganglionic parasympathetic fibers. They synapse in the ciliary ganglia with postganglionic parasympathetic fibers which innervate smooth muscle of the ciliary body and iris. Of the parasympathetic fibers to the eye, about 90 percent are said to innervate the ciliary musculature (accommodation, Chap. 12), while the remainder innervate the pupillary constrictor muscles of the iris diaphragm (miosis).

Functional Roles The precise roles of the extraocular muscles in eye movements are complex, with many actions depending upon the position of the eyeball within the orbit. The following is a summary:

1 The medial and lateral recti muscles rotate the eyeball around its vertical axis. The medial rectus is an adductor, which deviates the pupil inward toward the nose; the lateral rectus is an abductor, which deviates the pupil outward toward the temple. These muscles are antagonists.

2 The superior and inferior recti muscles rotate the eyeball around its transverse axis. With the eye rotated outward, the superior rectus is a pure elevator (pupil

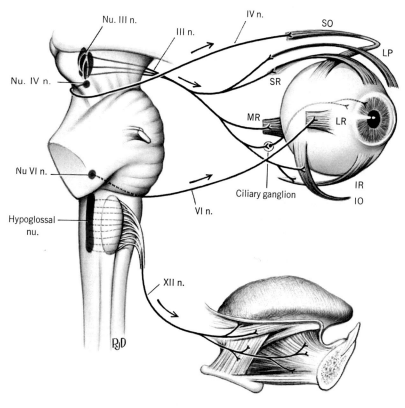

FIGURE 7-5
The cranial nerve nuclei and distribution of the oculomotor, trochlear, abducent, and hypoglossal nerves (III, IV, VI, and XII).

The extraocular muscles are indicated as follows: I.O., inferior oblique; I.R., inferior rectus; L.P., levator palpebral; L.R., lateral rectus; M.R., medial rectus; S.O., superior oblique; S.R., superior rectus.

directed upward), while the inferior rectus is a pure depressor (pupil directed downward). In other positions these muscles also have a role in adducting the eye.

3 The superior and inferior oblique muscles rotate the eyeball around its sagittal axis. With the eye directed inward, the superior oblique is a depressor and the inferior oblique is an elevator of the eye. With the eye directed outward, the superior oblique is an intorter of the eye (rotates on the sagittal axis), while the inferior oblique is an extorter of the eye. The superior rectus and inferior rectus act as intorter and extorter, respectively, when the eye is directed inward.

4 The levator palpebral muscles elevator the upper eyelids.

The movements of the eyes are precisely and delicately coordinated. *Conjugate movements* are those in which the eyes move in the same direction. On looking to the right, the lateral rectus of the right eye and the medial rectus of the left eye are the muscles involved in the movement. *Disjunctive movements* are those in which the eyes move in opposite directions. In close-up vision, the eyes converge. In this disjunctive movement the two medial recti contract and the two lateral recti relax. Conjugate and disjunctive movements are regulated and controlled by supranuclear (upper motor neuron) influences acting through circuits composed of interneurons.

The *trochlear nerve* originates from the small nucleus located in an indentation in the posterior margin of the medial longitudinal fasciculus at the level of the inferior colliculus (Fig. 8-9). The nucleus is actually a caudal extension of the oculomotor nucleus. The fibers from the nucleus of the trochlear nerve curve posterolaterally and caudally along the edge of the periventricular gray; all fibers cross the midline and emerge on the dorsal surface of the brainstem just caudal to the inferior colliculus (Fig. 1-8). The nerve courses through the sequence of rostral pons, along the under surface of the tentorium, lateral wall of the cavernous sinus, superior orbital fissure, and orbit before innervating the superior oblique muscle.

The *abducent* (*abducens*) *nerve* originates from the nucleus located in the floor of the fourth ventricle near the midline in the caudal pons (it forms the abducent or facial colliculus, Fig. 1-9). All its fibers have an ipsilateral course. They pass from the abducent nucleus anteriorly through the tegmentum before emerging from the brainstem just lateral to the pyramid at the pons-medulla junction (Figs. 1-6, 8-7). The nerve then continues forward through the sequence of cisterna pontis, lateral wall of the cavernous sinus, superior orbital fissure, and orbit before innervating the lateral rectus muscle.

Lesions The paralysis of one or more of the extraocular muscles results in diplopia (double vision) because of the faulty coordination of movements of the two eyes. A *complete lesion of an oculomotor nerve* results in the following: *1 ptosis*, or drooping, of the eyelid and inability to elevate the eyelid because of unopposed action of the orbicularis oculi muscle which closes the eyelid (innervated by N. VII); *2* dilated pupil (*mydriasis*) which is unresponsive to the light reflex because of interruption of the parasympathetic fibers and the unopposed activity of the intact sympathetic fibers to the iris diaphragm (Chap. 12); *3* loss of accommodation due to interruption of parasympathetic fibers; lens may be permanently adjusted for distant vision; and *4 external strabismus*, with the pupil directed laterally and downward (*divergent strabismus*) because of unopposed action of the lateral rectus and superior oblique muscles; the inability to direct the affected eye inward, upward, and downward. In this lower motor neuron paralysis of the third nerve, the subject turns his head away from the paralyzed side in an attempt to min-

imize the diplopia caused by the abnormal position of the involved eye.

A *complete lesion of the trochlear nerve* results in a vertical diplopia, head tilt, and limitation of ocular movement on looking down and in. Diplopia occurs when the subject turns his eyes in any direction except upward; the double vision is maximal when the pupils are turned down; this makes walking difficult, especially when walking downstairs. To align the eyes in order to minimize or eliminate the diplopia, the patient tilts his head to the shoulder on the side opposite the paralyzed muscle. Because the trochlear fibers decussate within the dorsal brainstem, the nucleus of the trochlear nerve is on the opposite side from the trochlear nerve itself; hence a lesion of a nucleus of the trochlear nerve is expressed in the contralateral eye.

A *complete lesion of the abducent nerve* results in a horizontal diplopia, with the ipsilateral eye adducted (convergent strabismus) because of the unopposed action of the normal medial rectus muscle. Abduction is limited. The diplopia is maximal when the subject attempts to gaze to the side of the lesion (because the eye with the paralyzed lateral rectus cannot be adequately abducted). It is minimal with gaze to the normal side, because the visual axis of the normal eye can parallel that of the affected eye.

TRIGEMINAL NERVE (N. V) (Figs. 7-6, 8-15)

The *trigeminal, or fifth cranial, nerve* is the main general sensory nerve, composed of GSA fibers conveying the modalities of pain, temperature, touch, and proprioception from the superficial and deep regions of the face. The regions innervated include the skin of the anterior scalp and face; mucous membrane of the mouth (including gum and tongue), nasal cavities and paranasal sinuses, teeth, and meninges. In addition, its masticator (motor) nerve, with SVE fibers, innervates muscles involved with mastication, swallowing, movements of the soft palate and auditory tube, and movements of the tympanic membrane and ear ossicles.

The trigeminal nerve emerges from the anterolateral surface of the midpons as two adjacent roots: the large sensory root and the small motor root. These roots course anteriorly on the floor of the posterior fossa, across the tip of the pet-

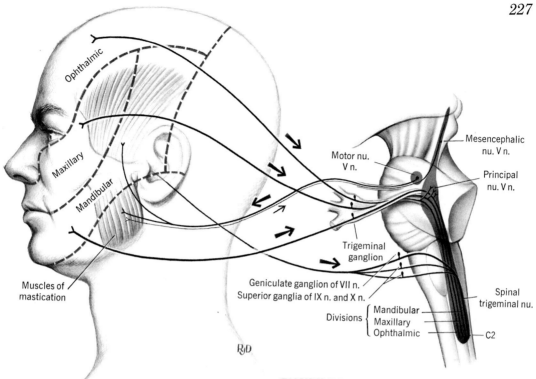

Ophthalmic

Maxillary

Mandibular

Muscles of mastication

Motor nu. V n.

Mesencephalic nu. V n.

Principal nu. V n.

Trigeminal ganglion

Geniculate ganglion of VII n.
Superior ganglia of IX n. and X n.

Divisions {
Mandibular
Maxillary
Ophthalmic
}

Spinal trigeminal nu.

C2

FIGURE 7-6
The cranial nerve nuclei and distribution of the trigeminal nerve (N. V).

Fibers of nerves VII, IX, and X from the region of the outer ear to the spinal nucleus of N. V are illustrated.

rous portion of the temporal bone into the middle cranial fossa, where it joins the massive trigeminal ganglia in the trigeminal cave. The latter is a cavity in the dura mater on the anterior surface of the petrosal bone. The internal carotid artery and the posterior aspect of the cavernous sinus are located medial to the trigeminal ganglion.

The unipolar neurons of the trigeminal ganglion (Gasserian ganglion, semilunar ganglion) give rise to the three large branches of the trigeminal nerve: the ophthalmic, maxillary, and mandibular nerves. The root fibers associated with these nerves are topographically represented within the sensory root. At the locale of emergence of the sensory root from the pons, the ophthalmic fibers are located caudally, the maxillary fibers in an intermediate position, and the mandibular fibers rostrally. In the region where the sensory root joins the trigeminal gan-

glion, the ophthalmic fibers are located medially, the maxillary in an intermediate position, and the mandibular fibers laterally. The motor root is generally located on the medial aspect of the sensory root; it courses laterally on the inferior aspect of the trigeminal ganglion before its fibers blend into the mandibular nerve.

Peripheral distribution The ophthalmic nerve passes forward in the dura mater on the lateral wall of the cavernous sinus and through the superior orbital fissure before entering the orbit. Branches of this nerve innervate the dura mater, including the tentorium, orbit, eye [including the cornea (e.g., corneal reflex)], upper eyelid, skin of the nose, forehead, and scalp back to a line between the ears, and the mucosa of the frontal, sphenoid, and ethmoid paranasal sinuses.

The maxillary nerve passes out of the skull through the foramen rotundum into the pterygopalatine fossa, where it becomes associated with the pterygopalatine ganglion (parasympathetic ganglion which receives preganglionic fibers from the facial nerve). The branches of the maxillary nerve innervate the dura of the middle cranial fossa, lower eyelid, skin of the temple, upper cheek, adjacent area of the nose and upper lip, mucous membranes of the upper mouth, nose, roof of pharynx, and maxillary, ethmoid, and sphenoid paranasal sinuses, and the gums, teeth, and palate of the upper jaw.

The mandibular nerve passes from the middle cranial fossa through the foramen ovale into the infratemporal fossa. One of its branches, the lingual nerve, is associated with the submandibular ganglion (parasympathetic ganglion) which receives preganglionic fibers from the chorda tympani of the facial nerve. Branches of the mandibular nerve supply the sensory innervation to part of the dura mater of the middle and anterior cranial fossa; teeth and gums of the lower jaw; oral mucosa of the cheek, floor of the mouth, and anterior two-thirds of the tongue; skin of the auricular temporal region, lower lip, external auditory meatus, tympanic membrane, and lower jaw; and the temporomandibular joint. The masticator nerve supplies the lower neuron innervation to *1* the four muscles of mastication (temporalis, masseter, and internal and external pterygoids), *2* the mylohyoid and anterior belly of the digastric muscles, and *3* the tensor tympani and tensor veli palatine muscles.

The jaw jerk is a two-neuron flexor reflex (similar to the extensor knee jerk), which involves the temporalis and masseter muscles. This reflex can be evoked by tapping the chin of the slightly opened mouth. The afferent limb of the reflex arc is composed of neurons of the mesencephalic nucleus of N. V, which convey influences from the neuromuscular spindles of these muscles to the motor nucleus of N. V. The lower motor neurons from the latter nucleus comprise the efferent limb, which innervates the muscles of mastication. The mylohyoid and anterior belly of the digastric muscles have a role in mastica-

tion and swallowing. During its contraction, the tensor tympani, through its pull on the malleus, tenses the tympanic membrane; this protects the tympanic membrane by dampening the amplitude of its vibration to loud noises. The tensor veli palatine muscle helps to prevent food from passing into the nasal pharynx by tensing the soft palate.

The branches of the trigeminal nerve are characterized by several special features.

1 Each of the three major branches—ophthalmic, maxillary, and mandibular—supplies a distinct dermatome of the head, face, and oral cavity (Figs. 7-6, 8-16). These three nerves show practically no dermatomal overlap, as do the nerves innervating the dermatomes formed by the spinal nerves.

2 Information from proprioceptive endings (e.g., neuromuscular spindles) in the extraocular muscles and muscles of facial expression are conveyed to the central nervous system by nerve fibers of the oculomotor, trochlear, abducent, and facial nerves, which join the trigeminal nerve. These fibers are presumed to have their cell bodies in the trigeminal ganglion and in the mesencephalic nucleus of the trigeminal nerve.

3 The lingual branch of the mandibular nerve contains gustatory fibers from the anterior two-thirds of the tongue. In fact, these fibers are facial rather than trigeminal nerve fibers. These taste fibers pass from the nucleus solitarius through the nervus intermedius and one of its branches, the chorda tympani, which joins the lingual nerve.

4 Many fibers of the autonomic nervous system join the branches of the trigeminal nerve. Among these are the postganglionic sympathetic fibers from the superior cervical ganglion, which leave the external carotid artery plexus and join each of the major branches of the trigeminal nerve. These fibers supply the sympathetic innervation to the sweat glands of the skin, the mucosal glands (mucous and serous) of the nasal and oral cavities, and the blood vessels.

5 Each of the three major branches of the trigeminal nerve is associated with a parasympathetic ganglion. The ophthalmic nerve receives postganglionic fibers from the ciliary ganglion, the maxillary nerve from the pterygopalatine ganglion, and the mandibular nerve from the submandibular and otic ganglia. Recall that preganglionic fibers to these ganglia are derived from the oculomotor nerve (ciliary ganglion), from the facial nerve (pterygopalatine and submandibular ganglia), and from the glossopharyngeal nerve (otic ganglion). The trigeminal nerve is actually the vehicle for the distribution of the postganglionic parasympathetic fibers to the smooth muscles of the eye and to the glands of the head (including the lacrimal gland and those of the nasal and oral mucosa).

Central projections The sensory root (portio major) of the trigeminal nerve enters the pons and divides into an ascending limb (which terminates in the principal nucleus of the trigeminal nerve) and a descending limb (which forms the spinal tract of the trigeminal nerve, N. V). The fibers of the sensory root of the trigeminal nerve rotate so that the fibers from the caudally located mandibular nerve become located posteriorly in the spinal tract of N. V, those from the rostrally located ophthalmic nerve become located anteriorly in the spinal tract of N. V, and those from the maxillary nerve become located in an intermediate position between the other two nerves (Fig. 7-6). The sensory root fibers consist of several types: *1* nonbifurcating ascending fibers to the principal sensory nucleus— these subserve touch, position sense, and two-point discrimination; *2* nonbifurcating descending fibers of the spinal tract of N. V—these subserve pain and temperature; and *3* bifurcating fibers each with an ascending branch to the principal sensory nucleus and a descending branch of the spinal tract of N. V—these subserve touch, position sense, and two-point discrimination. The descending fibers of the ophthalmic, maxillary, and mandibular nerves have collateral branches, which terminate throughout the spinal nucleus of N. V, and terminal branches, which descend as far caudally as the first two cervical spinal levels. The spinal nucleus of N. V is subdivided into *1* the rostrally located pars oralis, which receives tactile input from the head, mouth, and nose; *2* the intermediately located pars interpolaris, which receives input from cutaneous areas of the forehead, cheeks, and angle of the jaw; and *3* the caudally located pars caudalis, which receives

the modalities of light touch, pain, and temperature from the entire anterior part of the head.

In general, the pain and temperature modalities are conveyed from all trigeminal nerves via sensory root fibers which, after entering the pons, descend in the spinal tract of N. V as far caudal as the C2 spinal level. These fibers terminate in the spinal nucleus of N. V (pars caudalis and upper two cervical levels). The touch-pressure, position sense, and two-point discrimination modalities are conveyed via the sensory root fibers, which, after entering the pons, terminate in the principal nucleus and pars oralis of the spinal nucleus of the trigeminal nerve. Many collateral branches descend in the spinal tract before terminating in the spinal nucleus of N. V. Unconscious proprioceptive information (pressure and position sense) from the teeth, periodontal membrane, palate, muscles, and temporomandibular joint is conveyed to the mesencephalic nucleus of the trigeminal nerve. The motor nucleus of N. V is the nucleus of origin of the lower motor neurons which pass through the motor root and the mandibular nerve to the voluntary muscles innervated by N. V.

Lesions The interruption of all trigeminal fibers unilaterally results in anesthesia and loss of general senses in the region innervated by N. V and a lower motor neuron paralysis (weakness, fasciculations, loss of jaw jerk unilaterally and atrophy) of the jaw muscles. The sensory changes include loss of smarting effect in one nostril from the insensitivity of the nasal mucosa to ammonia and other volatile chemicals and loss of corneal sensation. The complete interruption of the sensory fibers from the cornea results in loss of the ipsilateral and contralateral (consensual) corneal reflex. The afferent limb of the corneal reflex (N. V) stimulates through interneurons both facial motor nuclei, whose lower motor neurons innervate the orbicularis oculi muscles of both eyes. The loss of proprioceptive input may result in the relaxation of the ipsilateral muscles of facial expressions (innervated by N. VII). The loss of the jaw jerk results from the interruption of both the afferent and efferent limbs of the reflex arc. Because of the action of the contracting pterygoid muscles on the normal side, the jaw, when protruded, will deviate and point to the paralyzed side. The patient may experience partial deafness to low-pitched sounds because of the paralysis of the tensor tympani muscle. The floor of the mouth on the paralyzed side exhibits flaccidity because of the paralysis of the mylohyoid muscle and the anterior belly of the digastric.

Sharp, agonizing pain localized in the area of distribution of one of the three branches of the trigeminal nerve is known as trigeminal neuralgia or *tic douloureux*. This condition of unknown cause may be accompanied by muscle twitchings during an episode. The stimulation of a region, called a *trigger zone*, may initiate an attack.

The supranuclear (upper motor neuron) influences upon the motor nucleus of N. V are outlined in Chap. 8. Unilateral supranuclear lesions usually do not impair trigeminal motor activity. This is because *1* crossed and uncrossed corticobulbar fibers and *2* crossed and uncrossed corticoreticular fibers (through interneurons) project to the motor nucleus of N. V.

FACIAL NERVE (N. VII) (Fig. 7-7)

The *facial, or seventh cranial, nerve* consists of the facial nerve proper with its lower motor neurons and the *nervus intermedius* with its sensory and parasympathetic components. The SVE fibers of the facial nerve proper convey motor impulses to the muscles of facial (*mimetic*) expression (i.e., those involved in closing the eyelids, frowning, smiling, whistling, wrinkling the forehead, puffing the cheek to blow up a balloon, and pursing the lips). Other muscles innervated by the facial nerve include the stapedius (controls the movements of the stapes) and the posterior belly of the digastric muscle (elevates hyoid bone). All the sensory neurons of the first order in the nervus intermedius have their unipolar cell bodies in the geniculate ganglion. This includes taste (SVA) from the anterior two-thirds of the tongue, GSA information from the back of the

external ear, and GVA input from the glands and other visceral structures of the face. The parasympathetic fibers (GVE) of the nervus intermedius, through their connections in the pterygopalatine and submandibular ganglia, exert influences on the lacrimal, nasal, oral, submaxillary, and sublingual glands and blood vessels.

The facial nerve emerges from the inferior lateral aspect of the brainstem at the pons-medulla junction just anterior to the vestibulocochlear nerve. The nervus intermedius is located between these two nerves. The three nerves pass successively through the cerebellopontine angle and internal auditory meatus. The facial nerve proper continues through the facial canal from which it emerges at the stylomastoid foramen; it then arborizes into branches which innervate the muscles of facial expression. Within the facial canal (distal to the geniculate ganglion), the facial nerve has three branches: the nerve to the stapedius muscle; the chorda tympani with its special (taste) and general visceral afferent fibers and preganglionic parasympathetic fibers to the submandibular ganglion (postganglionic fibers from this ganglion innervate the submandibular, sublingual, and other small salivary glands); and the nerve to the external auditory meatus and external ear (general somatic afferent).

The greater petrosal nerve is a branch of the nervus intermedius. It is composed of preganglionic parasympathetic fibers which synapse with postganglionic neurons in the pterygopalatine ganglion; the latter project influences to the lacrimal gland and the glands of the nasal cavity and palate. Some special (taste) and general visceral afferent fibers also pass through the greater petrosal nerve. Some postganglionic sympathetic fibers from the superior cervical ganglion leave the carotid plexus to join some branches of the facial nerve.

Central projections and connections The special visceral efferent fibers to the muscles of facial expression arise from the motor nucleus of the seventh nerve. After leaving the nucleus, the fibers take a hairpin course through the lower pons as they recurve as the internal genu around the nucleus of the abducent nerve before passing into the cerebellopontine angle. The preganglionic parasympathetic fibers from

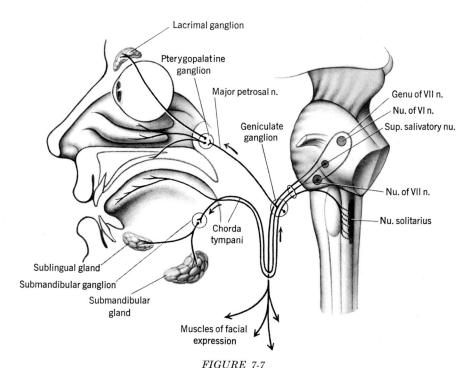

Lacrimal ganglion

Pterygopalatine ganglion

Major petrosal n.

Geniculate ganglion

Genu of VII n.

Nu. of VI n.

Sup. salivatory nu.

Nu. of VII n.

Nu. solitarius

Chorda tympani

Sublingual gland

Submandibular ganglion

Submandibular gland

Muscles of facial expression

FIGURE 7-7
The cranial nerve nuclei and distribution of the facial nerve (cranial nerve VII).

the superior salivatory nucleus pass via the nervus intermedius and its two branches: the chorda tympani to the submandibular ganglion, and the greater petrosal nerve to the pterygopalatine ganglion.

All afferent fibers associated with the nervus intermedius have their cell bodies (unipolar neurons) in the *geniculate ganglion.* The gustatory fibers from the anterior two-thirds of the tongue course through the chorda tympani primarily and at times through the greater petrosal nerve to the lateral and rostral aspects of the nucleus solitarius (called the *gustatory nucleus*). The general somatic afferent fibers from the external auditory meatus and back of the external ear course through the nervus intermedius and join the spinal tract of N. V before terminating in the spinal nucleus of N. V. General visceral afferent fibers from the visceral organs terminate in the nucleus solitarius.

Lesions A lesion interrupting the facial nerve (e.g., *Bell's palsy*) is primarily expressed as a

lower motor neuron paralysis of the muscles of facial expression. There is an abolition of both voluntary and reflex movements of the facial muscles. The paresis of Bell's palsy may occur suddenly (it is believed to be due to an edema of the nerve following rheumatoid infection of the nerve in the facial canal of the petrosal bone) and may be followed within a few months by a spontaneous recovery. On the ipsilateral side, the face is masklike, the forehead is immobile, the corner of the muscle sags, the nasolabial folds of the face are flattened, facial lines are lost, and saliva may drip from the corner of the mouth. The patient is unable to whistle or puff the cheek because the buccinator muscle is paralyzed. When the patient is smiling, the normal muscles draw the contralateral corner of the mouth up while the paralyzed corner continues to sag. Corneal sensitivity remains (N. V), but the patient is unable to blink or close the eyelid (N. VII). To protect the cornea from damage (e.g., drying), the eyelids are closed therapeutically or other measures are taken (e.g., patient wears eye mask, or lids are closed by sutures). Lacrimation on the lesion side may be impaired (fibers which pass through the greater petrosal nerve). There may be a reduction in the secretion of saliva (fibers which pass through the chorda tympani). Taste will be lost on the ipsilateral anterior two-thirds of the tongue (fibers which pass through the chorda tympani). An increased acuity to sounds (*hyperacusis*), especially to low tones, results from the paralysis of the stapedius muscle, which normally dampens the amplitude of the vibrations of the ear ossicles.

A *unilateral supranuclear lesion* of the upper motor neurons (corticobulbar and corticoreticular fibers) to the facial nucleus (see Chap. 8) results in a marked weakness of the muscles of expression of the lower part of the face on the side contralateral to the lesion. The frontalis muscle (which wrinkles the forehead) and the orbicularis oculi muscle (which closes the eyelid) are unaffected. The accepted explanation states that *1* bilateral upper motor neuron projections from the cerebral cortex influence the lower motor neurons innervating the frontalis muscle and orbicularis, and *2* only unilateral, crossed, upper motor neuron projections influence the lower motor neurons innervating the muscles of facial expression of the lower part of the face. Hence the contralateral muscles are deprived of upper motor neuron influences.

In some patients with unilateral supranuclear lesions, the contralateral, weak lower facial muscles are paralyzed to volitional influences but will contract to emotional or mimetic influences (jokes, distress). In *voluntary facial palsy* the deficits of facial movements are accentuated when the patient is consciously trying to contract these muscles. This voluntary facial palsy is apparently due to the interruption of the cortical influences conveyed by the corticobulbar and corticoreticular fibers. The mimetic (involuntary) influences are presumed to originate from such subcortical nuclei as the globus pallidus and thalamus. When the seventh nerve is deprived of these influences, the patient will have a *mimetic facial paralysis*. This may or may not be accompanied by a voluntary facial paralysis.

Note the distinction between a *lower motor (infranuclear) lesion* and an *upper motor (supranuclear) lesion* involving the muscles of facial expression. In a lower motor neuron paralysis these muscles on one-half of the face have a marked weakness; in an upper motor neuron paralysis only those muscles on the lower one-half of the face have a marked weakness.

VESTIBULOCOCHLEAR NERVE (N. VIII)
(Fig. 7-2 and Chap. 10)

The *vestibulocochlear (auditory, acoustic, or statoacoustic) or eighth cranial nerve* is actually two nerves. The *cochlear nerve* is associated with hearing (exteroception) and the *vestibular (stato-) nerve* is concerned with the state of equilibrium and orientation in three-dimensional space (proprioception). Both components are special somatic afferent. The bipolar cells of the cochlear nerve have their cell bodies in the spiral ganglion located within the spiral canal of the modiolus, and those of the vestibular nerve are in the vestibular ganglion located within the distal part of the internal auditory meatus.

After emerging from the lateral aspect of the pons-medulla junction, the vestibular root and the cochlear root join and pass laterally and slightly rostrally in the cerebellopontine angle and then through the internal acoustic meatus, accompanied, in part, by the facial nerve proper and the nervus intermedius. In the distal end of the meatus the nerve divides into cochlear and vestibular nerves. The cochlear nerve passes into the ganglion cells of the spiral ganglion lying within the spiral canal of the modiolus. The peripherally directed fibers ("dendrites") of the bipolar spiral ganglion cells pass through small canals within the bony spiral laminae to form a spiral sheet of fibers, which innervates the hair cells of the spiral organ of Corti. Within the spiral organ, the nerve fibers are unmyelinated. The vestibular nerve divides into two parts, each with its own ganglion: the superior part and inferior part of the vestibular ganglion. The distally directed fibers ("dendrites") of the bipolar vestibular cells are distributed as follows:

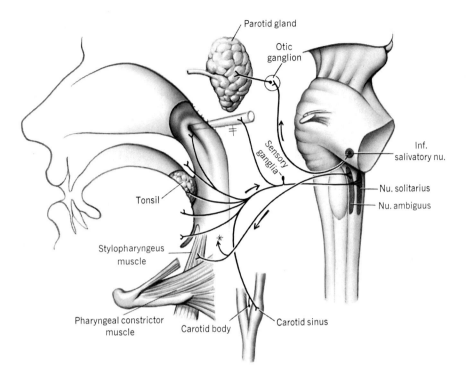

FIGURE 7-8

The cranial nerve nuclei and distribution of the glossopharyngeal nerve (N. IX).

This cranial nerve supplies the motor innervation to the stylopharyngeus muscle, the muscles (*) of the anterior and posterior pillars of the fauces, and possibly some superior pharyngeal constrictor muscle fibers (involved in deglutition). ‡Auditory tube.

1 the fibers of the superior part terminate in the receptor cells of the ampullae of the anterior and lateral semicircular canals, the macula of the utricle, and part of the macula of the saccule; 2 the fibers of the inferior part terminate in the receptor cells of the ampulla of the major part of the saccule and in the ampulla of the posterior semicircular canal; and 3 a small branch of the inferior part passes to the spiral ganglion of the cochlea; this branch is said to be composed of cochlear efferent fibers (Chap. 10). The vestibulocochlear nerve is the only nerve that terminates wholly within a bone (petrous portion of the temporal bone); all other cranial nerves emerge from the skull.

GLOSSOPHARYNGEAL NERVE (N. IX)
(Fig. 7-8)

The *glossopharyngeal, or ninth cranial, nerve* (from *glosso,* "tongue," and *pharynx,* "throat") is a mixed branchiomeric nerve composed of

1 special visceral afferent fibers conveying taste sensations from the posterior third of the tongue; 2 general somatic afferent fibers from the back of external ear and external auditory meatus; 3 general visceral afferent fibers from the *a* mucous membranes of tympanic cavity, auditory tube, palatoglossal arches, tonsil, soft palate, posterior third of tongue, and upper pharynx, and *b* pressoreceptors in the carotid sinus and chemoreceptors in the carotid body; 4 general visceral efferent fibers (parasympathetic) conveying visceromotor influences to the parotid gland; and 5 special visceral efferent fibers to the stylopharyngeus muscle (elevates

upper pharynx) and often to the muscles within the palatal arches and the upper pharyngeal constrictor muscle (involved with swallowing). The visceral afferent fibers have their unipolar cell bodies in the inferior (petrosal) ganglion, while the somatic afferent fibers have theirs in the superior ganglion.

The glossopharyngeal nerve emerges as five or six rootlets from the posterior lateral sulcus of the rostral medulla. These rootlets are located near the facial nerve and are in series to the caudally located rootlets of the vagus nerve. The rootlets of N. IX join to form the nerve, which passes, along with the vagus and accessory nerves, through the jugular foramen. It continues in an arc on the lateral aspect of the pharynx toward the region of the tonsils and soft palate.

The gustatory fibers from the taste buds are relayed by first-order neurons to the rostral and lateral regions of the *nucleus solitarius* (called *gustatory nucleus*). The presence or absence of taste sensations in the posterior third of the tongue can be evaluated clinically by the topical application of galvanic current in the tonsillar region. Normally an acid taste sensation is induced. The fibers conveying touch, pain, and temperature from the external ear, external auditory meatus, and tympanic cavity, and possibly from the region of the palatal arches and posterior third of the tongue, terminate in the spinal tract and nucleus of the fifth nerve, whereas those conveying tactile impulses terminate in the principal nucleus of the fifth nerve.

Specialized epithelioid cells are located within the carotid body at the carotid bifurcation and the aortic bodies (associated with the major thoracic arteries). These cells are arterial *chemoreceptors* which are stimulated by a decrease in the oxygen level, a rise in the carbon dioxide content, or a decrease in the hydrogen ion concentration in the arterial blood. General visceral afferent fibers convey influences from these chemosensitive cells via both the glossopharyngeal and vagus nerves. They terminate in the nucleus solitarius.

Stretch pressoreceptors are diffusely located within the adventitia of the carotid sinus at the carotid bifurcation, aortic arch, pulmonary tree, and in the atrium and ventricles of the heart. These *pressoreceptors* respond with changes in the intraarterial pressure. Nerve fibers of cranial nerves IX and X convey influences from the pressoreceptors centrally to the nucleus solitarius. The input from these chemoreceptors and pressoreceptors is integrated into the activity of the cardiovascular and respiratory centers in the medulla (*carotid reflex*). In addition, collaterals of the glossopharyngeal fibers terminate in the parasympathetic dorsal motor nucleus of the vagus nerve. Concomitant with a rise in the blood pressure, there is an increase in the frequency of impulses in the fibers innervating these stretch receptors. These influences appear to inhibit sympathetic activity and to facilitate parasympathetic vagal activity (reduction in the heart rate and arterial pressure). Following a pronounced lowering of blood pressure, there is a decrease in the frequency of impulses. This results in an increase in sympathetic and a reduction in parasympathetic discharges (an increase in the heart rate and arterial pressure).

The preganglionic parasympathetic fibers originate in the so-called *"inferior salivatory nucleus"*—a physiologically defined nucleus located just rostral to the dorsal vagal nucleus. The fibers from these cells course via the lesser petrosal nerve to the otic ganglion. The postganglionic parasympathetic cells in this ganglion give rise to secretomotor fibers to the parotid gland. Sympathetic fibers do not appear to innervate the parotid gland.

The special visceral efferent fibers of the glossopharyngeal nerve originate from the rostral portions of the *ambiguus nucleus*. The stylopharyngeus muscle is often said to be the only muscle innervated by the glossopharyngeal nerve. However, the palatal arch and superior pharyngeal constrictors are probably innervated by the glossopharyngeal nerve as well as the vagus nerve. This is indicated because following the interruption of N. IX, there may be a deviation of the pharynx, lowering of the palatal arches, and difficulty in swallowing.

Lesions Interruption of all fibers of the glossopharyngeal nerve results in the following symptoms: *1* loss of sensation, including taste, in the posterior third of the tongue and adjacent area; *2* unilateral loss of the *pharyngeal* (or

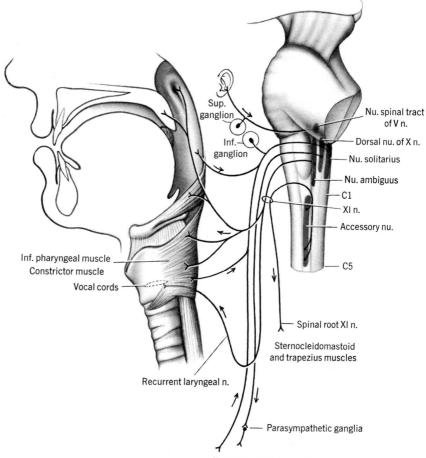

Sup. ganglion

Inf.- ganglion

Nu. spinal tract of V n.

Dorsal nu. of X n.

Nu. solitarius

Nu. ambiguus

C1

XI n.

Accessory nu.

C5

Inf. pharyngeal muscle
Constrictor muscle

Vocal cords

Spinal root XI n.

Sternocleidomastoid and trapezius muscles

Recurrent laryngeal n.

Parasympathetic ganglia

Thoracic and abdominal viscera

FIGURE 7-9
The cranial nerve nuclei and distribution of the vagus and accessory nerves (X and XI).

gag) reflex; *3* difficulty in swallowing (*dysphagia*); and *4* impairment of the *carotid reflex*. The *pharyngeal reflex* consists of the constriction of the pharyngeal musculature accompanied by the retraction of the tongue when the tonsillar region is stimulated; the afferent input to this reflex is conveyed via the glossopharyngeal nerve, while the efferent limb of the reflex arc is through the vagus and/or glossopharyngeal nerves. Thus the gag reflex may be accompanied by unilateral loss of the palatal and uvular reflexes with a deviation of the palate and uvula to the normal side (because

they are unopposed by the paralyzed muscles). *Glossopharyngeal neuralgia* (similar to trigeminal neuralgia) may be triggered by chewing or swallowing.

VAGUS NERVE (N. X) (Fig. 7-9)

The *vagus, or tenth cranial, nerve* is a mixed nerve with functional components similar to those of the glossopharyngeal nerve. A few special visceral afferent fibers with their cell bodies in the inferior ganglion relay influences from the taste buds on the epiglottis to the "gustatory" nucleus of the nucleus solitarius. Sensory information is also conveyed via general visceral afferent fibers (cell bodies in the inferior ganglion) from many sources to the nucleus solitarius. These sources include *1* the pharynx, esophagus, stomach and intestinal tract (to the left colic flexure), larynx, bronchi and lungs, and such organs as the liver, pancreas, and their ducts; *2* pressoreceptors in the aortic arch, atrium, and ventricles of the heart and in the pulmonary tree; and *3* chemoreceptors in the aortic bodies and major thoracic arteries. The influences from these structures may be interpreted as hunger pangs, fullness and distention of the abdominal viscera, and nausea (this information may also be conveyed to the spinal cord and its sensory pathways). They are also utilized by the visceral centers (e.g., cardiovascular and respiratory centers) in the medulla.

The general somatic afferent fibers from the back of the external ear and external auditory meatus pass through the spinal tract of N. V before terminating in the spinal nucleus of N. V.

The general visceral efferent fibers from the cells of the dorsal vagal nucleus in the medulla relay the parasympathetic influences via the vagus nerve to the heart and the smooth muscles and glands of the thoracic and abdominal viscera. These include the larynx, trachea and lungs, esophagus, gastrointestinal tract (to the left colic flexure), and associated glands and their ducts. The functional aspects of this innervation are discussed in Chap. 6.

The special visceral efferent fibers from the nucleus ambiguus of the medulla supply the lower motor neuron innervation to all the muscles of the soft palate (except the tensor veli palatini), pharynx (except the stylopharyngeus muscle), cricothyroid muscle, and all other intrinsic muscles of the larynx. Some of the palatal arch and pharyngeal constrictor musculature may be also innervated by fibers from the nucleus ambiguus which course through the glossopharyngeal nerve. The intrinsic muscles of the larynx and possibly some pharyngeal constrictor muscles are innervated by fibers from the nucleus ambiguus which pass through the cranial root of the accessory nerve before joining the vagus nerve. *In summary,* the SVE fibers of the vagus and cranial root of the accessory nerves are functionally involved with the movements of the soft palate, auditory tube (opening the lumen of the tube, e.g., to relieve pressure in the middle ear during rapid ascent in an elevator), pharynx, and larynx; these are associated with swallowing and regulating the laryngeal apertures during respiration and phonation.

The vagus nerve emerges as rootlets from the posterior lateral sulcus. The rostral rootlets are primarily sensory, and the caudal rootlets are primarily motor. These rootlets join and, along with the glossopharyngeal and accessory nerves, pass through the jugular foramen into the neck. After this the vagus nerve and its branches are distributed to structures in the neck, thorax, and abdomen. The spinal portion of the accessory nerve joins the vagus within and just distal to the jugular foramen. Small branches leave the vagus in the vicinity of the superior ganglia: one branch innervates the dura mater of the posterior fossa of the skull, and the other branch (auricular) innervates the cutaneous area in the back of the external ear and the floor of the external auditory meatus.

Lesions A complete unilateral lesion of the vagus nerve results in the following: *1* the flaccid soft palate produces a voice with a twang, and *2* swallowing is difficult (*dysphagia*) because of the unilateral paralysis of the pharyngeal constrictors; the pharynx is shifted slightly to the normally innervated side. Because of the unilateral paralysis of the palatal, uvular, and palatine arch musculature, the soft palate is elevated and the uvula deviates to the normal side during vocalization. A transient *tachycardia* (increased heartbeat) is a consequence of the interruption of some parasympathetic stimulation. After a unilateral lesion of the bulbar root fibers (inferior laryngeal nerve) of the accessory nerve, the ipsilateral vocal fold becomes fixed and partially adducted to the midline; the voice is hoarse (*dysphonia*) and reduced to a whisper. Bilateral lesions of the vagus nerves are rapidly fatal because the adducted vocal cords obstruct the flow of adequate amounts of air to and from the lungs. Asphyxia follows unless a tracheostomy is performed. Paralysis following lesions of vagal neurons may occur in *bulbar polimyelitis.*

ACCESSORY (SPINAL ACCESSORY) NERVE (N. XI)
(Fig. 7-9)

The *accessory, or eleventh cranial, nerve* arises as two roots: spinal and bulbar (cranial). The fibers (SVE) of the *spinal root* originate from cells located in the lateral portion of lamina IX of spinal segments C1 through C5 (Fig. 8-2). They course through the lateral funiculus and emerge as rootlets on the lateral side of the spinal cord between the dorsal and ventral roots. The rootlets join to form a common trunk which ascends within the vertebral canal on the posterior side of the denticulate ligament before passing through the foramen magnum. The rootlets of the *bulbar root* are actually composed of fibers (SVE) of the vagus nerve arising from the caudal portion of the nucleus ambiguus. The spinal and bulbar roots join and pass through the jugular foramen posterior to the jugular vein. Just distal to the jugular foramen the bulbar root rejoins the vagus nerve; its special visceral efferent fibers form the inferior (recurrent) laryngeal nerve which innervates the intrinsic muscles of the larynx. The spinal root descends into the neck in a posterocaudal direction to innervate the ipsilateral sternocleidomastoid and upper portions of the trapezius muscles. Motor fibers of the cervical segments which course via the cervical nerves of the cervical plexus supply the lower portions of the trapezius muscle.

Lesions A lower motor neuron paralysis is a consequence of the interruption of the accessory nerve. A unilateral lesion of the spinal root fibers is indicated by a weakness in the ability to rotate the head so that the chin points to the side contralateral to the lesion (paralyzed sternocleidomastoid muscle) and in a downward and outward rotation of the scapula accompanied by the flaring of the vertebral border of the scapula, a shoulder sag, and an upper extremity droop (paralyzed upper portion of the trapezius muscle). The head is readily held in its normal position. Although the chin can be pointed satisfactorily to the paralyzed side, it can be turned away from the affected side only to a limited degree. The effects of a lesion of the fibers of the bulbar root are noted with the vagus nerve.

HYPOGLOSSAL NERVE (N. XII)

The lower motor neuron fibers (GSE) of the *hypoglossal, or twelfth cranial, nerve* originate in the nucleus of the hypoglossal nerve, which is a 2-cm-long column of motor cells located underneath the floor of the fourth ventricle just lateral to the midline. It forms the bulge of the *hypoglossal trigone* (Fig. 1-9). The uncrossed nerve fibers pass ventrally through the tegmentum of the medulla lateral to the MLF, lateral lemniscus, and pyramid and medial to the inferior olivary nuclear complex. They emerge as 10 to 15 rootlets in the anterolateral sulcus. The rootlets join in the hypoglossal canal to form the hypoglossal nerve, which passes in an arc lateral to the pharynx to the root of the tongue. The nerve divides into branches which innervate the ipsilateral intrinsic muscles of the tongue, and the hypoglossus, styloglossus, and genioglossus muscles. Clinically, the chin to tongue muscle—the genioglossus—is important because the contraction of this pair results in the protrusion of the tongue.

Lesions Interruption of all the fibers of N. XII produces an ipsilateral lower motor neuron paralysis of the tongue. The fasciculations of the early stages are followed by the atrophy of the muscles, which results in a wrinkled tongue surface on the side of the lesion. When protruded, the tip of the tongue deviates to the paralyzed side. This deviation is due to the unopposed contraction of the contralateral genioglossus, which pulls the base of the tongue forward. Otherwise functional disturbances are minimal because many intrinsic tongue muscle fibers cross the midline. Bilateral lesions of the hypoglossal nerves result in an immobile tongue which can be displaced into the throat, interfering with respiration. Tracheotomy may be required.

PERIPHERAL GANGLIA ASSOCIATED WITH THE CRANIAL NERVES

Two types of peripheral ganglia are associated with the cranial nerves: *1 sensory ganglia,* which are the equivalent of the dorsal roots of the spinal nerves, and *2 parasympathetic ganglia* of the autonomic nervous system.

Sensory ganglia All the cell bodies of the sensory neurons of the spinal nerves are located in the spinal ganglia. In the case of each cranial nerve, the cell bodies of their sensory ganglia are usually located in one or more cranial ganglia (Fig. 7-1). Table 7-1 lists the cranial nerves and the name and location of the cell bodies of the peripheral sensory neurons. All sensory ganglia of the cranial nerves (except for the mesencephalic nucleus of the fifth nerve and the bipolar cells of the retina) are located outside the central nervous system (as are the spinal ganglia of the spinal nerves). The retina is considered to be a distal extension of the central nervous system.

Parasympathetic ganglia Within the head there are four parasympathetic ganglia where the preganglionic fibers (arising from cell bodies located within the brainstem) synapse with postganglionic neurons. These include the *ciliary ganglion* of the N. III, the *pterygopalatine and submandibular ganglia* of N. VII, and the *otic ganglion* of N. IX. The parasympathetic ganglia associated with the vagus nerve are the terminal ganglia located near or within the visceral organs of the thorax and abdomen.

CRANIAL NERVE NUCLEI WITHIN THE CENTRAL NERVOUS SYSTEM

The sensory neurons of the cranial nerves terminate and synapse within the brainstem in the sensory cranial nerve nuclei (Fig. 7-1). The motor nuclei of the cranial nerves are the location of cell bodies whose axons course through the cranial nerves to voluntary muscles or to parasympathetic ganglia (Figs. 7-3, 7-4). These nuclei are arranged in six longitudinal columns in the brainstem: *1 special somatic afferent, 2 general somatic afferent, 3 visceral afferent, 4 general somatic efferent, 5 general visceral efferent,* and *6 special visceral efferent.* The nuclei are illustrated in Figs. 8-2 through 8-11 and Atlas Figs. 1 through 25.

Special somatic afferent column This column includes the *four vestibular nuclei* and the *two cochlear nuclei* which are associated with the eighth cranial nerve. It is located in the dorsolateral tegmentum in the upper medulla and lower pons.

General somatic afferent column This column is located throughout the brainstem from the upper midbrain into the upper cervical spinal cord levels (in the lateral tegmentum of the pons and medulla and the dorsomedial tegmentum of the midbrain). The nuclei of this column include the *mesencephalic nucleus of the fifth nerve* (proprioception), *principal sensory nucleus* (chief, superior, or main sensory nucleus) of the fifth nerve located in the midpons (touch), and the *spinal (descending) nucleus of the fifth nerve* located in the lower pons, medulla, and upper cervical spinal cord (pain and temperature). All general somatic afferent fibers of the fifth, seventh, ninth, or tenth cranial nerves terminate in these nuclei. The mesencephalic nucleus of the fifth nerve is unusual, for it is actually composed of cell bodies of neurons of the first order. It may be considered as a portion of the trigeminal ganglion of the fifth cranial nerve displaced into the midbrain.

Visceral afferent column The visceral afferent column consists of the *nucleus solitarius*, located in the medulla just lateral to the dorsal vagal motor nucleus. The visceral senses conveyed by fibers of the seventh, ninth, and tenth cranial nerves terminate in this nucleus. This includes the impulses from taste endings (special visceral), pressoreceptors, and chemoreceptors (general visceral). All taste fibers are conveyed by the three cranial nerves (N. VII, N. IX, and N. X), and they terminate in this nucleus. The rostral portion of the solitary nucleus, called the gustatory nucleus, is involved with taste; the intermediate portion is a link in the cardiovascular reflex; and the caudal portion has a role in respiration.

General somatic efferent column Consisting of the *nucleus of the oculomotor nerve* (midbrain), *nucleus of the trochlear nerve* (lower midbrain), *nucleus of the abducent nerve* (lower pons), and *nucleus of the hypoglossal nerve* (medulla), this column is located in the dorsomedial tegmentum adjacent to the medial raphe and ventral to the central canal. These nuclei consist of the lower motor neurons to the voluntary muscles of the eye and the tongue.

General visceral efferent column   Also called the parasympathetic nuclear column, it includes the *accessory oculomotor nucleus (of Edinger-Westphal)* (midbrain), the *superior and inferior salivatory nuclei* (lower pons and upper medulla), and the *dorsal motor nucleus of the vagus nerve* (medulla). These nuclei tend to be located just lateral to the general somatic efferent column. The accessory oculomotor nucleus is the source of preganglionic neurons in the oculomotor nerve, the superior salivatory nucleus of preganglionic neurons in the facial nerve, the inferior salivatory nucleus of preganglionic neurons in the glossopharyngeal nerve, and the dorsal motor vagal nucleus of preganglionic neurons in the vagus nerve (Chap. 6). The salivatory nuclei are identifiable by their physiologic effects (stimulation evokes secretion), not by morphologic criteria.

Special visceral efferent column   Consisting of the *motor nucleus of the fifth nerve* (midpons), *motor nucleus of the facial nerve* (lower pons), and the *nucleus ambiguus* (medulla), this column is located in the middle of the tegmentum. The nuclei consist of the lower motor neurons to the branchiomeric (gill) arch musculature. The motor nucleus of the fifth nerve innervates the muscles of mastication (first arch), the motor nucleus of the seventh nerve innervates the muscles of facial expression (second arch), and the nucleus ambiguus innervates the pharyngeal (swallowing) and laryngeal muscles (vocalization) via the glossopharyngeal, vagus, and cranial roots of accessory nerves (third and fourth arches). Several other muscles innervated by these nerves include the tensor tympani muscle (fifth nerve) and stapedius muscle (seventh nerve, Chap. 10).

Bibliography

Brodal, A.: *The Cranial Nerves: Anatomy and Anatomicoclinical Correlations.* Blackwell Scientific Publications, Ltd., Oxford, 1965.

Cogan, D. G.: *Neurology of the Ocular Muscles.* Charles C Thomas, Publisher, Springfield, Ill., 1969.

Grant, J. C. B.: *An Atlas of Anatomy.* The Williams & Wilkins Company, Baltimore, 1972.

Romanes, G. J.: *Cunningham's Textbook of Anatomy.* Oxford University Press, New York and London, 1964.

Smith, R. Dale: The trematic interrelationships of the branchiomeric nerves. Acta Anat., 39:141–186, 1959.

CHAPTER 8
THE BRAINSTEM: MEDULLA, PONS, AND MIDBRAIN

The medulla, pons, and midbrain—the lower or infratentorial brainstem—are actually continuous structures (Fig. 8-1). They will be analyzed as a unit rather than as distinct entities. The major ascending and descending pathways in the brainstem are linked rostrally with the cerebrum, dorsally with the cerebellum, and caudally with the spinal cord.

Roof, ventricular cavity, tegmentum, and basilar portion

The brainstem may be considered to be organized as four longitudinally oriented structures: roof, ventricular cavity, tegmentum, and basilar portion (Figs. 1-2, 1-3, 8-2 through 8-11).

Roof The roof of the brainstem is located posterior to the ventricular cavity. The roof of the midbrain, called the *tectum* or *lamina quadrigemina*, is subdivided into the *pretectum* (rostral portion), paired *superior colliculi* of the optic system, and paired *inferior colliculi* of the auditory system. The colliculi are collectively called the *corpora quadrigemina*. The fourth cranial nerve emerges from the roof just caudal to the inferior colliculi. The cerebellum along with the superior and inferior medullary veli form the roof of the pons. The choroid plexus and the tela choroidea (layer of pia mater and ependyma) of the fourth ventricle form the roof of the medulla; the posterior columns and nuclei gracilis form the roof of the central canal of the caudal medulla.

Ventricular cavity The *ventricular cavities* include the cerebral aqueduct of the midbrain, the fourth ventricle of the pons and medulla, and the central canal of the caudal half of the medulla.

Tegmentum The tegmentum, which comprises the bulk of the brainstem, is located anterior to the ventricular canal. It may be subdivided into several structural-functional units, including *1* the ascending lemniscal pathways, *2* the reticular formation with its reticular nuclei and pathways, *3* the cranial nerves and their nuclei, *4* the "unconscious" proprioceptive systems, and *5* periventricular gray matter (called periaqueductal gray matter in the midbrain because it surrounds the cerebral aqueduct).

The *ascending lemniscal pathways* include the long ascending pathways which commence in the nuclei of the spinal cord and lower brainstem, terminate in nuclei of the higher brainstem and thalamus, and convey one or more sensory modalities. These pathways project their influences rostrally to the higher centers of the diencephalon and the cerebral cortex. In this context, the tracts of the lemniscal systems in the brainstem include the medial lemniscus (touch and deep sensibility), the spinothalamic tract (spinal lemniscus for pain and temperature), the trigeminothalamic tracts (trigeminal lemnisci for touch, pain, and temperature), and the lateral lemniscus (audition) (Figs. 8-2 through 8-11).

The *reticular formation* is the intricate neural network which forms most of the brainstem tegmentum. The *reticular system* is the functional system utilizing the reticular formation as its physical substrate. This widespread reticular system is not limited to the brainstem but is present throughout the central nervous system. The reticular formation is organized into reticular nuclei and into *1* ascending reticular path-

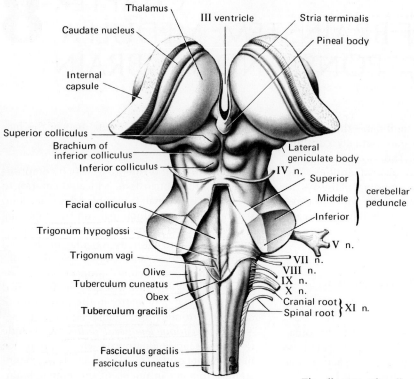

Thalamus
III ventricle
Stria terminalis
Caudate nucleus
Pineal body
Internal
capsule
Superior colliculus
Brachium of
inferior colliculus
Lateral
geniculate body
Inferior colliculus
IV n.
Superior
Middle } cerebellar peduncle
Facial colliculus
Inferior
Trigonum hypoglossi
V n.
Trigonum vagi
VII n.
Olive
VIII n.
Tuberculum cuneatus
IX n.
Obex
X n.
Tuberculum gracilis
Cranial root } XI n.
Spinal root
Fasciculus gracilis
Fasciculus cuneatus

FIGURE 8-1
Posterior surface of the brainstem.

ways and *2* descending reticular pathways. The brainstem portion of the reticular system is integrated with *1* the ascending reticular pathways involved with the relative state of alertness of the organism (sleep-wake pattern) and with some pain, and *2* the descending reticular pathways associated with the somatic and visceral motor activities expressed largely via the reticulospinal tracts and pathways. The major tract of the brainstem reticular formation is the central tegmental tract.

The *cranial nerves and their nuclei* include sensory and motor nuclei (Chap. 7). The sensory nuclei receive input from the cranial nerves, and the motor nuclei project output via motor fibers of the cranial nerves.

The *"unconscious" proprioceptive systems* in the brainstem are the nuclei and tracts associated with the vestibular system (Chap. 10) and with the pathways to the cerebellum (Chap. 9). The medial longitudinal fasciculus and the vestibulospinal tract contain fibers of the vestibular system. The spinocerebellar tracts, inferior, middle, and superior cerebellar peduncles, inferior olivary nuclear complex, lateral reticular nucleus, reticulotegmental nucleus, paramedial reticular nuclei, and red nucleus are functionally integrated with the cerebellum.

The *periventricular gray matter* (Figs. 8-2 through 8-11) is located in the immediate vicinity of the ventricular cavity. Within it is located the dorsal longitudinal fasciculus, a pathway of the autonomic nervous system (Chaps. 6 and 15).

Basilar portion The *basilar portion of the brainstem* comprises the *crura cerebri* of the midbrain, the *ventral pons* of the metencephalon, and the *pyramids* of the medulla (Figs. 8-2 through 8-11). The corticospinal tracts, cortico-bulbar fibers, corticopontine tracts, and ponto-cerebellar tracts form the basilar portion. The corticospinal tracts descend through the entire basilar portion before decussating in the lower medulla. The corticobulbar and corticoreticular fibers descend in the basilar portion before entering the tegmentum. The corticopontine tracts descend in the crura cerebri and terminate in the pontine nuclei of the pons proper. Pontocerebellar fibers cross over in the pons proper, pass through the middle cerebellar peduncle, and terminate in the cerebellar cortex. The *substantia nigra* is a large nuclear complex which is often included in the basilar portion of the midbrain. The *cerebral peduncles* comprise the tegmentum, substantia nigra, and crus cerebri (the midbrain without the tectum).

Transverse sections through the infratentorial brainstem

In the following account, the anatomic relations of the intrinsic structures of the infratentorial brainstem are briefly described in a representative series of transverse sections. These comprise a sequence of successively higher levels from the upper cervical segment through the upper midbrain.

FIRST CERVICAL SEGMENT OF THE SPINAL CORD
(Figs. 8-2, A-11)

The first cervical segment has several distinctive features. The fibers of the lateral corticospinal tract are located more medially than in the other spinal levels. Its location, abutting against the gray matter, indicates that the tract has not completed its decussation. The myelinated fibers of the *spinal tract* and the large *spinal nucleus of the trigeminal nerve,* which extend to the C2 level, are the equivalents to the posterolateral tract and substantia gelatinosa of the spinal cord. The fibers of the *spinal root of cranial nerve XI* originate in the anterolateral aspect of the anterior horn and pass posteriorly and then laterally before emerging from the lateral side of the spinal cord. Although the dorsal root is absent at C1, the ventral root of the first cervical nerve is present.

REARRANGEMENT OF STRUCTURES IN THE TRANSITION FROM THE SPINAL CORD TO THE MEDULLA (Figs. 8-2 through 8-5, A-1, A-2, A-11 through A-15)

The junctional zone where the spinal cord merges into the medulla is usually defined as being located at the foramen magnum. It is also stated to be at a slightly different site either just rostral to the ventral root of C1 or at the level of the decussation of the corticospinal tract.

Although the external topography of the medulla differs from that of the spinal cord, many similarities are present (Figs. 8-2 through 8-5).

1 The fasciculus gracilis is continuous rostrally with the *tuberculum gracilis* (*clava*), which is formed by the nucleus gracilis.

2 The fasciculus cuneatus is continuous with the *tuberculum cuneatus,* which is formed by the nucleus cuneatus.

3 The band of dorsal roots and posterolateral tract (zone of Lissauer) grades into the *trigeminal eminence* (*tuberculum cinereum*); the longitudinal line of this band is directed to the trigeminal roots, which emerge from the middle cerebellar peduncle of the pons. The *trigeminal eminence* is formed by the spinal tract and nucleus of the trigeminal nerve.

4 The longitudinal band of the ventral roots is represented in the medulla by the *rootlets of the hypoglossal nerve,* which emerge throughout the entire length of the anterior lateral sulcus of the medulla. The rostral continuation of this band comprises the sites of emergence of cranial nerve VI at the pontomedullary sulcus and of cranial nerve III into the interpeduncular fossa of the midbrain.

5 On the lateral aspect of the cervical spinal cord just posterior to the attachment on the denticulate ligament (halfway between the dorsal and ventral roots) is the longitudinal line formed by the sites of emergence of the rootlets and rostral course of the *spinal root of the accessory nerve* (*cranial nerve XI*). This is continuous rostrally along the lateral aspect of the medulla (posterior lateral sulcus) as the line formed by the emergence of the rootlets of the cranial part of N. XI and cranial nerves VII, IX, and X.

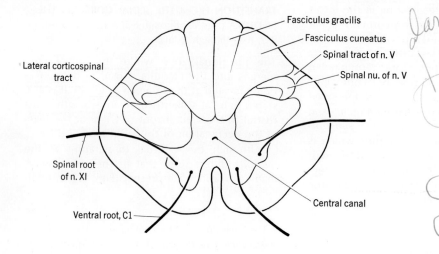

There are several other special topographic features of the medulla.

6 Each *pyramid* on the anterior aspect is located between the rootlets of cranial nerve XII and the midline. The pyramids are formed exclusively by the fibers of the corticospinal tract. In the caudal medulla is a series of ridges which traverse across the anterior median fissure; they represent the pyramidal decussation.

7 The *olive* is located between the rootlets of nerve XII and those of nerves IX and X. Deep to the olive is the inferior olivary nuclear complex.

8 The central canal of the spinal cord continues rostrally into the diamond-shaped fourth ventricle of the medulla and pons; the medullary portion of the ventricle is covered posteriorly by the tela choroidea (choroid plexus). The obex is a posterior midline site at the caudal end of the fourth ventricle.

9 The floor of the fourth ventricle has several eminences. Adjacent to the midline is the *trigonum hypoglossus*, which is formed by the nucleus of the hypoglossal nerve. Just lateral to the trigonum hypoglossi is the *trigonum vagi (ala cinerea)*, formed by the dorsal vagal nucleus (a parasympathetic nucleus) and the nucleus solitarius. On the caudolateral wall of the ventricle is a ridge called the *area postrema* (Chap. 11). The indentations on either side of the trigonum vagi constitute the inferior fovea, which represents the sulcus

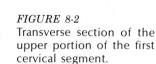

FIGURE 8-2
Transverse section of the upper portion of the first cervical segment.

limitans. The area vestibularis, an eminence formed by the vestibular nuclei, is located laterally.

Basic differences   The differences in structure between the spinal cord and the medulla are primarily the consequence of several major features.

1 The large size and lateral spread of the fourth ventricle are associated with the topographic differences between the derivations of the alar plate and the basal plate of the embryo. The structures which develop from the alar plate and basal plate are located dorsally and ventral to the sulcus limitans, respectively, in the spinal cord. In contrast, the derivatives of the alar plate and basal plate are located lateral and medial to the sulcus limitans (fovea), respectively, in the medulla.

2 These differences in orientation have several consequences. In the spinal cord, the sensory

nuclei (laminae) for the termination of the GSA and GVA fibers of the spinal nerves are located in the posterior horn dorsal to the sulcus limitans, while the motor nuclei or origin of GSE (alpha and gamma motor neurons) fibers and GVE (intermediolateral nucleus) fibers of the spinal nerves are located in the gray matter ventral to the sulcus limitans. In contrast, the nuclei of the cranial nerves differ. The sensory cranial nerve nuclei (nucleus solitarius, spinal nucleus of N. V, and vestibular nuclei) are located lateral to the inferior fovea, while the motor nuclei of the cranial nerves (dorsal vagal nucleus, nucleus ambiguus, and hypoglossal nucleus) are located medial to a plane from the inferior fovea to the posterolateral sulcus (Fig. 7-4).

3 Lamina VII and the fasciculi proprii of the spinal cord are presumed to be the equivalent of the expansive reticular formation of the brainstem.

4 The posterior column–medial lemniscus pathway undergoes a major shift in its location in the lower medulla. The posterior columns and their nuclei of termination (nuclei gracilis and cuneatus) are present dorsally throughout the spinal cord and lower medulla. The axons of the neurons of the second order course from these two nuclei (located dorsal to the central canal) in a curve, as the internal arcuate fibers, which cross the midline ventral to the central canal to form an ascending tract called the medial lemniscus. After passing through the brainstem, the medial lemniscus terminates in the ventral posterolateral nucleus of the thalamus.

5 The descending corticospinal fibers of the pyramid, which is located ventrally in the medulla, cross in the lower medulla (just caudal to the crossing of the internal arcuate fibers) as the pyramidal decussation. In this decussation most of the fibers course dorsally and laterally to the dorsal aspect of the lateral funiculus of the spinal cord to form the lateral corticospinal tract. The uncrossed fibers of the pyramid just descend into the anterior funiculus as the anterior corticospinal tract.

Basic similarities With some slight modifications, several structures have the same basic morphologic relations of one to the other and to the spinal cord and medulla. The *medial longitudinal fasciculus (MLF)* is located 1 ventral to the central canal of the spinal cord or fourth ventricle and cerebral aqueduct of the brainstem and 2 medially on either side of the midline. The spinothalamic tract, posterior and anterior spinocerebellar tracts, spinotectal tract, and spinal nucleus and tract of the trigeminal nerve are located as a group laterally in the spinal cord and medulla. Within the brainstem, the lateral spinothalamic tract is called the spinothalamic tract; it may be joined by some fibers of the anterior spinothalamic tract.

LEVEL OF THE PYRAMIDAL DECUSSATION
(Figs. 8-3, A-1, A-12)

The most distinguishing feature of this level is the crossing of 85 to 90 percent of the corticospinal fibers as the *pyramidal decussation*. It is composed of interdigitating descending fibers which decussate and course in a caudal and posterior direction to the dorsal aspect of the lateral funiculus of the spinal cord. Dorsal and ventral spinal roots are absent. Fibers of the *spinal root of N. XI* arise in the anterior horn and pass dorsally and then laterally before emerging on the lateral aspect of the medulla. The spinal tract of N. V is composed of fibers from cranial nerves V, VII, IX, and X which descend as far as C2; these fibers terminate in the spinal nucleus of N. V. The fasciculus gracilis is smaller than the fasciculus cuneatus; both fasciculi are in the same location as in the spinal cord. The *nucleus gracilis* is present; it is the nucleus of termination for the fibers of the fasciculus gracilis. The posterior and anterior spinocerebellar, spinothalamic, and spinotectal tracts have a relatively similar position as in the spinal cord. The medial longitudinal fasciculus and the anterior corticospinal tract pass on the ventrolateral side of the decussating pyramidal fibers. The *central reticular nucleus* of the medulla occupies the bulk of the reticular formation from the spinal cord–medulla junction to the midolivary level. In the medial part of the ventral gray matter of the caudal medulla is a rostral extension of the anterior horn (lamina IX) of the spinal cord; this nucleus, which gives rise to ventral root fibers of the first cervical nerves, is called the *supraspinal nucleus*.

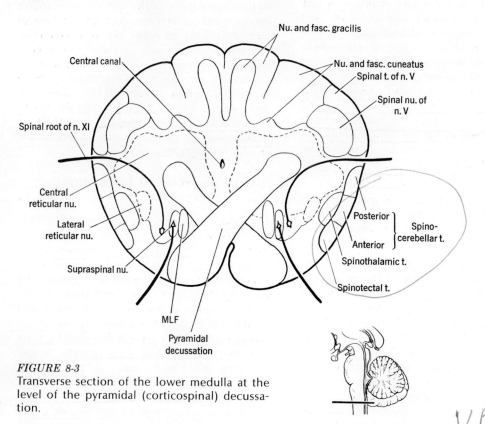

FIGURE 8-3
Transverse section of the lower medulla at the level of the pyramidal (corticospinal) decussation.

VPM

LEVEL OF DECUSSATION OF THE MEDIAL
LEMNISCUS (Figs. 8-4, A-2, A-13 through A-15)

The distinguishing feature of this level is the curve of the *internal arcuate fibers*, which, after arising from cells in the enlarged nuclei gracilis and cuneatus, sweep anteriorly in an arc and decussate across the midline to form the medial lemniscus of the opposite side. Upon entering the medial lemniscus, these fibers bend and ascend rostrally through the brainstem to the ventral posterolateral nucleus of the thalamus. The fasciculi gracilis and cuneatus are small because their ascending fibers terminate within the nuclei gracilis and cuneatus. The *spinal tract and nucleus of the trigeminal nerve* are displaced anteriorly. Some fibers arise from this nucleus and, with the internal arcuate fibers,

cross to the opposite side, ascending as the anterior trigeminothalamic tract to the ventral posteromedial nucleus of the thalamus. They are second-order neurons, conveying pain and temperature information derived from the trigeminal nerve, nervus intermedius, and glossopharyngeal and vagus nerves.

In addition to the spinal nucleus of N. V, four other cranial nerve nuclei are present at this level. The sensory *nucleus solitarius* (GVA and SVA) and the parasympathetic motor *dorsal vagal nucleus* (GVE) and the motor *nucleus ambiguus* (SVE) are involved with the vagus nerve, which emerges through the dorsolateral sulcus of the medulla. The former two nuclei are located anterior to the nucleus gracilis and medial to the internal arcuate fibers; the latter (nucleus ambiguus) is located in the middle of the teg-

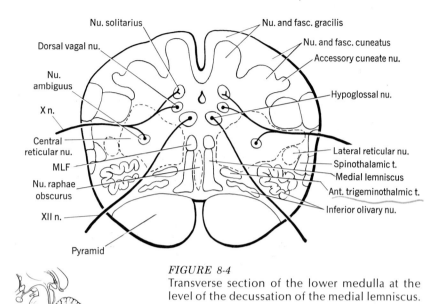

Nu. solitarius

Dorsal vagal nu.

Nu. ambiguus

X n.

Central reticular nu.

MLF

Nu. raphae obscurus

XII n.

Pyramid

Nu. and fasc. gracilis

Nu. and fasc. cuneatus

Accessory cuneate nu.

Hypoglossal nu.

Lateral reticular nu.
Spinothalamic t.
Medial lemniscus
Ant. trigeminothalmic t.
Inferior olivary nu.

FIGURE 8-4
Transverse section of the lower medulla at the level of the decussation of the medial lemniscus.

mentum just lateral to the internal arcuate fibers. Many of the fibers of the nucleus ambiguus from this level form the cranial root of the accessory nerve.

Anterior to the central canal on either side of the midline is the pair of *hypoglossal nuclei* (GSE); from each nucleus arises a hypoglossal nerve which passes through the medial tegmentum and emerges from the medulla between a pyramid and the olive (inferior olivary nuclear complex).

The ascending tracts located in the lateral medulla—comprising the posterior and anterior spinocerebellar, spinothalamic, and spinotectal tracts—occupy the same general location one to another as in the more caudal levels.

Three prominent cerebellar relay nuclei are the source of fibers which pass through the inferior cerebellar peduncle before terminating in the cerebellum. The *accessory cuneate nucleus* of the lower medulla, located lateral to the cuneate nucleus, is the homologue to the dorsal

nucleus of Clarke in the spinal cord; it receives proprioceptive input from the cervical and upper thoracic regions, especially the upper extremities, via uncrossed fibers ascending in the fasciculus cuneatus. The ipsilaterally projecting cuneocerebellar fibers from the accessory cuneate nucleus are the pathway from the upper extremity that is equivalent to the posterior spinocerebellar tract from the lower extremity. The *lateral reticular nucleus,* located anterolaterally in the vicinity of the spinothalamic tract, extends rostrocaudally at the level of the caudal two-thirds of the inferior olivary complex. This nucleus receives afferent input from the spinal cord via spinoreticular and collateral branches of spinothalamic fibers and from rubrobulbar fibers from the red nucleus of the midbrain. The nuclei of the *inferior olivary nuclear complex* are discussed further on under "Level of the middle third of the inferior olivary nucleus."

Of the descending tracts and fibers, the pyramids, composed of corticospinal fibers, are clearly demarcated. The anterior border of the medial longitudinal fasciculus (MLF) is not

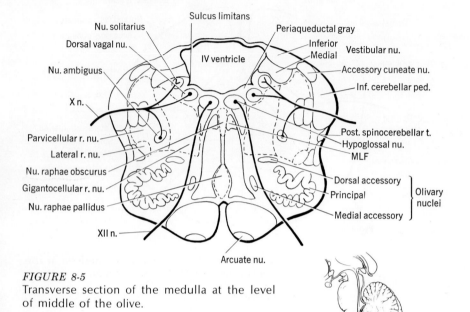

FIGURE 8-5
Transverse section of the medulla at the level
of middle of the olive.

clearly defined because its fibers overlap with
those of the medial lemniscus. At this level the
MLF is composed of *1* the pontine reticulospinal tract from the pars oralis and pars caudalis
of the pontine reticular nuclei, *2* the interstitiospinal tract from the interstitial nucleus of
Cajal, *3* the tectospinal tract from the midbrain
tectum, and *4* the vestibulospinal fibers from
the medial vestibular nucleus.

Just posterior to the inferior olivary nuclear
complex within the reticular formation are the
fibers of the rubrospinal tract from the red nucleus in the midbrain, the medullary reticulospinal tract from the nucleus reticularis gigantocellularis of the medulla, and the vestibulospinal
tract from the lateral vestibular nucleus. The
fibers of these tracts are intermingled with other
fibers; hence they are not clearly delineated.

Just rostral to this level are the *obex* and the
caudal extent of the fourth ventricle. The *reticular nuclei* include the nucleus raphae obscurus,
central reticular nucleus, and lateral reticular
nucleus; these belong to the raphae, central and
lateral nuclear groups, respectively (p. 259).

LEVEL OF THE MIDDLE THIRD OF THE INFERIOR OLIVARY COMPLEX
(Figs. 8-5, A-3, A-16)

The distinguishing features of this level are the
nuclei of the inferior olivary complex, fourth
ventricle, and cranial nerve nuclei. The *olivary
complex* comprises the phylogenetically new
principal inferior olivary nucleus and the phylogenetically old *dorsal and medial accessory
olivary nuclei.* The fibers from the inferior olivary complex decussate and pass successively
through the medial lemnisci, the vicinity of the
contralateral olivary complex, and the inferior
cerebellar peduncle before terminating in the
cerebellum. The accessory olivary nuclei and
principal inferior olivary nucleus have fibers
which project primarily to the vermis. The fibers
from the principal olivary nucleus terminate in
the contralateral cerebellar hemisphere. The
olivocerebellar fibers convey excitatory influences to the deep cerebellar nuclei and to the
entire cerebellar cortex. The input to the inferior
olivary complex is derived from the spinal cord,

cerebral cortex, deep cerebellar nuclei, red nucleus, and periaqueductal gray of the midbrain. The spino-olivary fibers ascend in the anterior funiculus and terminate in the accessory olivary nuclei; the existence of these fibers in man has been questioned. All the descending fibers to the olivary complex terminate in the principal inferior olivary nucleus. Originating from the frontal, parietal, temporal, and occipital lobes, the cortico-olivary fibers course with the corticospinal fibers before terminating bilaterally in the principal inferior olivary nuclei. The fibers from the red nucleus and periaqueductal gray descend in the central tegmental tract. From the dentate and interpositus nuclei of the cerebellum, fibers pass through the superior cerebellar peduncle, cross in the lower midbrain, and descend to the olivary nucleus in the descending limb of the superior cerebellar peduncle.

In the tegmentum anterior to the floor of the fourth ventricle is a row of cranial nerve nuclei. Two motor nuclei, located medial to the fovea (sulcus limitans), are the hypoglossal (GSE) and dorsal vagal (VE) nuclei. Two sensory nuclear groups, located laterally to the fovea, are the nucleus solitarius (GVA, SVA) and the medial and inferior vestibular (SSA) nuclei. The nucleus ambiguus (SVE) is a motor nucleus located in the middle of the tegmentum. The spinal nucleus of N. V is a sensory nucleus in the dorsolateral tegmentum. The vagus nerve is associated with the nucleus ambiguus, dorsal vagal nucleus, nucleus solitarius, and the spinal nucleus of N. V.

The *paramedian nuclei* and the nearby *arcuate* and *perihypoglossal nuclei* relay influences via the inferior cerebellar peduncles to the ipsilateral and contralateral halves of the cerebellum. The cells of the *raphe nuclei*—the *nucleus raphe obscurus, nucleus raphe pallidus*—contain serotonin (5-hydroxytryptamine). Fibers from these cells project to the spinal cord.

The *central reticular nuclear group* in the upper medullary levels is the *gigantocellular reticular nucleus,* which is located posterior to the inferior olivary complex. This large-celled nucleus occupies the medial two-thirds of the reticular formation as far rostral as the medullary-pontine junction. Input to this nucleus is derived largely from *1* widespread areas of the cerebral cortex via crossed and uncrossed corticoreticular fibers, *2* higher brainstem levels

via the central tegmental tract, *3* neurons from the parvicellular nucleus of the lateral nuclear group, and *4* spinoreticular fibers ascending in the anterolateral funiculus of the spinal cord. The output from this nucleus is projected *1* rostrally via the central tegmental tract to higher brainstem levels and the intralaminar nuclei of the thalamus and via the median forebrain bundle to the hypothalamus, and *2* caudally via the medullary (lateral) reticulospinal tract to the spinal cord. The reticular nucleus of the central group in the caudal medulla is called the ventral reticular nucleus.

The *lateral reticular group* comprises the *lateral reticular nucleus* and the *parvicellular reticular nucleus.* Input to the parvicellular reticular nucleus is derived largely from *1* widespread areas of the cerebral cortex via crossed and uncrossed corticoreticular fibers, *2* collateral fibers conveying influences from the auditory, vestibular, trigeminal, and visceral pathways, and *3* spinoreticular fibers from the spinal cord. The output from the parvicellular reticular nuclei is directed medially to the gigantocellular reticular nucleus.

Except for possible minor changes, the locations of the ascending and descending tracts and pathways are similar to those described under "Level of Decussation of the Medial Lemniscus." The posterior spinocerebellar tract is close to the inferior cerebellar peduncle, which it is about to join.

TANGENTIAL SECTION AT THE LEVELS OF THE GLOSSOPHARYNGEAL AND VESTIBULOCOCHLEAR NERVES (Figs. 8-6, A-4, A-5, A-17, A-18)

This medullary level is in the vicinity of the medullopontine junction; it is basically different from the midolivary level in several respects. The hypoglossal and dorsal vagal nuclei are absent. The *inferior salivatory nucleus* is a physiologically defined nucleus (related to secretion of the parotid gland) located just rostral to the dorsal vagal nucleus. The cranial nerve nuclei associated with the glossopharyngeal nerve comprise the nucleus solitarius, spinal nucleus of the trigeminal nerve, inferior salivatory nucleus, and nucleus ambiguus. The large inferior cerebellar peduncle (left side of the figure) is

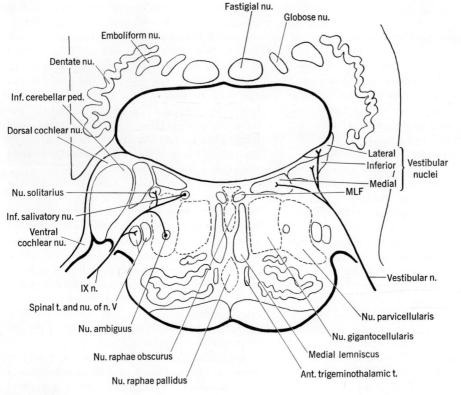

FIGURE 8-6
Transverse section (slightly oblique) of the
upper medulla at the level of the cochlear and
glossopharyngeal nerves (*left*) and the vestibular
nerve (*right*).

Section includes the cerebellum through the deep cerebellar nuclei.

illustrated as it passes (right side of the figure)
into the cerebellum. The *inferior cerebellar peduncle* comprises the following fibers passing to
the cerebellum: posterior spinocerebellar, cuneocerebellar, and olivocerebellar tracts, along with
fibers from such nuclei as the lateral reticular
and paramedian reticular nuclei. A portion of
the inferior cerebellar peduncle, called the juxtarestiform body, is composed of fibers associated with the vestibular system conveying influences to and from the vestibulocerebellum and
the fastigial nuclei of the cerebellum.

On the outer surface of the inferior cerebellar
peduncle are the dorsal and ventral cochlear
nuclei. The fibers of the cochlear nerve branch
in an organized sequence so that each fiber is
distributed in a precise pattern to both the dorsal and ventral cochlear nuclei. At a slightly
higher level the fibers of the vestibular nerve
pass at right angles among the fibers of the
inferior cerebellar peduncle on their way to the
four vestibular nuclei (the medial, inferior, and
lateral vestibular nuclei are illustrated).

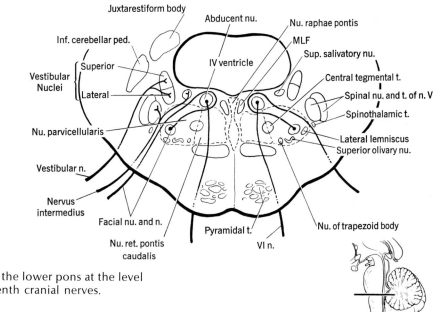

FIGURE 8-7
Transverse section of the lower pons at the level of the sixth and seventh cranial nerves.

The *reticular nuclei* at this level include the *nucleus raphe obscurus* and *nucleus raphe pallidus*, the *nucleus gigantocellularis* (a central reticular nucleus), and the *nucleus parvicellularis* (a lateral reticular group nucleus).

The four deep cerebellar nuclei, oriented in order from medial to lateral, are the fastigial, globose, emboliform, and dentate nuclei. The globose and emboliform nuclei are collectively called the nucleus interpositus. The fibers of the inferior cerebellar peduncle pass lateral to the dentate nucleus. The juxtarestiform body is located between the deep cerebellar nuclei and the lateral border of the fourth ventricle.

LEVEL OF NUCLEI OF SIXTH AND SEVENTH CRANIAL NERVES (Figs. 8-7, A-6, A-19)

The general pattern of organization at this level differs from that of the levels of the medulla primarily because of the massive size of the *ventral or basilar pons* relative to the *dorsal or*

tegmental pons. The *ventral pons* represents a modified, rostral continuation of the pyramids of the medulla. The *dorsal pons* represents the rostral continuation of the medulla exclusive of the pyramids. The boundary between the dorsal and ventral pons is a plane located just anterior to the medial lemniscus. The fourth ventricle is large.

The *ventral pons* is composed of *1* the longitudinally oriented corticospinal and corticobulbar tracts, and *2* the terminal branches of the corticopontine fibers, the pontine nucleus, and the transversely oriented pontocerebellar fibers. The latter course laterally, decussate, and pass through the middle cerebellar peduncle before terminating in the contralateral half of the cerebellum.

Except for a few significant modifications, the dorsal pons resembles the medulla. The medial longitudinal fasciculus (MLF) is still located anterior to the fourth ventricle and just lateral to the midline, while the spinal tract and nucleus of the trigeminal nerve are in the dorsolateral tegmentum. The medial lemniscus has shifted from a ventromedial tegmental location in the medulla to a ventral tegmental location in the pons. The *central tegmental tract* is prominent in the middle of the reticular formation.

The cranial nerve nuclei present at this level have their equivalents in the medulla. The *abducent nucleus* (GSE), *motor nucleus of the facial nerve* (SVE), and the *superior salivatory nucleus* (GVE) are located within the tegmentum in sites similar to those occupied within the medulla by the hypoglossal nucleus (GSE), nucleus ambiguus (SVE), and dorsal vagal nucleus (GVE), respectively. The *superior vestibular nucleus* (SSA) is found in the posterolateral tegmentum. The course of the fibers of the abducent and facial nerves is characteristic and significant. The lower motor neurons of the sixth nerve emerge from the abducent nucleus and pass ventrally through the medial tegmentum and basal pons lateral to the pyramidal tract before emerging medially at the pontomedullary junction. After leaving from the facial nucleus, the lower motor neurons form a bundle that follows a circuitous course. It passes posteromedially and ascends for a short distance medial to the abducent nucleus and posterior to the medial longitudinal fasciculus; at the rostral end of the abducent nucleus, the bundle turns laterally (as the internal genu of the facial nerve) and then continues anterolaterally through the lateral tegmentum and ventral pons before emerging at the cerebellopontine angle. The hillock in the floor of the fourth ventricle at the site of the abducent nucleus and the internal genu is called the facial or abducent colliculus. Fibers of the nervus intermedius are in close association with the facial nerve; they originate in the physiologically defined superior salivatory nucleus (GVE) or terminate in the spinal nucleus of N. V (GSA) and nucleus solitarius (SVA, GVA).

The upper motor neuron pattern of innervation is clinically significant. Bilateral upper motor neuron projections from the cerebral cortex via corticobulbar and corticoreticular fibers influence the lower motor neurons innervating the muscles in the upper part of the face and forehead (e.g., frontalis and orbicularis oculi). In contrast, unilateral upper motor neurons projecting from the contralateral cerebrum influence the lower motor neurons which innervate the muscles of the lower part of the face (i.e., buccinator and labial muscles). As a consequence, a unilateral lesion of the upper motor neurons to the facial nucleus results in paralysis of the muscles of facial expression in the contralateral part of the lower face; the other facial muscles are generally spared.

The trapezoid nucleus and superior olivary nuclei and fibers of the auditory pathways are located at this level. Decussating fibers of the trapezoid body are present in the vicinity of the medial lemniscus; these fibers collect in the ventrolateral tegmentum as the lateral lemniscus, which is located roughly posterior to the spinothalamic tract. Nuclei of the auditory pathways include the superior olivary nuclei and nuclei of the trapezoid body.

The reticular nuclei at this level and those of the lower pons caudal to the principal nucleus of the trigeminal nerve are the *nucleus raphe pontis* (a raphe nucleus), the *nucleus reticularis pontis caudalis* (a central reticular group nucleus), and the *nucleus parvicellularis* (a lateral reticular nucleus).

LEVEL OF THE TRIGEMINAL NERVE
(Figs. 8-8, A-7, A-20)

The characteristic features at this midpontine level are *1* the *principal sensory nucleus* and *motor nucleus of the trigeminal nerve*, and *2* the *superior cerebellar peduncle* on the lateral aspect of the narrowing fourth ventricle.

The *principal nucleus of N. V* is a nucleus of termination of the sensory root of the trigeminal nerve; other fibers of this root have their cell bodies in the *mesencephalic nucleus of N. V*, which is located lateral to the ventricle. The *motor nucleus of N. V*, located medial to the principal nucleus, contains the cell bodies of origin of the lower motor neurons of the motor root of the trigeminal nerve.

The *superior cerebellar peduncle* is composed of primarily cerebellar efferent fibers originating in the dentate, emboliform, and globose nuclei; these fibers decussate in the lower midbrain

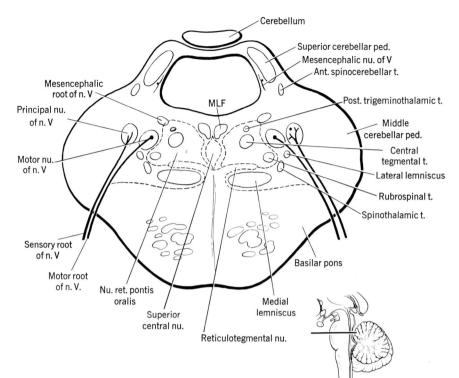

Cerebellum
Superior cerebellar ped.
Mesencephalic nu. of V
Ant. spinocerebellar t.
Mesencephalic root of n. V
Principal nu. of n. V
MLF
Post. trigeminothalamic t.
Middle cerebellar ped.
Motor nu. of n. V
Central tegmental t.
Lateral lemniscus
Rubrospinal t.
Spinothalamic t.
Sensory root of n. V
Basilar pons
Motor root of n. V.
Nu. ret. pontis oralis
Medial lemniscus
Superior central nu.
Reticulotegmental nu.

FIGURE 8-8
Transverse section of the midpons at the level of the entrance of the trigeminal nerve.

tegmentum and *1* ascend to the nucleus ruber and to the rostral intralaminar and ventrolateral thalamic nuclei, and *2* descend in the brainstem tegmentum to the reticulotegmental nucleus of the pons and the inferior olivary and paramedian nuclei of the medulla. The anterior spinocerebellar tract courses posteriorly in the superior cerebellar peduncle; its fibers terminate in the anterior vermal cortex. The roof of the fourth ventricle is covered by the superior medullary velum. Between the superior cerebellar peduncle and the fourth ventricle, extending from the rostral half of the principal nucleus of N. V to the level of the inferior colliculus, is a group of pigmented cells, the locus ceruleus (nucleus pigmentosus) (Fig. 8-9). These cells are noradrenergic neurons and have axons which are distributed to *1* the cerebellum and *2* the cerebrum. Although the pigment of these cells is brown it appears cerulean blue in the gross specimen.

The medial lemniscus has shifted somewhat laterally, and the spinothalamic tract and lateral lemniscus have shifted slightly dorsolaterally along the outer margin of the reticular formation. The medial longitudinal fasciculus, central tegmental tract, rubrospinal tract, and the structures of the basilar pons have the same topographic relations to one another as those described earlier under "Level of Nuclei of the Sixth and Seventh Cranial Nerves." The lateral lemniscus contains a small synaptic collection called the nucleus of the lateral lemniscus.

The *reticular nuclei* extending rostrally from this level into the isthmus of the midbrain are *1* the *superior central nucleus* (a raphe nucleus), *2* the *nucleus reticularis pontis oralis* and *locus ceruleus* (a central reticular group nucleus), and *3* the *reticulotegmental nucleus.* The latter is actually an extension of the pontine nuclei of the ventral pons into the tegmentum; as do the pontine nuclei, the reticulotegmental

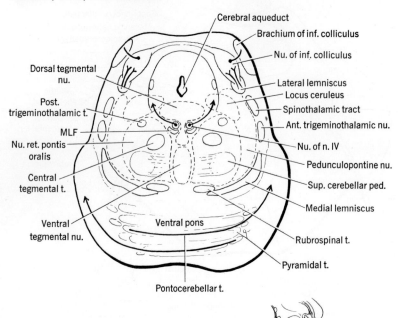

Cerebral aqueduct
Brachium of inf. colliculus
Nu. of inf. colliculus
Dorsal tegmental nu.
Lateral lemniscus
Locus ceruleus
Post. trigeminothalamic t.
Spinothalamic tract
Ant. trigeminothalamic nu.
MLF
Nu. of n. IV
Nu. ret. pontis oralis
Pedunculopontine nu.
Central tegmental t.
Sup. cerebellar ped.
Medial lemniscus
Ventral tegmental nu.
Ventral pons
Rubrospinal t.
Pyramidal t.
Pontocerebellar t.

nucleus projects its fibers to the cerebellum. The lateral reticular nuclear group is not represented in the midpontine level.

FIGURE 8-9
Transverse section of the lower midbrain at the level of the inferior colliculus and nucleus of the fourth cranial nerve.

LEVEL OF THE INFERIOR COLLICULUS
(Figs. 8-9, A-8, A-9, A-21, A-22)

The distinguishing features at this level include the inferior colliculus, the decussation of the superior cerebellar peduncle, and the ventral pons. The ventricular system is represented by the narrow *cerebral aqueduct* (*iter*).

The large *nucleus of the inferior colliculus* is a major processing station in the auditory pathways. It receives input from ascending auditory fibers of the lateral lemniscus and descending fibers from the medial geniculate body; it projects influences *1* rostrally to the medial geniculate body via the brachium of the inferior colliculus and to the superior colliculus, and *2* caudally to auditory nuclei via the lateral lemniscus. The nuclei of the inferior colliculi are interconnected by fibers of the commissure of the inferior colliculus. As a group, the medial lemniscus, spinothalamic tract, and lateral lem-

niscus have shifted laterally and dorsally along the outer margin of the reticular formation of the tegmentum. In this shift, the lateral lemniscus approaches the inferior colliculus; its fibers enter and terminate in the nucleus of the inferior colliculus. The rostrally projecting fibers from the nucleus form the brachium of the inferior colliculus, which is located in the dorsolateral tegmentum of the upper midbrain.

The small posterior trigeminothalamic tract from the ipsilateral principal nucleus of N. V is located in the tegmentum posterior to the central tegmental tract. The small anterior trigeminothalamic tract from the contralateral spinal and principal nuclei of N. V is located between the medial lemniscus and spinothalamic tract. The medial longitudinal fasciculus (MLF) is notched posteriorly by the nucleus of the trochlear nerve (GSE). The fibers of the trochlear nerve pass as

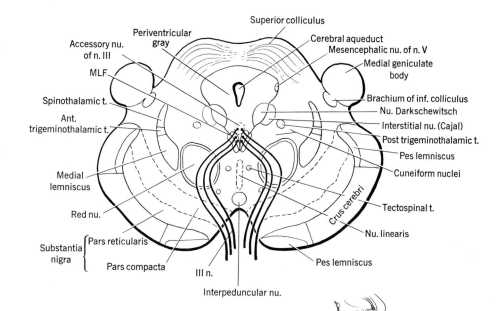

Accessory nu.
of n. III

Periventricular
gray

Superior colliculus

MLF

Spinothalamic t.

Ant.
trigeminothalamic t.

Medial
lemniscus

Red nu.

Substantia
nigra { Pars reticularis

Pars compacta

III n.

Interpeduncular nu.

Cerebral aqueduct
Mesencephalic nu. of n. V

Medial geniculate
body

Brachium of inf. colliculus

Nu. Darkschewitsch

Interstitial nu. (Cajal)

Post trigeminothalamic t.

Pes lemniscus

Cuneiform nuclei

Crus cerebri

Tectospinal t.

Nu. linearis

Pes lemniscus

FIGURE 8-10
Transverse section of the upper midbrain at the level of the superior colliculus and the third cranial nerve.

a dorsocaudally directed arc from this nucleus along the outer edge of the periaqueductal gray matter; they decussate completely in the superior medullary velum and emerge from the posterior tectum caudal to the inferior colliculus. The locus ceruleus is located deep to the inferior colliculus. The reticulotegmental nucleus is present in the anteromedial tegmentum.

The *reticular nuclei* at this level include *1* the *dorsal and ventral tegmental nuclei* (raphe nuclei), *2* the rostral portion of the *nucleus reticularis pontis oralis* and *locus ceruleus* (central reticular nuclei), and *3 pedunculopontine and cuneiform nuclei* (lateral reticular group nuclei). The dorsal tegmental nucleus (supratrochlear nucleus) is located dorsal to the trochlear nucleus in the periaqueductal gray matter; it receives input from the mamillary body. The ventral tegmental nucleus is present ventral to the medial longitudinal fasciculus; it is apparently a rostral extension of the superior central nucleus. The locus ceruleus (nucleus pigmentosus pontis) is the "blue place" located in the upper pons to lower midbrain between the mesencephalic nucleus of the trigeminal nerve and the medial longitudinal fasciculus. The pedunculopontine nucleus lies in the caudal midbrain lateral to the superior cerebellar peduncle

and medial to the medial lemniscus. This nucleus receives input from the precentral gyrus and the ipsilateral globus pallidus. It is the only infratentorial brainstem reticular nucleus which receives direct input from the globus pallidus.

SECTION THROUGH MIDBRAIN AT LOWER LEVEL OF THE SUPERIOR COLLICULUS
(Figs. 8-10, A-10, A-23, A-24)

The major characteristic features at this level are the *superior colliculus, nucleus of the oculomotor nerve, red nucleus, substantia nigra,* and *crus cerebri.*

The *superior colliculi* are paired laminated hillocks of the tectum, which are complex processing nuclei. Each superior colliculus should be referred to as cortex, because its neurons and their fibers are organized into laminae. Just rostral to the superior colliculus is a small area of nuclei called the pretectal area. The primary roles of the superior colliculi and pretectal area are in the light reflex, accommodation (focusing) reflex, and other responses to visual stimuli.

The *red nucleus* is a large oval nucleus in the medial tegmentum. It is composed of a caudal magnocellular part and a rostral parvocellular part. Some fibers of the superior cerebellar peduncle terminate within the nucleus, while others pass through and on its outer margins as a "capsule" on their way to the ventral lateral, ventral anterior, and some intralaminar thalamic nuclei. In the region between the two red nuclei is the dorsal and the ventral tegmental decussation. Cells in the deep layers of the superior colliculus give rise to the tectospinal tract; the fibers arc through the tegmentum and cross the midline as the dorsal tegmental decussation before descending as the spinotectal tract located anterior to the medial longitudinal fasciculus. The rubrospinal tract originates from cells in the caudal three-fourths of the red nucleus; its fibers cross as the ventral tegmental decussation before descending as the rubrospinal tract in the anterior tegmentum.

The *oculomotor nuclear complex* is located in a V-shaped region formed by the paired medial longitudinal fasciculi. The fibers of the oculomotor nerve arise in this nucleus, course anterior through the medial tegmentum, including the red nucleus, on their way to emerge as rootlets into the interpeduncular fossa.

The *substantia nigra* is located between the tegmentum and the crus cerebri. It is divided into a posterior pars compacta and an anterior pars reticularis. The large cells of the compact or black part contain melanin pigment and primary catecholamines; these cells synthesize and convey dopamine via nigrostriatal fibers to the neostriatum (caudate nucleus and putamen). The cells of the reddish-brown pars reticularis contain iron but no melanin pigment.

The *crus cerebri* is the basilar part of the midbrain. It is composed of descending cortico-fugal fibers which originate in the cerebral cortex. The corticospinal and corticobulbar fibers are located in the medial two-thirds of the crus; they are said to be somatotopically organized at this level with the head, upper extremity and lower extremity musculature influenced by nerve fibers arranged from medial to lateral within the crus. Frontopontine fibers are located in the medial portion, and the corticopontine fibers from the parietal, temporal, and occipital cortical areas are located in the lateral portion of the crus. The most medial and lateral portions of the crus may contain some corticobulbar fibers; each of these regions is called a pes lemniscus.

The medial lemniscus, anterior trigemino-thalamic tract, and spinothalamic tract have shifted to a slightly more dorsal location in the tegmentum. The brachium of the inferior colliculus (auditory tract) is located dorsolateral to the spinothalamic tract; it is heading to the medial geniculate body. The posterior trigemino-thalamic tract is located in the dorsomedial tegmentum. The interpeduncular nucleus is located in the midline just dorsal to the interpeduncular fossa.

In the roof of the cerebral aqueduct at the level of the posterior commissure is a sheet of modified ciliated ependymal cells called the subcommissural organ (Chap. 11).

Reticular nuclei at this level include *nuclei linearis* (raphe nuclei), *nucleus ruber,* which is considered to be a specialized central reticular nucleus, and *cuneiform nuclei* (lateral reticular nuclear group). Other nuclei include the *interpeduncular nucleus, mesencephalic nucleus of the trigeminal nerve, interstitial nucleus of Cajal,* and the *nucleus of Darkschewitsch.*

TRANSVERSE SECTION THROUGH JUNCTION OF MIDBRAIN AND THALAMUS (Figs. 8-11, A-25)

The midbrain structures illustrated are similar to those depicted in the previous level. The fibers of the brachium of the inferior colliculus are terminating in the medial geniculate body of the thalamus. The medial lemniscus and the spino-thalamic tracts will terminate just rostrally in the ventral posterolateral (VPL) nucleus of the thalamus. The optic tract is composed of fibers from the retinas of both eyes. Some fibers terminate in the lateral geniculate body of the thalamus.

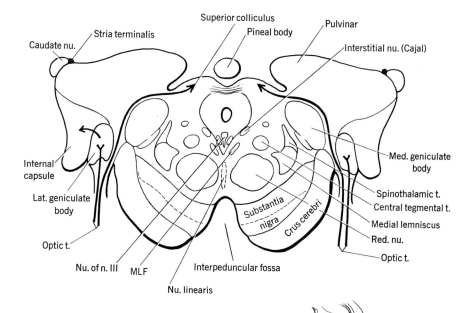

Caudate nu.
Stria terminalis
Superior colliculus
Pineal body
Pulvinar
Interstitial nu. (Cajal)
Internal capsule
Lat. geniculate body
Optic t.
Nu. of n. III   MLF
Nu. linearis
Interpeduncular fossa
Substantia nigra
Crus cerebri
Med. geniculate body
Spinothalamic t.
Central tegmental t.
Medial lemniscus
Red. nu.
Optic t.

The other fibers pass through the brachium of the superior colliculus before terminating in the superior colliculus. The pulvinar of the thalamus is located above the lateral geniculate body.

Concept of the reticular systems and the lemniscal systems

GENERAL CONCEPT

This classification is a means of conceptually dissecting the brainstem, as well as other parts of the central nervous system. However, the contrasting dichotomy implied in this characterization should not be considered absolute, for the structural and functional interrelations and interactions between the two systems are considerable and significant.

The *lemniscal systems* are characterized as the specific, oligoneuronal (parvoneuronal), oligosynaptic (parvosynaptic or paucisynaptic), phylogenetically more recent, compactly grouped systems which convey the signals of the conscious sensory modalities.

The *reticular system* (*reticular core*) is characterized as the nonspecific (aspecific, un-

FIGURE 8-11
Transverse section at the junction of the upper midbrain and diencephalon.

specific), multineuronal (polyneuronal), multisynaptic (polysynaptic), phylogenetically older, relatively diffuse tract systems that integrate and convey a great variety of ascending influences.

The lemniscal and reticular systems are composed of nuclei and tracts. The *lemniscal system* is called the specific system because its pathways convey those impulses of the specific conscious modalities ultimately recognized as pain, temperature, taste, audition, touch, discriminative touch, and appreciation of form, weight, and texture. The pathways associated with these senses are conceived of as having fewer sequences of neurons (oligoneuronal), fewer synapses (oligosynaptic), and somewhat more myelinated fibers (some fibers conduct faster) than are found in the reticular system. The specific systems are also characterized by point-to-point relays, by "secure" synaptic connections of the presynaptic neurons with the postsynaptic neurons, and by short latencies in the transmission times. These three characteristics are expressed by several observations. Stimuli from a spot (point) in the skin, mouth, joints, retina of the eye, or spiral organ of Corti of the ear project a limited number of neurons (points) in each of the relay nuclei of the pathway up to and including the primary sensory cortical area. This point-to-point relay from periphery to cerebral cortex is indicative of the secure connectivity within each pathway (Chap. 13). In addition, the relay of a minimal sequence of neurons (many with long myelinated axons) results in the short latency it takes from the time a stimulus is applied in the periphery until the evoked activity is indicated in the sensory cortex. The activity of the lemniscal systems is only slightly affected by anesthetics; these pathways readily transmit impulses when the subject is unconscious from an anesthetic. Although the lemniscal system is defined as an ascending system, several descending pathways may be considered to be "efferent lemniscal tracts." These are the corticobulbar, corticospinal, and corticopontine tracts. These pathways are oligoneuronal, oligosynaptic, phylogenetically more recent, and organized in compact bundles (as compared with descending reticular pathways).

In addition to their role in the conveyance of information associated with appreciation of the specific senses, the lemniscal systems also make significant contributions to behavioral activities. An animal with a cerebrum deprived of lemniscal stimulation exhibits little affect and facial expression. Emotional and associated autonomic reactions require the specific stimuli of the lemniscal systems. The cerebral cortex, particularly the neocortex, requires the input from the lemniscal pathways for many expressions of affect.

The *reticular system* is nonspecific (not primarily associated with the specific modalities). It is present throughout the central nervous system in spinal cord, brainstem, cerebellum, diencephalon, and cerebral hemispheres. The *reticular formation* is the anatomic substrate of much of the reticular system. In the spinal cord the reticular formation comprises some of the gray matter, the fasciculi proprii (spinospinalis) tracts, and spinoreticular tracts. Estimates suggest that as many as one-half of the neurons of the spinal gray matter are neurons of the spinal reticular formation. The spinoreticular fibers are essentially fibers of the fasciculi proprii which extend into the brainstem. The fasciculi proprii and the reticuloreticular fibers (central tegmental tract) are the reticular pathways of the spinal cord and brainstem, respectively.

In addition to the *reticuloreticular fibers*, the *central tegmental tract* also includes the rubrospinal fibers and ascending fibers from some brainstem reticular nuclei to certain thalamic nuclei (intralaminar nuclei and posterior thalamic region). The reticulospinal tracts are essentially reticuloreticular fibers which extend into the spinal cord. Many axons of the brainstem reticular neurons decussate before bifurcating into ascending and descending branches. This is a basis for the observations that some influences from the brainstem reticular formation are projected bilaterally. The reticular formation extends into the hypothalamus and into the thalamus as the intralaminar nuclei, reticular nucleus, and nuclei of the midline (nonspecific thalamic nuclei, Chap. 13). Some brainstem reticular nuclei project to the cerebellum. The axons of cells of the nonspecific thalamic nuclei probably do not project directly to the cerebral cortex. However, these nuclei generate activity which projects influences to widespread areas of the cerebral cortex. Through the neural networks of the reticular formation of the brainstem are conveyed those impulses associated with vaguely appreciated senses, such as poorly localized pain, neural activities associated with the arousal-sleep cycle, and affect behavior expressions. The effects of the reticular system are not actually random and indefinite but rather are organized and definite and hence, though mainly nonspecific, have some degree of specificity. These pathways have numerous neurons and many synaptic connections and consist essentially of unmyelinated and lightly myelinated fibers. The descending motor reticular pathways are the "extrapyramidal pathways" and the autonomic pathways that project their influences from the brainstem to the spinal cord as the reticulospinal tracts.

The nonspecific system is characterized by the lack of point-to-point relays, by the relative absence of "secure" synaptic connectivity of presynaptic neurons with postsynaptic neurons, and by long latencies in the transmission time. These three characteristics are expressed by several observations. Stimuli from many peripheral spots may exert their influences upon one neuron of the reticular system. This complex convergence does not permit point-to-point, secure relays. In addition, one peripheral spot may exert its influences upon many neurons. The multineuronal, multisynaptic connectivity results in the long latencies exhibited in the reticular pathways. The reticular system is extremely sensitive to even low levels of anesthesia.

RETICULAR FORMATION

The *reticular formation* is a column of neurons which extends as a continuum with minimal histologic variation through the length of the spinal cord, brainstem, and basal regions of the diencephalon and telencephalon. The boundaries of the reticular formation cannot be precisely delineated, because its constituent neurons are not generally grouped into compact nuclei or tracts. The most constant structural substrate of the reticular formation is the presence of *generalized or isodendritic neurons*—cells with long, sparsely branching dendrites (Ramón-Moliner and Nauta). Even the presence of this neuronal type is not always diagnostic, because it is also found in regions outside the classical reticular formation. The dendritic fields of one neuron overlap with those of other neurons; in addition, the fields are interlaced with the transit axons. Golgi type II cells are absent in the reticular formation. The axons of the reticular neurons bifurcate into a long ascending branch and a long descending branch; these branches with their collaterals are transit axons. The long branches form the pathway systems which convey the output of these cells rostrally and caudally. These pathways are diffuse systems which are interrupted by numerous synaptic connections and which are organized as orderly and precise linkages of neurons.

The following is a version of the extent of the reticular formation in the nervous system. In the spinal cord, the reticular formation is located in the intermediate zone (lamina VII), with extensions into parts of the anterior and posterior horns. The pathway of the spinal cord reticular formation is the fasciculus proprius. Rostrally it expands into the enlarged central region of the brainstem tegmentum, so that the brainstem reticular formation has been called the reticular core. The *nuclei of this reticular core of the medulla, pons, and midbrain* are arranged into three longitudinal columns (Fig. 8-12): the *raphe nuclei and paramedian reticular nuclear group*, which are located within, and adjacent to, the midline raphe, the *central reticular nuclear group*, which occupies the medial subcolumn of the brainstem reticular core, and the *lateral reticular nuclear group*, located in the lateral subcolumn of the reticular core. The central tegmental tract (fasciculus) is the pathway of the brainstem reticular core.

The *raphe nuclei* include *1* the *nucleus raphe obscurus, nucleus raphe pallidus, nucleus raphe magnus*, and *paramedian reticular nuclei* of the medulla; *2* the *nucleus raphe pontis, nucleus centralis superior, nucleus raphe dorsalis (dorsal tegmental nuclei or supratrochlear nucleus)*, and *ventral tegmental nucleus of the pons* (the latter two nuclei extend into the midbrain); and *3* the *nuclei linearis of the midbrain* (Figs. 8-3 through 8-11).

The *central reticular nuclear group* includes *1* the *nucleus reticularis centralis* and *nucleus reticularis gigantocellularis of the medulla*, *2* the *nuclei reticularis pontis caudalis and oralis and the reticulotegmental nucleus of the pons*, and *3* the *nucleus ruber of the midbrain*.

The *lateral reticular nuclear group* includes *1* the *nucleus reticularis parvicellularis* and *lateral reticular nucleus of the medulla*, *2* no nuclei in most of the pons, and *3* the *cuneiform nucleus* and *pedunculopontine tegmental nucleus of the midbrain*.

The nucleus ruber, locus ceruleus, and interpeduncular nucleus of the midbrain and the inferior olivary nuclear complex may be considered as specialized nuclei which are not usually classified as reticular core nuclei.

The most rostral extension of the reticular formation into the diencephalon and telencephalon may include *1* the midline nuclei, intralaminar nuclei, reticular nucleus, and part of the ventral anterior nucleus of the thalamus; *2* hypothalamus; *3* zona incerta of the ventral

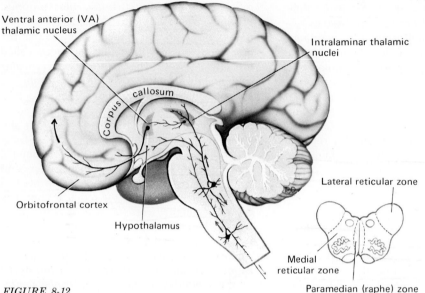

FIGURE 8-12
Ascending projections of the reticular pathway system.

In general, the multineuronal, multisynaptic relays of the brainstem reticular formation extend rostrally into two telencephalic regions: *1* posteriorly into the intralaminar, ventral anterior, and dorsomedial thalamic nuclear complexes, and *2* anteriorly into the subthalamic and hypothalamic complexes. The thalamic component projects, via the ventral anterior thalamic nucleus, to the orbitofrontal cortex.

The cross section through the brainstem (medulla) illustrates the division of the brainstem reticular formation into *1* a midline raphe or paramedian zone, *2* a medial reticular or "motor" zone, and *3* a lateral reticular or "sensory" zone.

thalamus; and *4* the septal nuclei and substantia innominata (located ventral to the globus pallidus) of the telencephalon. Some investigators include the subthalamic nucleus and globus pallidus in the reticular formation. The reticular pathways link *1* the midbrain with the hypothalamus and septal nuclei, and *2* the upper brainstem with the nuclei of the diencephalic reticular formation.

The brainstem reticular formation and its major rostral extension, the hypothalamus, have

been called the isodendritic core of the brain, because they are composed primarily of isodendritic neurons. The dendritic fields of isodendritic neurons overlap extensively. Differential specificity of function among these neurons within the isodendritic core is presumed to occur. Apparently the dendrites of each isodendritic neuron receive specialized inputs; these differ from the inputs received by the other isodendritic neurons.

BRAINSTEM RETICULAR SYSTEM

The brainstem reticular system is the phylogenetically ancient integrator, often called the "central core" (isodendritic core) of the mammalian brainstem. The cell bodies of the neurons of the reticular system are organized into groups throughout the reticular formation as the relatively diffuse brainstem reticular nuclei. The very long dendrites of each neuron are generally oriented in the transverse plane at right angles to the longitudinal axis of the brainstem, while the axon bifurcates into one long ascending branch and one long descending branch ori-

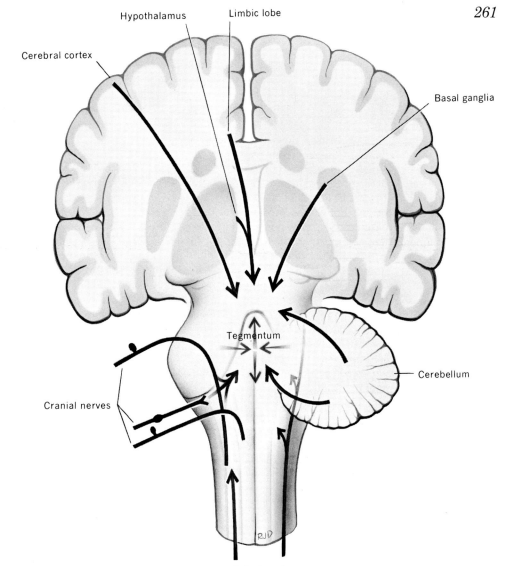

Hypothalamus

Limbic lobe

Cerebral cortex

Basal ganglia

Tegmentum

Cranial nerves

Cerebellum

Spinal cord

FIGURE 8-13
Input to the brainstem reticular formation.

Projections from the cerebrum and the spinal cord are directed to the lateral reticular zone. From this zone influences are conveyed to the medial reticular zone, as indicated by the arrows pointing toward the midline. From this medial zone neural influences are conveyed rostrally toward the cerebrum and caudally toward the spinal cord via the central tegmental tract. Other influences are projected laterally to the cranial nerve nuclei and the cerebellum.

ented parallel to the long axis of the brainstem (Fig. 8-12). Numerous collateral branches leave the main axonic branches. This organization permits a tremendous amount of interaction among the neurons of the system. Each neuron may receive synaptic input from over 4,000 other neurons (convergence), and, in turn, each neuron may have synaptic connections with over 25,000 other neurons (divergence).

The *input to the brainstem reticular system* is derived from many sources (Fig. 8-13). The ascending influences from the spinal cord include the spinoreticular tracts, the spinotectal tract, and the terminal and collateral branches of the spinothalamic tracts. The medial lemniscus does not have any branches which project into the reticular formation. All the sensory cranial nerves are sources of input. The brainstem reticular formation receives influences from visceral sources via the nucleus solitarius (facial, glossopharyngeal, and vagal nerves), from the vestibular and cochlear nuclei and their pathways, from the olfactory system via the median forebrain bundle, and from the visual system via cells of the superior colliculus. The input from the trigeminal system—its nuclei and pathways—is important; influences from this system have a significant effect on arousal. Descending influences from the cerebrum are derived from the corticobulbar and corticoreticular tracts, from collateral branches of the corticospinal tracts, and from projections from the basal ganglia, limbic lobe, and hypothalamus. Fibers from the cerebellum are included. The intrinsic tract of the reticular formation, called the central tegmental tract, is essentially a reticuloreticular tract consisting of the axons of the brainstem neurons. This reticuloreticular tract in the brainstem is more prominent than the propriospinal tract, its counterpart in the spinal cord. The descending portion of the central tegmental tract is located largely in the medial tegmentum, and the ascending portion in the lateral tegmentum. The lateral brainstem reticular formation is essentially an "affector," "sensory," or associative zone, receiving input primarily from higher centers (descending pathways), from spinal levels, and from trigeminal sources. The parvicellular reticular nucleus of the medulla and pons is an important reticular nucleus of this zone. This affector region projects its output to the medial brainstem reticular formation, which acts as an effector or motor zone.

The *output from the brainstem reticular system* is extensive because its axonic projections have diffuse connections; the full extent of its physiologic influences is somewhat unsettled (Fig. 8-14). Its ascending influences to the cerebral cortex and basal ganglia are largely directed to and through the thalamic intralaminar nuclei,

hypothalamus, and septal region. The mamillary peduncle (Chap. 11) is the main ascending pathway from the midbrain to the hypothalamus and septal region. Its descending influences are expressed via reticulospinal tracts upon the gamma and alpha motor neurons of the spinal cord. Many actions are exerted via the cranial nerves and via autonomic pathways upon the visceral output of the spinal cord and cranial nerves.

Ascending reticular system

The *functional role of the brainstem reticular system* is the subject of considerable comment. The reticular formation is a most significant integrating structure, for it is the region where impulses from the sensory modalities as well as from cerebral and cerebellar sources converge and interact. This region is able to modify the neural activity from these sources of stimulation and is capable of suppressing or enhancing the excitability of many neurons, thus inhibiting, facilitating, or modifying the transmission of neural information even through the specific pathways. The stimulation of the brainstem reticular formation may heighten pain sensibility. Through its neural networks the reticular system may utilize slight shifts of the excitatory and inhibitory interplay to direct input into any of the numerous responses without in any way altering the neuroanatomic substrate. This implies a functional lability of paramount significance. The reticular system is probably crucial in evoking the myriad nuances that may result from a single stimulation such as a sound, including the range of responses from no reaction to an intense attraction or repulsion.

The reticular system is involved with the range of behavioral expressions, from animations of alertness and attention to the "passiveness" of sleep. Deprivation of the ascending reticular influences may produce sleep. Depending in part on the state of the animal, stimulation of the midbrain reticular formation may induce sleep or awakening. A *sleep center* may be present in the reticular formation of the lower pons–upper medulla. Thus it has been postulated that sleep is produced *1* actively by the stimulatory activity of this sleep center in the lower brainstem (*active reticular deactiva-*

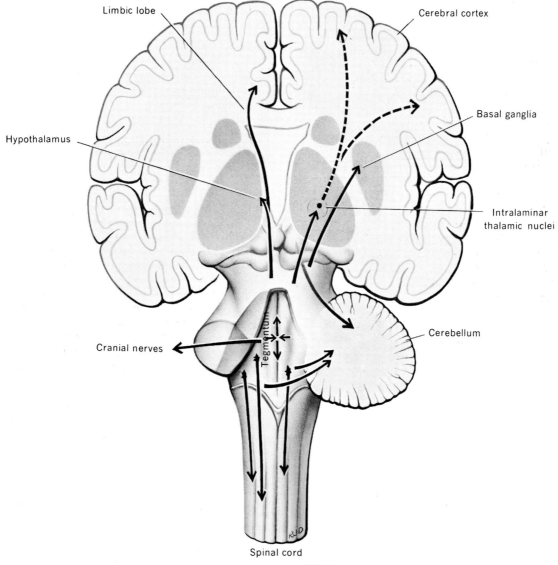

Limbic lobe

Cerebral cortex

Hypothalamus

Basal ganglia

Intralaminar
thalamic nuclei

Tegmentum

Cranial nerves

Cerebellum

Spinal cord

FIGURE 8-14
Output from the brainstem reticular formation.

The output is directed from the medial reticular zone *1* rostrally to the hypothalamus and intralaminar and other nuclei of the thalamus (Fig. 8-12) and from these structures to the limbic lobe and cerebral cortex, *2* laterally to the cerebellum and cranial nerve nuclei, and *3* caudally to the spinal cord via the reticulospinal tracts and descending autonomic pathways.

tion), or *2* passively by the suppression of the influences of the ascending reticular system (*passive reticular deactivation*). A permanent coma, following a brain injury, is probably the result of damage to the reticular formation (deprivation of ascending influences) within the ascending reticular pathways. A lesion in the lower brainstem may result in a deep coma whereas a lesion in the upper brainstem reticular formation may result in a less deep coma which is not as deep.

The ascending reticular system has been implicated in the neural integrative mechanisms associated with many facets of behavioral activities, including emotion, perception, motivation, drive, wakefulness, sleep, and habituation. *Habituation* is the neural mechanism whereby the organism becomes inattentive to monotonously repeated stimuli, as when a student falls asleep during a dull lecture. It refers to decreased sensitivity to a repeated stimulus pattern. In contrast, *adaptation* is the decreased sensitivity to a continuing stimulus. The reticular system may have a role in reducing the impact of stimuli upon the cerebral cortex. An example would be the relative unawareness of a driver to traffic noises that persist.

Ascending lemniscal pathways

PAIN AND TEMPERATURE PATHWAYS

(Lateral Column–Spinal Lemniscal Pathways; Protopathic Pathway and Trigeminal Lemniscus)

From the body The *lateral spinothalamic tract* conveying the pain and temperature modalities from regions innervated by the spinal cord (Fig. 5-14) is located in the lateral column (spinal cord) and lateral tegmentum of the brainstem, where it is called the *spinothalamic tract* (*spinal lemniscus*). This *lateral column–spinal lemniscus tract* terminates in the ventral posterolateral nucleus of the thalamus (Chap. 13). The spinothalamic tract attenuates as it ascends, for many of its fibers terminate in the brainstem reticular formation (including the lateral reticular nucleus of the medulla) and in the roof of the midbrain (spinotectal tract).

Other pain fibers ascend parallel to the spinothalamic tract near the medial lemniscus, in the brainstem reticular formation (*spinoreticular-thalamic pathway*), and in the periventricular gray matter. Deep pain and visceral

pain are apparently associated with these diffuse pathways. The association of the primitive pain modality and the phylogenetically old ascending reticular system is geared to the basic self-preservation drive of the organism.

From the head The pain and temperature fibers from the head are conveyed chiefly via the fifth cranial nerve (with some contribution from the seventh, ninth, and tenth cranial nerves).

The fibers of the first-order neurons with cell bodies in the trigeminal ganglion of the fifth nerve enter the midpons and descend as the ipsilateral spinal tract of the fifth nerve as far down as the second or third cervical spinal cord level (Fig. 8-15). They terminate in the caudal third of the spinal (descending) nucleus of the fifth nerve (subnucleus caudalis). The spinal tract and nucleus of the fifth nerve have as their functional and anatomic equivalents the posterolateral tract of Lissauer and the substantia gelatinosa of the spinal cord. The fibers from the mandibular branch of the fifth nerve are located in the dorsal aspect of the spinal tract and terminate in the lower medulla level; those of the ophthalmic branch are located in the ventral aspect of the spinal tract and terminate in the second and third cervical levels; and those of the maxillary branch are located in the middle of the spinal tract and terminate largely in the first cervical level. The neurons of the spinal nucleus of the fifth nerve project fibers of the second order which decussate and ascend in the medial lemniscus or in the adjacent ventral tegmentum as the *anterior tract* (quintothalamic tract, anterior trigeminothalamic tract, and trigeminal lemniscus) and terminate in the ventral posteromedial nucleus of the thalamus. Some secondary ascending trigeminal fibers are incorporated in the ascending reticular pathways. In addition, the primary afferent fibers of the trigeminal nerve extend (many via the spinal tract of the fifth nerve) to the brainstem reticular formation, nucleus solitarius, motor nucleus of the fifth nerve, and motor nucleus of the seventh nerve. The input from the fifth nerve into the functional activity of the reticular system is crucial to the maintenance of the arousal state (Chap. 13). The bilateral representation of the general senses of the head in the cerebral cortex may result from the presence of uncrossed ascending trigeminal fibers.

(Posterior Column–Medial Lemniscal
Pathway and Central Trigeminal Tracts;
Epicritic Pathways)

From the body The *medial lemniscus* is the brainstem tract of the *posterior column–medial lemniscus* pathway (Fig. 5-15). The fibers (neurons of the first order) of the fasciculus gracilis and fasciculus cuneatus (posterior column) of the spinal cord terminate in the nuclei gracilis and cuneatus, respectively, in the lower dorsal medulla. Axons from the neurons in these nuclei cross over the midline of the medulla just dorsal to the pyramids as the internal arcuate fibers and then ascend as the medial lemniscus. The medial lemniscus, found at all levels of the brainstem, gradually shifts laterally and then dorsally as the tract ascends, until it terminates in the ventral posterolateral nucleus of the thalamus. This tract does not contribute collateral fibers to the reticular formation.

From the head. Tactile discrimination in the face and head in front of the ears, including the nasal and mouth cavities, is transmitted by sensory fibers in the fifth nerve to the principal sensory nucleus of the fifth nerve, located in the lateral tegmentum of the pons (Fig. 8-15). This principal sensory nucleus is the cranial equivalent of the nuclei gracilis and cuneatus of the spinal pathways. Both nuclei contain neurons of the second order of the touch and deep sensibility pathways; the former nucleus receives input from the head and the latter two nuclei receive input from the body. Some neurons in this trigeminal nucleus project fibers that decussate in the pons and ascend in the medial lemniscus as the anterior trigeminal tract and terminate in the ventral posteromedial nucleus of the thalamus. Other neurons project uncrossed fibers that ascend in the dorsal tegmentum as the *posterior trigeminal tract* to the ventral posteromedial nucleus of the thalamus. These uncrossed ascending fibers convey influences from the mandibular nerve.

The proprioceptive input from the head, especially from the muscles of mastication, teeth, and gums and the voluntary eye muscles, is probably carried mainly by fibers of the fifth cranial nerve with their cell bodies (neurons of the first order) in the mesencephalic nucleus of the fifth nerve. These fibers project their axons into the reticular formation and to the motor nucleus of the fifth nerve for the jaw reflexes, involving the muscles of mastication. This nucleus is unique, for it is the only nucleus within the brain that is actually composed of spinal (sensory) root ganglion neurons (like the spinal root ganglion, it has no synapses). The equivalence of the two-neuron extensor reflex in the arc of the spinal cord and of the flexor jaw reflex is apparent.

The ascending pathways from the spinal cord conveying *light touch* are incorporated in either the crossed *anterior spinothalamic tract* or the uncrossed *posterior columns* of the spinal cord. The anterior spinothalamic tract joins and ascends through the brainstem with the medial lemniscus and possibly with the lateral spinothalamic tract. The light-touch fibers in the posterior columns ascend in the posterior column–medial lemniscus pathway to the higher centers (thalamus and cerebral cortex). Light-touch impulses from the head may be conveyed after synapsing in the principal sensory nucleus of the fifth nerve as crossed fibers in the medial lemniscus or as the uncrossed fibers in the dorsal tegmentum (*posterior trigeminal tract*). These ascending fibers terminate in the ventral posteromedial nucleus of the thalamus.

TASTE PATHWAYS

"Taste," in its colloquial usage, is equated with flavor, and flavor is the complex subjective perceptive quality which is the composite of several sensations, including smell, texture, temperature, "common chemical sense," and even pain. Flavor is also influenced by sight, feel, and sounds. Receptors in the oral and nasal cavities are utilized in the "taste" perceptions involved in the evaluation and appreciation of the smells of aromatic spices, of the texture of liquids and solids, of the temperature of foods, of the astringency of a persimmon ("puckering" results from the competition for the moisture in the mouth), of the "chemical heat," of the buccal pain of hot Mexican chili, and of the tang of many cheeses. The sight or the sound of a frying

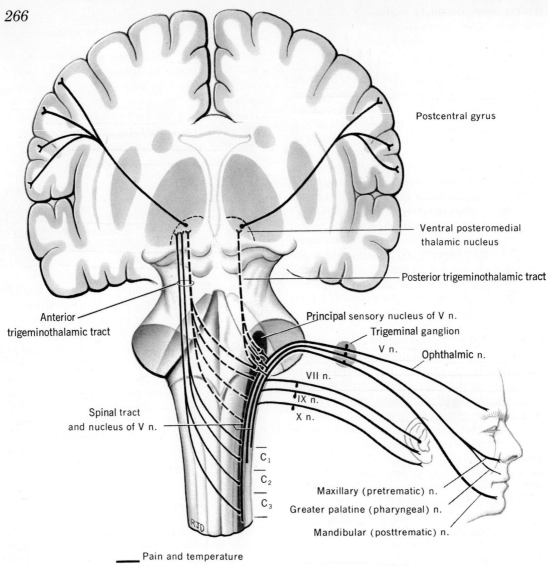

Postcentral gyrus

Ventral posteromedial
thalamic nucleus

Posterior trigeminothalamic tract

Principal sensory nucleus of V n.

Trigeminal ganglion

V n.

Ophthalmic n.

VII n.

IX n.

X n.

Anterior
trigeminothalamic tract

Spinal tract
and nucleus of V n.

C₁

C₂

C₃

RJD

Maxillary (pretrematic) n.

Greater palatine (pharyngeal) n.

Mandibular (posttrematic) n.

—— Pain and temperature

--- Tactile

FIGURE 8-15
General somatic sensory pathways from the
head in front of the ears.

These pathways consist of *1* first-order neurons of
cranial nerves V, VII, IX, and X, which pass through the
spinal tract of the fifth nerve and terminate in the
principal sensory nucleus and spinal nucleus of the fifth
nerve; *2* second-order neurons, which either decussate and ascend as the contralateral anterior trigeminothalamic tract, or ascend as the ipsilateral posterior
trigeminothalamic tract; and *3* third-order neurons,
which project to the "head region" of the postcentral
gyrus.

This figure illustrates the older concept that the
various components of the spinal tract of N. V descend
to different levels: *1* fibers from the ophthalmic nerve
descend as far as the third cervical level, *2* fibers from
the maxillary division descend as far as the first cervical
level, and *3* fibers from the mandibular nerve and
cranial nerves VII, IX, and X descend as far as the caudal
medulla. The recent concept that fibers from all nerves
descend as far as the second cervical level is illustrated
in Fig. 7-6.

steak can modify taste sensations. Even a "water sense" is indicated; distilled water applied to the taste buds may evoke discharges in "taste nerve fibers."

It is normally impossible to perceive pure taste without sensing an overlay of smell, because true taste is a much cruder and less sensitive senation than smell; taste thresholds are significantly higher than smell thresholds. For example, estimates indicate that some 20,000 times more molecules are needed to induce a taste sensation than a smell sensation. This explains why it is that when we taste, we invariably also smell.

In man, taste sensations can be obtained following appropriate stimulation of the taste receptors in the tongue, palate, and pharynx. To utilize all his taste receptors, the wine taster swishes the wine in his mouth and swallows slowly. Four taste modalities are generally recognized in man: salt, sweet, sour, and bitter. Each of these modalities can be sensed in each of these regions. Salt and sweet are perceived most acutely on the tongue, while bitter and sour are perceived most acutely on the palate. Bitter and sour are definitely but mildly tasted on the tongue and pharynx, while salt and sweet are mildly tasted on the palate and pharynx. Many taste sensations cannot even be described in terms of these four "elementary taste sensations." Among these are the taste qualities of numerous spices, fruits, and vegetables. In fact a truly objective classification of the tastes has not been developed; probably there are no primary taste qualities. All are chemically induced sensations. Salt taste is maximally perceived on the sides of the tongue, probably by the stimulation from chloride (Cl^-) and sulfate (SO_4^-) ions. Sour taste is maximally sensed part way back on the tongue by the stimulation of the hydrogen (H^+) ions of acids. Sweet is optimally perceived at the tip of the tongue, where sugars react with the fatty substances in the taste ending. Bitter is tasted mainly at the back of the tongue.

The true taste qualities in man are derived from the stimulation of taste buds. Each brandy-snifter-shaped taste bud contains upward of 25 neuroepithelial taste cells. In addition, other less-differentiated cells, called "sustentacular cells," act as reserve cells to replenish the taste cells when they die out. The receptor taste cells are continuously turning over. Each mature taste cell is replaced every 200 to 300 hr. A degenerated neuroepithelial cell can be replaced rapidly, usually within 10 hr. If the nerve fibers to a tastebud are cut, the taste bud atrophies and disappears. After the nerve regenerates and reinnervates the tongue epithelium, the taste buds redifferentiate. The distal tip of each taste cell extends as a surface specialization of microvilli into the small taste pit which is continuous with the oral cavity through the gustatory pore. The solutions containing sapid substances, either as ions or as dissolved molecules, enter the pore into the pit to interact with receptor sites on the taste cells. All substances must be in solution in order to be tasted. The proximal ends of the taste cells are in synaptic contact with nerve endings of the "taste" nerves.

The receptor sites are probably located on the surface of the microvilli. Not only does each taste cell have many different types of receptor sites, but the proportion of different types varies from taste cell to taste cell. Hence each gustatory cell can respond to several stimuli. No evidence indicates that a specific gustatory cell responds to but one group of stimuli (e.g., one cell for salts; another cell for hydrogen ion concentration). Another factor may regulate the types of stimuli that have access to the receptor sites. The proteins on the cell membrane surface may act to open or close gates of the membrane to different types of potential gustatory stimuli.

The exact mechanisms by which a taste cell is stimulated are not known, although many theories have been proposed. Each taste bud, and possibly each taste cell, responds to more than one of the classical taste qualities. No structural differences in the 10,000 taste buds or in the taste cells of the young adult have been revealed. The taste cells stimulate the taste nerve fibers. Structurally each neuroepithelial cell in a taste bud is innervated by the nerve fibers of several nerve cells; and several neuroepithelial cells in a taste bud are innervated by the branches of one neuron. Functionally, each neuroepithelial cell apparently responds to several taste qualities; and each neuron from a taste bud also responds to several taste qualities. The taste buds of man may well respond to as many as 10,000 different chemicals, of which many do not occur naturally. Discrimination by taste can be made between the dextro and levo forms of some amino acids. The numerous nuances of true taste are the result of transmission via many patterns of afferent impulses in the various nerve fibers and of processing in the nuclei of the taste pathways, the situation being comparable to the transmission of the qualities of sound (Chaps. 10, 13). The variations in the intensity of taste are transmitted by the differences in the frequency of firing of nerve impulses. Adaptation is rapid, usually in seconds or minutes.

A decrease in the sensitivity of taste with age is paralleled by the decrease in the total number of taste buds after the age of 40. A human baby has more than 10,000 taste buds, including some even on the palate and pharynx. This large number explains, in part, why babies dislike spiced foods and prefer bland baby food. The latter is probably tasty to them. Elderly people use spices, sugar, and salt more liberally to make food more tasty for their jaded gustatory sense by stimulating the lesser number of taste buds present. For example, the young adult can taste sugar in concentration about one-third (0.4 percent sugar) that of elderly adults (1.2 percent sugar). The center of the tongue, with only a few taste buds, is relatively taste blind.

Taste impulses are conveyed from the anterior two-thirds of the tongue by the fibers of the chorda tympani branch of the facial nerve and from the posterior third of the tongue, palate, and pharynx by fibers in the branches of the glossopharyngeal and vagus nerves. The sensory nerves in this region terminate either in the taste buds or as free nerve endings in the connective tissues and epithelium other than taste buds. Many of the free nerve endings are of terminals of general sensory fibers of the trigeminal nerve. The taste buds on the anterior two-thirds of the tongue are located on the free surface of the fungiform papillae, with each papilla containing from one to eight taste buds (Fig. 8-16). These *fungiform papillae,* which are scattered singly, are especially numerous near the tip of the tongue. In the region of the V-shaped sulcus terminalis is a linear series of 10 to 12 large *circumvallate papillae;* they cover a portion of the posterior third of the tongue. The numerous taste buds on each papilla are generally located along the sides of the papilla facing the moat surrounding the structure. In man, taste buds are also present on the surface of the hard and soft plate, pharynx, and larynx.

The taste fibers of the facial, glossopharyngeal, and vagus nerves pass into the medulla and terminate in the rostral and lateral portions of the nucleus solitarius; this portion is called the *nucleus gustatorius.* The taste neurons of the second order have axons which probably ascend as uncrossed fibers in association with the medial lemniscus and reticular formation to their termination in the most medial portion of the ventral posteromedial (VPM) nucleus of the thalamus. It is possible, but not proved, that some fibers of the gustatory pathways from the nucleus solitarius to the thalamus cross and ascend in association with the contralateral medial lemniscus (Fig. 8-16). Tertiary fibers from the VPM nucleus pass through the posterior limb of the internal capsule and terminate in the lower end of the postcentral gyrus (opercular region of the parietal lobe) and possibly in the cortex of the insula and superior temporal gyrus.

The ability to taste certain chemicals has a hereditary basis. Some individuals have a taste blindness to certain substances that other individuals can taste. One such compound is phenolthiourea (PTC), which is tasteless to some and bitter to others. Two-thirds of males are tasters and one-third are nontasters. Some taste abnormalities are known to be associated with the alteration of the body metabolism as a consequence of the action of certain chemical substances. Miracle fruit, a tropical fruit found in Southeastern United States, will, after being eaten, modify taste perception drastically. Foods, which formerly tasted sour and bitter, will then taste sweet.

Taste may have a role in the preservation of life itself. A rat without its parathyroid glands will die unless it ingests quantities of calcium salts. A parathyroidectomized rat selects calcium or calcium-containing foods from a mixed diet. By increasing its intake of calcium, the rat maintains its blood calcium at a level essential to life. This same animal with his "taste nerves" severed

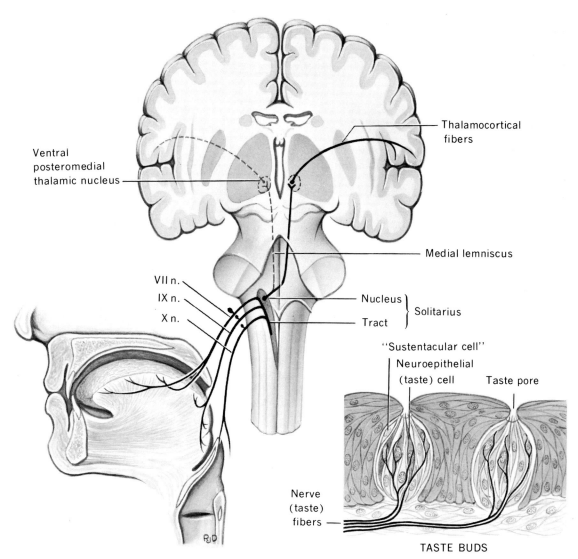

Ventral posteromedial thalamic nucleus

Thalamocortical fibers

Medial lemniscus

VII n.
IX n.
X n.

Nucleus } Solitarius
Tract }

"Sustentacular cell"
Neuroepithelial (taste) cell
Taste pore

Nerve (taste) fibers

TASTE BUDS

FIGURE 8-16
The taste (gustatory) pathway.

The taste pathway is composed of *1* first-order neurons of cranial nerves VII, IX, and X which pass through the solitary fasciculus and terminate in the solitary nucleus; *2* second-order neurons which decussate as the internal arcuate fibers, ascend in the medial lemniscus, and terminate in the ventral posteromedial nucleus of the thalamus; and *3* third-order neurons (thalamocortical fibers) which project to the inferior aspect of the postcentral gyrus. Some investigators claim that the taste pathways project to the ipsilateral thalamus.

does not select sufficient quantities of calcium out of the same mixed diet. As a result, its blood calcium level drops, tetany results, and death follows. A rat without its adrenal glands will die within a few days unless it ingests extra sodium chloride. An adrenalectomized rat will drink a solution of sodium chloride in preference to plain water, and in such quantities as to maintain good health for months. This same rat with its "taste nerves" severed loses its ability to discriminate between a saline solution and plain water. As a consequence it does not selectively drink the saline solution in sufficient quantities to maintain life. The animal soon dies. An adrenalectomized rat with taste perception intact is so specific in its salt preferences that it will select a sodium chloride solution and neglect available potassium chloride solutions or calcium chloride solutions. This predilection for salt is related to the searching out of salt licks by wild herbivorous animals living on salt-deprived vegetation.

AUDITORY PATHWAY (LATERAL LEMNISCUS) AND VESTIBULAR PATHWAYS

The nuclei and other structures contributing to the lateral lemniscal pathways of the auditory system and those contributing to the medial longitudinal fasciculus, vestibulospinal tract, and the cerebellar connections of the vestibular system are discussed elsewhere (Chap. 10).

Monoamine pathways of the central nervous system

Several pathways have been identified and described in chemical as well as anatomic terms. The neurons of these pathways contain one of the following monoamines: norepinephrine, 5-hydroxytryptamine (serotonin, 5-HT), and dopamine. These monoamines are present in the cell bodies, axons, and endings of these neurons. Hence, they are collectively called *monoamine (aminergic, monoaminergic) neuronal pathways* (Figs. 8-17, 8-18). Evidence indicates that these monoamines and their precursors and associated enzymes are presumably synthesized in the cell bodies of neurons and distributed in monoamine vesicles via axoplasmic flow to the nerve terminals. These putative neurotransmitters are also synthesized in axon terminals. Neurons with norepinephrine comprise the *noradrenergic pathways* (Fig. 8-17); those with serotonin, the *serotoninergic pathways* (Fig. 8-18); and those with dopamine, the *dopaminergic pathways* (Fig. 8-18).

The cell bodies of the neurons comprising the aminergic pathways have been identified in limited regions of the infratentorial brainstem and hypothalamus. With respect to the brainstem, the cell bodies of the *noradrenergic neurons* are localized in the tegmentum of the pons and medulla (apparently they are absent in the midbrain tegmentum); those of the *serotoninergic neurons* are found in the raphe nuclei; and those of the *dopaminergic neurons* are restricted to the substantia nigra and to regions surrounding the interpeduncular nucleus of the midbrain. The aminergic pathways within the central nervous system may be classified into several groups: *1* descending noradrenergic (NA) pathway, *2* descending serotoninergic (5-HT) pathway, *3* ascending noradrenergic (NA) pathway, *4* NA pathways from the locus ceruleus, *5* ascending serotoninergic (5-HT) pathway, and *6* dopaminergic (DA) pathway.

DESCENDING NORADRENERGIC (NA) PATHWAY AND DESCENDING SEROTONINERGIC (5-HT) PATHWAY (Figs. 8-17, 8-18)

The descending aminergic pathways originating in the medulla and terminating in the spinal cord include the *NA and the 5-HT pathways*. The NA fibers originate from cells in the ventrolateral part of the reticular formation of the caudal medulla; the 5-HT fibers originate from cells of the raphe nuclei of the medulla. Many of the NA fibers and 5-HT fibers descend in the anterior funiculus and ventral part of the lateral funiculus and then terminate in the anterior horn of the spinal gray matter. Other NA and 5-HT fibers descend in the dorsal part of the lateral funiculus and then terminate in the posterior horn and the intermediolateral nucleus of the spinal cord.

ASCENDING NORADRENERGIC (NA) PATHWAY (Fig. 8-17)

Ascending NA fibers originate from cells of the brainstem reticular nuclei located *1* in the ventrolateral medulla, *2* in the lower pons dorsal and lateral to the superior olivary nuclei, and *3* in the upper pons ventral to the superior cerebellar peduncle. These fibers ascend as *"the ventral NA pathway"* within the medial and ventromedial brainstem reticular formation and

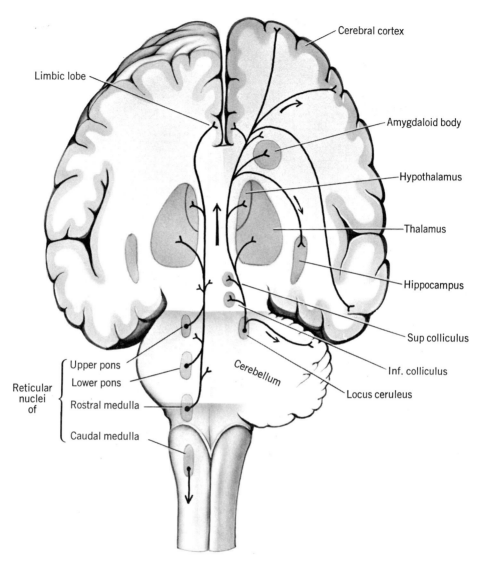

Limbic lobe

Cerebral cortex

Amygdaloid body

Hypothalamus

Thalamus

Hippocampus

Sup colliculus

Inf. colliculus

Locus ceruleus

Cerebellum

Reticular nuclei of
{ Upper pons
Lower pons
Rostral medulla
Caudal medulla

FIGURE 8-17
Noradrenergic pathways.

medial forebrain bundle of the hypothalamus. The fibers of this pathway terminate as nerve endings in the lower brainstem, mesencephalon, and cerebrum. Some of the structures in which these fibers terminate include the dorsal vagal nucleus and nucleus solitarius of the medulla, some reticular nuclei and periaqueductal gray matter of the midbrain, hypothalamus, thalamus, and limbic lobe.

The ascending pathway on the left originates from the medullary and pontine reticular nuclei and terminates in the cerebrum. The descending pathway on the left originates from medullary reticular nuclei and terminates in the spinal cord. The projections from the locus ceruleus on the right course *1* via the lateral pathway to the cerebellum and *2* via the ascending pathway to the midbrain and cerebrum.

272

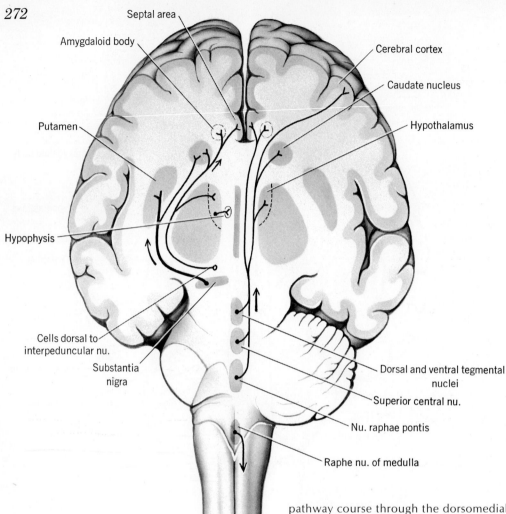

Septal area

Amygdaloid body

Cerebral cortex

Caudate nucleus

Putamen

Hypothalamus

Hypophysis

Cells dorsal to interpeduncular nu.

Substantia nigra

Dorsal and ventral tegmental nuclei

Superior central nu.

Nu. raphae pontis

Raphe nu. of medulla

FIGURE 8-18
The dopaminergic pathways (*left*) and the serotoninergic (5-HT) pathway (*right*). These pathways are described in the text.

NA PATHWAYS FROM THE LOCUS CERULEUS
(Fig. 8-17)

The *locus ceruleus* is composed entirely of catecholamine-containing cell bodies, which contain norepinephrine. These cells give rise to the ascending pathway to the cerebrum called the *dorsal NA pathway*, and the *lateral pathway* to the cerebellum. The fibers of this ascending

pathway course through the dorsomedial brainstem reticular formation. At the midbrain-diencephalic junction the fibers join those of the ventral NA pathway in the medial forebrain bundle (see Chap. 15) and then continue to the cerebral cortex and hippocampus. This *dorsal pathway* is composed primarily of uncrossed fibers; a few of the fibers are crossed. These fibers from the locus ceruleus project directly as an ascending monosynaptic pathway (without interposed relay nuclei) to many regions of the brain, especially in the diencephalon and telencephalon. These include some brainstem nuclei such as the inferior and superior colliculi, thalamic nuclei, hypothalamus, amygdaloid body, septal area, hippocampus, and wide areas of the cerebral cortex. The terminals of NA fibers are present in all laminae of the cerebral cortex.

The fine fibers of the *lateral pathway* course through the ipsilateral superior cerebellar peduncle to all parts of the cerebellar cortex. Evidence indicates that these fibers exert inhibitory influences upon the distal segments of the dendritic tree of the Purkinje cells (Siggins et al., 1971). It is likely that each cell body in the locus ceruleus has axonal branches, one of which terminates in the cerebellum and another in the cerebral cortex; in addition, collateral branches terminate in the midbrain colliculi, thalamus, and hypothalamus. These axons from one cell, which terminate monosynaptically in such diverse regions, may exert influences simultaneously in both the cerebral and cerebellar cortices (Olsen and Fuxe, 1971). Increased activity may result in desynchronization of the electroencephalograph (Chap. 16), behavioral arousal, and alerting of the cerebral cortex. This NA system may have an important role in the induction of paradoxic sleep (Chap. 16).

ASCENDING SEROTONINERGIC (5-HT) PATHWAY
(Fig. 8-18)

The cell bodies of the raphe nuclei of the pons and lower midbrain (nucleus raphe pontis, superior central nucleus, and dorsal and ventral tegmental nuclei) have high concentrations of serotonin. Axons originating from these cell bodies form the ascending serotonin (5-HT) pathway. It ascends through the medial brainstem reticular formation and ventral part of the medial forebrain bundle, from which it divides into a *lateral component*, which courses through and terminates in the hypothalamus, amygdala, and cerebral cortex; and a *medial component*, which courses through and terminates in the septal nuclei and cingulate cortex.

These raphe nuclei are, in some way, related to various aspects of behavior and to the sleep-wake cycle. Total insomnia occurs when these raphe nuclei are destroyed or when the serotonin stores are depleted by the drug reserpine. In contrast, an increase in the brain serotonin level decreases the sensitivity to pain.

DOPAMINERGIC (DA) PATHWAY (Fig. 8-18)

The cell bodies of the compact zone of the substantia nigra and of the region dorsal to the interpeduncular nucleus have high concen-

trations of dopamine (DA). The axons originating in the compact zone ascend successively through the globus pallidum and internal capsule to the neostriatum (caudate nucleus and putamen). This *nigrostriatal DA system* is integrated in the basal ganglia circuits (Chap. 14). Some DA fibers from the substantia nigra terminate in the amygdala. The fibers originating from the cells dorsal to the interpeduncular nucleus ascend within the medial forebrain bundle and terminate in the hypothalamus, amygdala, and other portions of the limbic lobe. Some dopaminergic neurons project to the hypophysis.

According to Ungerstedt, bilateral focal lesions of the DA fibers to the hypothalamus in the rat result in an animal that will not eat or drink and is apparently insensitive to pain.

Structures associated with the cerebellum

TEGMENTAL CONNECTIONS

A number of major structures in the brainstem tegmentum are involved with the input and output of the cerebellum (Chap. 9). The nuclei and tracts associated with the inferior cerebellar peduncle include 1 vestibular pathways to and from the archicerebellum (Figs. 9-7 and 10-10), 2 the posterior spinocerebellar tract from the spinal cord, and 3 nerve fibers from the inferior olivary nuclei (olivocerebellar tract), accessory cuneate nucleus, and the paramedian reticular nuclei in the medulla (reticulocerebellar tract) to the cerebellar cortex (Fig. 9-7). The cerebellum receives influences from the lower extremity via the posterior spinocerebellar tract and from the upper extremity via fibers from the accessory cuneate nucleus (Fig. 5-12). Fibers from the reticulotegmental nucleus of the pons pass through the middle cerebellar peduncle to the entire vermis except for the nodulus. The nuclei and tracts associated with the superior cerebellar peduncle include: input via the anterior spinocerebellar tract from the spinal cord; and outflow via 1 ascending fibers to the nucleus ruber (a reticular nucleus) and the ventrolateral and intralaminar nuclei of the thalamus, and 2 descending fibers of the descending division of the superior cerebellar peduncle to the reticulotegmental nucleus of the pons (Fig. 8-8), paramedian reticular nuclei of the medulla (Fig. 8-14), and the inferior olivary nuclear complex (Fig. 8-5).

Corticoreticular fibers from the cerebral cortex project to the paramedian reticular nuclei and lateral reticular nucleus of the medulla and the reticulotegmental nucleus of the pons.

BASILAR CONNECTIONS

The *corticopontine tracts* arise from all lobes of the cerebral cortex and descend through the internal capsule and the crus cerebri before terminating by synapsing with the ipsilateral pontine nuclei (Fig. 9-5). The frontopontine fibers from the frontal lobe are located in the anterior limb of the internal capsule and the medial part of the crus cerebri. The parieto-occipitopontine fibers are located in the posterior limb of the internal capsule and in the lateral part of the crus cerebri. The corticopontine tracts are a link in the corticopontocerebellar pathways (Chap. 9). The pontine nuclei give rise to axons which decussate (a few fibers are uncrossed) as the pontocerebellar tract that passes through the middle cerebellar peduncle before terminating in the neocerebellum.

Descending pathways: input to brainstem reticular formation (Fig. 8-13)

The descending pathways of the brainstem reticular system receive input from many sources. Its motor activities are expressed via influences exerted upon the somatic and visceral (autonomic) effectors. The sources of neural input to this system include the ascending reticular system, collateral fibers from some ascending lemniscal pathways (except the medial lemniscus), and descending direct and indirect pathways from higher centers (hypothalamus, globus pallidus, thalamus, and cerebral cortex). Many influences from subcortical cerebral centers are conveyed to the cerebral cortex, from which they are projected via corticoreticular fibers to the brainstem reticular formation. The *reticulo-reticular fibers (central tegmental fasciculus)* constitute the brainstem intrareticular integrating pathway.

Descending somatic tracts from brainstem reticular formation

Reticulospinal tracts (Fig. 8-19) The two descending pathways from the brainstem reticular formation to the spinal cord comprise the pontine (medial) reticulospinal tract and the medullary (lateral) reticulospinal tract. The *pontine reticulospinal tract* arises in the nuclei reticularis oralis and caudalis and descends as an uncrossed tract adjacent to and within the medial longitudinal fasciculus through the entire length of the spinal cord. Its fibers terminate in the medial part of the anterior horn (lamina VIII and adjacent parts of lamina VII). The *medullary reticulospinal tract* originates in the nucleus gigantocellularis of the medulla. Its fibers are primarily uncrossed; they descend in the anterolateral funiculus and terminate primarily in lamina VII of all levels of the spinal cord. A major input to these tracts is derived from the motor (area 4), premotor (area 6), and somesthetic (areas 3, 1, and 2) areas of the cerebral cortex.

These *corticoreticular fibers* descend in the vicinity of the corticospinal tracts and terminate bilaterally (with slighly more crossed than uncrossed fibers) in the nucleus reticularis pontis oralis and nucleus reticularis gigantocellularis. As a total unit, these pathways should be called corticoreticulospinal pathways. The fibers of the reticulospinal tracts are presumed to terminate upon interneurons of laminae VII and VIII, which, in turn, influence gamma (and also alpha) motor neuron activity, especially that related to posture and muscle tone.

Stimulation of the medullary reticular formation generally inhibits the myotatic reflexes and extensor muscle tone (a rigid limb in the decerebrate animal becomes flaccid) and movements evoked by cerebral cortical stimulation (cortically induced movements). In the normal animal, this medullary component tends to inhibit antigravity muscle tone and facilitate flexor

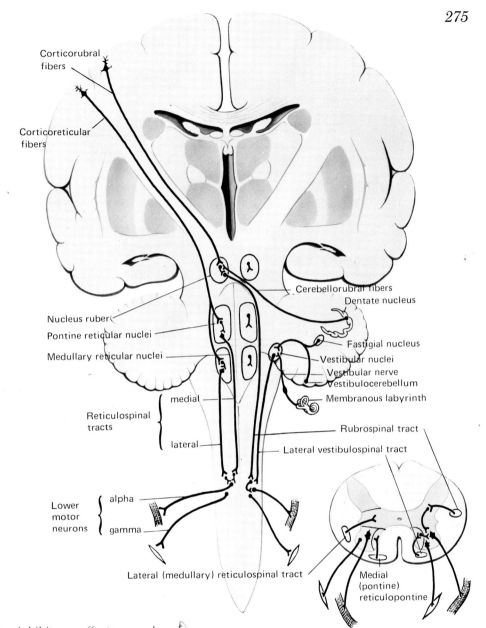

Corticorubral
fibers

Corticoreticular
fibers

Cerebellorubral fibers
Dentate nucleus

Nucleus ruber
Pontine reticular nuclei
Medullary reticular nuclei

Fastigial nucleus
Vestibular nuclei
Vestibular nerve
Vestibulocerebellum
Membranous labyrinth

medial

Reticulospinal
tracts

lateral

Rubrospinal tract

Lateral vestibulospinal tract

Lower
motor
neurons

alpha

gamma

Lateral (medullary) reticulospinal tract

Medial
(pontine)
reticulopontine

muscle tone. Inhibitory effects are largely evoked from the medullary reticular formation and are mediated via the medullary reticulospinal fibers. Facilitatory effects are largely evoked by stimulation of the pontine reticular formation (increased muscle tone); these are mediated via pontine reticulospinal tracts. The response evoked by these stimulations is produced by the activity of antagonistic muscle groups (e.g., flexors and extensors) through re-

FIGURE 8-19
Descending motor pathways to the spinal cord, including the reticulospinal tracts (cortico-reticulospinal pathways), rubrospinal tracts (corticorubrospinal pathways), and vestibulo-spinal tracts.

ciprocally organized interneuronal intrinsic circuits within the spinal cord. In the normal animal, the pontine component has the opposite effect from the medullary component. Reticulospinal tracts convey influences involved with respiratory movements and with activities of the autonomic nervous system. Those fibers which terminate upon neurons of the ascending pathways have a role in the processing and biasing of sensory input.

Vestibulospinal tracts and medial longitudinal fasciculus The (*lateral*) *vestibulospinal tract* from the lateral vestibular nucleus passes from the lateral vestibular nucleus through the lateral medullary tegmentum and anterolateral funiculus of the spinal cord. This uncrossed tract exerts facilitatory influences upon muscle tone, especially the extensor musculature, associated with posture and maintenance of equilibrium. The *medial longitudinal fasciculus (MLF)* is a bundle of fibers, mainly involved with reflexes of the vestibular system (Fig. 10-10). These reflexes include movements of the eyes (vestibulomesencephalic and associated fibers) and neck movements for maintaining position of the head in space (medial vestibulospinal tract, Fig. 10-10). The MLF contains some descending interstitiospinal descending fibers of unknown function from the interstitial nucleus of Cajal of the midbrain.

Rubrospinal and tectospinal tracts The *rubrospinal tract* originates in both large and small neurons of the nucleus ruber, decussates in the midbrain as the ventral tegmental decussation, and extends through the entire length of the spinal cord (Figs. 5-25, 5-29, 8-19, A-10). The nucleus ruber, actually a nucleus of the reticular formation, receives input from the cerebellum (dentatorubral tract) and cerebral motor cortex (uncrossed corticorubral tract). As a total unit, this pathway is called the corticorubrospinal tract. The rubrospinal tract exerts facilitatory influences on the tone of flexor musculature.

The *tectospinal tract* originates in the deep layer of the superior colliculus, decussates in the midbrain as the dorsal tegmental decussation, and extends through the spinal cervical region (Figs. 5-25, 5-29, A-10). This tract, a component of the medial longitudinal fasciculus, is presumed to be involved with postural movements initiated by visual stimuli.

DESCENDING AUTONOMIC PATHWAYS

The autonomic pathways in the brainstem may be thought of as a complexly organized interacting, multineuronal network with certain tegmental regions acting as focal or nodal sites. The autonomic nervous system acts not alone but in concert with the somatic nervous system, also represented in the reticular formation.

The descending influences of the autonomic nervous system are derived primarily from diffuse pathways from the hypothalamus. Other cerebral structures, including the cerebral cortex, basal ganglia, and the thalamus, direct their effects essentially through connections in the hypothalamus (Chap. 11). The hypothalamic output to the brainstem is conveyed via *1* the dorsal longitudinal fasciculus and diffuse fibers located in the periventricular gray, terminating primarily in the dorsal tegmental nucleus of the lower midbrain, and *2* the median forebrain bundle and mamillotegmental tract, terminating largely in the midbrain tegmentum (Chap. 15). The multineuronal nets of the reticular formation (reticuloreticular tract) convey the influences to the rest of the brainstem. The dorsal longitudinal fasciculus has indirect connections with the parasympathetic dorsal vagal nucleus of the medulla.

The descending autonomic pathways from the hypothalamus and the cerebellum also interact in the brainstem reticular formation with the input from the peripheral viscera (via the cranial nerves, especially the vagus nerve) and with the various ascending influences and modulating feedbacks from the spinal cord. These complex patterns in the reticular formation are organized for the regulation of many visceral functions.

Many vital activities are mediated through the brainstem by "centers" definable largely by physiologic criteria. These "centers" project their influences *1* to the spinal cord via reticulospinal fibers and *2* to the body, largely, but not exclusively, through the parasympathetic and sympathetic outflows (Chap. 6). The ventromedial tegmentum of the medulla contains an *inhibitory cardiovascular center* and an *inspiratory respiratory center;* the lateral tegmentum of the medulla and lower pons contains an *excitatory cardiovascular center;* and the dorsolateral tegmentum contains the *salivatory centers* and an *expiratory respiratory center.*

These medullary respiratory centers are responsible for the rhythmic discharges which result in the spontaneous respiratory cycle. Anatomically, the two respiratory centers overlap. A neuronal group in the rostral pontine tegmentum is called the *pneumotaxic center.* This area is presumed to exert inhibitory influences on neurons of the medullary inspiratory center and lower pontine apneustic center. The pontine pneumotaxic center acts to prevent sustained inspiration. The arrest of respiration in the inspiratory phase is called apneusis. In the caudal pontine tegmentum is a neuronal group called the *apneustic center.* When released from the influences of the pneumotaxic center, the activity of the cells of the apneustic centers produces *apneusis.* This apneustic center is presumed to be facilitatory to respiration, when uninhibited; normally it receives inhibitory influences from the vagal nerves and the pneumotaxic centers.

Each of these bilateral centers is composed of scattered neuronal groups, which are not delineated as morphologically discrete nuclei. These centers are involved in the following phenomena. Stimulation of the ventromedial tegmentum may result in a deceleration of the heartbeat, a lower blood pressure and an inspiratory (inhalation) phase of the respiratory cycle. Stimulation of the lateral tegmentum may result in an acceleration of the heartbeat and a higher blood pressure, and stimulation of the dorsolateral tegmentum may evoke salivation, vomiting (*vomiting center*), and the expiratory phase (exhalation) of the respiratory cycle. The area postrema of the medulla (Figs. 11-6, A-15) may have a role in certain vomiting (emetic) reflexes; the area may be a chemoreceptor which acts upon the vomiting center (Chap. 11).

Input from peripheral receptors to the respiratory and cardiovascular centers of the brainstem is derived from *1* the *pressoreceptors* located in the lung (stretch receptors), in the atrium and ventricle of the heart, in the carotid sinus in the vicinity of the carotid bifurcation, and in the walls of the aorta and its major branches (monitors of the blood pressure); and *2* the *chemoreceptors* in arterial receptors located in the carotid body (innervated by the glossopharyngeal nerve), the aortic bodies, the roots of the main thoracic arteries (innervated by the vagus nerve), and the medulla (called *central receptors*). The stretch (Hering-Breuer) reflex is an activity initiated by pulmonary pressoreceptors; it is protective to the lungs. When the lung is inflated, these receptors are stimulated to convey influences which act to inhibit inspiration. In contrast the pressoreceptors of the deflating lungs initiate activity which results in stimulating inspiration. Pain, heat, or cold may excite an increase in respiration (e.g., spanking a newborn infant). The pressoreceptors in the heart, aorta, and carotid sinus can influence vasomotor (cardiovascular) centers in the medulla, which have a role in regulating cardiovascular activity.

The chemoreceptors of the carotid and aortic bodies are stimulated to increase their rate of discharge by a lowered P_{O_2}, elevated P_{CO_2}, and increased hydrogen ion concentrations (H^+) in their arterial blood supply. These bodies have a high rate of blood flow passing through them. They are rugged receptors, which drive respiration. They remain active even when the chemoreceptors within the central nervous system are depressed by anesthetics or shock. Some neurons within the ventrolateral tegmentum of the medulla act as central chemoreceptors. They respond to an increase in P_{CO_2} primarily through the hydrogen ions of the carbonic acid. Carbon dioxide is known as a most sensitive and potent stimulant to respiration; this activity is mediated largely through these central chemoreceptors. The CO_2 in cerebrospinal fluid, which readily diffuses through the pia-glial membrane, is another source of carbonic acid. Pulmonary chemoreceptors are either nonexistent or not important.

The parasympathetic nuclei include the accessory oculomotor nucleus of Edinger-Westphal of the oculomotor nerve, the salivatory nuclei of the facial and glossopharyngeal nerves, and the dorsal vagal nucleus of the vagus nerve.

CORTICOBULBAR AND CORTICORETICULAR PATHWAYS TO CRANIAL NERVE MOTOR NUCLEI

The corticobulbar fibers transmit impulses from the cerebral cortex to the motor nuclei of the cranial nerves. The precise course of these upper motor neuron fibers has not been fully documented. The pathway commences in the lower aspect of the precentral gyrus (area 4) and other cerebral cortical areas such as 8 and 44. Direct stimulation of these cortical areas produces movements of cranial nerve-innervated muscles. A topographic representation of the head is present in area 4 (Chap. 16). The corticobulbar fibers descend in order through the genu of the internal capsule, the middle of the crus cerebri of the midbrain, and the pons proper. These fibers enter into the brainstem tegmentum to interact with interneurons that innervate the lower motor neurons of the cranial nerves. Because practically all the corticobulbar fibers terminate on interneurons in the reticular formation, they are often called corticoreticular pathways. The "aberrant" corticobulbar fibers have a similar course until they reach the upper midbrain. In the brainstem these fibers take variable paths through the tegmentum, which may account for the margin of safety from limited injury of these pathways.

The corticobulbar pathways consist of both crossed and uncrossed fibers, so that many cranial nerve nuclei receive both a crossed and an uncrossed upper neuron innervation. In general, all the cranial nerve motor nuclei are innervated by crossed corticobulbar fibers. In addition, many nuclei are innervated by a significant number of uncrossed corticobulbar fibers.

In this account, *direct corticobulbar fibers* convey influences from the cerebral cortex directly, without interruption, to the lower motor neurons of the cranial nerves (Fig. 8-20). The *indirect corticobulbar (corticoreticular) fibers* convey influences from the cerebral cortex to brainstem interneurons, which, in turn, innervate the lower motor neurons of the cranial nerves (Fig. 8-20). This is comparable to the process in which some *corticospinal fibers* ter-

minate and synapse directly with lower motor neurons, while others terminate and synapse with spinal interneurons that, in turn, synapse with lower motor neurons (Chap. 5). In effect, direct corticobulbar projections are associated with those nerves which innervate muscles which contract somewhat independently from the others of the group (e.g., control of a few of the muscles of facial expression).

The cranial nerves which innervate the extraocular muscles of the eye (cranial nerves III, IV, and VI), the muscles of the pharynx and soft palate (swallowing), and larynx (cranial nerves IX, X, and cranial root of XI) are innervated by both uncrossed and crossed indirect corticobulbar fibers (Fig. 8-20). Apparently the lower motor neurons of these cranial nerves do not receive direct corticobulbar innervation.

The cranial nerve nuclei that innervate the muscles of mastication (cranial nerve V), the muscles of facial expression (cranial nerve VII), and the muscles of the tongue (cranial nerve XII) are innervated by both uncrossed and crossed direct and indirect corticobulbar fibers (Fig. 8-20). These nuclei receive bilateral upper motor neuron influences. The spinal nucleus of cranial nerve XI (mainly to the sternocleidomastoid muscle) is presumably innervated by uncrossed (not crossed) direct corticobulbar fibers. The relative number of crossed and uncrossed direct corticobulbar fibers may vary from individual to individual.

The direct corticobulbar innervation of the motor nucleus of the seventh nerve differs from the above in a way that is clinically significant. The neurons of the facial nucleus innervating the muscles of the upper part of the face (forehead, eyelids) receive a substantial number of crossed and uncrossed fibers. Those neurons of the facial nucleus innervating the muscles of the lower part of the face (lips, nose, and cheek) receive crossed direct corticobulbar fibers almost exclusively (i.e., they receive few, if any, uncrossed fibers).

Paralysis of the voluntary muscles of the head may result from the interruption of cranial nerve fibers (lower motor neurons) or of the corticobulbar tracts (upper motor neurons). A lower motor neuron paralysis results when the cranial nerve fibers to a muscle group are transected. An upper motor neuron paralysis is not necessarily a consequence of the unilateral interrup-

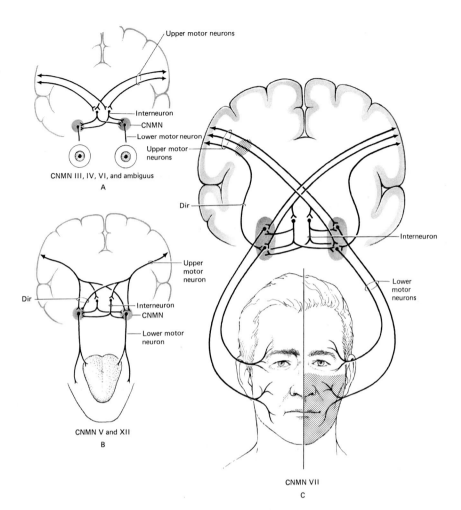

CNMN III, IV, VI, and ambiguus
A

CNMN V and XII
B

CNMN VII
C

tion of a significant number of upper motor neurons. Muscles innervated by the cranial nerves that have bilateral cortical representation generally do not show any signs of paralysis, while those with only a crossed unilateral representation show signs of upper motor neuron paralysis on the contralateral side. The consequences of damage to the corticobulbar pathways to the facial nucleus may be expressed with several variations. A unilateral lesion of the corticobulbar tracts to the facial nucleus may result in an upper motor neuron paralysis of the lower facial muscles of the contralateral side and a complete sparing of the upper facial muscles. The affected muscles may not respond to voluntary stimulation (*central facial palsy*) but may respond to an emotional stimulus (*mimetic palsy*); e.g., the patient cannot smile when asked to smile but can smile when told a joke. The facial muscles may respond to voluntary stimulation but not to emotional stimulation, or vice versa. The precise neural mechanisms involved in these diverse expressions are unknown.

FIGURE 8-20
The three groups of cranial nerve motor nuclei (CNMN) according to their upper motor neuron (UMN) innervation.

(A), *CNMN III, IV, VI, and Ambiguus.* The UMNs exert influences through direct bilateral projections to interneurons, which, in turn, innervate the lower motor neurons (LMN) of these motor nuclei. (B), *CNMN V and XII.* The UMNs exert influences both through (1) indirect bilateral projections to interneurons and (2) direct (Dir) bilateral projections to the LMNs of these motor nuclei. (C), *CNMN VII.* The UMNs exert influences through indirect bilateral projections to LMNs. *Of importance,* (1) the LMNs innervating muscles of upper face and forehead receive direct (Dir) bilateral UMN projections and (2) the LMNs innervating muscles of lower face receive predominantly direct crossed UMN projections. The UMN lesion (shaded) results in a paralysis limited to muscles of contralateral lower face (shaded).

DESCENDING CORTICOBULBAR (CORTICONUCLEAR) FIBERS FROM CORTEX TO NUCLEI OF ASCENDING PATHWAYS

Influences from the cortex on the nuclei of the ascending pathways are important in neural processing (Chap. 16). These descending corticonuclear pathways terminate in the nuclei gracilis and cuneatus of the posterior column-medial lemniscus pathway, in the trigeminal nuclei of the brainstem, in the nuclei of the auditory pathways, and in the nucleus solitarius (Chaps. 13 and 16). The descending influences are mainly inhibitory; they have a role in the sharpening effect by enhancing the signal and reducing the noise accompanying the signal (Chap. 10).

CORTICOSPINAL TRACT

The *corticospinal (pyramidal) tract* is composed of motor fibers from the cerebral cortex passing through the basilar portion of the brainstem on their way to the spinal cord (Fig. 5-24). Throughout the brainstem course numerous collateral branches which leave the main axon and terminate in the reticular formation. The corticospinal tract is located in the middle two-thirds of the crus cerebri of the midbrain, in fascicles among the pontine nuclei of the pons proper, and in the pyramid of the medulla. Most of its fibers (85 to 90 percent) cross over in the lower medulla as the decussation of the pyramidal tract (Chap. 5, Figs. 5-24 and 8-3).

Cranial nerves and their nuclei

Some basic structural and functional aspects of the cranial nerves are outlined in Chap. 7.

The *general somatic efferent cranial nerves* (oculomotor, trochlear, abducent, and hypoglossal nerves) have their nuclei of origin adjacent to the midline, ventral to the cerebral aqueduct and fourth ventricle, and adjacent to the medial longitudinal fasciculus. The *oculo-motor nuclear complex*, including the parasympathetic accessory oculomotor nucleus of Edinger-Westphal and the several subdivisions of the somatic efferent nuclei, is located in the midbrain. Each oculomotor nerve consists mainly of uncrossed and a few crossed fibers that pass through the medial tegmentum and leave the brainstem in the interpeduncular fossa. Each *trochlear nucleus*, located in the lower midbrain, gives rise to the trochlear nerve that curves dorsally through the edge of the periaqueductal gray, decussates in the roof, and then emerges from the midbrain tectum. Each *abducent nucleus*, located in the lower pons, gives rise to the uncrossed abducent nerve, which passes through the medial brainstem and emerges at the pontomedullary junction. Each elongated *hypoglossal nucleus*, located in the medulla, gives rise to the uncrossed hypoglossal nerve which emerges from the brainstem as a series of rootlets in the anterior lateral sulcus between the pyramid and the olive.

The *vestibulocochlearis nerve* enters the dorsolateral aspect of the upper medulla. The *four vestibular nuclei* (superior, medial, lateral, and inferior) are located in the dorsolateral tegmentum in the lower pons and the upper medulla. The *dorsal and ventral cochlear nuclei* are located on the external aspect of the inferior cerebellar peduncle in the upper medulla.

The *visceral arch*, or the *branchiomeric cranial* nerves, emerge from the brainstem on its lateral aspect; the trigeminal nerve leaves in the pons; and the facial, glossopharyngeal, vagus, and spinal accessory (cranial portion) nerves leave in a line (posterior lateral) along the entire medulla just dorsal to the olive. The *nuclei of the trigeminal nerve* form a column extending throughout the entire brainstem and upper two cervical levels of the spinal cord. The *mesencephalic nucleus of the fifth nerve*, located in the lateral periaqueductal gray of the midbrain, is an elongated nucleus receiving proprioceptive impulses from the head. The *motor nucleus of the fifth nerve* is located in the lateral tegmentum of the midpons just medial to the principal sensory nucleus of the fifth nerve. The trigeminal nerve sends descending fibers in the lateral tegmentum as the spinal tract of the fifth nerve as far down as the second cervical spinal cord level. These fibers terminate along its entire course in the adjacent *spinal nucleus of the fifth nerve.* The caudal third of the nucleus is concerned with pain, temperature, and light touch. The oral two-thirds of the nucleus, which projects to the reticular formation, probably supplies unspecific trigeminal input to the reticular system.

Three cranial nerve nuclei are associated with the facial nerve. The *motor nucleus of the facial nerve,* located in the midtegmentum in the low pons, projects its fibers dorsomedially to the medial aspect of the nucleus of the abducent nerve, where they hook around the nucleus as the genu of the facial nerve and continue ventrolaterally through the tegmentum to their exit from the brainstem at the lateral pontomedullary junction (Figs. 7-7, A-5, A-6, A-19, A-20). Parasympathetic fibers from the *superior salivatory nucleus* in the lateral tegmentum join the facial nerve. The visceral afferent fibers, including those of taste, enter the fasciculus and *nucleus solitarius* (rostral half of the nucleus in the middorsal tegmentum of the medulla). The fasciculus solitarius is a bundle of descending fibers from cranial nerves VII, IX, and X (the cell bodies are in the sensory ganglia of these nerves).

The cranial nerve nuclei associated with the glossopharyngeal nerve, vagus nerve, and the cranial part of the accessory nerve are the nucleus solitarius, dorsal nucleus of the vagus nerve, and inferior salivatory nucleus (all located in the medullary dorsal tegmentum), the spinal nucleus of the fifth nerve (located in the lateral tegmentum), and the nucleus ambiguus (located in the medullary central tegmentum). The taste and general visceral sensory fibers in these nerves enter and descend in the fasciculus solitarius before terminating in the *nucleus solitarius.* The *spinal nucleus of the fifth nerve* receives the few general somatic sensory fibers from the facial nerve, glossopharyngeal nerve, and vagus nerve. The *inferior salivatory nucleus* supplies the parasympathetic fibers to the glossopharyngeal nerve, and the dorsal vagal nucleus supplies the parasympathetic fibers to the vagus and spinal accessory nerve. The *nucleus ambiguus* supplies the motor innervation of the glossopharyngeal and vagus nerves to the pharyngeal (swallowing), palatal, and laryngeal muscles (vocal cords).

Functional considerations and lesions in the brainstem

In general, the tracts passing through and within the brainstem are oriented in a longitudinal plane parallel to the long axis of the brainstem (e.g., spinal trigeminal tract, medial lemniscus, and pyramidal tract). The cranial nerves course through a coronal plane perpendicular to the long axis (e.g., facial nerve). These orientations should be kept in mind in the following account.

Lesions of the following pathways within the brainstem result in signs on the opposite side of the body and back of the head because they are crossed tracts: spinothalamic (decussates in the spinal cord), medial lemniscus (decussates in the low medulla), and corticospinal (decussates in the low medulla). In their courses through the brainstem, *1* the spinothalamic tract is located in the lateral tegmentum, *2* the medial lemniscus shifts as it ascends from its location in the anteromedial tegmentum in the medulla to the posterolateral tegmentum in the midbrain before terminating in the ventral posterior lateral thalamic nucleus, and *3* the corticospinal tract descends through the anterior and anteromedial aspects of the basilar part of the brainstem.

A unilateral lesion of the auditory pathway (lateral lemniscus and brachium of the inferior colliculus) results in the diminution of hearing in both ears, but is more marked in the opposite ear (each auditory pathway conveys influences from both ears, but mainly from the contralateral ear). A lesion of the anterior trigeminothalamic tract (i.e., a lesion above the level where the fibers cross in the medulla) is accompanied by loss of pain and temperature sense on the forehead, face, nasal cavity, and oral cavity on the opposite side.

Because the cranial nerves are oriented at right angles to the long axis of the brainstem, they can be helpful in localizing the level of a lesion. Nerves III (midbrain), VI (pons-medulla junction), and XII (medulla) emerge on the anterior aspect of the brainstem in close proximity to the massive corticospinal tract. Injury to one of these nerves and the corticospinal tract results in an *alternating hemiplegia*. A lesion to the nerve is accompanied by a lower motor neuron paralysis on the same side, and a lesion to the corticospinal tract by an upper motor neuron paralysis on the opposite side of the body (i.e., a lesion of the corticospinal tract rostral to the level of its decussation).

The branchiomeric nerves (cranial nerves V, VII, IX, X, and XI) pass close to the spinothalamic tract before emerging on the lateral side of the brainstem. Injury to one of these nerves and the spinothalamic tract results in *1* sensory loss of the region and a lower motor neuron paralysis of the muscles innervated by that nerve, and *2* loss of pain and temperature sense on the opposite side of the body and back of the head due to the interruption of the decussated fibers of the spinothalamic tract.

Cranial nerves III, IV, VI are exquisitely integrated to ensure that the eyes move together; these are called conjugate or coordinated movements. The isolated action of any extraocular muscle does not normally occur.

Blood supply The sequence of vertebral arteries, basilar artery, and posterior cerebral arteries forms the main trunk system supplying arterial blood to the medulla, pons, midbrain, cerebellum, and posterior medial cerebrum (Fig. 1-25). The paired vertebral arteries ascend along the anterolateral aspect of the medulla and join at the pons-medulla junction to form the medial basilar artery, which ascends and then divides in the midbrain region into the paired posterior cerebral arteries. Branches of these arteries supply the brainstem in patterns which may be conceptually summarized as follows: in a general way, the paramedian branches are distributed to a medial zone on either side of the midsagittal plane, the short circumferential branches to an anterolateral zone, and the long circumferential branches to a posterolateral zone and to the cerebellum (Fig. 8-21).

Medial zone of the medulla (Fig. 8-22*A*). The occlusion of an anterior spinal artery and its paramedian branches to the medial zone of the medulla may be the cause of a lesion which involves the hypoglossal nerve (N. XII), corticospinal tract of the pyramid, and medial lemniscus. This *alternating hemiplegia* combines a lower motor neuron paralysis of the tongue on the ipsilateral side (N. XII) with an upper motor neuron paralysis and a loss of discriminatory general senses (medial lemniscus) on the contralateral side of the body. During the first few weeks after the lesion, the ipsilateral half of the tongue will fasciculate (denervation sensitivity); later the muscles atrophy, and that side of the tongue appears wrinkled. When protruded, the tongue deviates to the paralyzed side, primarily because of the unopposed action of the contralateral genioglossus muscle. The contralateral side of the body exhibits the signs of an upper motor neuron paralysis (corticospinal tract) and loss of position, muscle, and joint sense, impaired tactile discrimination, and loss of vibratory sense (medial lemniscus), because the lesion interrupts these tracts above the level of their decussation.

Posterolateral medulla (Fig. 8-22*B*) The occlusion of the posterior inferior cerebellar artery (a long circumferential artery) may be the cause of this lesion, which results in the syndrome of the posterior inferior cerebellar artery (lateral medullary syndrome). Damage to the following structures will produce the symptoms: spinothalamic tract, spinal trigeminal tract and nucleus, fibers and possibly nuclei associated with the glossopharyngeal, vagal, and spinal portions of accessory nerves (including the nucleus ambiguus, dorsal vagal nucleus, and fasciculus and nucleus solitarius), part of the reticular formation, portions of the vestibular nuclei, and some fibers of the inferior cerebellar peduncle. The symptoms include

1 Loss of pain (*analgesia*) and temperature sense (*thermoanesthesia*) on the opposite side of the body including the back of the head (crossed spinothalamic tract)

2 Loss of pain and temperature sense on the same side of the face and nasal and oral cavities in all three trigeminal divisions (uncrossed spinal trigeminal tract and nucleus)

3 Difficulty in swallowing (*dysphagia*) and a voice that is hoarse and weak (damage of nucleus ambiguus produces a lower motor neuron paralysis of the ipsilateral

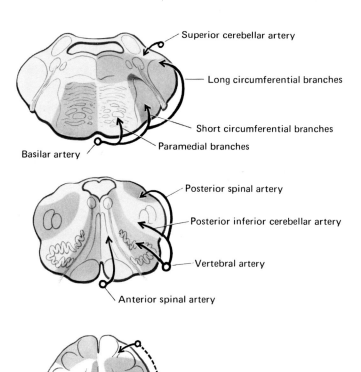

Superior cerebellar artery

Long circumferential branches

Short circumferential branches

Paramedial branches

Basilar artery

Posterior spinal artery

Posterior inferior cerebellar artery

Vertebral artery

Anterior spinal artery

FIGURE 8-21
The patterns of arterial supply of the branches of the basilar artery within the pons (*upper*), mid-medulla (*middle*), and caudal medulla (*lower figure*).

pharyngeal and laryngeal muscles; the normal palatal muscles will deviate the uvula to the normal side)

4 Loss of gag reflex on the ipsilateral side and absence of sensation on the ipsilateral side of the fauces (glossopharyngeal nerve). A transient tachycardia (increase in heartbeat) may result from sudden withdrawal of some parasympathetic innervation; compensatory mechanisms, including influences from the contralateral vagus nerve, will restore the normal heartbeat. The absence of visceral afferent stimulation from some visceral receptors (e.g., carotid body and carotid sinus) to the solitary nucleus is compensated for by the input from similar receptors to the normal contralateral side. The interruption of fibers passing through the inferior cerebellar peduncle results in some signs of cerebellar malfunction on the ipsilateral side of the body—including hypotonia, asynergia, and poorly coordinated vol-

untary movements (Chap. 9). Irritation of the vestibular nuclei may be expressed by nystagmus or a deviation of the eyes to the ipsilateral side. Horner's syndrome on the same side may occur if many descending fibers of the autonomic nervous system to the thoracic sympathetic outflow are damaged. The tactile and discriminative general senses from the face are normal because the principal sensory nucleus of N. V and its ascending pathways are above the lesion.

Region of the cerebellopontine angle (cerebellopontine angle syndrome) The slowly growing acoustic neuroma, which originates from neurolemmal cells of the vestibular nerve in the vicinity of the internal auditory foramen, may extend into the junctional region of the cerebellum, pons, and medulla near the emergence of cranial nerves VII and VIII, known as the *cerebellopon-*

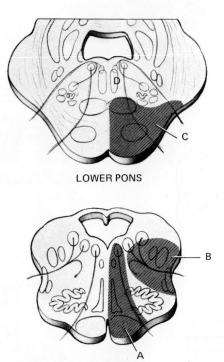

LOWER PONS

MEDULLA

FIGURE 8-22
Sites of lesions in the lower brainstem, as described in the text.

In the medulla, the lesions are located in the medial zone (*A*) and in the posterolateral zone (*B*). In the lower pons, the lesions are located in the medial and basal portion (*C*) and in the medial longitudinal fasciculus (*D*).

tine angle. In the early stages, symptoms are referable to the eighth cranial nerve; they include tinnitus followed by progressive deafness on the lesion side, and abnormal labyrinthine responses such as tilting and rotation of the head with the chin pointing to the lesion side. Later the tumor exerts pressure upon the brainstem and damages the fibers of the inferior and middle cerebellar peduncles, spinothalamic tract, spinal trigeminal tract, and facial nerve.

The cerebellar signs which result from the involvement of the cerebellar peduncles include coarse intention tremor, dysmetria, moderate ataxic gait, adiadochokinesis, and others on the lesion side (Chap. 9). The loss of pain and temperature sense on the ipsilateral side of the face, oral cavity, and nasal cavity, and on the contralateral side of the body are a consequence of damage to the spinal trigeminal tract and the spinothalamic tract, respectively. Injury to the facial nerve may result in a lower motor paralysis of the muscles of facial expression (Bell's palsy), hyperacusis, and loss of taste on the anterior two-thirds of the tongue ipsilaterally (Chap. 7).

Medial and basal portion of the caudal pons (Fig. 8-22*C*) The occlusion of paramedian and short circumferential branches of the basilar artery may result in damage to the following structures within the confines of the lesion: abducent nerve (N. VI), facial nerve (N. VII), pyramidal tract, medial lemniscus, and medial longitudinal fasciculus. The interruption of the fibers of N. VI (lower motor neurons) and the pyramidal tract (upper motor neurons) results in an *alternating abducent hemiplegia.* The transection of N. VI produces a horizontal diplopia (double vision) because of the paralysis of the lateral rectus muscle (an abductor), as a consequence of which the image of an object falls upon noncorresponding portions of the two retinas and is seen as two objects. The diplopia is maximal when the patient attempts to gaze to the lesion side. When the ipsilateral lateral rectus muscle, which is innervated by N. VI, is paralyzed, the subject's ability to abduct the eye (i.e., direct the pupil toward the temple) is impaired. The signs occurring from damage to the corticospinal fibers, seventh nerve, and medial lemniscus are discussed above, and the medial longitudinal fasciculus is discussed below.

Medial longitudinal fasciculus (Fig. 8-22*D*) A unilateral lesion of the medial longitudinal fasciculus (MLF) rostral to the nucleus of the abducent nerve results in a disturbance of conjugate horizontal eye movements (abduction and adduction) called internuclear ophthalmoplegia. This lateral-gaze paralysis is characterized by an impaired adduction of the ipsilateral eye and nystagmus of the abducting contralateral eye on gaze to the side opposite the lesion. It is due to the damage of the fibers which interconnect and integrate, during lateral gaze, the contraction of the contralateral lateral rectus muscle (abductor innervated by N. VI) and the ipsilateral medial rectus muscle (adductor innervated by N. III). The weakness of the ipsilateral medial rectus muscle is due to the absence of influences derived from the ascending fibers in the MLF. These fibers cross at the level of the abducent nucleus. The horizontal diplopia is most marked during maximal lateral gaze to the contralateral side, because the paralyzed ipsilateral medial rectus muscle is unable to adduct the eye. Lateral gaze to the side of the lesion is essentially conjugate, because the pathways integrating the contractions of the ipsilateral lateral rectus muscle and the contralateral medial rectus muscle are intact.

Lateral half of the midpons The structures within the region of the lesion (Fig. 8-23A) include the trigeminal nerve, spinothalamic tract, lateral lemniscus, and middle cerebellar peduncle. Damage to the trigeminal nerve (N. V) results in *1* the absence of all general senses (anesthesia) on the ipsilateral side of the face, forehead, nasal cavity, and oral cavity, including absence of corneal sensation and corneal reflex; and *2* a lower motor neuron paralysis of the muscles of mastication, with the chin deviating to the lesion side on opening of the mouth. If the lesion is extensive enough to include the corticospinal tract, the combination of the pyramidal tract and N. V produces an *alternating trigeminal hemiplegia.* The lesion of the lateral lemniscus may be followed by a diminution of audition, which is more marked on the opposite side (the lateral lemniscus is composed of fibers conveying some auditory influences from the same side but mainly from the opposite side). Interruption of pontocerebellar fibers may be expressed with some cerebellar signs on the same side (Chap. 9) including hypotonia, coarse intention tremor, and tendency to fall to the side of the lesion.

Basal region of the midbrain The occlusion of paramedian branches and short circumferential branches of the basilar and posterior cerebral arteries may produce a *Weber's syndrome* (Fig. 8-23B), which is a consequence of damage to the oculomotor nerve (N. III), the corticospinal tract, and a variable number of corticobulbar and corticoreticular fibers. The interruption of all the fibers in the oculomotor nerve results in

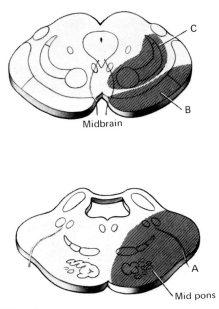

FIGURE 8-23
Sites of lesions in the pons and midbrain, as described in the text.

In the midpons, the lesion is located laterally (*A*). In the superior collicular level of the midbrain, the lesions are located in the basal region (*B*) and in the midbrain tegmentum (*C*).

signs restricted to the ipsilateral eye, including drooping of the eyelid (ptosis, or inability to raise the eyelid because of paralysis of the levator palpebral muscle), diplopia, external strabismus (squint) due to unopposed contraction of the lateral rectus muscle, inability to elevate, depress, or adduct the eye, and a fully dilated pupil (the normally acting sympathetic influences are unopposed because of absence of the parasympathetic influences conveyed by the damaged parasympathetic fibers of N. III). The consensual light reflex to the contralateral eye is normal (Chap. 12). An alternating hemiplegia is a consequence of the lower motor neuron paralysis of the oculomotor nerve and the upper motor neuron paralysis of the contralateral side of the body from the damage to the corticospinal tract.

The unilateral interruption of the corticobulbar and corticoreticular (indirect corticobulbar) fibers results in only minimal, if any, effects upon the muscles innervated by the cranial nerves except for the contralateral muscles of facial expression of the lower part of the face. In general, the motor nuclei of the cranial nerves (except for the neurons of the facial nucleus innervating the lower part of the face) receive upper motor neuron influences from both halves of the cerebrum. Hence supranuclear unilateral lesions interrupting the upper motor neurons to these motor nuclei do not produce upper motor neuron paralysis of the muscles innervated by these nerves, except for the weakness of the contralateral muscles of facial expression of the lower part of the face. In some individuals, the interruption of the upper motor neurons results in a tongue and jaw which deviate to the side contralateral to the lesion; the explanation for this observation is that these patients have few, if any, upper motor neurons originating in the ipsilateral cerebral cortex.

The bilateral, diffuse involvement of the corticobulbar and corticoreticular fibers results in a *pseudobulbar palsy.* In this syndrome there is a bilateral paralysis or weakness without atrophy of many muscles innervated by cranial nerves. The muscle groups affected control chewing, swallowing, speaking, and breathing. Unrestrained crying and laughing occur in many subjects with pseudobulbar palsy. These emotional outbursts may be related to release from influences derived from the cerebral cortex and subcortical centers in the telencephalon and diencephalon.

Upper midbrain tegmentum A unilateral lesion in the midbrain tegmentum (Fig. 8-23*C*) limited to the region including the fibers of the oculomotor nerve, red nucleus, superior cerebellar peduncle, medial lemniscus, and spinothalamic tract results in *Benedikt syndrome.* The damage to the red nucleus and the fibers of the superior cerebellar peduncle (decussated dentatorubral and dentatothalamic fibers) results in such signs of cerebellar damage as coarse intention tremor, adiadochokinesis, cerebellar ataxia, and hypo-

tonia on the contralateral side of the body (Chap. 9). Experimental evidence indicates that no signs in this syndrome are definitely attributable to a lesion of the red nucleus. The injury to the third cranial nerve results in a lower motor neuron paralysis of the ipsilateral extraocular muscles and in a dilated pupil (mydriasis) from absence of parasympathetic influences (see "Basal Region of the Midbrain," above). The interruption of the crossed spinothalamic tract, anterior trigeminothalamic tract, and medial lemniscus results in the loss of sense of pain, temperature, light touch, vibratory sense, pressure touch, and other discriminatory senses on the opposite side of the body and head. The retention of touch and other discriminatory senses on the contralateral side of the head may occur when the uncrossed posterior trigeminothalamic tract is intact.

Cranial nerves of brainstem A *lesion of one oculomotor nerve* results in outward deviation of the ipsilateral eye, drooping of the upper eyelid (ptosis), and a dilated pupil of the eye (unopposed action of sympathetic innervation because of lack of parasympathetic innervation). *Lesion of one trochlear nerve* results in impaired ability to turn the eye downward; *lesion of one abducent nerve* results in an inwardly turned eye (internal strabismus), because of pull of the medial rectus muscle unopposed by the paralyzed lateral rectus muscle. Double vision is a consequence of paralyzed eye muscles because the visual images on the two eyes are not properly fused. The patient turns and tilts his head to one side to minimize and prevent the diplopia (thereby fusing the images by causing the visual axes of the eyes to become parallel to each other). A *lesion of one hypoglossal nerve* results in an ipsilateral paralysis of the tongue muscles; because the tongue is pulled forward when protruded, it will deviate to the paralyzed side when voluntarily protruded (the paralyzed side acts as a pivot).

Lesions of the corticospinal tract at the levels where the oculomotor nerve (midbrain level) or the abducent nerve (pontomedullary junction) or the hypoglossal nerve (medulla) emerges on the ventral aspect of the brainstem may be combined with the interruption of one of these cranial nerves. This combination of the interruption of an uncrossed cranial nerve and the corticospinal tract (and a portion of tegmentum to include other motor tracts) may result in an *alternating hemiplegia*—an ipsilateral lower motor paralysis of the muscles innervated by the cranial nerve and the contralateral upper motor neuron paralysis of the muscles on the opposite side of the body.

A *lesion of the trigeminal nerve* results in the complete loss of the general senses of pain, temperature, touch, and proprioception on the ipsilateral side of the head and in the lower motor neuron paralysis of the muscles of mastication (when voluntarily protruded, the jaw deviates to the paralyzed side). The *functional interruption of the facial nerve* results in the total paralysis of the ipsilateral muscles of facial expression and in the loss of taste on one side of the anterior two-thirds of the tongue. This paralysis (*Bell's palsy*) is expressed as the ipsilateral sagging of the face, inability to close the eyelid (the patient may wear an eyemask to prevent drying out of the cornea), and drooping of the side of the mouth (saliva may drip from the corner of the mouth). Many patients with Bell's palsy recover after several months. The face is actually drawn to the normal side by the contraction or tone of unaffected muscles of facial expression.

Impairment of the nucleus ambiguus and its efferent fibers in the glossopharyngeal and vagus nerves results in difficulty in swallowing (dysphagia) and in forming vocal sounds (dysphonia). A nasal quality of sounds (dysarthria) and hoarseness may follow.

Bibliography

Andén, N. E., A. Dahlström, K. Fuxe, K. Larsson, L. Olson, and U. Ungerstedt: Ascending monoamine neurons to the telencephalon and diencephalon. Acta Physiol. Scand., 67:313–326, 1966.

Anderson, F. D., and C. M. Berry: Degeneration studies of long ascending fiber systems in the cat brain stem. J. Comp. Neurol., 111:195–229, 1959.

Beidler, L. M. (ed.): Taste, in *Handbook of Sensory Physiology*, vol. IV, sec. 2, pp. 1–410. Springer-Verlag, Berlin and New York, 1971.

Brodal, A.: *The Reticular Formation of the Brain Stem: Anatomical Aspects and Functional Correlations*. Charles C Thomas, Publisher, Springfield, Ill., 1957.

Hassler, O.: Arterial pattern of the human brain stem. Neurology, 17:368–375, 1967.

Jasper, H. H., and L. O. Proctor (eds.): *Reticular Formation of the Brain*. Little, Brown and Company, Boston, 1958.

Kruger, L.: A critical review of theories concerning the organization of the sensory trigeminal nuclear complex of the brain stem, in R. Dubner and Y. Kawamura (eds.), *Oral-Facial Sensory and Motor Mechanisms*, pp. 135–158. Appleton-Century-Crofts, Inc., New York, 1971.

Massion, J.: The mammalian red nucleus. Physiol. Rev., 47:383–436, 1967.

Olszewski, J., and D. Baxter: *Cytoarchitecture of the Human Brain Stem*. S. Karger, Basel, 1954.

Ramón-Moliner, E., and W. J. H. Nauta: The isodendritic core of the brain stem. J. Comp. Neurol., 126:311–336, 1966.

Siggins, G. R., B. J. Hoffer, A. P. Oliver, and F. E. Bloom: Activation of a central noradrenergic projection to cerebellum. Nature, 233:481–483, 1971.

Taber, E.: The cytoarchitecture of the brain stem of the cat. I. Brain stem nuclei of cat. J. Comp. Neurol., 116:27–70, 1961.

Ungerstedt, U.: Stereotaxic mapping of the monoamine pathways in the rat brain. Acta Physiol. Scand., Suppl., 367:1–48, 1971.

CHAPTER 9
CEREBELLUM

The cerebellum has an essential role in the co-ordination of group muscle activities. It is not the initiator of motion but acts *1* as a monitor of on-going dynamics of stretch and tension within the muscular system, and *2* as the great modulator and control system of motor activities. The cerebellum plays no part in the appreciation of conscious sensations or in intelligence.

The cerebellum is integrated with the vestibular system in the maintenance of muscle tone and equilibrium, and with other motor systems in such phasic movements as locomotion. This suprasegmental structure functions primarily in smoothing out and synchronizing the delicate timing between the muscles of a group, and between groups of muscles, whether the activities are at the reflex, automatic, or conscious level. A patient with a cerebellar lesion is capable of carrying out the general outlines of movements, but each movement is usually executed with an inadequacy of the finer muscular coordination.

In common with neural structures that are derived from the embryonic alar plate, the cerebellum is basically a somatic afferent organ, often called the *head ganglion of proprioceptive and exteroceptive systems*. The cerebellum receives and processes unconscious afferent stimuli from general proprioceptive (primarily from receptors in muscles, joints, and tendons) and exteroceptive receptors in the body and from the vestibular, auditory, and visual systems. This information is then utilized by the motor systems. For example, the performance of skilled movements initiated by the cerebral cortex is dependent, in part, on the extensive interconnections of the cerebrum with the cerebellum.

Gross divisions of the cerebellum

Several general schemas of dividing the cerebellum are useful (Figs. 9-1, 9-2). The classic subdivisions of the cerebellum into numerous lobes and lobules is not described in this account, for they are based on descriptive criteria with little or no known special functional significance.

The cortex of the cerebellum is the thin layer of gray which covers it. Deep to the cortex is the medullary core of white matter, which consists of fibers projecting to and from the cerebellar cortex. Deep in the medullary core are four pairs of the deep cerebellar nuclei (Fig. A-5): fastigii, globosus, emboliformis, and dentatus (from medial to lateral). These nuclei consist of neurons that project the cerebellar output to other portions of the brain.

The cerebellum is connected to the brainstem by the three cerebellar peduncles or pillars: the inferior cerebellar (restiform body), the middle cerebellar (brachium pontis), and the superior cerebellar (brachium conjunctivum). The *inferior cerebellar peduncle* is the bridge between the medulla and the cerebellum, with fibers projecting both to and from the cerebellum. The *middle cerebellar peduncle* is the bridge between the pons and the cerebellum, with fibers projecting to the cerebellum. The *superior cerebellar peduncle* is the bridge between the midbrain and the cerebellum, with fibers largely projecting from the cerebellum toward the midbrain and the thalamus.

LONGITUDINAL SUBDIVISIONS

Classically, the cerebellum is divided into two large bilateral *cerebellar hemispheres* and the

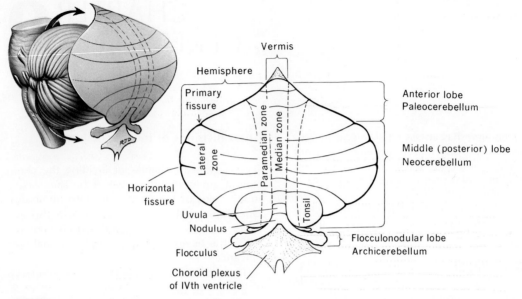

FIGURE 9-1
The surface of the cerebellum after it is un-
folded and laid out flat.

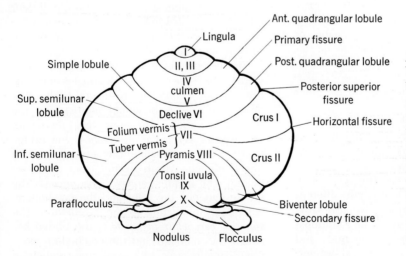

FIGURE 9-2
The fissures and lobules of
the cerebellum.

Regions of the vermis are designated by Roman numerals. In
this figure, the paleocerebellum
(anterior lobe) is located rostral
to the primary fissure, and the
archicerebellum (flocculonodular lobe) lies caudal to the posterolateral fissure. The neocerebellum is located between the
primary fissure and the posterolateral fissure.

narrow median *vermis*. This older longitudinal
schema may be modified into a modern version
(Fig. 9-2), based on the relation of the cerebellar
cortex and the deep cerebellar nuclei. The median zone includes the *vermal cortex (vermis)*
and the nucleus to which it projects, the nucleus
fastigii. Each intermediate zone includes the
paravermal (paramedial) cortex and the nuclei
to which it projects, the nucleus interpositus
(nucleus globosus and nucleus emboliformis).

Each *lateral (hemispheric) zone* includes the bulk of each cerebellar hemisphere and the nucleus to which it projects, the nucleus dentatus. The median zone has a role in the movements of the trunk and extensor muscle tone through the vestibular system. The paramedian (paravermal) zone has a role in ipsilateral movements through its influences on flexor muscle tone. The lateral or hemispheric zone has a functional role in muscle coordination, largely through connections with the nucleus ruber, thalamus, and cerebral cortex.

TRANSVERSE SUBDIVISIONS

The cerebellum may be divided into three transverse divisions: archicerebellum, paleocerebellum, and neocerebellum (Figs. 9-1, 9-2). These lobes, based partially on phylogenetic criteria, are not defined in precisely the same way by different investigators. The *archicerebellum* consists of the paired flocculi of the hemispheres and the unpaired nodulus of the vermis. This *flocculonodular lobe* is phylogenetically the oldest lobe of the cerebellum. It is actually a specialized portion of the somatic afferent column that is dominated by direct, indirect, and feedback connections with the vestibular system. It receives direct input via fibers from the vestibular nerve and the medial and inferior vestibular nuclei. The archicerebellum subserves a significant role in muscle tone, equilibrium, and posture through its influences of the trunk muscles.

The *paleocerebellum* consists of most of the vermis and of the superior (anterior) aspect of the cerebellar hemispheres in front of the primary fissure. This phylogenetically old lobe is primarily associated with the proprioceptive (spinocerebellar, cuneocerebellar, and rostral spinocerebellar tracts) and the exteroceptive input from the head and body, including some from the vestibular system. It has a significant role in the regulation of muscle tone.

The *neocerebellum* consists of the main bulk of the cerebellar hemispheres and part of the vermis. This phylogenetically new lobe (essentially a mammalian structure) is primarily associated with the neocortex of the cerebrum, pontine nuclei, and the principal inferior olivary nucleus of the medulla. Input is also derived from visual, auditory, and cutaneous senses. It has an essential role in the muscular coordination of phasic movements.

The cerebellar cortex

FOLIA

The cerebellar surface is corrugated into numerous parallel, long "gyri" called *folia* (Fig. 9-3). The folia are separated from one another by cerebellar fissures that are equivalent to the sulci of the cerebral cortex. Although the cerebellum is much smaller than the cerebrum, its total cortical surface area, because of the increased surface formed by the folia, is actually three-fourths that of the cerebral cortex. Only 15 percent of the cerebellar cortex is exposed to the outer surface, whereas 85 percent faces the sulcal surfaces between the folia. The branching of the white matter and the treelike appearance of the folia in sections of the cerebellum at right angles to the long axis of the folia suggested the name *arbor vitae.* All folia have the same histologic structure.

CYTOARCHITECTURE AND INTRINSIC CEREBELLAR CIRCUITS

The cerebellar cortex is organized in a precise geometrically ordered pattern. Its neuronal elements are oriented along axes resembling a Cartesian coordinate system; some neurons are arranged in planes perpendicular to the long axis of a folium (stellate cells, basket cells, and dendritic arborization of the Purkinje cells), while the granule cell and its axonal branches are oriented in a plane parallel to the long axis of a folium (Fig. 9-3). Knowledge of this geometric organization is fundamental to an understanding of the cerebellar circuits.

The cerebellar cortex is divided into three layers: the *inner or granular layer* in which are located the cell bodies of granule cells and the glomeruli; the thin *middle layer* composed of the cell bodies of the Purkinje cells; and the *outer or molecular layer* in which are located the stellate and basket cells. Deep in the cerebellum are the cerebellar nuclei: *fastigii, em-*

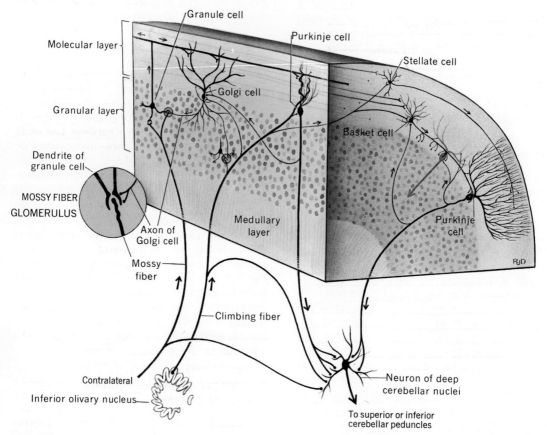

FIGURE 9-3
The neuronal organization within a cerebellar folium.

Right, transverse section through a folium; *left,* longitudinal section (long axis). The nerve processes of the stellate cells, basket cells, and Purkinje cells are oriented parallel to the transverse plane; the axonal branches of the granule cells are oriented parallel to the longitudinal plane. Note the mossy-fiber glomerulus (insert) and climbing-fiber glomerulus (*). The main circuits (thick lines) exerting excitatory influences on the Purkinje cells include *1* mossy fiber→granule cell→Purkinje cell; *2* climbing fiber→granule cell→ Purkinje cell; and *3* climbing fiber→Purkinje cell. The Golgi cells, stellate cells, and basket cells are interneurons integrated into circuits exerting inhibitory influences on the main circuits. The climbing-fiber glomerulus was described by Chan-Palay and Palay.

boliform, globose, and dentate. The *emboliform and globose nuclei* are collectively known as the *nucleus interpositus.* The cerebellum is constructed of *1* two types of input axons: climbing fibers and mossy fibers; *2* five types of intrinsic neurons: granule cells, stellate cells, basket cells, Golgi type II cells, and Purkinje cells; and *3* one type of output neuron: cells of the cerebellar nuclei. Some Purkinje cells are output neurons projecting to the lateral vestibular nucleus.

The number of neurons of the cerebellar cortex is enormous. In fact more neurons are present in the cerebellar cortex than in the cerebral cortex. In man, there are as many as 100 billion granule cells, 200 million stellate and basket cells, and 30 million Purkinje cells. The fibers within the cerebellar cortex are unmyelinated.

Input fibers The *climbing fibers* originate from cells of the inferior olivary complex (olivocerebellar fibers) and other brainstem nuclei. The main unmyelinated branches of these fibers "climb" and coil around the dendrites of a Purkinje cell; they make axodendritic synapses with the smooth (nonspinous) portions of the dendrites. Collateral branches of the climbing fibers synapse with all other neuronal cell types of the cerebellum, including neurons of the deep cerebellar nuclei, granule cells, Golgi cells, stellate cells, and basket cells.

The *mossy fibers* originate from many nuclei of the brainstem and spinal cord; they course to the cerebellum via spinocerebellar, cuneocerebellar, vestibulocerebellar, and pontocerebellar tracts and other small tracts. Each of the mossy fibers branches many times before terminating in hundreds (or even thousands) of mossy-fiber rosettes. Each *rosette* is the central element of a *cerebellar glomerulus* (cerebellar island). Each *glomerulus* is composed of *1* one mossy-fiber rosette, *2* dendritic terminals of many granule cells, and *3* axonic terminals of several Golgi cells. The basic functional units of a glomerulus (Fig. 9-3) are considered to be *1* two presynaptic elements—the mossy-fiber rosette and several axonic terminals of Golgi cells—and *2* one postsynaptic element—dendrites of many granule cells. Each glomerulus is ensheathed by the lamella of a glial cell. Another type of glomerulus receives its input from a climbing fiber instead of a mossy fiber (Chan-Palay and Palay).

INTRINSIC NEURONS

Each *granule cell* has from four to five short dendrites; each dendrite terminates in a different glomerulus. Thus each granule cell receives input from several mossy fibers (an average of four). The unmyelinated axon of each granule cell extends from a cell body, located in the granular layer, into the molecular layer, where it bifurcates as a T into two branches, which extend for about 2 mm in opposite directions *parallel to the long axis of a folium;* these so-

called parallel fibers have synaptic connections with the spines of the Purkinje cell dendrites and the dendrites of the stellate, basket, and Golgi cells. The synapses between the parallel fibers and the dendrites of these neurons are called *"cross-over" synapses.* As many as 300,000 parallel fibers pass through the dendritic tree of each Purkinje cell, making about 60,000 to 120,000 synapses with each Purkinje cell (each parallel fiber does not synapse with each Purkinje cell it traverses). Each parallel fiber passes through the planes of about 500 Purkinje cells.

The *stellate (outer stellate) cells* and the *basket (inner stellate) cells* are interneurons, located within the molecular layer; their dendritic and axonal processes are oriented in a plane perpendicular to the long axis of a folium. These neurons receive input from the climbing and parallel fibers and collaterals of Purkinje cells; they project their output to the Purkinje cells. The axons of the stellate cells terminate upon the dendrites (axodendritic synapses) of a number of Purkinje cells. The axons of a basket cell terminate in arborizations around the cell bodies (axosomatic synapses) of about 10 Purkinje cells and as terminal collaterals on the dendrites of Purkinje cells (axodendritic synapses). Each Purkinje cell receives input from many stellate and basket cells.

Each *Golgi cell* has a cell body in the granular layer and a dendritic tree which arborizes in all planes through the granular and molecular layers. A Golgi cell receives input from the parallel, climbing, and Purkinje cells and conveys output to thousands of glomeruli.

The *Purkinje cells* are the sole output neurons of the cerebellar cortex. Their espalier-like dendritic trees arborize within the molecular layer *in a plane perpendicular to the long axis of a folium.* Each Purkinje cell receives input from about 80,000 granule cells and from stellate, basket, and other Purkinje cells. The main axon of each cell makes terminal synaptic connections with the neurons of the deep cerebellar nuclei or of the lateral vestibular nucleus. Each has recurrent axonal collateral branches which synapse with stellate, basket, Golgi, and other Purkinje cells.

OUTPUT NEURONS

The output cells of the cerebellum are located in the fastigial, emboliform, globose, and dentate nuclei. They receive input from climbing and mossy fibers and axons of the Purkinje cells. Their axons course to the brainstem and thalamus via the superior cerebellar peduncle and juxtarestiform body. These axons do not have collaterals which project to the neurons of the cerebellar cortex.

INTRINSIC CIRCUITRY (Fig. 9-3)

Although the input fibers convey excitatory influences to the cerebellum, the *entire output of the cerebellar cortex is inhibitory*. Of the five neurons with cell bodies in the cerebellar cortex, four exert inhibitory influences—they act to reduce the excitability of the neurons on which their axons synapse. These *inhibitory neurons* include the stellate, basket, Golgi, and Purkinje cells. The excitatory cortical neuron is the granule cell. The role of the inhibitory intracortical neurons—Golgi, stellate, and basket cells—is to regulate and focus (a process called *sharpening of the focus* or *focusing effect*) the excitatory influences conveyed by the input fibers upon the Purkinje cells. The entire output of the cerebellar cortex is inhibitory because the inhibitory Purkinje cells are the sole output neurons of the cerebellar cortex. This should not be equated with the final output of the cerebellum, which is conveyed to the rest of the brain by the excitatory neurons of the deep cerebellar nuclei.

The *climbing fibers* exert monosynaptic excitatory influences upon the Purkinje cells. The resulting excitation is so powerful that it is difficult for the influences from the stellate and basket cells to inhibit the Purkinje cells completely from exerting some inhibitory influences upon the output neurons of the deep cerebellar nuclei. These *output neurons of the deep cerebellar nuclei normally convey excitatory influences* from the cerebellum; the degree of this excitatory activity can be reduced by the inhibitory influences from the Purkinje cells. The output neurons of the deep cerebellar nuclei generate their excitatory activity *1* by excitatory influences received from the collaterals of climbing and mossy fibers, and *2* by a pacemaker mechanism which generates action potentials "spontaneously" without extrinsic excitatory sources. In effect, the degree of the frequency of the output of action potentials to the rest of the brain is modulated by the inhibitory activity of the Purkinje cells upon the deep cerebellar nuclei.

The inhibitory activity of the Purkinje cells is regulated and focused by the inhibitory and excitatory inputs received following the activity of the other neuronal circuits within the cerebellum. These will be outlined. The excitatory climbing fibers stimulate the inhibitory stellate and basket cells to exert inhibitory influences upon the Purkinje cells. This inhibition from the stellate and basket cells partially suppresses the excitatory activity resulting from the facilitatory influences exerted by the climbing fibers on the Purkinje cells. The mossy fibers, through their rosettes within the glomeruli, excite the granule cells to exert facilitatory influences via the parallel fibers upon the stellate, basket, Purkinje, and Golgi cells. In effect, granule cells convey *1* excitatory influences directly to the Purkinje cells through the *"cross-over" synapses*, and *2* inhibitory influences indirectly to the Purkinje cells by facilitating the inhibitory stellate and basket cells. The latter circuit of the mossy fibers to granule cells to stellate and basket cells to Purkinje cells is a *feed-forward (or on-going) inhibitory control system*.

The excitatory influences conveyed by the granule cells can be modulated by a *negative feedback control circuit* which helps to sharpen the focus by conveying inhibitory influences upon the granule cell dendrites within the glomeruli. This circuit is composed of granule cell to Golgi cell to granule cell dendrite in a glomerulus; the granule cell facilitates the Golgi cells to convey inhibitory influences (via an inhibitory presynaptic element of the glomerulus) to the granule cells. The Golgi and granule cells can also be facilitated by collateral branches from the climbing fibers. Additional inhibitory influences can be exerted upon these cortical neurons by collaterals of the Purkinje cell axon, which synapse with the stellate, basket, Golgi, and other Purkinje cells. Some inhibitory influences are conveyed from the locus ceruleus

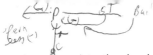

(noradrenergic neurons) to the dendrites of the Purkinje cells (Chap. 8).

The intracerebellar circuits do not initiate or stop the operation of the system. Rather they act by altering the level of operation of the cerebellum.

The cerebellar peduncles and pathways

CEREBELLAR AFFERENT CONNECTIONS

There are approximately three times as many cerebellar afferent fibers as cerebellar efferent fibers. Each of the cerebellar peduncles (Fig. 1-7) contains afferent fibers projecting to the cerebellar cortex (Figs. 9-4 through 9-7).

The *inferior cerebellar peduncle* (restiform body) conveys "unconscious" exteroceptive and proprioceptive information to the cerebellum from the spinal cord, medulla, and vestibular system. The *posterior spinocerebellar tract* projects ipsilaterally in the paleocerebellum (lobules I to IV) and the caudal vermis. The *cuneocerebellar fibers* from the lateral cuneate nucleus terminate in lobule V of the ipsilateral vermis. The *lateral reticular nucleus* receives input from the spinoreticular, spinothalamic, and rubrobulbar (red nucleus) fibers and projects its output to the neocerebellum. This nucleus is somatotopically organized, with the rostral and caudal parts receiving input from the upper and lower extremities, respectively. The *paramedian reticular nuclei of the medulla* are integrated in a cerebello-brainstem reticular-cerebellar feedback circuit. The *accessory inferior olivary nuclei (paleo-olive)* receive input from the spinal cord, nucleus ruber, and periaqueductal gray of the midbrain; they relay their output to the vermis. In man, these nuclei may not receive any direct spinal input. The *principal olivary nucleus (neo-olive)* receives its input from frontal, parietal, temporal, and occipital cortex of both sides, red nucleus, periaqueductal gray matter, and cerebellum; in turn, the medial part of this nucleus projects to the vermis, whereas the main bulk of the neo-olive projects to the neocerebellum. In addition to terminating in all parts of the cerebellar cortex, olivocerebellar fibers project to the deep cerebellar nuclei. It is possible that this nucleus is not the major source of climbing fibers.

The input from the vestibular system to the cerebellum is conveyed via the *juxtarestiform body of the inferior cerebellar peduncle.* Some direct (first-order) vestibulocerebellar fibers are distributed to the ipsilateral archicerebellum (nodulus, uvula, and flocculus). Secondary vestibular fibers from the medial and inferior vestibular nuclei are distributed bilaterally, but mainly ipsilaterally, to the nodulus, uvula, and flocculus and, additionally, to the fastigial nuclei.

The *middle cerebellar peduncle* (brachium pontis) conveys information primarily from the pons. The pontocerebellar tract projects fibers from the pontine nuclei primarily to the contralateral neocerebellum (with some to the contralateral paleocerebellum). A few projections are also conveyed from the pontine nuclei to the ipsilateral neocerebellum. Fibers from the reticulotegmental nucleus pass through the middle cerebellar peduncle on their way to most of the vermis.

The *superior cerebellar peduncle* (brachium conjunctivum) has only a few afferent fibers. The anterior spinocerebellar tract projects from the spinal cord to the contralateral paleocerebellum (lobules I to IX). A tectocerebellar tract is presumed to project from the midbrain tectum to the ipsilateral neocerebellum; apparently it represents input from the auditory system (inferior colliculus) and from the optic system (superior colliculus) to the audiovisual area (Fig. 9-8). Trigeminocerebellar fibers to the neocerebellum convey general afferent stimuli from the head. Noradrenergic fibers from the locus ceruleus pass via the superior cerebellar peduncle and white matter before terminating in the cerebellar cortex.

CEREBELLAR EFFERENT CONNECTIONS

No direct cerebellospinal pathways exist. The influences from the cerebellum on motor activity are mediated through indirect pathways. The efferent pathways of the inferior cerebellar peduncle are associated primarily with the vestibular system (archicerebellum and the nuclei fastigii); those of the superior cerebellar peduncle,

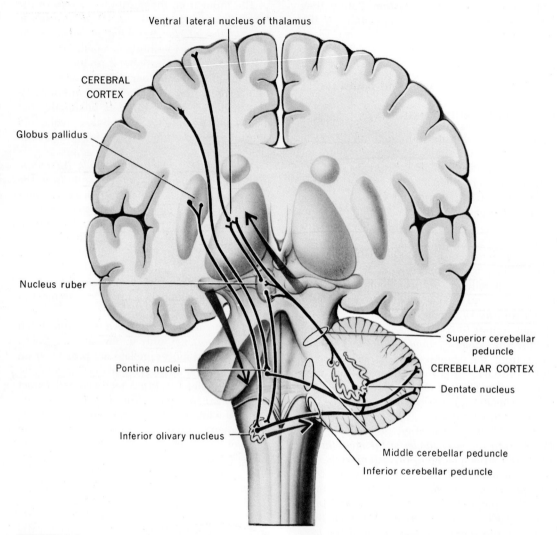

FIGURE 9-4
Neocerebellar connections with the cerebrum and some brainstem nuclei.

A feedback loop from the cerebrum to cerebellum to cerebrum is indicated in the following sequence: cerebral cortex→pontine nuclei→neocerebellar cortex→deep cerebellar nuclei→nucleus ruber→ventral lateral thalamic nucleus→cerebral cortex. Another loop is the sequence of cerebellar cortex→deep cerebellar nuclei→nucleus ruber→inferior olivary nucleus →neocerebellar cortex.

primarily with the neocerebellum and paleocerebellum (dentate, emboliform, and globose nuclei). Efferent fibers are not present in the middle cerebellar peduncle.

The cerebellar cortex projects its influences (all inhibitory) via Purkinje cell axons to the deep cerebellar nuclei and to the lateral vestibular nucleus. The *vermal cortex* projects directly to the fastigial nuclei and lateral vestibular nuclei. The *paravermal cortex* projects primarily to the interposed nuclei (globose and emboli-

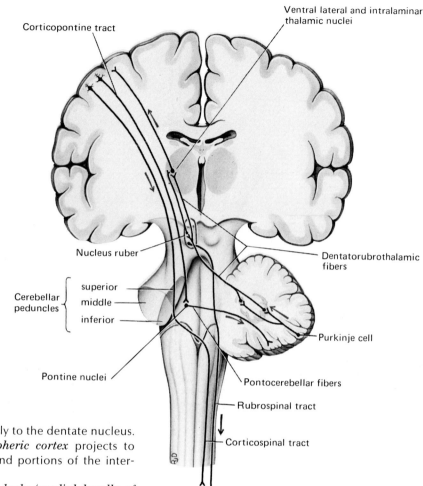

Corticopontine tract

Ventral lateral and intralaminar thalamic nuclei

Nucleus ruber

Dentatorubrothalamic fibers

Cerebellar peduncles
- superior
- middle
- inferior

Purkinje cell

Pontine nuclei

Pontocerebellar fibers

Rubrospinal tract

Corticospinal tract

form nuclei) and slightly to the dentate nucleus. The *cerebellar hemispheric cortex* projects to the dentate nucleus and portions of the interposed nuclei.

The *juxtarestiform body (medial bundle of the inferior cerebellar peduncle)* consists of fibers associated with the vestibular system, archicerebellum, and nuclei fastigii. The fibers from the fastigial nuclei project via two pathways by way of the juxtarestiform body to all the vestibular nuclei and the brainstem reticular formation: an uncrossed direct fastigiovestibular tract and a crossed and uncrossed uncinate fasciculus (Figs. 9-7, 10-11). The *uncinate fasciculus (hooked bundle)* is a bundle of fastigiovestibular fibers which arch rostrally around the superior cerebellar peduncle before joining the juxtarestiform body. These fastigiovestibular fibers exert facilitatory influences upon ipsilateral extensor muscle tone. The fastigioreticular projec-

FIGURE 9-5
Neocerebellar connections with the cerebral cortex, thalamus, nucleus ruber, and pontine nuclei.

Note *1* the sequence of cerebellum→nucleus ruber→ thalamic nuclei→cerebral cortex, and *2* the connections of this sequence with the corticospinal tract, rubrospinal tract, and corticopontine-pontocerebellar pathway.

tions probably influence the medullary reticulospinal pathways.

The *superior cerebellar peduncle* consists primarily of the efferent fibers from the dentate,

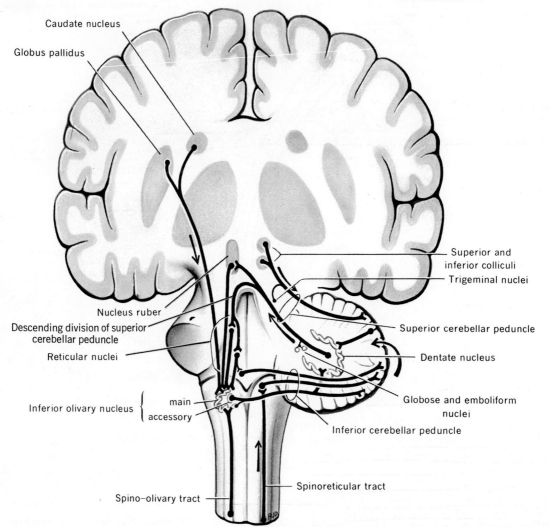

Caudate nucleus

Globus pallidus

Superior and
inferior colliculi

Trigeminal nuclei

Nucleus ruber

Descending division of superior
cerebellar peduncle

Superior cerebellar peduncle

Reticular nuclei

Dentate nucleus

Inferior olivary nucleus { main
accessory

Globose and emboliform
nuclei

Inferior cerebellar peduncle

Spinoreticular tract

Spino–olivary tract

FIGURE 9-6
Neocerebellar connections with the brainstem
and basal ganglia.

Some input to the cerebellum is conveyed from *1* the
brainstem reticular nuclei and inferior olivary nucleus
via the inferior cerebellar peduncle, and *2* the midbrain via the superior cerebellar peduncle. Note the
feedback circuit of cerebellum→nucleus ruber, reticular nuclei, and inferior olivary nucleus of the brain-
stem→cerebellum via the inferior cerebellar peduncle.

emboliform, and globose nuclei (dentate nucleus used to designate efferent tracts) via the
dentatorubral, dentatothalamic, and dentato-
reticular fibers. The entire outflow completely
crosses over in the lower midbrain as the decussation of the superior cerebellar peduncle. Most
fibers from the dentate nucleus project rostrally
to the ventral lateral thalamic nucleus and the
rostral intralaminar (reticular) nuclei of the thalamus with some fibers to the rostral third of the
nucleus ruber. The globose and emboliform
nuclei project mainly to the caudal two-thirds
of the nucleus ruber.

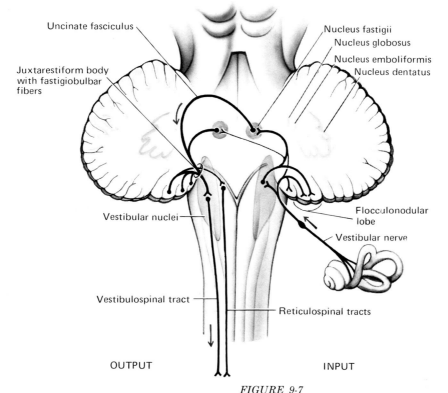

Uncinate fasciculus

Juxtarestiform body
with fastigiobulbar
fibers

Nucleus fastigii
Nucleus globosus
Nucleus emboliformis
Nucleus dentatus

Vestibular nuclei

Flocculonodular
lobe

Vestibular nerve

Vestibulospinal tract

Reticulospinal tracts

OUTPUT

INPUT

FIGURE 9-7
Cerebellar connections of the vestibulocerebellum (archicerebellum and fastigial nucleus) with the vestibular nerve and vestibular nuclei.

Some efferent fibers from the dentate and interposed nuclei, after crossing in the decussation of the superior cerebellar peduncle, project caudally as the descending division of the superior cerebellar peduncle. These fibers terminate in the reticulotegmental nucleus, paramedian reticular nuclei of the medulla, and inferior olivary nuclear complex. These fibers and nuclei are integrated into feedback systems projecting back to the cerebellum. The fibers of the reticulotegmental nucleus course through the middle cerebellar peduncle and terminate in the vermis (except for the nodulus). The paramedian reticular nuclei of the medulla also receive a major input from the corticoreticular systems; the fibers from these nuclei pass through the ipsilateral inferior cerebellar peduncle before terminating in the vermis. The fibers of the inferior olivary nuclear complex cross and pass through the inferior cerebellar peduncle and terminate in the contralateral neocerebellum.

GENERAL OVERALL CIRCUITRY

The neuronal circuits to and from the cerebellum are *1* the source of the polysensory input to the cerebellum, *2* output from the

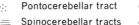
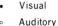

:·: Pontocerebellar tract   • Visual
≡ Spinocerebellar tracts   ○ Auditory
⫴ Vestibulocerebellar t.   ⁄⁄ Tactile

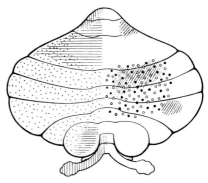

FIGURE 9-8
Projection areas on the cerebellar cortex that receive influences from outside the cerebellum. (*Adapted from Snider.*)

cerebellum, and *3* links in complex feedback loops.

Polysensory input The unconscious polysensory input projects to the cerebellar cortex and deep cerebellar nuclei. The impulses derived from these various sources are projected to regions of the cerebellar cortex designated as the somatosensory, visual, auditory (audiovisual), and vestibular areas (archicerebellum). These zones have been mapped by electric recordings subsequent to the stimulation of peripheral receptors and other regions of the nervous system. The exteroceptive sensors, including tactile endings, retina, and cochlea, and the proprioceptive sensors, including general peripheral endings and the vestibular labyrinth, project influences to these cerebellar areas. The tactile endings project influences to the several somatotopically organized somatosensory areas of the ipsilateral neocerebellum (Fig. 9-8). In the rostral neocerebellar cortex is a somatotopic representation of the entire body plan, while in each of the bilateral caudal areas is a somatotopic representation of the ipsilateral half of the body. There is a large overlap of somatic inputs. Each small region receives inputs from many sources. The general proprioceptive endings have an essentially similar representation in these somatosensory areas. Most of these influences are conveyed via the spinocerebellar tracts, trigeminocerebellar tracts, and pathways utilizing the accessory cuneate nucleus and the lateral reticular nucleus of the medulla. Somatotopic projections from the cerebral somesthetic cortex are also represented in these somatosensory areas. Photic and click stimuli send influences, via the optic pathways and auditory pathways, to the midbrain tectum and from there through tectocerebellar connections to the coextensive audiovisual area of the neocerebellar cortex (Fig. 9-8). Vestibular influences are conveyed to the archicerebellum in the vestibular pathways (Chap. 10).

Output In a general way, the output of the cerebellum, except for the feedback loops, may be conceived as being integrated into three pathway systems involved with somatic motor activity.

1 The *cerebellar vermal zone,* including the flocculonodular lobe through its main connections with the fastigial and vestibular nuclei, exerts its influences via the vestibulospinal tracts upon spinal reflexes (Fig. 9-7). This system has a role in facilitating extensor muscle tone.

2 The *cerebellar paravermal zone,* through its main connections with the ipsilateral nucleus interpositus and contralateral nucleus ruber, exerts its influences via the crossed rubrospinal tract upon spinal reflexes (Fig. 9-5). This system has a role in facilitating flexor muscle tone on the side ipsilateral to the paravermal zone.

3 The *cerebellar hemispheric zone* (*neocerebellum*), through its connections with the dentate nucleus and the ventral lateral (VL) nucleus of the thalamus, exerts powerful effects upon the motor cortex (Figs. 9-4, 9-5). In turn this input from the cerebellum to the motor cortex influences the activity of the corticospinal, corticorubrospinal, and corticoreticulospinal systems. These pathways are essential in the coordination of somatic motor activity.

Feedback loops The cerebellum is integrated into a number of circuits and feedback loops (Figs. 9-3 through 9-7).

1 The *intracerebellar loops* include *a* the recurrent inhibitory pathway of granule cells to Golgi cells back to the dendrites of the granule cells in the glomeruli (negative feedback loops); *b* the inhibitory pathways of granule cells via basket cells and stellate cells to the Purkinje cells (feed-forward or on-going inhibitory control circuits); and *c* pathway of the recurrent collaterals of Purkinje cells back to cerebellar interneurons and either to the same or other Purkinje cells (Fig. 9-3).

2 The *vestibular-archicerebellar loop* (Figs. 9-7, 10-11) includes the connections from the vestibular nerve and vestibular nuclei to the archicerebellum and fastigial nuclei, and the output from the latter through the juxtarestiform body to the vestibular nuclei and reticular nuclei of the brainstem. This loop is an integral part of the vestibular system (Chap. 10).

3 The *cerebrocerebellar loop* (Figs. 9-4, 9-5) interconnects the cerebrum and the cerebellum.

It includes, in order, the corticopontine tracts (from wide areas of the cerebral cortex to the ipsilateral pontine nuclei), the mainly crossed pontocerebellar tracts to the contralateral cerebellar cortex, the Purkinje cell axons of the cerebellar cortex to the deep cerebellar nuclei, and the dentatorubrothalamic cortical pathway that projects to the cerebral cortex. The latter pathway has neural processing stations in the nucleus ruber and ventral lateral thalamic nuclei of the opposite side (crossing occurs at the decussation of the superior cerebellar peduncle) before projecting topically to the cerebral motor cortex. This circuit interrelates the cerebral cortex of one side and the cerebellar cortex of the opposite side, and it is a significant system in phasic locomotor activities. Volitional movements initiated in the cerebrum utilize this feedback system to modulate coordinated movements. The corticopontine and pontocerebellar tracts are the pathways by which the auditory, visual, general somesthetic, and motor areas of the cerebral cortex transmit their influences to the cerebellum. Much of the cerebral neocortex evolved together with the cortex of the neocerebellum.

4 The *cerebello-brainstem reticular-cerebellar loop* (Figs. 9-4, 9-6) includes, in order, *a* the lower brainstem nuclei—reticulotegmental nucleus, paramedian reticular nuclei of the medulla, and inferior olivary nuclear complex, *b* the projections from these nuclei to the deep cerebellar nuclei and the cerebellar cortex, *c* the projections from the cerebellar cortex to the deep cerebellar nuclei, and *d* completing the loop, the fibers of the descending division of the superior cerebellar peduncle to these brainstem reticular nuclei. Some fibers in the descending division project directly from some deep cerebellar nuclei to the inferior olivary nuclear complex.

These "loops" should be thought of not as self-contained circuits but rather as sequences of tracts which are indicative of the complexities of the interconnections of the cerebellum with other centers of the brain. Of significance are the numerous influences upon these loops from other centers and the influences of these loops upon other centers. For example, collaterals from the corticospinal tract have connections with the ventral lateral nucleus of the thalamus, nucleus ruber, pontine nuclei, lateral reticular nucleus, and inferior olivary nuclear complex.

Functional aspects of the cerebellum

The cerebellum is the great modulator subserving the coordination of groups of muscles (synergy). Its significant background role is expressed in the simple and complex movements associated with standing, walking, sitting, running, and dextrous finger and hand manipulations. The cerebellum smooths out the actions of muscle groups by delicately regulating and grading muscle tensions. It has been conceived as an organ which is continuously receiving input from the neuromuscular and Golgi tendon sensors in the muscles and tendons regarding the moment-to-moment status of the tension within the muscular system. This information is utilized by the motor pathway systems. This constant monitoring is essential because the cerebellum does not store or retain information on this input from the periphery for more than a fraction of a second; rather, it assembles information on the on-going status of the muscular system.

The cerebellum acts as a servomechanism in a negative feedback system, functioning to prevent oscillations (tremor) during motion and thereby maintaining stability in a movement (Chap. 3). Marked injury to the cerebellum releases other regions of the nervous system from cerebellar influences. The resulting *release phenomena* illustrate the loss of the effects of the negative feedback system. In the motion of moving the upper extremity to touch an object with the tip of the finger, an intention tremor results, with the extremity oscillating in a series of rhythmic movements as the object is approached. This resembles the automatic pilot and automatic antiaircraft control system, in which each correction is followed by an overshoot. In normal cerebellar activity the negative feedback activity reduces the overshoot to insignificance.

The unconscious *polysensory input* from the tactile, proprioceptive, vestibular, auditory, visual, and visceral sources is processed by the cerebellum and utilized in the activities of the cerebellum. Although a localization of input to the cerebellar cortex is demonstrable, all regions of the cerebellum contribute to the general cerebellar activity. The functional expression of the cerebellum is channeled into *1* equilibration and tonus, and *2* voluntary movements. Equilibration and tonus are utilized in the static and postural activities of standing, sitting, and balancing. *Muscle tone* (hypotonus and hypertonus) is influenced and modified by the archicerebellum and paleocerebellum. The facilitation of extensor muscle tone is mediated through connections with the lateral vestibular nucleus (vestibulospinal tract) and reticular nuclei of the brainstem (medullary reticulospinal tract); its inhibition is mediated through connections with other reticular nuclei. The phasic or locomotive movements involved in the voluntary movements are mediated largely through the cerebrum-to-neocerebellum-to-cerebrum feedback circuit, with the corticospinal tract as the major pathway for the expression of the neocerebellum. The paravermal cortex is particularly involved with facilitatory influences on extensor muscle tone, whereas the vermal cortex has a role in flexor muscle tone.

Cerebellar dysfunction

Lesions of the cerebellum or of its input or its output result in a characteristic constellation of symptoms expressed on the motor side. The disturbances are actually the result of the activity of other units (such as the lateral ventral thalamic nucleus) of the nervous system that are functionally intact. These functional units are released (*release phenomenon*) from cerebellar influences. Following lesions of the cerebellum, volitional motor activity usually results in an excess of motion.

NEOCEREBELLAR LESIONS

Dysfunction of the neocerebellum produces a complex of clinical disorders. These symptoms are primarily the result of the release of cerebellar influences on the thalamic nuclei, for neocerebellar symptoms are abolished or reduced by lesions in the ventral lateral thalamic nucleus and intralaminar nuclei of the thalamus. The tendon reflexes are diminished (*hypotonia*), this effect being expressed at times as a pendular knee jerk that swings freely back and forth. The muscles are weak and flabby, and tire easily (*asthenia*). The horizontally extended forelimb will gradually drift downward when the eyes are closed because the proprioceptive sense from the extremity is not being used properly. *Asynergia*, or loss of muscular coordination, is revealed by jerky, puppetlike movements, including *decomposition of movement, dysmetria, past pointing, adiadochokinesis,* and the *rebound phenomenon.*

The *decomposition of movement* is the breaking up of the movement into its component parts, as in the finger-to-nose test. Instead of a smooth, coordinated flow of movement in bringing the tip of the finger of the extended upper extremity to the nose, each joint of the shoulder, elbow, wrist, and fingers may flex independently (puppetlike) in an almost mechanical fashion.

Dysmetria, or the inability to gauge or measure distances accurately, results in the overshooting of the intended goal by consistently pointing to the lesion side of the object (past pointing).

Adiadochokinesis is impaired ability to execute alternating and repetitive movements, such as supination and pronation of the forearm, in rapid succession with equal excursions. The limb on the lesion side will perform the movements more slowly and clumsily.

The *intention or action tremor* is expressed during the execution of a voluntary movement. It is absent or diminished during rest. These tremors are particularly noted at the end of the movement (terminal tremor).

The *ataxic gait,* or the asynergic activity elicited during walking, is a staggering gait resembling that of drunkenness. (The cerebellum is sensitive to alcohol and to slight circulatory impairment.) The ataxia is due to incoordination of the trunk and proximal shoulder and pelvic girdle muscles. A tendency to veer or to fall to the side of the lesion is apparent. To counteract the unsteadiness, the patient will stand or walk with legs far apart (broad-base stance).

The loss of the normal check of an antagonist over an agonist muscle results in the *rebound phenomenon.* When the actively flexed forearm, held within a few inches of the face, is suddenly released, the open hand does not hit the face in the normal individual (normal rebound), because the antagonistic extensor muscles check the flexor muscles immediately. The patient with a cerebellar lesion will hit his face because the antagonist muscles contract too late.

A *scanning speech,* or *dysarthria,* is a result of the incoordination of the muscles used in speaking. The speech is hesitating, slurred, and explosive in quality, with a telegram-staccato pace (pauses in the wrong places). Nystagmus does not occur following a cerebellar lesion.

ARCHICEREBELLAR LESIONS

Lesion of the flocculonodular lobe may result in ataxia of the trunk muscles without any signs of tremor or hypotonia. There are bilateral disturbances of locomotion and equilibrium. Children with nodular lobe tumors (archicerebellum) have a tendency to fall backward, sway from side to side, and walk with a wide base. They may be unable to maintain equilibrium or an upright balance. This *truncal ataxia* resembles the walk of a drunkard; there is staggering accompanied by a tendency to fall to the side or backward. An experimental animal with ablated nodulus is not subject to motion sickness and can swim upright under water. An animal without semicircular canals of the vestibular system is unable to swim upright under water (Chap. 10).

PALEOCEREBELLAR LESIONS

No definite data are available to define the symptoms of a paleocerebellar lesion in man. There is a probable increase in extensor muscle tone and postural reflexes so as to resemble decerebrate rigidity. The experimental ablation of the entire anterior lobe in animals produces a decerebrate rigidity.

GENERAL COMMENT

Unilateral cerebellar lesions have homolateral effects. The symptoms are expressed on the same side because the pathways from the cerebellum decussate and integrate with systems that in turn cross over to the side of the original cerebellar output, before exerting their effects. For example the crossed dentatorubrothalamo-cortical ascending pathways have connections with the contralateral nucleus ruber, thalamus, and cerebral cortex. The rubrospinal and corticospinal tracts are crossed descending tracts. In effect the cerebellum exerts its influences primarily through a *double crossing* of *1* the ascending fibers of the superior cerebellar peduncle and *2* the descending fibers of the corticospinal tract.

Lesions of the cerebellum result in inadequacy of certain responses and general symptoms. The disturbance is expressed in the constellation of symptoms and neurologic signs previously noted. Small lesions may produce no symptoms or only transient symptoms, whereas large lesions produce severe symptoms. The cerebellum possesses a good margin of physiologic safety; with time the neurologic symptoms attenuate and the resulting compensation markedly reduces the severity of the deficits. The reasons for this phenomenon are not fully known but are probably related to the polysensory input which is integrated in a cortex that is similar throughout. The reduction of certain input is compensated for by other input sources that become adequate for effective activity. Cerebellar cortical lesions are notable for being associated with attenuating deficits and reduction in severity of the symptoms with time, whereas damage to the deep cerebellar nuclei or superior cerebellar peduncle is accomplished by similar but lasting (nonattenuating) and more enduring deficits.

Bibliography

Eager, R. P.: Modes of termination of Purkinje cell axons in the cerebellum of the cat, in R. Llinás (ed.), *Neurobiology of Cerebellar Evolution and Development,* pp. 585–601. American Medical Association, Chicago, 1969.

Eccles, J. C., M. Ito, and J. Szentágothai: *The Cerebellum as a Neuronal Machine.* Springer-Verlag, New York, 1967.

Fields, W. S., and W. D. Willis: *The Cerebellum in Health and Disease.* Warren H. Green, Inc., St. Louis, 1970.

Fox, C. A., and R. S. Snider (eds.): The Cerebellum. Prog. Brain Res., 25:1–335, 1967.

Larsell, O., and J. Jansen: *Cerebellum: The Human Cerebellum, Cerebellar Connections and Cerebellar Cortex.* University of Minnesota Press, Minneapolis, 1972.

Llinás, R. (ed.): *Neurobiology of Cerebellar Evolution and Development.* American Medical Association, Chicago, 1969.

Nieuwenhuys, R.: Comparative anatomy of the cerebellum, in C. A. Fox and R. S. Snider (eds.), The Cerebellum. Prog. Brain Res., 25:1–93, 1967.

Palay, S. L., and V. Chan-Palay: *Cerebellar Cortex. Cytology and Organization.* Springer-Verlag, Berlin, 1974.

CHAPTER 10
THE EAR, AUDITORY SYSTEM, AND VESTIBULAR SYSTEM

The ear consists of two functional units: the acoustic apparatus, concerned with the exteroceptive sense called hearing, and the vestibular apparatus, concerned with the special proprioceptive sense involved with posture and equilibrium. The former is innervated by the *cochlear nerve*, the latter by the *vestibular nerve*. These two nerves are collectively known as the *vestibulocochlear, auditory, statoacoustic,* or *eighth cranial nerve*.

The labyrinths

The sensory receptors of the cochlear system and the vestibular system are located in a complex of canals and vesicles called the *membranous labyrinth* (Figs. 10-1 and 10-2). The tube of this membranous labyrinth is filled with a fluid called *endolymph*. The membranous labyrinth is in turn surrounded by canals and vesicles filled with a fluid called *perilymph*. The entire complex is encased by a rigid box called the *bony labyrinth*. The endolymph and the perilymph, which have different chemical compositions and electrical potentials, are not continuous with each other. An analogous model would be a closed tube encased by another tube. The inner tube would be the membranous labyrinth containing the endolymph (Fig. 10-2). The outer tube is within the bony labyrinth. The perilymph fills the cavity of the outer tube and surrounds the inner tube (Fig. 10-2).

The *membranous labyrinth* consists of the three semicircular ducts, utricle, and saccule which are associated with the vestibular system, and the cochlear duct (scala media) which is associated with the auditory system (Fig. 10-3). Each semicircular duct is in open communi-

cation at each end of the utricle. By definition, the semicircular ducts are bounded by the membranous labyrinth, and the semicircular canals by the bony labyrinth; the ducts are erroneously called canals. Each semicircular duct has one bulbous portion, the ampulla.

There are six specialized sensory epithelial receptor areas in contact with the terminal endings of the eighth cranial nerve. These are the three cristae ampullae (one in the ampulla of each semicircular canal), one macula utriculi, one macula sacculi, and a long ribbonlike spiral organ of Corti in the cochlea.

Within the bony labyrinth of the auditory system are three ducts: the scala vestibuli, scala tympani, and cochlear. The ducts, arranged in parallel, ascend in a spiral $2\frac{3}{4}$ times around the bony core, or modiolus.

The cochlear duct of the membranous labyrinth extends between the two scalae. Its roof is the vestibular (Reissner's) membrane, adjoining the scala vestibuli. Its floor is the basilar membrane, bordering the scala tympani. Resting on the basilar membrane is the spiral organ of Corti, the organ of hearing. The surface of the spiral organ is bounded by the reticular membrane (Fig. 10-3). The last two membranes together with the spiral organ itself comprise the cochlear partition. The term cochlea refers to the cochlear duct, with the spiral organ of Corti and the scalae vestibuli and tympani.

The cochlear duct, like the entire membranous labyrinth, is filled with endolymph. The reticular membrane prevents endolymph from entering the spaces of the spiral organ. The scalae vestibuli and tympani, like the rest of the bony labyrinth, are filled with perilymph.

The vestibular organs lie superiorly in the inner ear; the cochlea lies inferiorly.

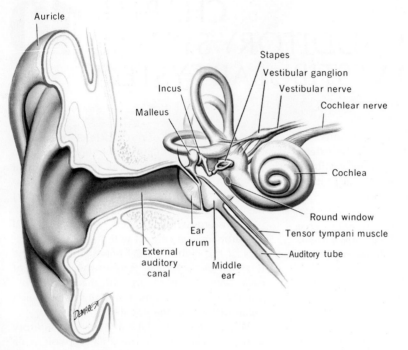

FIGURE 10-1
External ear, middle ear,
and inner ear. (Right ear
viewed from the front.)

The auditory system

OUTER EAR AND MIDDLE EAR

Airborne vibrations may be perceived as sounds
by our auditory system or as vibrations by our
sense of "touch." The vibrations that are heard
are conveyed successively through the outer ear,
middle ear, and inner ear before reaching the
sensory receptors of the spiral organ of Corti
(Fig. 10-1). Sounds can also reach the ears
through solids or liquids.

The *outer ear* consists of the auricle and the
external acoustic meatus (auditory canal); it
ends at the oval-shaped tympanic membrane
(eardrum). The canal acts as a resonator, especially at the frequencies of greatest acuity (2,000
to 5,500 cycles per second), and as a buffer
against temperature and humidity changes
which can alter the elasticity of the drum. The
tympanic membrane is a thin, slightly stiff cone
(like a paper-cone loudspeaker) sensitive to air-

borne vibrations. The remarkable sensitivity of
the tympanic membrane offers an example of
extreme biologic miniaturization, for air movements in ordinary conversation produce inward
and outward displacements of the membrane of
about the diameter of the hydrogen atom.

Because the threshold of hearing is low, the
transfer of the vibratory energy from the com-
pressible atmospheric air (low impedance) to
the incompressible perilymphatic fluid (high
impedance) of the inner ear must be accomplished without any appreciable loss of energy.
The impedance matching device that effects this
efficient energy transfer includes the sequence
from the tympanic membrane to the solid levers
(ear bones), to the liquid perilymph, to the
(solid) sensory hair cell receptors in the spiral
organ of Corti. The device works at 99.9 percent
transmission efficiency. The ear is considered a
more efficient energy converter than the eye.

The *middle ear (tympanic cavity)* is a small
chamber located between the tympanic mem-

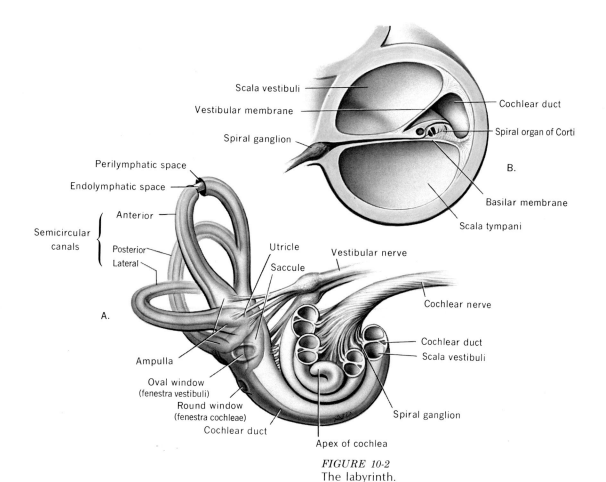

Scala vestibuli
Vestibular membrane
Spiral ganglion
Cochlear duct
Spiral organ of Corti
B.
Basilar membrane
Scala tympani

Perilymphatic space
Endolymphatic space
Anterior
Semicircular canals
Posterior
Lateral
Utricle
Saccule
Vestibular nerve
Cochlear nerve
Cochlear duct
Scala vestibuli
A.
Ampulla
Oval window
(fenestra vestibuli)
Round window
(fenestra cochleae)
Cochlear duct
Apex of cochlea
Spiral ganglion

FIGURE 10-2
The labyrinth.

A Right labyrinth, from the front. The perilymphatic space is located between the bony labyrinth and the membranous labyrinth. The endolymphatic space is located within the membranous labyrinth, which includes the three semicircular ducts, utricle, saccule, and cochlear duct.

B Cross section through the cochlea. The scala vestibuli and scala tympani are connected through a passage called the helicotrema, located at the apex of the cochlea.

brane and the inner ear. The three ear ossicles (malleus, incus, and stapes) are located in the middle ear, which is continuous with the throat via the auditory (eustachian, pharyngotympanic) tube (Fig. 10-1).

The ear bones of the middle ear form the lever chain extending from the tympanic membrane to the inner ear. The bones are the malleus (hammer), incus (anvil), and stapes (stirrup), in that order. The oval foot of the stapes fits into the oval window (fenestra vestibuli in the bony labyrinth) which is the site of the functional contact between the stapes and the perilymph of the inner ear. The efficiency of the energy transfer from the tympanic membrane to the oval window is enhanced *1* by the arrangement of the connective tissue fibers within the

tympanic membrane, and *2* by the fact that the tympanic membrane has an area which is about 18 times greater than that of the oval window. This areal difference accounts for the great hydraulic piston thrusts of the stapes on the peri-

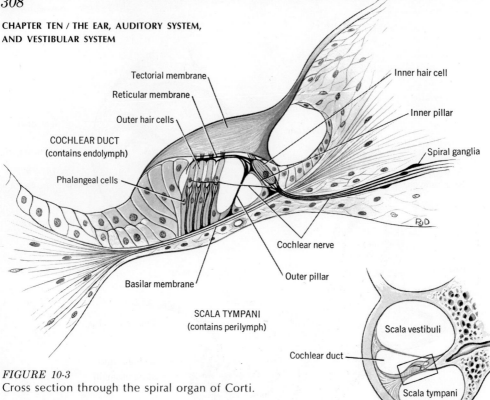

FIGURE 10-3
Cross section through the spiral organ of Corti.

lymph (even though the total force exerted in the tympanic membrane and the oval window are about equal). The lever action of the ear ossicles contributes only slightly to the energy transfer. Therefore the middle ear is an efficient transformer; it converts the large-amplitude, low-force vibrations of the sound in the air at the tympanic membrane to the low-amplitude, large-force vibrations at the oval window.

These bony levers are important; airborne vibrations are almost impossible to hear when these ear ossicles are fused and become immobilized. This condition, called *otosclerosis,* also occurs following the formation of new bone around the round window. Use of a hearing aid, which utilizes bone conduction, can make hearing essentially normal in persons with fused bony ossicles. In hearing by bone conduction, the vibrations are conducted through the bones of the skull (bypassing ear ossicles) to the cochlea. Bone conduction plays little part in hearing ordinary sounds, except by adding resonance

and body to one's voice. This is why our voice sounds different to us than to others, and why a tape recording of our voice sounds different from our voice when we are speaking.

Protection against loud sounds is afforded by the two tiny muscles that are inserted into two of the ear ossicles—the tensor tympani muscle into the malleus, and the stapedius muscle into the stapes. The tensor tympani and the stapedius muscles are innervated, respectively, by branches of the trigeminal and facial nerves. Their contractions have a dampening effect, especially to intense sounds, by exerting tension on the malleus and stapes. In addition, weak sounds may be magnified and amplified as much as 50 times by decreasing the tension on the ear ossicles by the relaxation of these muscles. The tensor tympani regulates the stiffness of the tympanic membrane. In effect, these muscles increase the range of loudness we hear through dampening and magnification. The contraction of these muscles provides a protective mechanism, producing a significant attenuation of cochlear excitation for frequencies less than 1,000 cycles per second. This attenuation can reach 40 decibels. This *auditory reflex* is analogous to the pupilloconstrictor reflex of the eye to bright and dim light.

The middle ear is connected to the pharynx through the auditory (eustachian) tube. Discomfort from the differential pressure on the tympanic membrane results from changing atmospheric pressures (e.g., during ascent or descent in an elevator). This discomfort can be alleviated by opening the auditory tube by swallowing movements, because this permits the atmospheric pressure in the pharynx to force air to enter (or leave) the middle ear cavity and equalize the atmospheric pressure on the outside of the tympanic membrane. The air pressure within the middle ear would not be maintained without the presence of an auditory tube; the pressure would fall because gases within enclosed body cavities are naturally absorbed by the vascular system.

INNER EAR

The vibrations of the stapes are converted at the oval window into pressure waves in the perilymph of the inner ear. These pressure waves travel up through the perilymph of the scala vestibuli to the helicotrema at the apex of the cochlea and, along the way, are transmitted across the vestibular membrane to the endolymph of the cochlear duct. After passing through the helicotrema, the vibrations travel down the perilymph of the scala tympani and are transmitted to the basilar membrane and the spiral organ of Corti, and finally to the thin resilient membrane of the round window at the base of the cochlea. This membrane at the round window accommodates the vibratory motions of the perilymph originally generated at the oval window. The inward (or outward) thrust of the stapes is accompanied, after a fraction of a second, by the outward (or inward) compensatory movement of the membrane at the round window.

The spiral organ of Corti and the basilar membrane are attached on either side of the bony labyrinth, along the entire 35-mm length

of the cochlear coil. The membrane gradually widens as it ascends; it broadens from 0.08 mm wide at the base to 0.52 mm at the apical end. The spiral organ of Corti is an organized complex of supporting cells and hair cells (Fig. 10-3). The hair cells (neuroepithelial sensory end organs) are arranged in rows along the length of the coil. The number of rows of outer hair cells varies from three in the basal coil and four in the middle coil to as many as five in the apical coil. The inner hair cells are in a single row. There are about 3,500 inner hair cells and 20,000 outer hair cells.

Although differences exist between the inner and outer hair cells, the similarities are important. Both have bristlelike *sensory hairs* (Fig. 10-4), which are specialized microvilli; these sensory hairs, or stereocilia, are similar to those of the vestibular hair cells described later in the chapter and shown in Fig. 10-9. Each outer hair cell has from 80 to 100 sensory hairs, while each inner hair cell has from 40 to 60 sensory hairs. They are arranged in each hair cell in rows that form the letter W or U, with the base of the letter directed laterally (Fig. 10-5). The tips of many hairs are embedded within and firmly bound to the tectorial membrane or one of its specialized portions. The tectorial membrane is an acellular protein structure similar to epidermal keratin. One of its specialized portions, on its undersurface, is *Hardesty's membrane.* The tips of many hairs of the outer hair cells are embedded within it. Another specialized area on the underside of the tectorial membrane is *Hensen's stripe.* The tips of many of the hairs of the inner hair cells may be in contact with it.

Because the basilar membrane and the rigid tectorial membrane are hinged to different sites, a shearing (tangential) motion develops when these structures vibrate, and as a result the sensory hairs of the hair cells are displaced. The hairs are probably stiff levers that do not bend. Rather, the stiff bundle of hairs of a cell may depress or elevate the basal body (Fig. 10-4). This distortion of the basal body region is presumed to be the event that triggers the generation of the receptor potential. The basal body is a remnant of a kinocilium like that associated with

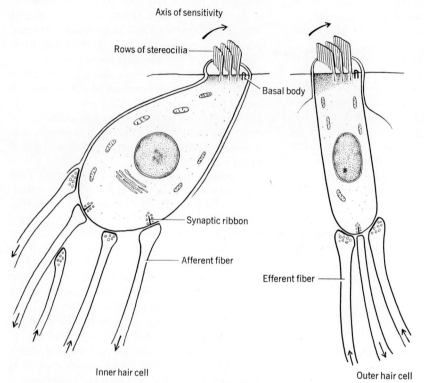

FIGURE 10-4
The hair cells of the spiral organ of Corti.

The axis of sensitivity of a cochlear hair cell is in the direction of the basal body. (*After Wersäll, Flock, and Lundquist.*)

the hair cells of the vestibular receptors (see Fig. 10-9). (A kinocilium is a true cilium, not a microvillus.)

The hair cells are the mechanoreceptors in which transduction of the mechanical energy of the sound waves into the generator potentials of the cochlear nerve endings occurs. The response in the hair cell and nerve terminals is graded. Each hair cell is innervated by several neurons. The nerve terminals of the myelinated cochlear nerve fibers are naked fibers (unmyelinated and without neurolemma cell sheaths) that conduct with decrement. In total,

there are about 23,500 hair cells in the spiral organ of Corti and approximately an equal number of neurons in the cochlear nerve of man.

The nature of the perilymph and endolymph may be significant in the genesis of the receptor and action potentials. The *perilymph* resembles an ultrafiltrate of blood similar in composition to other extracellular fluids, including the cerebrospinal fluid. Perilymph has high Na^+ and low K^+ concentrations. In contrast, endolymph resembles intracellular fluids in having high K^+ and low Na^+ concentrations. The site and process of perilymph generation is not resolved.

The *endolymph* within the cochlea is located in the cochlear duct, including the space between the tectorial membrane and reticular membrane of the spiral organ of Corti. Note that the sensory hairs of the hair cells are bathed in endolymph. Endolymph is produced, and its

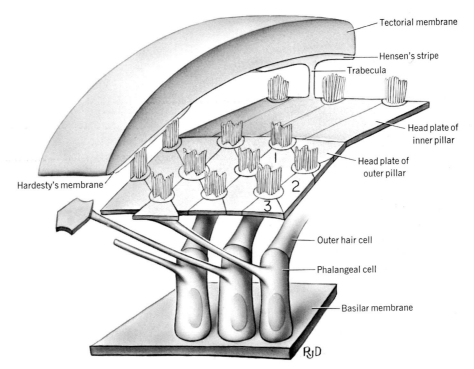

Tectorial membrane

Hensen's stripe

Trabecula

Head plate of inner pillar

Head plate of outer pillar

Hardesty's membrane

Outer hair cell

Phalangeal cell

Basilar membrane

RjD

FIGURE 10-5
The spiral organ of Corti viewed from the outer rim of the tectorial membrane.

The tips of the long hairs of the outer hair cells are embedded in the tectorial membrane; those of the inner hair cells probably are not. Along with the head plates of the inner and outer pillars, the expanded phalanges (1, 2, 3) of the processes of the phalangeal cells form the bulk of the reticular membrane. (*From Rivera-Dominquez, Agate, and Noback*, Brain Research, *Elsevier, Amsterdam, The Netherlands, 1974.*)

ionic composition maintained, by active transport and secretion from blood plasma.

A fluid called *cortilymph* is in the spaces of the spiral organ of Corti between the reticular membrane and the basilar membrane and surrounding the hair cells and unmyelinated nerve fibers. Cortilymph resembles perilymph, not endolymph; it has high Na^+ and low K^+ concentrations. The ionic composition of cortilymph is maintained by the basilar membrane acting as a "sieve" for ions passing from the perilymph of the scala tympani; in contrast, the reticular membrane acts as an ionic barrier preventing exchange between the endolymph and cortilymph. The high Na^+ and low K^+ concentrations of cortilymph form a normal physiologic ionic environment for the excitable cells; the rich K^+ levels of the endolymph would be incompatible with the generation and transmission of excitatory impulses.

Because the spiral organ of Corti has no blood vessels of its own, its oxygen supply is presumably precarious. Most of its nourishment

apparently comes via the cortilymph from the perilymph. Short periods of diminished oxygen supply are in part compensated for by the high concentration of enzymes in the cortilymph. These enable anaerobic glycolysis to satisfy the organ's energy needs.

A relationship exists between the pitch of a tone (frequency of vibration) and the region of maximal vibratory displacement of the basilar membrane. The highest tones (high pitch, high frequency, and short waves) are "heard" at the base of the cochlea near the stapes, and the lowest tones (low pitch, low frequency, and long waves) are "heard" at the apex. The basilar membrane acts as a low-pass filter (i.e., high frequencies are filtered out), and thus low frequencies progress farther along the membrane than do higher ones.

The *tonotopic localization* described above formed the basis of the *place theory* of Helmholtz, in which the basilar membrane is considered a string resonator like the strings of a harp, with a specific place on the basilar membrane vibrating for each tone. However, it now seems likely that the basilar membrane is not a string resonator; it appears to exert no tension in any direction. Yet it displays a stiffness gradient from the base to the apex, the membrane being 100 times more compliant at the apex than at the base. It vibrates as a unit with the vestibular (Reissner's) membrane.

The *traveling-wave,* or *telephone, theory* of Rutherford was based on the thesis that the entire basilar membrane vibrates to a degree for each tone. The displacement of the membrane "travels" continuously up the cochlea from the base to the apex.

The modern *duplex theory* combines elements of the place theory and the traveling-wave theory. The vibrating stapes sets up traveling waves successively in the perilymph and basilar membrane. For each tone, the wave height of the vibrating basilar membrane, as it moves up the cochlea, increases to a maximum and then drops off rapidly. Each site of maximal displacement of the basilar membrane is correlated with a specific frequency of a sound wave. The sites of lesser displacement along the basilar membrane have as yet unknown functional roles that are probably associated with some of the qualities of each tone.

Loudness or intensity discrimination depends on the length of the basilar membrane set into maximal motion (amplitude of vibration); a longer portion activates more receptors and, in turn, more neurons than a short one. Musical sounds, chords, and harmonics are the result of the several frequencies vibrating in simple numeric oscillations. These are rhythms. Noises and background sounds are the result of frequencies not in periodic oscillation. These may be unpleasant discords.

The human ear is used most often at frequencies ranging from 300 to 3,000 cycles per second, the approximate range of the human voice (middle C is 256 cycles per second). Man is most sensitive to vibration of about 2,000 cycles per second, with little useful hearing occurring below 50 or above 16,000 cycles per second, although some individuals can hear sounds with frequencies of from 16 to 30,000 cycles per second. High frequencies are best perceived in early childhood, with a gradual decrease with age, a loss that may be related to a change in the stiffness of the basilar membrane. Vibrations can be sensed as vibrations of the joints (vibratory sense) when the stem of a vibrating tuning fork is placed in contact with the joint.

The input codes conveyed by the fibers in the cochlear nerve are significant to loudness and to pitch. The loudness code is related to the frequency of nerve impulses (up to a maximum of 1,000 per second) transmitted in each nerve fiber. The arrangement is not that each sound is conveyed by only one specific fiber in the cochlear nerve; neither does each sound stimulate the firing of all the fibers of the nerve. Rather, the code for a sound is transmitted over the cochlear nerve by a compromise between these two extremes. Apparently the pitch code for each of the many thousands of different pitches heard by man is relayed via the cochlear nerve by different combinations of nerve fibers. One theory suggests that the outer hair cells are involved with the initial processing that results in loudness or volume discrimination, and that the inner hair cells are involved in pitch discrimination. The auditory input is conveyed via the cochlear nerve. It averages about 1 million or so impulses per second.

The detection of the location of a sound depends primarily on the differences in the time of the arrival of the sound to the two ears. The source of the sound is directly in front, behind, or above when the sound reaches each ear with the same intensity. Sound location is based on the capacity of the subject to detect interval differences as small as 10 milliseconds ($\frac{1}{100}$ of a second) in the arrival of a sound at the two ears. It is difficult to localize a sound heard only by one ear.

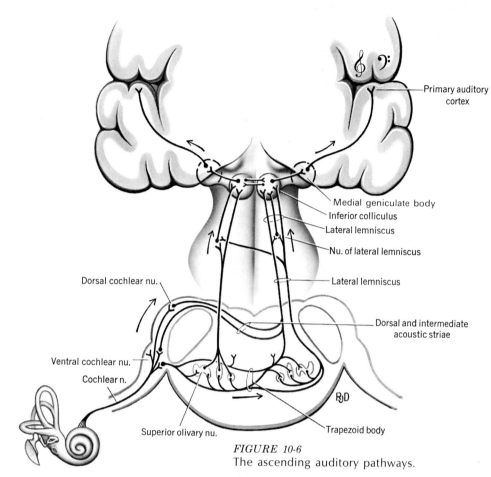

FIGURE 10-6

The ascending auditory pathways.

The cross section is through the upper medulla.

AUDITORY PATHWAYS

General features The ascending pathway of the auditory system is composed of sequences of neurons which are organized both in series and in parallel. Some neurons extend from one nucleus to the next, the neurons forming "sequences in series," whereas other neurons, arranged in parallel, extend from one nucleus and bypass a nucleus before terminating in another nucleus. This organization does not permit a precise designation of second-order, third-order, and fourth-order neurons. In general, the following sequence may be considered as basic (Fig. 10-6):

1 Neurons of the first order, with cell bodies in the spiral ganglion of the cochlear nerve, extend from the spiral organ of Corti and terminate centrally in the dorsal and ventral cochlear nuclei.

2 Neurons of the second order, with cell bodies in the dorsal and ventral cochlear nuclei, extend from these nuclei and ascend as crossed fibers in the lateral lemnisci to the inferior colliculus.

3 Neurons of the third order, with cell bodies in the inferior colliculus, have axons which pass through the brachium of the inferior colliculus to the medial geniculate body (parvocellular or dorsal portion) of the thalamus.

4 Neurons of the fourth order, with cell bodies in the medial geniculate body, pass from there via the auditory (geniculocortical) radiations to the primary auditory cortex (transverse temporal gyri of Heschl, areas 41 and 42).

Several nuclei are intercalated in the auditory pathways between the cochlear nuclei and the inferior colliculus. These include the superior olivary nuclei, the nucleus of the trapezoid body, and the nucleus of the lateral lemniscus. These nuclei receive input from the cochlear nuclei, interconnect with one another, and project to the inferior colliculus (Fig. 10-6).

The cochlea converts the acoustic signals into neural signal codes that are then further processed within the nuclear stations along the auditory pathways. As previously noted, there is a linear spatial distribution from the base to the apex of the cochlear coil in the selective responsiveness of the spiral organ of Corti to different frequencies (tone). In this sense *frequency coding* of auditory input is basically initiated and determined in the spiral organ. This tonotopic organization within the spiral organ is preserved within the cochlear nuclei and inferior colliculi. A neuron within these processing stations has a characteristic frequency response to a tone of a certain frequency. According to the standard interpretation, this highly systematic tonotopic organization is apparently not maintained in the medial geniculate body and the primary auditory cortex.

Recent studies suggest that the tectal component (inferior colliculus), thalamic component (medial geniculate body), and cerebral cortical component of the auditory pathway may be composed of two subsystems, the core subsystem and the fringe subsystem. The *core subsystem* consists of the central nucleus of the inferior colliculus, portions of the medial geniculate body, and regions of the auditory cortex. This subsystem is considered to be the direct auditory pathway, which is tonotopically organized in some degree throughout its course. The *fringe subsystem* consists of the capsule of the inferior colliculus, part of the medial geniculate body, and peripheral regions of the auditory cortex. This subsystem receives input from nonauditory as well as auditory sources and is less tonotopically organized at successive higher levels. The details of these subsystems in man and other primates are incompletely understood.

Specific features The displacement of the sensory hairs of the hair cells produced by the shearing motion generates the receptor potentials. These potentials are responsible for the so-called cochlear microphonics. The neurons of the cochlear nerve have their bipolar cell bodies in the spiral ganglion, which forms a spiral following the inner portion of the cochlear coil.

The nerve fibers of the cochlear nerve comprise a homogeneous nerve population of lightly myelinated axons 4 to 6 μm thick. The unmyelinated dendritic terminal branches of each neuron synapse directly with from several to many hair cells. The central axons of the cochlear nerve terminate in the ventral and dorsal cochlear nuclei, which are located on the lateral surface of the inferior cerebellar peduncle.

Each of the fibers of the cochlear nerve bifurcates into branches which are precisely distributed within each cochlear nucleus in a tonotopic organization. Fibers from the basal cochlear coil (high tones) terminate in the dorsal part of both cochlear nuclei, and those from the apical cochlear coil (low tones) terminate in the ventral part of both cochlear nuclei.

The neurons of the cochlear nuclei have axons which project to several nuclei of the same and/or the opposite sides, as follows (Fig. 10-6):

1 The fibers from the dorsal cochlear nucleus decussate through the posterior tegmentum as the *dorsal acoustic stria,* ascend in the contralateral lateral lemniscus, and terminate in the nucleus of the lateral lemniscus and the inferior colliculus.

2 The fibers from the dorsal part of the ventral cochlear nucleus pass dorsal to the inferior cerebellar peduncle, decussate through the intermediate tegmentum as the *intermediate acoustic stria,* ascend in the contralateral lateral lemniscus, and terminate in the nucleus of the lateral lemniscus and the inferior colliculus.

3 The fibers from the ventral cochlear nucleus pass through the anterior tegmentum as the large *ventral acoustic stria* (part of the trapezoid body); these fibers *a* terminate in the ipsilateral and contralateral reticular formation, superior olivary nuclei, and nuclei of the trapezoid body, and *b* ascend in the contralateral lateral lemniscus and terminate in the contralateral nucleus of the lateral lemniscus and the inferior colliculus. The decussating fibers of the ventral acoustic stria and from the superior olivary and trapezoid nuclei are collectively called the trapezoid body.

The *superior olivary* and *trapezoid body nuclei* give rise to third-order fibers, which ascend in both lateral lemnisci to the nucleus of the lateral lemniscus and the inferior colliculus.

The cochlear nuclei give rise to contralateral, not ipsilateral, second-order neurons.

The *nucleus of the lateral lemniscus* projects to the inferior colliculus. Commissural fibers interconnect the inferior colliculi and other neural levels, including the cerebral cortex. The inferior colliculus projects fibers rostrally to the parvocellular portion of the medial geniculate body via the brachium of the inferior colliculus. *Fibers from the medial geniculate body* pass via the sublenticular portion of the posterior limb of the internal capsule to the transverse gyri of Heschl (area 41 and 42) as the auditory radiations.

The *inferior colliculus* is actually a cortical structure (laminated gray matter on a surface) consisting of four layers. The two deep layers receive their inputs from the ascending lateral lemniscus; the two superficial layers receive their inputs from the descending auditory pathways. This laminated cortex is organized to relate and to process a diversity of inputs to a variety of outputs. This is a structural expression for neural integration.

It is important to note that most of the influences from an ear are projected to the cerebral cortex via the cochlear nuclei of the same side and the contralateral auditory pathways (lateral lemniscus, brachium of inferior colliculus, and auditory radiations). Some influences are projected via the ipsilateral auditory pathways. These bilateral inputs to the auditory cortex contribute to the ability to localize sounds in space.

In addition the ascending auditory pathways have significant connections with the brainstem reticular system, with the cerebellum, and with many additional areas of the cerebral cortex.

The auditory pathways to the cortex are not

analogous to telephone circuits. At all levels neurons receive synaptic connections from many other neurons and each neuron, in turn, has synaptic connections with many (50 to 100) other neurons (one neuron projects to many neurons and many neurons converge on one neuron). These complex arborizations at some nuclear stations are arranged in topically organized patterns. Processing of the auditory input occurs in each of the nuclei in the auditory pathways. Some auditory consciousness, including recognition of pitch, may occur at thalamic and inferior collicular levels in man.

More neurons are found at each successive nucleus along the auditory pathways. Many more fibers ascend from each nucleus than enter from below (not counting terminal arborizations). One estimate indicates that in a man the following ratio exists: 1 neuron of the cochlear nerve to 3 in the cochlear nuclei to 13 in the nucleus of the inferior colliculus to 14 in the medial geniculate body to over 100 in the primary auditory cortex (area 41).

DESCENDING EFFERENT FIBERS WITHIN THE AUDITORY PATHWAYS

Parallel to the ascending fibers of the auditory pathways are *centrifugal (descending) fibers* (Fig. 10-7). These centrifugal projections comprise *1 corticogeniculate fibers,* from temporal cortex to medial geniculate body; *2 corticocollicular fibers,* from temporal cortex to the inferior colliculus; *3 geniculocollicular fibers,* from the medial geniculate body to the inferior colliculus; *4 collicular efferents,* from the inferior colliculus to the nuclei of the superior olivary complex and lateral lemniscus and to the dorsal and ventral cochlear nuclei; and *5* the *efferent cochlear bundle* of fibers, from the superior olivary complex to the hair cells of the spiral organ of Corti.

The efferent cochlear bundle consists of many crossing fibers, together termed the *olivocochlear bundle,* and of fewer uncrossed fibers, comprising the *peduncle of the olive.* The olivocochlear bundle originates in the medial accessory superior olivary nucleus and passes near the abducent nucleus before leaving the brainstem

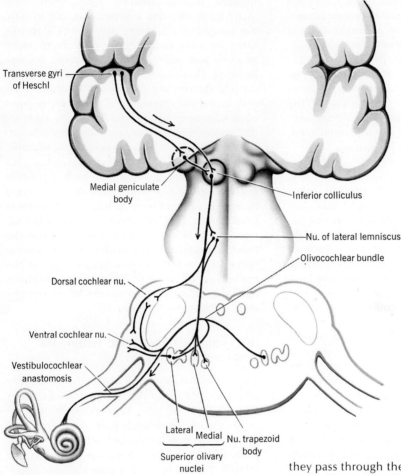

Transverse gyri
of Heschl

Medial geniculate
body

Inferior colliculus

Nu. of lateral lemniscus

Olivocochlear bundle

Dorsal cochlear nu.

Ventral cochlear nu.

Vestibulocochlear
anastomosis

Lateral Medial Nu. trapezoid
body

Superior olivary
nuclei

FIGURE 10-7
The descending auditory pathways.

The fibers of the olivocochlear bundle emerge from the medulla through the vestibular nerve and then pass via the vestibulocochlear anastomosis into the cochlear nerve.

within the contralateral vestibular nerve. The peduncle of the olive arises in the principal superior olivary nucleus and joins the ipsilateral vestibular nerve. The fibers course through the vestibular nerve to the labyrinth region, where they pass through the *vestibulocochlear anastomosis (Oort's bundle)* to the cochlear nerve.

These centrifugal fibers are integrated in the feedback control of auditory input. They are involved with processing and sharpening the ascending auditory influences by channeling the essential neural information (*signal*) and inhibiting and suppressing unwanted neural activity (*noise*). The fibers of the efferent cochlear bundle convey inhibitory influences directly to the hair cells. This is an example of the regulation and control by the central nervous system of peripheral sensory receptors. Stimulation of these cochlear efferent fibers suppresses the activity of the afferent fibers of the cochlear nerve.

The fact that the impulses from the ear largely ascend on the opposite side of the brain explains why sounds perceived by the right ear result in neural activity in the auditory cortex of the left cerebral hemisphere. Lesions interrupting the ascending auditory pathways result not in complete deafness in either ear but rather in diminished hearing, especially on the opposite side. The bilateral composition of the auditory projections helps to explain these findings. Total deafness is a consequence of complete bilateral lesions of the cochlear nerves, cochlear nuclei, or the cochlear partition of both ears.

Although meaningful conscious hearing requires the neural activity of the cerebral cortex, the cortex is not essential for the auditory reflexes. "Listening" and reacting to cochlear input can take place with only the lower brain stations intact. A decorticate animal (one without a cerebral cortex) or even a decerebrate animal (one without a cerebrum) will respond to sounds; a sound can induce a decerebrate cat to mew and to turn its head toward the sound, which may not be subjectively heard. The nucleus of the inferior colliculus and the brainstem reticular formation may be the integrative center for this reflex.

The ascending and descending fibers and the several nuclei of the auditory pathways are involved with complex integrative mechanisms. The anatomic expressions of *1* one neuron synapsing with many other neurons, *2* many neurons converging on one neuron, *3* descending pathways among the ascending auditory pathways, *4* cross connections, and *5* the increasing number of neurons as the pathway ascends are indicative of the complex neuronal networks forming the substrates for physiologic mechanisms involved in hearing.

Cruder responses to various frequencies are primarily the function of the first station, the spiral organ of Corti. The transmission of stimuli from the spiral organ of Corti to the cerebral cortex is far more than just the relaying of neural impulses to the cortex. Fine discrimination of pitch, timbre, intensity of sound, and volume are the products of complex processing and interactions in and among the various nuclear stations in the auditory pathways. *Pitch coding* is in part a function of the combination of neurons stimulated and conducting and the frequency of neural impulses.

Active processing in the nuclei of the auditory pathways accounts for such contrasting expressions as the dampening and even loss of the conscious perception of extraneous background noises and the heightened awareness of sounds demanding attention. The filtering out of background noises and the enhancement and intensification of attention-directing sounds are expressions of the *focusing effect* (*sharpening effect, lateral inhibition, or mutual inhibition*), which is the equivalent of the simultaneous brightness-contrast effect in the visual system (Chap. 12). Theoretically the vibration produced by the flow of blood in the ear should be heard, but it is not. Blood flow can be heard as a hum when we concentrate and tense the jaw muscles, or magnify the sounds with the cupped hand (sea shell) over the ear. Usually these "weak, unheard" vibrations are filtered out, in part, by lateral inhibition in the nuclei of the ascending pathways. In theory, a sound may commence to ascend by several subpathways. The optimal path is sustained and reinforced, and the others are inhibited along the way.

The vestibular system

The information required by the nervous system to control posture and equilibrium is obtained from three afferent sources: the eyes, the general proprioceptive receptors throughout the body, and the vestibular membranous labyrinth. The vestibular system is actually the special proprioceptive system that functions especially to maintain equilibrium, to direct the gaze of the eyes, and to preserve a constant plane of vision (head position), primarily by modifying muscle tone. The specific receptors in the membranous labyrinth that sense the critical stimuli are the *cristae in the ampullae of the semicircular ducts, the macula of the utricle,* and *the macula of the saccule.*

The cristae of the semicircular ducts are organs of *angular acceleration;* they are bidirectional accelerometers monitoring angular acceleration and deceleration, i.e., change in the direction of movements of the head. The macula of the utricle and possibly of the saccule are organs of gravitation; these position recorders respond to *linear acceleration* (i.e., movement of the head in a straight line—forward, backward, up, or down), gravitational forces, and tilting of the head. The role of the macula of the saccule is unknown; destruction of the saccule in animals produces no obvious defects in locomotion or equilibrium. The macula of the saccule may be an organ of vibration monitoring low-frequency vibrations.

VESTIBULAR MEMBRANOUS LABYRINTH

The *three semicircular ducts* are arranged at right angles to one another in the three orthogonal planes, as are the three sides in the corner of a cube (Figs. 10-1, 10-2, and 10-8). The lateral (horizontal) duct is in the horizontal plane when the head is tilted forward at an angle of 30°. The posterior (vertical) duct forms a 55° angle with the midsagittal plane of the head. The inferior (anterior) duct is at right angles to the posterior duct. The lateral ducts of the two ears are in the same plane. The anterior duct of one side is parallel to the posterior duct of the opposite side. Each duct is but 0.1 mm in diameter and 10 to 15 mm long.

The ampulla (1 mm in diameter) of each duct contains the crista ampullaris, which is the sensory receptor. The crista contains hair cells and supporting cells. The cupula, a gelatinous wedge in which the hairs of the hair cells are embedded, acts like a swinging door. The hinge is the crista, and the free-swinging edge of the cupula brushes against the curved wall of the ampulla. Any movement of the endolymph pushes the cupula and consequently bends the hairs, thereby setting up transduction. The semicircular ducts are sensors detecting the movements involved with the change of direction of the head (angular movement or angular rotation) associated with acceleration and deceleration.

The crista of each duct is stimulated by the rotation of the head in its own plane. Although

the hair cells can quickly detect the direction of acceleration by the deflection of the sensory hairs, it takes roughly 15 sec for the velocity of the endolymph to attain that of the ducts. Once the endolymph is rotating at a speed equal to that in the ducts, the endolymph and ducts rotate at similar speeds. The *cupula-endolymph system* acts like a dampened spring-loaded torsion pendulum. The cupula and hairs return to their resting position after acceleration and deceleration ceases when endolymph and ducts move at the same speed. The cristae are especially geared to detect the common *angular movements*—those which are transient and end abruptly. The movement in one directly results in a discharge of a greater number of impulses than in the resting rate, while a movement in the opposite direction results in a discharge of a lesser number of impulses than in the resting rate.

Rotation as slow as 2° per second can be recognized and interpreted as direction. The semicircular ducts do not sense movement at slow uniform speeds, because the duct and the endolymph move at the same rate. During an angular (not straight-line) movement the ducts move with the head, but through inertia the endolymph lags and thereby forces the cupula of the ampulla to bend in a direction opposite to that in which the head moves. When the head stops quickly, the momentum of the endolymph forces the cupula to move in the direction of the original head movement (i.e., to reverse the bend of the hairs). In an analogous situation, a car rider (endolymph) is thrown back in the seat as the car accelerates and is thrown forward when the car suddenly stops. In a specific movement the stimulated crista is the one associated with the duct in the plane of the motion. Endolymph can set up currents if it is warmed or cooled by placing a warm or cold tube in the outer ear. Such caloric tests are used diagnostically to test vestibular function.

A ridge or macula composed of hair cells and supporting cells is the receptor in the utricle and in the saccule. The hairs are embedded in the gelatinous mass containing minute concretions of calcium carbonate and protein (ear dust, otoliths, statoconia, or otoconia) located near the tips of the hairs. The long axis of the macula in the utricle is oriented in the horizontal plane, and that of the macula in the saccule is in a

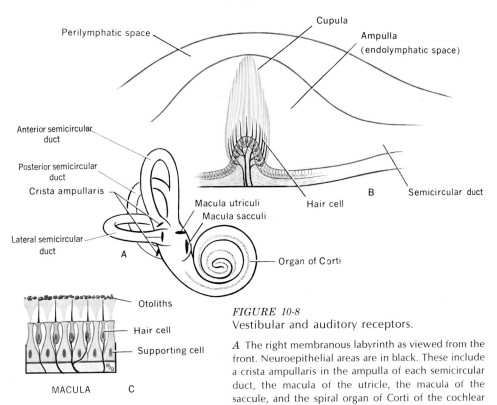

CRISTA AMPULLA

Perilymphatic space

Cupula

Ampulla
(endolymphatic space)

Anterior semicircular
duct

Posterior semicircular
duct

Crista ampullaris

Lateral semicircular
duct

A

Macula utriculi
Macula sacculi

Hair cell

B

Semicircular duct

Organ of Corti

Otoliths

Hair cell

Supporting cell

MACULA   C

FIGURE 10-8
Vestibular and auditory receptors.

A The right membranous labyrinth as viewed from the front. Neuroepithelial areas are in black. These include a crista ampullaris in the ampulla of each semicircular duct, the macula of the utricle, the macula of the saccule, and the spiral organ of Corti of the cochlear duct.

B The crista ampullaris of an ampulla. Note that the free border of the crista is in contact with the wall of the ampulla.

C The macula. Note that the tips of the hairs of the hair cells are in contact with the otoliths embedded in the gelatinous mass.

vertical plane parallel to the sagittal plane and facing laterally. The weight of the otoliths responds to the pull of gravity, thereby bending the hairs of the receptive hair cells. The utricle acts as a plumb line reacting to gravity and to linear (straight-line) acceleration and deceleration, as during a sudden rise or drop in an elevator. When the elevator commences to rise, one automatically flexes the knees; when the elevator commences to drop, one automatically extends the knees. The utricle and saccule are gravity organs that sense these linear phenomena.

The *macula utriculi* is maximally stimulated when the head is bent either forward or backward, and is minimally stimulated when the head is erect. The *macula sacculi* is said to be maximally stimulated when the head is bent to

the side. The utricle and the saccule are not such efficient static sensors in man as they are in other animals. The failure of these sensors to function reliably explains why an airplane pilot, when flying through clouds in a small plane without instruments, may fly upside down without realizing it. The delayed response of a standee in a bus to a sudden stop by the bus has been attributed to the delay of the utricle in registering the deceleration. The vomiting reflex may be initiated by utricular stimulation.

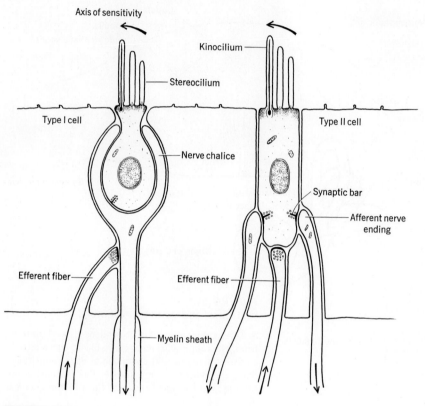

FIGURE 10-9

Schematic drawing of type I and type II vestibular hair cells in the maculae of the saccule and
utricle and in the crista ampullaris of each semicircular duct.

The afferent nerve envelops the hair cell in a cuplike
ending. The axis of sensitivity of a vestibular hair cell
is in the direction of the kinocilium. (*After Wersäll.*)

HAIR CELLS

The hair cells are specialized receptor cells of
vestibular sense organs; they act as transducers
characterized by a high degree of directional
sensitivity, wide dynamic range, and slow adaptation and high sensitivity to mechanical stimulation. Two types of sensory hairs are present in
the hair cells: *stereocilia*, which are modified
microvilli; and *kinocilia*, which are modified

cilia. Each hair cell has about 70 stereocilia
(called sensory hairs) and one kinocilium. The
hairs are arranged in parallel rows. At one side
of the cell is the long kinocilium and the row
of longest sensory hairs; the length of the hairs
in a row decreases successively with increasing
distance from the kinocilium. This is known as
a morphologic polarization. When the hairs deviate toward the kinocilium, the hair cell tends
to depolarize; when they deviate in the opposite
direction, a hyperpolarization of the hair cells
follows.

The vestibular sensory receptors consist of
two types of sensory cells and some supporting
cells (Fig. 10-9). The *sensory cell type I* is a
flask-shaped cell with a round base and constricted neck enclosed by a chalice-shaped
afferent nerve ending. Vestibular efferent fiber

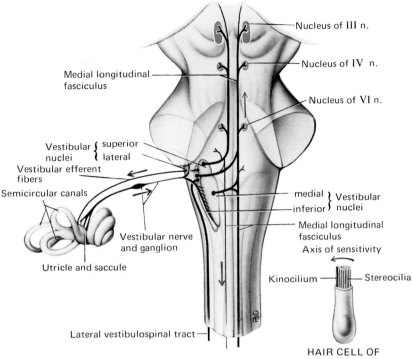

Nucleus of III n.

Nucleus of IV n.

Nucleus of VI n.

Medial longitudinal fasciculus

Vestibular nuclei { superior lateral

Vestibular efferent fibers

Semicircular canals

Vestibular nerve and ganglion

Utricle and saccule

medial } Vestibular
inferior } nuclei

Medial longitudinal fasciculus

Axis of sensitivity

Kinocilium — Stereocilia

Lateral vestibulospinal tract

HAIR CELL OF VESTIBULAR SYSTEM

synapses are associated with the afferent nerve ending.

The *sensory cell type II* is a cylindric columnar cell with a basally located synaptic region. Several afferent and efferent nerve terminals synapse with the hair cell. Within both types of hair cell are synaptic bars, which resemble synaptic ribbons in the retinal neurons. Each vestibular end organ has synaptic connections with both afferent and efferent fibers. With respect to the location of the stereocilia, the kinocilium of each hair cell of the crista ampullaris of the lateral semicircular duct is oriented on the utricle side, while the kinocilium of each hair cell of the anterior and posterior semicircular ducts is oriented toward the semicircular duct (away from the utricle).

VESTIBULAR PATHWAYS

The vestibular tracts consist of suprasegmental pathways that are distributed to the brainstem, spinal cord, and cerebellum (Figs. 10-10 and

FIGURE 10-10
Vestibular pathways comprising the vestibular nerve, vestibular nuclei, medial longitudinal fasciculus, and lateral vestibulospinal tract.

The connections of the vestibular system with the vestibulocerebellum are illustrated in Fig. 9-7.

10-11). The "sensation of dizziness and the associated vague feelings" may be projected via the medial longitudinal fasciculus to the posteromedial ventral nucleus of the thalamus; and finally via thalamocortical fibers to the temporal cortical area just rostral to the auditory cortex, area 41.

The 19,000 nerve fibers of each vestibular nerve have their cell bodies in the vestibular (Scarpa's) ganglion near the membranous labyrinth. The *vestibular ganglion* is divided into the pars superior and pars inferior. The nerves from the receptors of the anterior and lateral semicircular ducts and the utricle have their cell bodies in the pars superior; the nerves from the

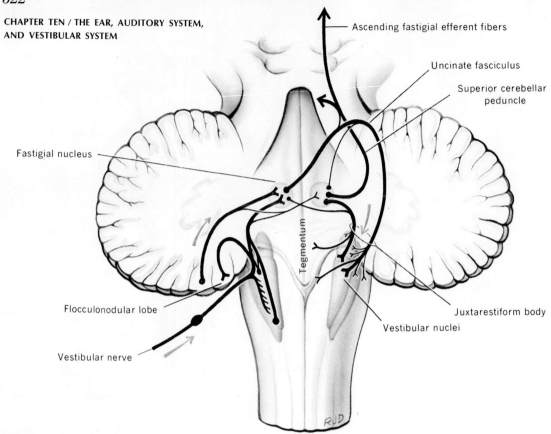

Ascending fastigial efferent fibers

Uncinate fasciculus

Superior cerebellar
peduncle

Fastigial nucleus

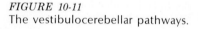

Tegmentum

Flocculonodular lobe

Juxtarestiform body

Vestibular nuclei

Vestibular nerve

FIGURE 10-11
The vestibulocerebellar pathways.

Left, input to the cerebellum; *right,* output from the
cerebellum.

posterior semicircular duct and the saccule have
their cell bodies in the pars inferior.

The primary vestibular fibers from the vestibular nerve pass into the upper medulla deep
to the inferior cerebellar peduncle, bifurcate
into short ascending and descending branches,
and terminate in specific regions in each of the
four vestibular nuclei—lateral, medial, superior,
and inferior—in the upper lateral medulla; and
mainly in the nodule of the archicerebellar cortex (flocculonodular lobe). Although there are
precise anatomic patterns in the cytoarchitecture and in the fiber connections in each of
these vestibular nuclei, the four nuclei may be
considered as a single functioning unit.

The primary vestibular fibers from the cristae
of the semicircular ducts are distributed mainly
to portions of the superior and medial vestibular
nuclei, whereas the primary vestibular fibers
from the maculae of the utricle and saccule
terminate mainly in portions of the medial and
inferior vestibular nuclei. They receive input
primarily from the labyrinth and the archicerebellum. Influences from the fastigial nuclei to
the vestibular nuclei are facilitatory; those from
the cerebellar cortex (vermis and flocculonodular lobe) are inhibitory. The vestibular nuclei
project *secondary vestibular fibers* to *1* the
upper brainstem (pons and midbrain) via the
medial longitudinal fasciculus, *2* cervical spinal
segments via the medial longitudinal fasciculus
(medial vestibulospinal tract), *3* the full length
of the spinal cord via the (lateral) vestibulospinal tract, *4* the archicerebellum and fastigial

nucleus of the cerebellum via the juxtarestiform body (medial part of the inferior cerebellar peduncle), 5 brainstem reticular formation, and 6 hair cells of the maculae and crista of the membranous labyrinth via the vestibular nerve as the vestibular efferent fibers. All contralateral projections from the vestibular nuclei to the medial longitudinal fasciculus decussate at the level of the vestibular nuclei. The *medial longitudinal fasciculus* is composed of many ascending and descending fibers from the vestibular nuclei; this association bundle is important because it conveys influences which integrate the vestibular system with the movements of the eyes, head, and neck.

The ascending vestibular pathway is presumed to project via the magnocellular part of the medial geniculate body (apparent thalamic vestibular processing nucleus) to the "head region" of areas 1 and 3 of the postcentral gyrus of the cerebral cortex.

EYE MOVEMENTS AND THE MEDIAL LONGITUDINAL FASCICULUS

The functional interaction of the vestibular receptors resulting in eye movements is mediated by ascending fibers that project from the vestibular nuclei to the *medial longitudinal fasciculus* of the same and the opposite side and ascend to the midbrain. The superior vestibular nucleus projects ascending uncrossed fibers, the inferior and medial vestibular nuclei project both crossed and uncrossed fibers, and the lateral vestibular nucleus projects largely crossed fibers via the medial longitudinal fasciculus. This pathway is appropriately called the *"vestibulomesencephalic pathway."* Its connections with the nuclei of cranial nerves III, IV, and VI form a basis of many coordinated (conjugate) eye movements. The synchronized movements of both eyes to the side, upward, or downward are mediated by means of this pathway.

Stimulation of the nerve innervating the crista ampullaris of the lateral semicircular duct on one side results in lateral conjugate deviation of the eyes to the contralateral side. For example, facilitatory influences from the left side produce contractions of the lateral rectus muscle of the right eye and the medial rectus muscle of the left eye.

Stimulation of the nerves innervating the cristae ampullaris of both anterior semicircular ducts results in the elevation of both eyes by the contraction of the superior rectus and inferior oblique muscles of both eyes.

Stimulation of the nerves innervating the cristae ampullaris of both posterior semicircular ducts results in the depression of both eyes by the contraction of the superior oblique and inferior rectus muscles of both eyes.

These ocular responses indicate that the vestibular projections to the nuclei of the extraocular muscles are precise. The most potent vestibular projections are directed primarily to horizontal eye movements (lateral and medial recti muscles); the effect of vestibular influences upon the movements of elevation and depression of the eyes are minimal. Each crista seems to have preferential connections with two extraocular muscles.

The *interstitial nucleus of Cajal* and the *nucleus of Darkschewitsch* are midbrain nuclei located in the ventrolateral periaqueductal gray at the level of the oculomotor nucleus. Fibers from the interstitial nucleus of Cajal descend (some cross in the posterior commissure) bilaterally in the medial longitudinal fasciculus; they terminate in the oculomotor, trochlear, and medial vestibular nuclei of the brainstem and in laminae VII and VIII of the spinal cord. Lesions of these nuclei may result in impaired vertical eye movements (elevation and depression). The nucleus of Darkschewitsch, the role of which is unknown, does not project fibers through the medial longitudinal fasciculus.

The phenomenon of nystagmus is related to the imbalance of synchronized impulses from vestibular sources. *Nystagmus* refers to the rhythmic to-and-fro movements of the eyes, with a rapid movement in one direction followed by a slow movement in the opposite direction. This forms the basis for the whirling sensation that follows after rapidly spinning in one direction and suddenly stopping. The impulses from the vestibular source stimulate the eye movements, and the visual impulses from the eyes, in turn, create the conscious spinning sensation (vertigo).

Nystagmus in the normal individual has the following basis. As the head and body pivot and circle, the eyes attempt to fix on an object in space (slow component); as the head and body continue to circle, the eyes snap quickly in the direction in which the head is circling (fast or quick component or compensatory movement). The action is similar to what happens when one is watching telegraph poles from a moving train—the fast component is in the direction in which the train is moving. These eye movements repeat throughout the duration of the circling. By convention, *nystagmus is named by the direction of the fast component.* Following a sudden stop after spinning, the direction of the nystagmus is reversed (postrotatory nystagmus), because the semicircular ducts stop when the head stops, but the endolymph, with its momentum, continues to move, thereby pushing the cupula and hairs of the hair cells in the opposite direction from that of the spin. In relation to the original direction of the spin, the postrotatory nystagmus is associated with the following features: a fast component and the sensation of turning (vertigo or dizziness), which are in the opposite direction; a slow component, tendency to fall, past pointing, and direction of movement of endolymph, which are in the same direction. *Past pointing* is the phenomenon of missing an object when reaching to touch it. The plane in which the head is held during a spin will determine whether the nystagmus is horizontal, oblique, vertical, or rotary.

HEAD AND BODY MOVEMENTS AND THE VESTIBULAR SYSTEM

The vestibular nuclei project crossed and uncrossed fibers (largely from the medial vestibular nucleus and the inferior vestibular nucleus) that descend in the medial longitudinal fasciculus. This pathway, often referred to as the medial vestibulospinal pathway, terminates in the cervical segments of the spinal cord. It conveys influences inhibitory to extensor tonus.

The vestibular nuclei, particularly the lateral vestibular nucleus, project uncrossed fibers to all levels of the spinal cord via the (lateral) vestibulospinal tract which is somatotopically orga-

nized. The dorsocaudal portion of this nucleus projects to lumbosacral spinal levels, and the rostroventral portion to the cervical spinal levels. Some influences from the archicerebellum are directed through the lateral vestibular nucleus to the lateral vestibulospinal tract and to the lower motor neurons in the spinal cord. The lateral vestibular nucleus is regarded as a displaced cerebellar nucleus because, aside from the deep cerebellar nuclei, it is the only nucleus receiving direct input from the Purkinje cells of the cerebellar cortex. This somatic pathway has a role in the muscular activities of the body and extremities associated with postural movements and balance. These vestibulospinal pathways exert facilitatory influences upon extensor tonus through both the alpha and the gamma motor neurons of the spinal nerves. In addition, spinovestibular fibers project ascending influences to the vestibular nuclei from the spinal cord.

VESTIBULAR CONNECTIONS WITH THE CERE-BELLUM AND WITH THE RETICULAR FORMATION

Primary fibers of the vestibular nerve and secondary fibers mainly from the inferior and medial vestibular nuclei pass through the juxta-restiform body (medial portion of the inferior cerebellar peduncle) and course as mossy fibers mainly to the ipsilateral flocculonodular lobe and uvula (Fig. 10-11). The *flocculonodular* lobe and the adjacent cerebellar cortex are often called the *vestibulocerebellum.* In addition, fibers from these vestibular nuclei project to the fastigial nuclei. The maculae of the utricle and saccule are the major source of vestibular input to the cerebellum. Influences from these receptors are conveyed to the inferior and medial vestibular nuclei. The Purkinje cells of the vestibulocerebellum and vermis relay inhibitory influences to the fastigial nuclei and the lateral vestibular nucleus. The fastigial nuclei project fibers conveying excitatory influences to parts of each vestibular nucleus and to the reticular formation (lateral reticular nucleus and nucleus reticularis pontis caudalis). The vestibular nuclei probably receive most of their input from the cerebellum.

The vestibulocerebellum exerts its influences primarily on the coordination of the axial muscles of the neck and vertebral column in balance and posture through *1* the lateral vestibular nucleus and lateral vestibulospinal tract, *2* the medial vestibular nucleus and the medial vestibulospinal tract, and *3* the caudal pontine reticular nucleus and the pontine reticulospinal tract. Collateral fibers from the vestibular pathway system to the pontine and medullary reticular formation are integrated into the activities of the reticular system. These connections to the reticular formation may be involved in producing the nausea, vomiting, and sweating which result from stimulation of the vestibular system.

VESTIBULAR EFFERENT PATHWAY TO THE MEMBRANOUS LABYRINTH

Efferent fibers from the brainstem pass through the vestibular nerve and terminate in the vestibular receptors of the membranous labyrinth. The nuclei of origin and the role of these vestibular efferent fibers are controversial. They may arise from cells in the reticular formation and vestibular nuclei. Some fibers terminate directly on sensory cells type II and on the afferent fibers innervating sensory cells type I (Fig. 10-9). These fibers are similar to the efferent fibers of other systems, including the cochlear efferent fibers. These vestibular efferent neurons probably exert inhibitory influences and ameliorate the effects of motion sickness and its aftersensations and nystagmus.

FUNCTIONAL FEATURES OF THE VESTIBULAR SYSTEM

The influences from the labyrinth have significant roles in the maintenance of head and neck position and body posture. The tightrope walker relies on vestibular and other proprioceptive cues to sustain his performance. A cat held up in the air, back down and feet up, turns with incredible speed and lands on his feet when dropped. Labyrinthine activity is critical to this complex maneuver. When the cat is released, its neck musculature reacts to vestibular stimulation by twisting the head to the normal position of eyes parallel to the ground. Differential tension is now exerted on the neck muscles of the two sides. The resulting proprioceptive imbalance of these muscles sends impulses that activate the spinal reflexes that twist the trunk to its normal relation with the neck. The se-

quence repeats, and finally the hindquarters are properly positioned. The rapid sequence from head to tail is initiated by the vestibular sensors. A falling man does not respond so rapidly nor so deftly. We utilize the less effective cues from the visual and the proprioceptive receptors for our righting reflexes. A cat can right himself by utilizing vestibular cues or visual cues exclusively.

Labyrinth activity is integrated into many natural postures, actions, and positions, as seen in the boxer's pose, with the left arm and forearm partially flexed, the right upper extremity cocked and forearm partially flexed, left thigh and both legs partially flexed, and the right thigh partially extended; the performance of the high diver, who utilizes the position and movements of his head and neck as the key to his dive, the rest of his body following naturally; or the coordination of a runner or marcher, who uses all four extremities rhythmically.

Vertigo dizziness or the sensation associated with lack of equilibrium involves the subjective sense of rotation, either of the surroundings or of the person. It is a cardinal sign of labyrinthine and vestibular dysfunction. Vertigo may occur in the normal subject; excessive stimulation of the semicircular ducts gives the sensation of vertigo, with objects appearing to move in a circular pattern because of compensatory movements of the eyes (nystagmus). In vestibular disease nystagmus occurs; it is a consequence of influences conveyed from the vestibular system via the medial longitudinal fasciculus to the extraocular muscles.

The pirouetting ballet dancer prevents vertigo by periodically snapping her head as she breaks up, as far as her head is concerned, the continuous movement of the spin. This minimizes the flow of the endolymph. In addition she learns to compensate by practice, and completes the pirouette by coming to a broad-based stance.

Dizziness, headache, nausea, and vomiting are symptoms of motion sickness (seasickness, carsickness, and airsickness). *Motion sickness* is primarily due to the excessive stimulation of the utricle and saccule. The vestibulocerebellar projections are involved; following the removal of the flocculonodular lobe, experimental animals do not show evidence of motion sickness. The conflict of sensory cues from the labyrinth, the body, and the eye may contribute. Deaf-mutes, who lack labyrinthine receptors, do not experience motion sickness. Drugs like Dramamine raise the threshold of vestibular stimulation and thereby help to prevent motion sickness. Because the labyrinth is not functional during the first year of life, infants do not get motion sickness.

Ménière's disease is a disorder probably resulting from an abnormal circulation of the vestibular endolymph. *Tinnitus* (ringing in the ear), violent attacks of vertigo, pallor, vomiting, nausea, and increased respiration occur. The cristae ampullaris are entirely normal. Symptoms of Ménière's disease may be partially alleviated by pharmaceutic agents that block motion sickness.

Man is not so dependent on his vestibular system as on his visual and general proprioceptive systems. Injury to the labyrinths, the vestibular nuclei, or the vestibular pathways may result in nystagmus, tendency to fall to one side, past pointing, and some difficulty in maintaining erect posture. However, these symptoms will attenuate and finally disappear as other proprioceptive cues are more fully utilized. Astronauts experience motion sickness, including nausea, dizziness, and unsteadiness, during the first few days of exposure to the weightlessness of outer space, and again for a few days after returning to earth and its gravitational forces.

Loss of both labyrinths is not followed by vertigo or nystagmus. Normal locomotion and posture will then require the utilization of visual cues. The difficulties of walking and performing postural movements will lessen with time, but walking, for example, will always be accomplished with a broad base. A swimmer who has lost the use of his labyrinths may navigate down instead of up to reach the surface unless he receives adequate visual cues.

Bibliography

Békésy, G. von: *Experiments in Hearing*. McGraw-Hill Book Company, New York, 1960.

Brodal, A., O. Pompeiano, and F. Walberg: *The Vestibular Nuclei and Their Connections, Anatomy and Functional Correlations*. Charles C Thomas, Publisher, Springfield, Ill., 1962.

De Reuck, A. V. S., and J. Knight (eds.): *Hearing Mechanisms in Vertebrates*, Ciba Foundation Symposium. Little, Brown and Company, Boston, 1968.

Engström, H., H. Ades, and A. Anderson: *Structural Pattern of the Organ of Corti*. Almqvist and Wiksell, Stockholm, 1966.

Fields, W., and B. Alvord (eds.): *Neurological Aspects of Auditory and Vestibular Disorders*. Charles C Thomas, Publisher, Springfield, Ill., 1964.

Iurato, S. (ed.): *Submicroscopic Structure of the Inner Ear*. Pergamon Press, New York, 1967.

Lim, D. J.: Fine morphology of the tectorial membrane: Its relationship to the organ of Corti. Arch. Otolaryngol., 96:199–215, 1972.

Moskowitz, N.: Comparative aspects of some features of the central auditory system of primates, in J. M. Petras and C. Noback (eds.), Comparative and Evolutionary Aspects of the Vertebrate Central Nervous System. Ann. N.Y. Acad. Sci., 167:357–369, 1969.

Rasmussen, G. L., and W. F. Windle (eds.): *Neural Mechanisms of the Auditory and Vestibular Systems*. Charles C Thomas, Publisher, Springfield, Ill., 1961.

Spoendlin, H.: The innervation of the organ of Corti. J. Laryngol., 81:717–738, 1967.

Stein, B. M., and M. B. Carpenter: Central projections of portions of the vestibular ganglia innervating specific parts of the labyrinth in the rhesus monkey. Am. J. Anat., 120:281–318, 1967.

Strominger, N. L.: The origins, course and distribution of the dorsal and intermediate acoustic striae in the rhesus monkey. J. Comp. Neurol., 147:209–234, 1973.

Tonndorf, J.: Cochlear mechanics and hydrodynamics, in J. V. Tobias (ed.), *Foundations of Modern Auditory Theory*, vol. 1, pp. 203–254. Academic Press, Inc., New York, 1970.

——— and S. M. Khanna: Submicroscopic displacement amplitudes of the tympanic membrane (cat) measured by a laser interferometer. J. Acoust. Soc. Am., 44:1546–1554, 1968.

Whitfield, I. C.: *The Auditory Pathway*. The Williams & Wilkins Company, Baltimore, 1967.

Wilson, V. J.: Physiological pathways through the vestibular nuclei. Int. Rev. Neurobiol., 15:27–82, 1972.

CHAPTER **11**
HYPOTHALAMUS

Location and general function

The hypothalamus is the phylogenetically ancient region which forms the base of the diencephalon. It is flanked medially by the third ventricle and laterally by the subthalamus. It is bordered rostrally by the lamina terminalis, dorsally by the anterior commissure and the hypothalamic sulcus (which extends from the interventricular foramen of Monro to the cerebral aqueduct of Sylvius), and caudally by the midbrain. Its ventral part consists (from the rostral aspect to the caudal) of the preoptic region, optic chiasma, median eminence, hypophysis, tuber cinereum, and the mamillary bodies (Fig. 11-1). The median eminence is a subdivision of the tuber cinereum.

The hypothalamus has a vast array of functional correlates in both the visceral and the somatic sphere in its mere 4-Gm mass. It functions in two broad areas: the maintenance of a relatively constant internal body environment (homeostasis), and behavior patterns. For example, the hypothalamus has *1* a homeostatic role in the regulation of body temperature, and *2* a role in behavioral expressions ranging from calm to rage and in such feeling patterns as hunger, thirst, and sexual affect.

Neuroanatomy of the hypothalamus

NUCLEI OF THE HYPOTHALAMUS

The *hypothalamus* may be anatomically divided into four areas, arranged from the lamina terminalis to the midbrain: the *preoptic area* (telencephalic portion), the *supraoptic area* dorsal to the optic chiasma, the *tuberal area* dorsal to the tuber cinereum, and the *mamillary area* dorsal to and including the mamillary bodies.

Each area may be schematically subdivided into three zones of nuclei arranged mediolaterally into *a* the *periventricular zone* adjacent to the third ventricle, *b* the *medial zone,* and *c* the *lateral zone.* In the following schema the letters *a, b,* and *c* correspond to the zones as lettered above; only some of the hypothalamic nuclei in these zones are noted. The *preoptic area* includes *a* the periventricular zone, *b* the medial preoptic zone, and *c* the lateral preoptic zone. The *supraoptic area* includes *a* the periventricular zone, *b* the paraventricular nucleus and other nuclei of the medial hypothalamic zone, and *c* the supraoptic nucleus and other nuclei of the lateral hypothalamic zone. The *tuberal (infundibular) area* includes *a* the periventricular zone, *b* the dorsal medial and the ventral medial nuclei, and *c* the nuclei of the lateral zone. The *mamillary area* includes *a* the periventricular zone, *b* the nuclei of the mamillary body, and the posterior hypothalamic zone, and *c* the lateral hypothalamic zone.

BASIC CIRCUITS OF THE HYPOTHALAMUS

General The neural circuits associated with the hypothalamus are numerous and complex. The named fiber pathways have reciprocal connections with widespread regions of the cerebrum and the brainstem. These intricate interrelations, in which are intercalated numerous synaptic stations, are consistent with the multifaceted functions of the hypothalamus. In addition, extensive intrahypothalamic connections exist.

In general, the hypothalamus is thought of as deriving its major input either directly or indirectly from the nonspecific reticular system and little, if any, input from the specific lemniscal system (Chap. 8). The sites of hypothalamic input and output include the brainstem reticular

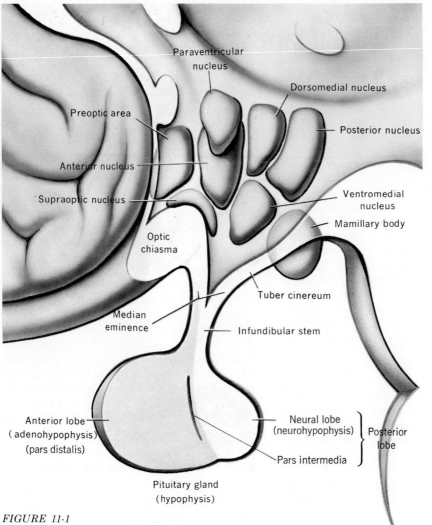

Paraventricular
nucleus

Dorsomedial nucleus

Preoptic area

Posterior nucleus

Anterior nucleus

Supraoptic nucleus

Ventromedial
nucleus

Mamillary body

Optic
chiasma

Tuber cinereum

Median
eminence

Infundibular stem

Anterior lobe
(adenohypophysis)
(pars distalis)

Neural lobe
(neurohypophysis)

Posterior
lobe

Pars intermedia

Pituitary gland
(hypophysis)

FIGURE 11-1
Some hypothalamic nuclei and the hypophysis.

The hypothalamus is composed of four nuclear areas: *1* nuclei of the preoptic area (telencephalic region); *2* nuclei of the supraoptic or anterior area, including the paraventricular nucleus, anterior nucleus, and supraoptic nucleus; *3* nuclei of the tuberal or middle area, including the dorsomedial and ventromedial nuclei; and *4* nuclei of the mamillary or posterior area, including the posterior nucleus and the mamillary body.

formation, the limbic lobe (including the hippocampus and the amygdaloid body), neocortex, thalamus, and the olfactory system. Significant neural and vascular connections are made with the hypophysis.

Many of the basic anatomic features of the hypothalamus (e.g., isodendritic neurons) are similar to those of the brainstem reticular formation. Thus the hypothalamus is considered to

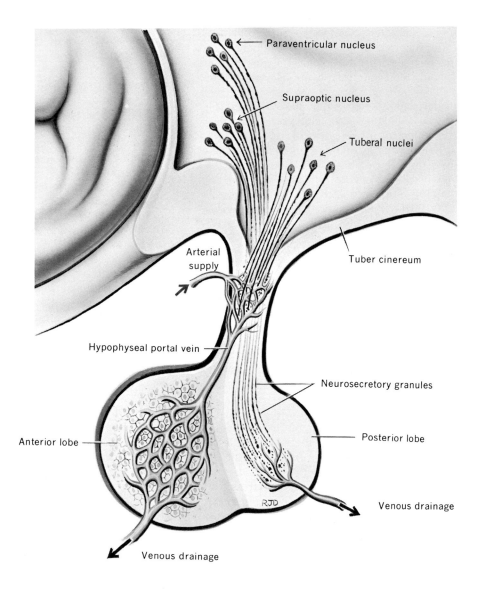

Paraventricular nucleus

Supraoptic nucleus

Tuberal nuclei

Arterial supply

Tuber cinereum

Hypophyseal portal vein

Neurosecretory granules

Anterior lobe

Posterior lobe

Venous drainage

RJD

Venous drainage

FIGURE 11-2

The hypothalamohypophyseal tract and the hypophyseal portal vein.

Neurosecretions are transported via nerve fibers of the hypothalamohypophyseal tract from the supraoptic and paraventricular nuclei to the posterior lobe of the hypophysis; they are conveyed from this lobe via the bloodstream. Other neurosecretions, elaborated in other hypothalamic nuclei, are conveyed via the hypophyseal portal vein to the anterior lobe of the hypophysis.

thalamus (a few fibers from the retina may also project to the hypothalamus). The input from the olfactory system to the hypothalamus is not involved with the subjective interpretation of odors but rather with behavior and emotional expression (Chaps. 6 and 15).

c Fibers from the orbitofrontal neocortex (cortico-hypothalamic fibers) and septal nuclei may pass along with the medial forebrain bundle to the lateral hypothalamus (Fig. 11-4).

be a rostral extension of the reticular formation, especially that of the medial midbrain tegmentum and the periaqueductal gray matter. The preoptic area of the hypothalamus and the septal regions of the telencephalon are the most rostral extensions of the reticular formation. This may be called the septopreoptico-hypothalamic component of the reticular formation.

Most of the ascending sensory input is derived from the multisynaptic pathways of the mesencephalic reticular formation and from the thalamic reticular nuclei (tegmentohypothalamic pathways, medial forebrain bundle, dorsal longitudinal fasciculus, and thalamohypothalamic pathways). The major fiber connections with the limbic lobe are mediated through the median forebrain bundle, fornix system, and stria terminalis pathway (Chap. 15). The influences from the neocortex are relayed either directly to the hypothalamus or indirectly via the limbic lobe or the thalamus.

The effector role of the hypothalamus is mediated via neural pathways and via endocrine (humoral, hormonal, or neurosecretory) agents. The pathways of the autonomic nervous system (primarily) and the somatic motor system are both instrumental in the expression of hypothalamic activity. Behavioral and psychic manifestations are mediated via the pathways to the limbic lobe and neocortex. The neurosecretions elaborated in the hypothalamus are the humoral agents that influence *1* the anterior lobe of the hypophysis (pituitary gland) via the hypophyseal (hypothalamic-hypophyseal) portal blood vessels (Figs. 11-2, 11-3); and *2* the neurohypophysis via the supraopticohypophyseal pathways (Figs. 11-2, 11-3).

In brief, the hypothalamus is strategically located between the cerebrum and the brainstem and spinal cord.

PATHWAYS OF THE HYPOTHALAMUS

Input (Fig. 11-4) The *input to the hypothalamus* is conveyed via *1* ascending fibers from the brainstem tegmentum and periaqueductal gray matter, *2* descending fibers from the forebrain, and *3* other sources. Most of these fibers are

accompanied by fibers projecting influences in the opposite direction. These fiber groups are thus reciprocally directed.

1 The *ascending fibers from the brainstem to the hypothalamus* include the following: fibers originating in the dorsal and ventral tegmental nuclei pass in the mamillary peduncle to the lateral mamillary nucleus; fibers originating in the periaqueductal gray matter pass in the dorsal longitudinal fasciculus of Schütz to several hypothalamic nuclei; fibers originating in the midbrain tegmentum pass in the medial forebrain bundle to the lateral hypothalamus; and the ascending catecholamine pathways (Chap. 8) and fibers from a number of brainstem tegmental and raphe nuclei (Fig. 8-12).

The *input to these brainstem tegmental nuclei and the periaqueductal gray matter* is derived from *a* cerebral levels largely through descending fibers accompanying the ascending fibers (reciprocal connections), and *b* ascending fibers from the nuclei of the lower brainstem tegmentum (ascending reticular pathways). In turn, these pontine and medullary reticular nuclei receive their input from *a* spinal levels via spinoreticular fibers and collaterals of the spinothalamic tract, and *b* brainstem levels via cranial nerves and their nuclei. Many ascending signals from the nucleus solitarius are relayed to the hypothalamus.

2 The *descending fibers from the forebrain* include:

a Fibers of the fornix originating in the hippocampus and the septal nuclei of the limbic system and terminating in the medial hypothalamus (preoptic region, anterior hypothalamus, and medial mamillary nucleus). The hippocampus is a significant channel for sensory and neocortical input to the hypothalamus (Fig. 11-4).

b The olfactory system is the only sensory system with relatively direct access to the hypothalamus; influences are relayed primarily from the amygdaloid body and the primary olfactory cortex (Chapter 15). Fibers from the pyriform cortex, olfactory tubercle, and amygdaloid body project to the medial hypothalamus via the stria terminalis and ventral amygdalofugal pathway (Figs. 11-4, 15-3). Influences from the primary olfactory cortex project to the lateral hypothalamus indirectly via the medial forebrain bundle.

c The septal nuclei and area are sources of input to the hypothalamus (Fig. 11-4).

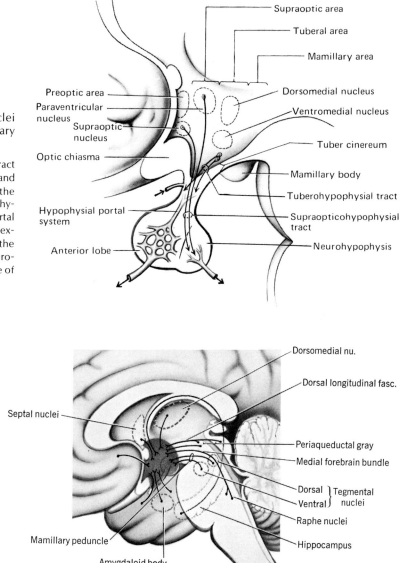

FIGURE 11-3
Some hypothalamic nuclei and the hypophysis (pituitary gland).

The supraopticohypophyseal tract extends from the supraoptic and paraventricular nucleus to the capillary bed of the neurohypophysis. The hypophyseal portal system is a vascular network extending from the base of the hypothalamus and upper neurohypophysis to the anterior lobe of the hypophysis.

FIGURE 11-4
The major tracts conveying input to the hypothalamus.

d Some thalamohypothalamic fibers from the magnocellular portion of the dorsomedial nucleus and midline thalamic nuclei pass to the lateral hypothalamus and rostral portions of the amygdaloid body. (The dorsomedial nucleus has reciprocal connections with the prefrontal neocortex.) The several possible routes from the neocortex to the hypothalamus are important as the channels by which the affective states of one's being can elicit the unconscious autonomic responses and endocrine activities.

3 The *blood vascular system* conveys influences to which the hypothalamus may respond. These include hormones, temperature of the blood, and osmolality of the blood plasma.

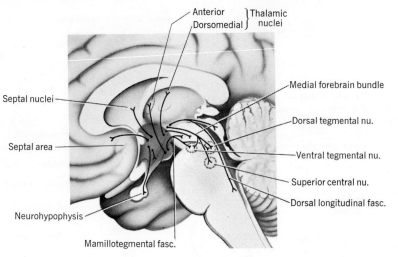

Septal nuclei

Medial forebrain bundle

Septal area

Dorsal tegmental nu.

Ventral tegmental nu.

Superior central nu.

Neurohypophysis

Dorsal longitudinal fasc.

Mamillotegmental fasc.

FIGURE 11-5
The major tracts convey-
ing output from the hypo-
thalamus.

Output (Fig. 11-5) The *output from the hypothalamus* is conveyed via *1* ascending fibers to
the forebrain, *2* descending fibers to the midbrain, and *3* pathways of fibers and blood vessels to the hypophysis (endocrine effector projections).

1 The *ascending fibers from the hypothalamus
to the forebrain* include the following: *a* Fibers
originating from the lateral hypothalamus pass
with the medial forebrain bundle to the septal
region, septal nuclei, and olfactory tubercle.
These fibers are integrated in the limbic pathways (Chap. 15). *b* Fibers originating from the
medial mamillary nucleus course via the mamillothalamic tract to the anterior thalamic nuclear
group. Reciprocally connecting fibers are included in this tract, which is a link in the so-
called Papez circuit of the limbic pathways
(Chap. 15, Fig. 15-4). *c* Several hypothalamic
nuclei are reciprocally connected via periventricular fibers with the magnocellular portion of the dorsomedial thalamic nucleus. This
suggests a functional relation to the prefrontal
cortex (Chap. 16), which has reciprocal connections with the parvocellular portion of the dorsomedial nucleus.

2 The *descending fibers from the hypothalamus
to the midbrain* are paralleled by ascending
fibers as reciprocally connecting pathways.
Some of these fibers are incorporated in the
pathways of the limbic system, discussed in
Chap. 15. Many of these descending fibers are
the significant links in the activity of the autonomic nervous system. In general, the medial
hypothalamic system is involved through the
hypophysis with neuroendocrine functions. The
lateral hypothalamic system and its major pathway, the medial forebrain bundle, are associated
with visceral (autonomic nervous system) and
somatic (somatic nervous system) responses.
This lateral system is interconnected with the
medial system.

Fibers originating in the lateral hypothalamic
form the medial forebrain bundle, which terminates primarily in paramedian cell groups of the
midbrain tegmentum (limbic midbrain area of
Nauta), and in several mesencephalic raphe
nuclei—superior central nucleus and the dorsal
and ventral tegmental nuclei. The fibers of the
mamillotegmental fasciculus from the mamillary
bodies descend in the midbrain tegmentum and
terminate in the dorsal and ventral tegmental
nuclei. Some fibers terminate in the lateral mid-

brain tegmentum. These descending hypothalamic pathways are the most rostral links conveying hypothalamic influences to the peripheral neurons of the autonomic nervous system. Interneurons convey influences to the accessory oculomotor nucleus. A second link in this descending autonomic pathway extends from these mesencephalic nuclei to the rhombencephalic tegmentum, which contains the nuclei of origin of the pontine reticulospinal and medullary reticulospinal tracts. These are the third in the chain of linkages to the interneurons of the spinal gray matter which synapse with the preganglionic autonomic neurons.

The medial hypothalamus is interconnected by reciprocally connected fibers of the dorsal longitudinal fasciculus of Schütz with the ventral half of the periaqueductal gray matter of the midbrain and the dorsal tegmental nucleus. From this mesencephalic source, other fibers convey influences caudally to rhombencephalic reticular nuclei and, probably, to such parasympathetic nuclei as the dorsal vagal nucleus and the superior and inferior salivatory nuclei of the seventh, ninth, and tenth cranial nerves.

3 Neurons in the medial basal hypothalamus, including the median eminence, apparently synthesize neurohormones called *hypothalamic releasing hormones* (RH) or releasing factors. These neurohormones are transported from the cell bodies in the tuber cinereum as neurosecretory substances via axons of the so-called *tuberohypophyseal tract* (*tuberoinfundibular tract*), which terminates in pericapillary loops in the median eminence and the infundibular stem. This region is known as the *hypophysiotropic* or *neurohaemal area*, where the neurally derived hypothalamic releasing hormones are released and transferred to the *hypophyseal portal system.*

The hypophysiotropic area and the hypophysis receives its blood supply from several arteries. A pair of *inferior hypophyseal arteries* from the internal carotid arteries furnishes the blood supply to the neurohypophysis (neural lobe, infundibular process) and, to a lesser degree, to the sinusoids of the anterior lobe. Several *superior hypophyseal arteries* from each internal carotid artery and posterior communicating artery of the circle of Willis form a capillary plexus in the pars tuberalis, median eminence, and infundibular stem (Fig. 11-3). This *capillary plexus* collects into the hypophyseal portal veins, which, in turn, arborize into the sinusoidal capillary plexus of the pars anterior. In essence, these portal veins are intercalated between the capillaries of the former and the sinusoidal capillaries of the latter. Functionally, this *hypophyseal portal system* is the neurovascular bridge or link between the hypothalamus of the brain and the pars anterior of the hypophysis, an endocrine gland. This portal system forms a conduit by which hypothalamic releasing hormones (hypophysiotropins, hypophysiotropic factors) are conveyed from the tuber cinereum and infundibular stem to the anterior lobe of the hypophysis. The *venous drainage* of the pars anterior and pars nervosa is via hypophyseal veins that drain into the cavernous sinus.

The hypophyseal portal system is the vascular pathway through which the neural language from the hypophysiotropic area, in the form of releasing hormones (RH) is transferred and conveyed to the pars anterior to trigger the endocrine language of the pituitary gland. More specifically, the hypothalamic nerve fibers of different types liberate the releasing hormones from these nerve endings into the capillary plexuses of the median eminence and infundibular stem; these hormones are conveyed through the hypophyseal portal vessels to the adenohypophysis, where they stimulate or inhibit the release of a number of the hypophyseal hormones. The *hypothalamic hormones* known to control the release of pituitary hormones include corticotropin RH, thyrotropin RH, leuteinizing hormone RH, follicle-stimulating hormone RH, growth hormone RH, prolactin RH, and melanocyte-stimulating hormone RH. Other hormones include the growth hormone (release)-inhibiting hormone, prolactin (release)-inhibiting hormone, and melanocyte-stimulating hormone (release)-inhibiting hormones.

The *hypothalamic-hypophyseal* (*supraoptico-hypophyseal*) *tract* is a bundle of about 50,000 to 100,000 unmyelinated fibers originating in the supraoptic and paraventricular nuclei of the hypothalamus. Its fibers pass through the median eminence and infundibular stalk and terminate in palisades around the capillaries of the neurohypophysis. The cells of these nuclei are neurosecretory cells, which synthesize the neurohypophyseal hormones *oxytocin* and *vasopressin* (*antidiuretic hormone, ADH*). These hormones are incorporated into dense-core vesicles, which are transported down the axonal fibers by *axoplasmatic flow* to the nerve endings. The neurosecretory material accumulates within the axoplasm of these fibers as the so-called *Herring bodies*. These axon terminals contain granules about 2,000 Å in diameter and synaptic-like vesicles about 400 Å in diameter. The *vasopressin* and oxytocin are probably formed in the supraoptic and paraventricular nuclei. The neurohypophysis serves as both a storage and release center for these hormones. They pass through the neurolemma, perivascular space, and fenestrated endothelium into the capillaries, which drain into the systemic circulation. Evidence indicates that vasopressin is also released into the hypophyseal portal system and conveyed to the pars anterior where it exerts an influence on the activity of this gland.

REFLEX ARCS OF THE HYPOTHALAMUS

The hypothalamus is integrated into a number of complex reflex arcs, many of which vary considerably from the classic reflex arcs. Several examples follow.

Neural reflex arc utilizing a peripheral receptor
To perform its role as a modulator of the rate of the heartbeat, the hypothalamus utilizes the classic reflex arc patterns. The peripheral receptors in the carotid sinus and the aorta (Chap. 6) relay stimuli via the glossopharyngeal nerve and brainstem tegmentum to the hypothalamus, which in turn projects efferent impulses to the cardiovascular centers in the medulla and eventually by the vagus nerve (autonomic nervous system) to the heart.

Neural reflex arc utilizing an intrinsic hypothalamic receptor
To permit the hypothalamus to perform in its role as the integrator of body temperature, an intrinsic receptor within the hypothalamus monitors the temperature of the blood flowing through the capillaries of the hypothalamus itself. The efferent arms of this arc include *1* descending autonomic pathways to the sweat glands and peripheral blood vessels, and *2* descending somatic pathways to the trunk musculature (used in panting).

Neurohumoral reflex
This arc utilizes both the *nervous system* (*neuro-*) and the *blood vascular system* (*humoral*). To perform its role in water metabolism, the hypothalamus utilizes an intrinsic hypothalamic receptor to monitor the osmotic pressure of the blood flowing through the brain. This receptor is stimulated to put forth a neurosecretion which is conveyed via the neural pathways to the neurohypophysis, where it is released into the blood system and conveyed to its target structures in the kidney. Further examples of this type of reflex arc are noted further on in this chapter under "Hypothalamus and the Hypophysis."

In the analyses of the functional roles of the hypothalamus below, it should be borne in mind that the reflex arcs are integrated into negative-feedback, closed-loop servomechanisms (Chap. 3). The nervous system and the endocrine system have reciprocal interrelationships. Not only does the nervous system modify the functional activities of the endocrine glands, but the endocrine system, acting through the hormones in the blood circulation, influences the nervous system. This effect of the endocrine system on the nervous system may be expressed through both *1* the secretory activity of the hypophysis, and *2* the behavioral patterns of the animal. For example, female sex hormones in the bloodstream may act upon hypothalamic receptors, which, in turn, "secrete" pituitary-releasing hormones (factors) into the hypophyseal portal system. These factors influence the secretory activity of the anterior lobe of the hypophysis. When the blood titer of a sex hormone is elevated, the reacting hypothalamus can act to depress the secretion of gonadotropic hormones by the hypophysis; when the titer is low, the hypothalamus can act to elevate the secretion of gonadotropic hormones. The seasonal behavioral activity of mammals "in heat" or "in rut" appears to be determined, at least in part, by the response of the central nervous system to the stimulation of gonadal hormones.

Functional role of the hypothalamus

HYPOTHALAMUS AND THE AUTONOMIC NERVOUS SYSTEM

The hypothalamus has a significant role in the regulation of autonomic activities. Essentially it acts as a modulator (Chap. 3), influencing the autonomic centers in the brainstem and spinal cord. For example, anxiety generates neocortical activity that may be projected to the hypothalamus. In turn, the hypothalamic output to the cardiovascular integrative center in the medulla has a modulatory effect which may increase the rate and force of the heartbeat and raise the blood pressure.

The anterior (anterolateral) hypothalamus has an excitatory parasympathetic (inhibitory to sympathetic activity) role. The stimulation of this region may produce a decrease in the force and rate of the heartbeat, decrease of the blood pressure, dilatation of the visceral blood vessels, increase in peristalsis and digestive juice secretion in the alimentary canal, constriction of the pupil of the eyes, sweating, and increased salivation. Activity in this region produces a *parasympathetic (vagal) tone.* As a consequence, lesions of this region often result in the production of sympathetic effects. Stimulation may also produce somatic responses such as panting (increased activity of the voluntary muscles of the chest).

The posterior (posteromedial) hypothalamus has an excitatory sympathetic role. The stimulation of this region may produce an increase in the force and rate of the heartbeat, increase in blood pressure, decrease in peristalsis and in secretion of digestive juices into the alimentary canal, dilation of the pupil, and erection of hair. Stimulation of this region often results in the production of a *sympathetic tone.* A lesion in this region may reduce both the sympathetic and parasympathetic effects of the hypothalamus upon other centers, because in addition to

destroying the hypothalamic "sympathetic" centers, the lesion interrupts the caudally projecting pathways from the "parasympathetic" centers. In addition, stimulation of the posterior hypothalamus may produce such somatic activities as shivering, running, and struggling.

Vertebrates, including man, may have a small pathway of retinohypothalamic fibers which convey information from the retina to the hypothalamus. Through this pathway, influences from light stimulation exert a physiologic role in the activity of the hypothalamus and the hypophysis (*photoneuroendocrine system*), especially in nonmammalian vertebrates. In many lower vertebrates, differences in light intensity, acting through this pathway, may alter the degree of pigmentation in the skin through the melanophore pigment cells. In man and mammals the precise role of this pathway is obscure. Evidence suggests that this pathway may have a role in some of the metabolic activities of the organism (e.g., light may influence water balance and carbohydrate balance). The daily cycle of light and dark and the seasonal variations of this daily cycle may exert a role on the reproductive cycle. Drastic experimental modification of the light and dark environment of rats may produce demonstrable changes in their estrous cycles, uteri, ovaries, hormonal levels, sexual drives, and psychic behavioral patterns. The diurnal light-dark rhythm of the environment ("external clock") may thus act through the eye, the hypothalamicohypophyseal system, and the hypothalamicoautonomic system to correlate some internal cycles ("internal clocks," circadian systems). Other aspects of this subject are noted later on in the chapter, under "Pineal Body."

HYPOTHALAMUS AND TEMPERATURE REGULATION

The hypothalamus has an essential role in the maintenance of body temperature within the narrow ranges vital to warm-blooded animals. Impairment of hypothalamic activity may give rise to either a hyperthermia (hyperpyrexia) or a hypothermia, because the hypothalamus contains the integration center for the homeostatic regulation of temperature. More specifically, the hypothalamus houses the thermal receptors that monitor the blood temperature and the *thermostat* that regulates the heat-producing and the heat-conserving control systems. Thermal receptors may be located in the preoptic area. The specific function of the hypothalamus is to utilize its monitor for making the continual fine adjustments which maintain a constant body temperature. In addition the cerebral cortex (conscious recognition), after processing the environmental information from peripheral sensors in the skin, for example, operates to effect crude adjustments against environmental heat and cold (use of clothes, furnaces, and air conditioners).

The anterior hypothalamus contains a region which acts to prevent a rise in body temperature. It operates to activate those processes which favor heat loss, including vasodilatation of cutaneous blood vessels, sweating (evaporation of water for cooling), and panting. Destruction of the "heat-dissipating region" may result in a highly elevated body temperature (hyperthermia). Animals with this condition may survive in a cold environment, for they can then dissipate excess heat; however, they are hyperthermic in normal and warm environments. An animal with a lesion in the rostral hypothalamus cannot lose heat efficiently; death may result from hyperthermia even at room temperature.

The posterior hypothalamus contains a region which triggers those activities concerned with heat production and heat conservation. These include the metabolic heat-producing systems (oxidation of glucose), vasoconstriction especially of cutaneous blood vessels, erection of hair (goose pimples), and shivering. Destruction of this region may produce a cold-blooded mammal (poikilothermic) that cannot sustain a uniform body temperature. Such a lesion destroys not only the heat-conservation center but also the caudally projecting pathways from the heat-dissipating center.

Pyrogenic substances produced in some diseases affect the hypothalamus. A fever, known as *neurogenic hyperthermia*, results.

HYPOTHALAMUS AND FEEDING RESPONSES

The primitive drive to ingest food for the survival of the organism is generally associated with true hunger. A more sophisticated urge to ingest food is called *appetite*, which is a drive regulated largely by the cerebral cortex. Appetite does not necessarily have any relationship to the need for food for survival. The stimulus for appetite comes from such diverse sources as stomach distention, glucose concentration in the blood, and such psychic associations as the smell, sight, and taste of food.

The hypothalamic region involved with feeding responses has been called the *appestat*, with the ventral medial hypothalamic nucleus called the *satiety center* and the lateral hypothalamic nucleus called the *hunger, or feeding center.* Stimulation of the ventral median nucleus inhibits the animal's urge to eat. Destruction of this nucleus produces an animal exhibiting decreased physical activity and a voracious appetite (not true hunger) with a two- to three-fold increase in food intake. The animal becomes excessively obese. Stimulation of the lateral hypothalamic nucleus induces the animal to eat, whereas its destruction produces an animal that refuses to eat until severe emaciation or death from starvation ensues.

These hypothalamic nuclei apparently respond to the blood glucose levels. When the level is low, the hypothalamus discharges impulses to the brainstem. Such responses as salivation, gastric contractions, chewing motion, and swallowing reflexes follow. Stimuli from the cerebrum (orbital cortex, hippocampus, and amygdaloid body) to the hypothalamus influence feeding responses. Animals with lesions in the postorbital cortex have a low food intake; those with frontal lobe lesions may have an increased food intake. Animals with small lesions of the amygdaloid body may experience transient aphagia; those with large lesions may experience hyperphagia.

HYPOTHALAMUS AND THE HYPOPHYSIS (PITUITARY GLAND)

The hypothalamus (Table 11-1; Figs. 11-2, 11-3) exerts its influences on the hypophysis and thus on endocrine activity. These influences utilize

1 the neural pathway to the pars nervosa of the pituitary gland (*hypothalamo-hypophyseal tract*), and *2* the combination of a neural pathway and a vascular route to the adenohypophysis (*tuberoinfundibular tract* and *hypophyseal portal system*). It is in the pars nervosa and adenohypophysis that the neurosecretions and hormones are released into the systemic circulation. In addition, these hypothalamic influences are regulated by reciprocal interactions from more peripherally located structures (hypophysis and endocrine glands) through negative- and positive-feedback control systems.

The *hypophysis* is divided into the adenohypophysis, derived embryologically from the oral ectoderm, and the neurohypophysis, derived from neural ectoderm. The *adenohypophysis* consists of the pars tuberalis; the pars anterior, which is the largest subdivision of the hypophysis; and the pars intermedia, which is a lamina located adjacent to the pars nervosa. The *neurohypophysis* comprises the median eminence, which is a continuation of the tuber cinereum of the hypothalamus; the infundibular stem; and the pars nervosa, which is the distal end of the neurohypophysis. The pars intermedia and pars nervosa form the *posterior lobe*. The *infundibulum* of the neurohypophysis consists of the median eminence of the tuber cinereum and the infundibular stem; it is a ventral projection of the hypothalamus.

The *hypothalamic-neurohypophyseal system* displays features of an endocrine gland and the nervous system: a locus for the formation of secretory products (nuclei), a route for transporting the products (nerve tract), and an end organ for the storage and release of the hormonal secretions. These hormones are the octapeptides vasopressin (antidiuretic hormone,

ADH) and oxytocin. *Vasopressin* has roles in the regulation of water balance through its action in the kidney as the antidiuretic hormone and in the contraction of the smooth muscles in the walls of small blood vessels (it raises blood pressure). *Oxytocin* causes the contraction of uterine smooth muscle during coitus and during parturition, and the contraction of the myoepithelial cells of the mammary gland alveoli; this mediates the milk ejection reflex (response to suckling in lactating mammals). (See "Regulation of Water Balance," below.)

The hypothalamus influences the adenohypophysis through the *hypophyseal portal system*. Commencing as a capillary bed in the hypothalamus (median eminence of the tuber cinereum), this portal blood system collects into several main channels before arborizing as a capillary (sinusoidal) bed in the anterior lobe of the hypophysis. This portal system reaches its highest state of development in man and the other higher mammals. No neural connections exist between the hypothalamus and the anterior lobe of the hypophysis. In fact the anterior lobe has been described as a gland without an innervation, yet under the control of the nervous system (through the hypophyseal portal system).

The hypophyseal portal system may be thought of as the final common pathway to the anterior lobe. The secretion of the humoral agents into this portal system is stimulated (or inhibited) by neural and humoral input to the hypothalamic neurons, which, in turn, project axons to the capillary bed in the median eminence. The pituitary-releasing hormones (or

TABLE 11-1
Divisions of the hypophysis (Fig. 11-1)

Adenohypophysis	Pars tuberalis	
	Pars anterior (pars distalis, anterior lobe)	
	Pars intermedia (intermediate lobe)	
Neurohypophysis	Pars nervosa (neural lobe)	Posterior lobe
	Infundibulum (neural stalk)	Infundibular stem / Median eminence of the tuber cinereum

their precursors) may be liberated from axon terminals at the neurovascular contacts (synapses) in the median eminence; the nerve terminals on these capillaries are filled with presynaptic vesicles. These vesicles probably contain the neurosecretions that are liberated into the portal system through which they are conveyed to the anterior lobe. In addition, inhibiting hormones are also produced in the hypothalamus and transported via the hypophyseal portal system to the anterior lobe.

The structural and functional (neurohypophyseal hormones) relations of the hypothalamus and the neurohypophysis are discussed above, under "Pathways of the Hypothalamus."

These activities are indicative of the role of the hypothalamus in the integration of the nervous system and the endocrine system. Although seemingly different, these two systems show many basic similarities in their role in the regulatory processes of the organism. The nervous system is the rapidly reacting coordinator; the endocrine system is the slower, more general integrator. The distance between the site of origin of the chemical transmitter (neurosecretions and hormones) and its site of action (synapse) are only several hundred angstrom units in the nervous system; the distances are much longer in the endocrine system (the bloodstream is interposed between the endocrine organ and the target organ). Temporally, the nervous system acts in the time scale of milliseconds, and the endocrine system in hours and days. The nervous system and the endocrine system are functionally linked both in the suprarenal medulla (Chap. 6) and in the hypothalamic-hypophyseal complexes.

The synthesis and release of many hypothalamic-releasing hormones may be regulated and influenced through several feedback mechanisms to the neurons in the basal hypothalamus. Both negative (inhibitory) and positive (stimulatory) feedback mechanisms have been demonstrated. These include *1* the hormones synthesized and released in the peripheral target glands (e.g., estrogens, testosterone, corticoids) and fed back to the basal hypothalamus, *2* the tropic hormones synthesized and released by

the adenohypophysis (e.g., follicle- and thyrotropin-stimulating hormones) are also fed back to the basal hypothalamus, and *3* the releasing hormones released in the tuber cinereum may feed back to the neural receptors of the hypothalamus involved with regulating the synthesis of releasing hormones.

REGULATION OF WATER BALANCE

The hypothalamus contains the integration center concerned with the regulation of water balance. In fact, this most highly vascularized region in the brain is essentially an osmoreceptor sensitive to the osmotic pressure (concentration of sodium chloride level) of the blood in the capillaries that bathe these nuclei. As a consequence, this general region has been called the "drinking center." An animal with a lesion in the region of the ventral median nucleus and the lateral hypothalamic area may consume little water even when dehydrated, while an animal with this region stimulated will consume prodigious amounts of water even when already "saturated" with it.

Other stimuli may influence water intake. The stimulation of peripheral receptors in the mouth resulting from dryness of the mucous membranes creates the sensation of thirst. The sight of beverages and the smell of aromatic coffee can produce psychic responses that affect fluid consumption.

The role of the hypothalamus in water metabolism is focused on the supraoptic nucleus and paraventricular nucleus, the hypothalamohypophyseal pathways, and the posterior lobe. The supraoptic and paraventricular nuclei respond to the variations in the osmotic pressure of the blood.

Hyperosmotic blood is present during dehydration of the water stores of the body, stimulates *osmoreceptor* cells of the hypothalamus to initiate the sequence that releases the *antidiuretic hormone (ADH)* into the bloodstream from the supraoptic nucleus proper and from the storage depots in the neurohypophysis. In turn, the ADH acts upon the kidney (distal convoluted tubules) to increase the reabsorption of water back into the bloodstream. Water is thereby conserved, not excreted in the urine. Thirst also follows, with an increased water intake by drinking.

If the blood is hypotonic, as in a hydrated animal, ADH is not released. Water is not conserved, because it is reabsorbed in lesser quantities by the kidney tubules. Normally only 1 to 2 liters of urine is excreted each day because 14 to 18 liters is reabsorbed into the bloodstream each day, largely by the distal convoluted tubules. The more ADH released, the more water is conserved; the less ADH released, the more water is excreted. A man with a lesion of the supraoptic nuclei drinks excessive amounts of water to quench his thirst, because the lack of ADH may result in the excretion of 15 to 25 gal of urine per day (diabetes insipidus).

HYPOTHALAMUS AND THE ANTERIOR LOBE OF THE HYPOPHYSIS

The hypothalamus acts as a regulatory center capable of modifying the secretory activity of the anterior lobe through hypothalamic neurosecretions (pituitary hormone–releasing hormones) which are transported via the blood vessels of the hypophyseal portal system to the anterior lobe. These humoral (blood-conveyed) substances activate the secretion of such anterior lobe hormones as growth hormones, gonadotropins (ovary and testis), corticotropin (suprarenal cortex), and thyrotropin (thyroid gland); these pituitary hormones are then conveyed through the bloodstream to their target organs.

Ovulation (extrusion of the ovum from the ovary) in the cat offers an example of a physiologic process which is influenced by the nervous system acting through the hypothalamus and the hypophysis. The activity generated in the limbic lobe cortex following sexual excitement stimulates the hypothalamus to secrete luteinizing hormone–releasing hormone (factor) into the hypophyseal portal circulation. The resulting release of luteinizing hormone by the anterior lobe into the systemic bloodstream induces ovulation in the ovary.

The interplay and interdependence between the nervous system and the endocrine system are illustrated in the maintenance of lactation. The sucking of the mother's nipple by the infant results in the generation of neural impulses from tactile receptors which are conveyed by peripheral nerves to the spinal cord and ultimately to the mother's hypothalamus (tuberal region), where neurosecretions are released into the hypophyseal portal system. This neurosecretion stimulates the anterior lobe to release the hormone lactogen into the bloodstream. In turn, the lactogen activates the cells of the mammary gland to secrete milk. The distended mammary gland apparently feeds back information to the paraventricular nucleus of the hypothalamus, which acts via the hypothalamohypophyseal tract, upon the neurohypophysis. The resulting release of oxytocin by the posterior lobe into the circulation stimulates the myoepithelial cells of the mammary glands, resulting in their contraction and the ejection of milk from the glandular cells into the ducts of the mammary gland, so that the infant may successfully suckle its mother's milk. The cycle is thereby completed and sustained.

HYPOTHALAMUS IN EMOTION AND BEHAVIOR

The behavioral patterns associated with our emotional experiences are of two general types: *subjective "feelings," or inward expression* and *objective physical expressions,* or *consummatory behavior.* The subjective aspects of emotion, from depression to euphoria, are more intimately bound up with the cerebral cortex. Many of the physical expressions are largely mediated through the hypothalamus and the autonomic nervous system under the influences of the cerebral cortex, limbic system (Chap. 15), thalamus, and brainstem. Many of these objective expressions are recognizable as the enhanced activity of the autonomic nervous system. They include alterations in the heartbeat (palpitations) and the blood pressure, blushing and pallor of the face, dryness of the mouth, clammy hands, dilatation of the pupil (glassy eye), disturbances of secretory activity and motility of the digestive system, cold sweat, tears of happiness or sadness, and changes in the concentration of the blood sugar. Some of the expressions of emotional stress that utilize the somatic nervous system include such voluntary muscle activities as facial grimaces, shrugging of the shoulders, and the movements accompanying nervousness, crying, escaping, and fighting.

The primitive expressions of emotional behavior may be evoked by ablating or stimulating portions of the hypothalamus. Bilateral destruction of the ventromedial nuclei (or stimulation of the dorsomedial nuclei) can transform a gentle animal into one exhibiting varying degrees of wildness. If mildly provoked, an animal whose hypothalamus has been injured may attack savagely and hiss, or may attempt to escape. Such an animal exhibits a *sham (simulated) rage*, for when the provoking stimulus is removed, the animal immediately becomes seemingly placid. In a sham rage, an animal demonstrates objective signs of rage but does not have the corresponding subjective feelings. Some investigators claim that the provoked rage is not a true sham rage for these outbursts are often directed at a specific object or goal and are not actually aimless. Stimulation of the hypothalamus in man is said to evoke changes in the blood pressure and rate of heartbeat without any psychic manifestations.

An animal with portions of its new and old cerebral cortices removed exhibits the explosive behavior patterns of sham rage. Under these conditions, the sham rage is a form of *release phenomenon* as the hypothalamus, autonomic nervous system, and other regions are released from the regulatory influences of the cortex. In a decorticate cat, for example, a mildly noxious stimulus, such as pinching the tail, may evoke such sympathetic effects as pupillary dilation, elevated blood pressure and faster heartbeat, piloerection, and such somatic effects as arching of the back, snarling, and striking with protracted claws. The entire reaction ceases immediately when the tail pinching is stopped.

The hypothalamus has a central role in many expressions associated with sexual behavior. The sources of powerful influences upon the hypothalamus are the olfactory system, neocortex, limbic system, and hormones. Many of the functional aspects of these influences are obvious. The output from the hypothalamus for these expressions utilizes primarily *1* the descending autonomic pathways, and *2* the hypophyseal portal system to the hypophysis in order to mobilize the autonomic nervous and endocrine systems.

HYPOTHALAMUS AND THE SLEEP-WAKE CYCLE

The hypothalamus is associated with the state of awakeness, but precisely how this structure is integrated into the sleep-wake cycle is not known. In contrast to the agitated reactions of the "sham rage" evoked in an animal with a tuberal lesion, the bilateral ablation of the regions dorsolateral and caudal to the mamillary bodies produces a tame, apathetic, and often somnolent monkey or cat. Stimulation of the hypothalamus of the cat may induce drowsiness and sleep. The ascending reticular activating system which projects to the hypothalamus and the diffuse projections from the hypothalamus to the cerebral cortex are among the neural substrates for the sleep-wake cycle.

HYPOTHALAMUS AND THE "PLEASURE" AND "PUNISHING" CENTERS

The region of the lateral hypothalamus in the median forebrain bundle near the feeding center is incorporated into the "pleasure-center" complex discussed in Chap. 15. Electric stimulation of this area drives the animal to seek more of such stimulation. The medial hypothalamus is integrated into the "punishing-center" complex (Chap. 15). Electric stimulation of this area is apparently unpleasant, because the animal attempts to avoid further stimulation.

Some clinical considerations

Degenerative changes of the hypothalamo-hypophyseal tract result in a deficiency of the antidiuretic hormone (vasopressin, ADH); this condition may be accompanied by *diabetes insipidus, polydipsia* (compulsive water drinking), and *polyuria* (excessive excretion of urine). Some lesions of the hypothalamus, often in the region of the tuber cinereum, give rise to severe gastric disturbances, associated with erosion, ulceration, and hemorrhaging in the mucosa of the stomach; this condition may involve areas involved with the secretion of hydrochloric acid in the stomach preparatory to the ingestion of food.

Lesions in the tuberal region, including the adjacent ventral medial nuclei, result in *adiposo-*

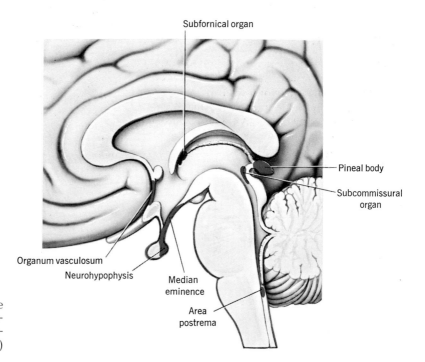

Subfornical organ

Pineal body

Subcommissural organ

Organum vasculosum

Neurohypophysis

Median eminence

Area postrema

FIGURE 11-6
Midsagittal view of the brain illustrating the location of the circumventricular organs. (*After Weindl.*)

genital dystrophy—characterized by obesity and gonadal atrophy. The obesity is a consequence of the damage to the ventral medial nuclei; the gonadal atrophy is probably due to the malfunctioning of the tuberoinfundibular tract, which is involved with the releasing hormone system. Tuberal lesions may give rise to hyperglycemia and disturbances in heat regulation.

The circumventricular organs of the central nervous system (Fig. 11-6)

Adjacent to the median ventricular cavities (third ventricle, cerebral aqueduct, and fourth ventricle) are several specialized regions called *circumventricular organs.* The common vascular, ependymal, and neural organization of these structures differs from that found in typical brain tissue. They are referred to as "being in the brain but not of it." In humans, the circumventricular organs include *1* the median eminence of the

tuber cinereum, the neurohypophysis, and the pineal body, which are considered to be sites of neuroendocrine activity, and *2* the organum vasculosum of the lamina terminalis, subfornical organ, subcommissural organ, and the area postrema (Fig. 11-6), the functional roles of which have not, as yet, been clearly defined. The ependymal cells of the circumventricular organs and choroid plexus are nonciliated.

MEDIAN EMINENCE OF THE TUBER CINEREUM

The *median eminence of the tuber cinereum* is that portion of the floor of the third ventricle where the releasing and inhibiting hormones are released from the axon terminals into the capillary loops of the hypophyseal portal system. In essence, it is the site of a neurovascular link between the nervous system and the adenohypophysis. The secretion of the releasing hormones from the axon terminals may be influenced by a system of dopaminergic and noradrenergic neurons.

NEUROHYPOPHYSIS

As previously noted, the *neurohypophysis* is the site for the storage and release of vasopressin and oxytocin, which are synthesized in the supraoptic and paraventricular nuclei. The nerve terminals of the supraopticohypophyseal tract containing these neurohormones are intermingled among cells called pituicytes, which are modified glial cells.

PINEAL BODY

The *pineal body, or epiphysis cerebri,* in mammals is a midline cone-shaped structure located in the caudal epithalamus just above the midbrain tegmentum. Descartes called the pineal body, "the seat of the soul." It is a highly vascular organ consisting of parenchymal cells (*pineocytes*), astrocyte-like glial cells and calcareous granules (corpora arenacea). The parenchymal cells have processes which terminate on the basal lamina of the perivascular space surrounding the fenestrated capillaries. It is probable that the only innervation to the pineal body is by postganglionic sympathetic fibers from the superior cervical ganglion. Vesicles are present in the nerve endings and the parenchymal cells. These vesicles contain melatonin, serotonin, and other "pineal hormones," and norepinephrine.

Evidence suggests several roles for the pineal body. The pineal "hormones" exert influences upon preoptic and hypothalamic neurons. The route of hormone transport from the pineal body to the effector neurons may be via the blood vascular system or the cerebrospinal fluid within the third ventricle. These neurons, in turn, are the vehicles by which some of the neuroendocrine activity of the pineal body influences diurnal and seasonal reproductive activity. This role of the pineal body is performed by modulating the release of gonadotropin-releasing hormone from the median eminence in response to influences received by the pineal body from diurnal and seasonal changes. This role is significant in animals which breed seasonally. In addition, the pineal "hormones" have

roles in gonadal development by inhibiting the maturation of the gonads.

The pineal body of mammals is presumed to be influenced by light via an indirect pathway (Moore et al.) from the eyes. The neural pathway includes the sequence of retina, accessory optic tract via optic nerve, chiasm, and tract to the midbrain tegmentum, medial forebrain bundle to the hypothalamus, descending multineuronal autonomic pathway to the upper thoracic intermediolateral cell column, and postganglionic and preganglionic (superior cervical ganglion) neurons to the pineal body. Through this complex pathway light may regulate pineal body activity. Pineal body activity is increased and gonadal development is inhibited in mammals deprived of light (because of blindness or long-term exposure to the dark).

A direct retinohypothalamic tract has been suggested as a possible route by which light may influence hypothalamic activity.

ORGANUM VASCULOSUM OF THE LAMINA TERMINALIS

The *organum vasculosum* (*supraoptic crest, "prechiasmatic gland"*) is a highly vascular region of the lamina terminalis. Structurally it is similar to the median eminence. Its loops of fenestrated capillaries are surrounded by wide, fluid-filled perivascular spaces. The role of this structure is unknown. The organum vasculosum may be functionally related to the adjacent preoptic region of the hypothalamus.

SUBFORNICAL ORGAN

The *subfornical organ* (*intercolumnar tubercle*) is an elevation located between the diverging columns of the fornix at the level of the interventricular foramina (of Monro). It is partially covered by choroid plexus. This organ may be a neuroendocrine structure. Its sinusoid and glomerular loops are supplied by adjacent blood vessels. The nerve endings synapsing with the parenchymal cells of the organ have synaptic vesicles which may contain acetylcholine. Two of the many suggested functional roles for this organ are: *1* it may be involved in osmoregulation (drinking), and *2* it may have an effect on the circulation of the choroid plexus analogous to that of the juxtaglomerulus apparatus of the kidney.

SUBCOMMISSURAL ORGAN

The *subcommissural organ* is located in the roof of the cerebral aqueduct just rostral and ventral to the posterior commissure and fairly close to the pineal body. It is composed of specialized ependymal cells and some associated glial cells in a capillary bed of nonfenestrated endothelium. The ependymal cells are secretory. They release a product directly into the ventricular fluid, which condenses to form Reissner's fiber—a neutral mucopolysaccharide protein complex. Reissner's fiber can be traced through the cerebral aqueduct, fourth ventricle, and central canal of the spinal cord to the coccygeal levels. Although the functional role of the subcommissural organ is unknown, several proposals include thermoregulation, regulation of water and electrolyte balance, and responses to change in illumination.

AREA POSTREMA

The *area postrema* is one of a pair of small rounded eminences on either side of the fourth ventricle just rostral to the obex at the junction of the ventricle and the central canal (Figs. 11-6, A-15). The area is deep to the nonciliated ependymal cell lining the ventricle. It is composed of modified neurons (its parenchymal cells), astrocyte-like cells, and rich overlapping arterial and sinusoidal network. The synaptic terminals within the area postrema are derived from the nucleus solitarius and from ascending spinal fibers. It is possible that the area postrema monitors certain changes in the composition of the blood and, in addition, releases neurosecretory substances into the systemic circulation. This would be in line with some of the suggested functional roles ascribed to other circumventricular organs. These include the regulation of blood pressure and functioning as a chemoreceptor for CO_2 in the regulation of respiration; these roles may be expressed through nearby medullary areas involved with blood circulation and respiration. The area postrema or an adjacent region of the medulla may act as an osmosensitive zone or a chemoreceptor emetic trigger zone involved with the vomiting reflex.

Bibliography

Ganong, W. F., and L. Martini (eds.): *Frontiers in Neuroendocrinology.* Oxford University Press, New York and London, 1969, 1971, 1973.

Harris, G. W., and B. T. Donovan (eds.): *The Pituitary Gland.* University of California Press, Berkeley, 1966.

Haymaker, W., E. Anderson, and W. J. H. Nauta: *The Hypothalamus.* Charles C Thomas, Publisher, Springfield, Ill., 1969.

Hess, W. R.: *The Functional Organization of the Diencephalon.* Grune & Stratton, Inc., New York, 1958.

Knigge, K. M., D. E. Scott, and A. Weindl (eds.): *Brain-Endocrine Interaction. Median Eminence: Structure and Function.* Karger, Basel, 1972.

Martini, L., M. Motta, and F. Fraschini: *The Hypothalamus.* Academic Press, Inc., New York, 1971.

Moore, R. Y., A. Heller, R. K. Bhatnager, R. J. Wurtman, and J. Axelrod: Central control of the pineal gland: visual pathways. Arch. Neurol., 18:208–218, 1968.

Olds, J.: Hypothalamic substrates of reward. Physiol. Rev., 42:554–604, 1962.

Schally, A. V., A. Arimura, and A. J. Kastin: Hypothalamic regulatory hormones. Science, 179:341–350, 1973.

Scharrer, E., and B. Scharrer: *Neuroendocrinology.* Columbia University Press, New York, 1963.

Sutin, J.: The periventricular stratum of the hypothalamus. Int. Rev. Neurobiol., 9:263–300, 1966.

Szentágothai, J., B. Flerko, B. Mess, and B. Halasz: *Hypothalamic Control of the Anterior Pituitary.* Akademiai Kiado, Budapest, 1968.

Weindl, A.: Neuroendocrine aspects of circumventricular organs, in W. F. Ganong and L. Martini (eds.), *Frontiers in Neuroendocrinology.* Oxford University Press, New York and London, 1973.

Wurtman, R. J., J. Axelrod, and D. E. Kelly: *The Pineal.* Academic Press, Inc., New York, 1968.

CHAPTER **12**
THE OPTIC SYSTEM

Sight is our most dominant sense; we live primarily in a visual world. The rods and cones in the retinas of the eyes comprise about 70 percent of the receptors of the entire body. About one-third of all the afferent nerve fibers projecting information to our central nervous system are the approximately 2 million nerve fibers in both optic nerves.

Out of the engulfing sea of radiation in the electromagnetic spectrum, from the minute gamma rays one million-millionth micron in length to radio waves several miles in length, *our eyes are sensitive only to that narrow band of radiation known as the visual spectrum of from 400 nanometers (millionth part of a millimeter) to 700 nanometers (from blue to red).* We do not see in or beyond the infrared band, because our visual receptors cannot be stimulated by these wavelengths. The *ultraviolet radiations from 365 to 400 nanometers are capable of being "seen" but are normally absorbed by the lens.* An individual without a lens (*aphakic*) can literally see in ultraviolet light. In one respect we are fortunate that the entire electromagnetic spectrum does not supply the stimulus energy to produce a visual image. Otherwise we would literally see everything. Because our sense of sight is restricted to but one-seventieth of the spectrum, we are selective. If we perceived all radiation we should be in a perpetual daylight; even at night we would not see the stars for the glare. Man has devised instruments (radios and oscilloscopes) that are capable of bringing invisible forms of radiation (e.g., radio waves) to our selective receptors (e.g., radio to our auditory sense, oscilloscope to our visual sense).

Some of the waves outside the visual spectrum may affect an organism. The invisible short-wave radiation can induce a chemical reaction in living tissues—ultraviolet light can produce a sunburn, and the ionizing radiation of x-rays and cosmic rays can damage tissues. Infrared rays, at the other end of the spectrum, can be felt as heat. Ultraviolet rays and infrared rays can be seen if presented to the eye in very high intensities.

It is essential to understand that the optic system performs in several areas: *1* light and dark, *2* color, *3* image reproduction or form vision, *4* visual acuity, *5* spatial or depth sense, *6* motion perception or resolution of images in time, *7* appreciation of brightness or intensities of light, and *8* recognition and comparison of images with previous experience.

The visual process may be subdivided into five phases: *1* the refraction of the light rays and the focusing of images on the retina, *2* the transduction of light quanta by photochemical activity into nerve impulses, *3* the processing of neural activity in the retina and the transmission of coded impulses through the optic nerve, *4* the processing in the brain culminating in perception, and *5* the reflexes associated with the visual system (e.g., accommodation).

Anatomy of the eye

The eye is a sphere that is analogous to the common camera obscura (Fig. 12-1). It is constructed to perform both optical and sensory functions. Its optical role is to gather light rays and to focus them onto the retina. To do this, the eye has *1* a variable aperture system—the iris and its opening, the pupil—which regulates the amount of light passing to the retina, and *2* a lens system—cornea and lens—which produces a two-dimensional image of the object on the retina. Its sensory roles are to respond to and to process environmental influences and to

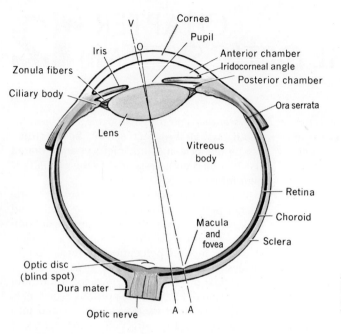

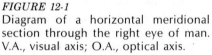

FIGURE 12-1
Diagram of a horizontal meridional section through the right eye of man. V.A., visual axis; O.A., optical axis.

transmit coded messages to the brain. These roles are performed by the retina. The fibers of the optic nerve, which originate in the retina, convey the output of the retina to the brain. The sclera corresponds to the frame of the camera; the pigment epithelium of the retina and the choroid layer correspond to the black interior lining of the camera; the cornea and lens to the camera lenses; the aqueous humor of the anterior and posterior chambers and the vitreous humor of the vitreous body to the air spaces within the camera; the iris corresponds to the diaphragm; the pupil to the opening in the diaphragm; the eyelid to the lens cap; and the retina to the film. The television camera is an even better analogue; it not only focuses light and forms coded messages of images but also relays these messages to "transmitters."

The eye is composed of three coats: the *outer or fibrous tunic* comprises the *sclera* and *cornea;* the *vascular tunic, or uveal tract (uvea),* consists of the *choroid, ciliary body,* and *iris;* and the *inner tunic, or retina,* includes the photosensitive portion in the back of the eye, the unpig-

mented epithelium of the ciliary body, and the pigmented epithelium of the posterior iris (Figs. 12-1, 12-2). In describing the anatomic locations within the eye, the terms *outer* and *inner* are used with reference to the center of the eye. Thus the fibrous tunic is an outer layer and the retina is an inner layer. The same terms apply to the retinal structures (e.g., the rods and cones are "outer" to the bipolar cells). The transparent biconvex *lens* is located behind the iris and the pupil. It is suspended by fine "guy ropes" called the *zonular fibers,* which are anchored in the 70 or more ciliary processes of the ciliary body located in the vicinity of the corneoscleral junction. The ocular chamber is the fluid-filled space between the cornea and vitreous body, which is partially divided by the iris into an anterior chamber and a posterior chamber. Both chambers are filled with clear watery fluid called the *aqueous humor.* The *anterior chamber* is located between the cornea, iris, and front of the lens; the *posterior chamber* is bounded by the iris, ciliary body, lens, and vitreous body. The large *vitreous chamber* is located between the poste-

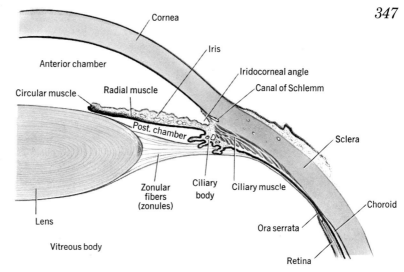

FIGURE 12-2
Horizontal meridional section through a portion of the human eye.

rior surface of the lens and ciliary body and the posterior wall of the eyeball. This chamber, comprising about five-sixths of the eye, is filled with a transparent gelatinous material.

The adult human eyeball is roughly a globe of approximately 24 mm in diameter and 6.5 ml in volume; it consists of the segments of two spheres which are unequal in size. The smaller sphere comprises the anterior one-sixth of the eyeball; this forms the *corneal curve.* The larger sphere comprises the posterior five-sixths; its outer coat forms the *scleral curve.* The anterior segment has a greater curvature than the posterior segment. The anterior pole is located in the center of the corneal curve, and the posterior pole in the center of the scleral curve. The *geometric (anatomic) axis* is a line from the anterior pole through the posterior pole. The *optical axis* is a theoretic line passing through the center of the optical centers of the principal refracting surfaces of the cornea and lens (Fig. 12-1). The *visual axis* forms a line passing from the fixation point (center of the object in focus) through the nodal point near the posterior surface of the lens and the fovea centralis (spot of most acute vision). The optical axis differs from the visual axis because the lens is decentered slightly downward and nasally with respect to the optic axis. This decentration does not alter the visual role of the eye.

Two planes—the vertical and horizontal meridians—are important. The plane of the *vertical meridian* passes through the fovea and divides the eye into a *nasal (medial)* and a *temporal (lateral)* half. The plane of the *horizontal meridian* passes through the fovea centralis and divides the eye into upper and lower halves. The planes divided the eye into four quadrants—*upper nasal, upper temporal, lower nasal,* and *lower temporal quadrants.* The associated divided retinal segments are respectively called the *nasal hemiretina, temporal hemiretina, upper nasal retinal quadrant, etc.*

The retina near the posterior pole of the eye is modified into three concentric regions (Fig. 12-1), namely, the *central part of the retina* (5 to 6 mm in diameter), the *macula or macula lutea* (3 mm in diameter), and the *fovea centralis (central fovea,* 0.4 mm wide). The *macula, or yellow spot,* has a yellowish color because of the carotinoid and xanthophyll pigments in the neurons of the region. The *fovea centralis* is a small, funnel-shaped pit in the macula, formed by the spreading and deviation of the inner layers of the retina from the center of the region. Cones are the only photoreceptors found in this region of most acute vision. Medial to the macula is the *blind spot,* where no image is registered. This is the site of the nerve head at the emergence of the optic nerve; it is called the *optic disk.* This bulging disk has a central depression or excavation. A precise positional

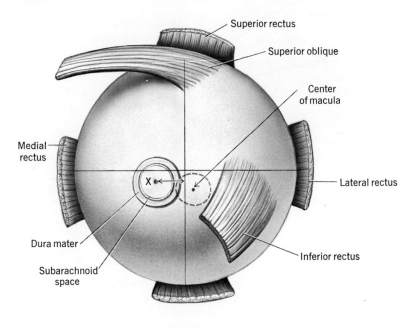

Superior rectus
Superior oblique
Center of macula
Medial rectus
Lateral rectus
Dura mater
Inferior rectus
Subarachnoid space
X

FIGURE 12-3
A posterior view of the right eye.

The horizontal and vertical meridians are indicated by the two lines which intersect at the posterior pole of the eye. The center of the optic nerve is 3 mm nasal to the posterior pole of the eye and 1 mm below it. The center of the macula is located 1 mm temporal to the posterior pole and 1.8 mm below it. The circular outline of the 3-mm-diameter macula lutea is indicated by the broken-line circle. (*Adapted from Hogan, Alvarado, and Weddell.*)

relationship exists among the posterior pole, fovea centralis, and optic disk. The fovea centralis is about 1 mm temporal and 1.8 mm inferior to the posterior pole (Fig. 12-3). The center of the optic disk is located 3 mm nasal and 1 mm inferior to the posterior pole. The blind spot can be located in the following way: place two large dots a few inches apart on a piece of paper, close the left eye, and continually focus on the left dot with the right eye. Move the head toward (or away from) the paper. Note that while you are looking at the left dot, the right dot is not seen at a certain distance from the paper. At this distance the right dot is focused on the blind spot. The blind spot is located in the lower nasal retinal quadrant, which means that it appears in the upper temporal quadrant of the visual fields (see "Fields of Vision and the Retina," later on in this chapter).

The optic nerve is surrounded by the meninges and their spaces up to the junction of the nerve with the eye (Figs. 12-1, 12-3). The dura mater is continuous with the sclera. Because the subarachnoid space surrounds the optic nerve, changes in the cerebrospinal fluid pressure can be registered in the optic disk. A high cerebrospinal fluid pressure, such as one caused by a space-occupying lesion, exerts a force which is transmitted to the optic nerve and everts the central depression of the optic disk to produce a *swollen optic disk* or *choked disk.* The retina and optic disk can be observed with an ophthalmoscope, an instrument which enables a doctor to look into the eye. In such an examination of a patient with a choked disk, the living retina appears red (because of vessels in the choroid layer) except for the pale, circular swollen optic disk. This result of an increased intracranial pressure is also called *papilledema.*

The collagenous *corneoscleral tunic* is a slightly elastic skeleton of the eye, which, with the help of the intraocular pressure, maintains the shape of the eye. It is comparable to a balloon filled with a fluid. This tough coat is composed of 94 percent sclera and 6 percent cornea. The sclera, or white of the eye, is relatively avascular. It is structurally continuous with the cornea. The boundary between the opaque sclera and the transparent cornea is called the limbus. Of the lenses of the eye, the cornea is nonadjustable, whereas the lens is adjustable.

The *transparency of the cornea* results from *1* the regularity of its epithelial surface, *2* its avascularity, *3* the organizational pattern of its collagen and ground substance, and *4* the chemical composition and the state of hydration of its stroma. The basis for this transparency is considered to be wholly physiologic and not anatomic, because no histologic differences are observable in the light microscopy of the corneal and scleral stroma. Its optical homogeneity is primarily maintained by the metabolic activity of its cells, which are continually pumping out interstitial fluid against the normal tendency of the cornea to become hydrated. In this way the cornea is kept in a deturgescent state. In contrast, the sclera possesses a higher water content. The sclera can become transparent if it is partially dehydrated locally. Following the cessation of the metabolic pumping, after death, the cornea becomes opaque. The sensitivity of the cornea is due to the rich and extensive innervation by sensory fibers of the ophthalmic division of the trigeminal nerve.

The cornea is most resistant to infection; because of the mitotic potential of its surface epithelium, it can effectively heal penetrating wounds. The cornea is one of those few structures that can be readily transplanted (*corneal transplants*) from the eye of a donor to the eye of a host. This resistance of the cornea to rejection when in the host is related to several factors, chiefly its avascularity, including the absence of lymphatics, and the barrier effect of the aqueous humor supplying its metabolic needs. In the transplants that "take," the epithelial surface cells are quickly lost; within days the layers are replaced by the migration and mitotic activity of cells from the host. Apparently the intrinsic cells of the bulk of the cornea (substantia propria) may survive for years; ultimately they are replaced by the host tissue.

The *choroid layer* is the highly vascularized, richly black-pigmented layer of the uveal tract, extending forward about two-thirds of the distance toward the pupil. It is coextensive with the photoreceptive retina, which it supplies with nutriment and oxygen. The pigment absorbs light.

The *ciliary body* is located between the *ora serrata* (anterior edge of the photoreceptive retina) and the corneoscleral junction (Fig. 12-3). It subserves three roles: accommodation, production of the aqueous humor of the anterior and posterior chambers, and restoration of the mucopolysaccharides of the vitreous body.

The delicate adjustment altering the shape and thereby the refractive power of the lens is called *accommodation*. This adjustment results from the state of contraction of the ciliary muscles—the circular muscle, radial muscle, and meridional muscle—which have a role in adjusting the tension exerted on the lens through the zonular fibers comprising the suspensory ligaments of the lens. The precise manner in which the ciliary body regulates the curvature of the lens is often misunderstood. When the eye is relaxed, as in viewing distant objects, the ciliary muscles are relaxed; in this state the tension exerted by the ring of the ciliary body through the ciliary processes on the zonular fibers is maximal and, as a result, the lens is flattened. To view objects close to the eye (near vision) a rounder lens is necessary, so that the light rays will be refracted more. To accomplish this, the ciliary muscles contract and pull the ciliary body slightly forward and inward, narrowing the ring of the ciliary body and thereby reducing the tension on the zonular fibers. Because the lens has an inherent elasticity, it rounds up on its own when the tension is reduced. The refraction of light is greater with a rounder lens; this occurs with the shift of one's gaze from a distant to a close object.

The *lens* is a transparent biconvex disk with an elliptical shape. It is surrounded by a thin *lens capsule*. The lens is held in position and suspended by hairlike zonular fibers which extend in a radial pattern from the lens capsule to the ciliary body. Nourishment and oxygen for the lens are derived from the aqueous and vitreous humors. The cells constituting the lens have a metabolic role in maintaining its optical transparency. The reduction in the nutritional status and metabolic efficiency of the lens cells is an expression of normal aging. One consequence is a decrease in the accommodation power of the lens in middle age (see discussion of presbyopia, below). Poor nourishment of the lens during various metabolic and aging diseases can lead to opacities, or cataracts. For example, abnormal sugar metabolism, as in diabetes, may have an effect on the vitality of the lens, resulting in the development of cataracts. *Cataracts* are the presumed consequence for all who reach extreme old age. The lens continues to grow throughout life, with the addition of new cells at the lens equator. The lens has no nerve supply.

The *muscular iris* surrounds the pupil, resulting in an adjustable optic diaphragm which is a variable aperture. Dilating or constricting the iris causes the pupil to be enlarged or reduced, thereby regulating the amount of light passing into the depths of the eyeball (see "The Visual Reflexes," further on). As compared to the f-stop in a camera, the eye operates in the range of f2 to f22. The pupillary size is increased by the radial muscle cells of the iris (contraction of these muscles results in a pupillary dilation), and is decreased by the circular muscle cells of the iris (contraction results in pupillary constriction). The posterior epithelial layer of the iris (iridial portion of the retina) is pigmented. The bulk of the iris is composed of a loose, pigmented, highly vascular connective tissue. The color of the eye is related to the amount of pigment in the melanocytes of the iris. Blue eyes have a slight amount of pigment; brown eyes have a moderate amount; and black eyes a great amount. The red of the eyes of an albino is produced by the blood in a pigmentless iris. The blue color results from stromal absorption of long wavelengths, with the blue waves returning to the observer's eyes.

The anterior and posterior chambers are filled with *aqueous humor*—a thin watery fluid which is essentially an ultrafiltrate of blood resembling cerebrospinal fluid. It is largely responsible for the intraocular pressure, and provides such essential nourishment as oxygen, glucose, and amino acids for the avascular lens and cornea. The aqueous humor is formed primarily by the ciliary body, passes into the posterior chamber, and slowly circulates through the pupil to the anterior chamber. At the *iridocorneal (filtration) angle* at the lateral circular border of the anterior chamber, it leaves through the spaces of a trabecular meshwork before diffusing through a thin, nonperforated wall of tissue into the *canal of Schlemm* (an aqueous vein) which drains into the veins of the blood system (Fig. 12-2). The aqueous humor flows from the posterior chamber to the anterior chamber, not in the reverse direction, because of the ball-valve effect produced by the contact of the pupillary margin with the lens.

Glaucoma results when there is too much aqueous humor, usually caused by a defective drainage by the outflow channels at the iridocorneal angle. Under such conditions, the intraocular pressure increases above its normal 15 to 20 mm above atmospheric pressure, which, if untreated, can result in destructive effects on the retina.

The maintenance of the eye as an optical instrument is due in part to the pressures exerted by the blood and aqueous humor; when these pressures drop at death, a partial collapse of the eye occurs. The cornea receives its main, but insufficient, supply of oxygen for its metabolic requirements from the aqueous humor. Additional oxygen is obtained by diffusion from the air in contact with the cornea. The metabolic activity of the cornea is impaired if the cornea is unable to maintain some intermittent contact with the air.

The large *vitreous chamber,* occupying about five-sixths of the eye, is filled with a transparent gelatinous material which is a hydrated mucoprotein enmeshed in some collagenous fibrils. Except for the addition of collagen and hyaluronic acid, the chemical composition is similar to that of the aqueous humor. It contains no blood vessels, and its few cells may be microglia from the retina. The vitreous humor is formed by the ciliary body; it provides a passageway for the nourishment of the lens and possibly of the retina. The turnover of the vitreous water is rather rapid; approximately one-half the vitreous water is replaced every 10 to 15 min. The slow movement of "fibrous" materials in the vitreous body is supposed to be the source of stimulus for the common experience of threads and spots floating before the eyes.

To visualize a clear image, the environmental field must be focused on the retina. In order to reduce a large field to a small image on the retina, the light entering the eye is refracted by the cornea and lens. As already mentioned, the *cornea acts as the nonadjustable lens,* whereas the *lens proper acts as the adjustable lens of the eye.* The refraction actually occurs at the interfaces between *1* the air and cornea, *2* cornea and aqueous humor, *3* aqueous humor and lens, and *4* lens and vitreous body. Most of the refraction occurs at the air-cornea interface because the *refractive power (index)* is much greater at the air-cornea interface than at the cornea–aqueous humor, aqueous humor–lens, and lens–vitreous humor interfaces.

The *normal eye (emmetropic eye)* accommodates perfectly, so that the environmental field is in focus on the retina.

In *farsightedness (hypermetropia, hyperopia)* the image is in focus behind the retina (i.e., the ciliary muscles are relaxed). Two reasons may lead to this condition: *1* the eyeball is too short, the distance from the cornea to the retina being less than in the normal eye, or *2* the cornea and lens do not refract light sufficiently for the image to focus on the retina. The ciliary muscles are said to be well developed in hyperopic eyes. Farsightedness is corrected by using a third lens, i.e., eyeglasses with a convex lens (Fig. 12-4).

In *nearsightedness (myopia),* the image is in focus in front of the retina (in the vitreous body). Two reasons are possible: the eyeball is too long, or the cornea and lens are too powerful and refract the light too much. The ciliary muscles are said to be poorly developed in myopic eyes. Nearsightedness is corrected by a concave lens (Fig. 12-4).

The inherent elasticity of the lens is progressively reduced with age. This reduction is expressed by a gradual decrease in the ability of the lens to assume a spherical shape. Near vision is made more difficult, so that the need for glasses for near focusing becomes most marked by middle age. This decrease in the refractive power of the lens until it is almost nonaccommodating is known as *presbyopia.* This condition is corrected with convex lenses. Subjects

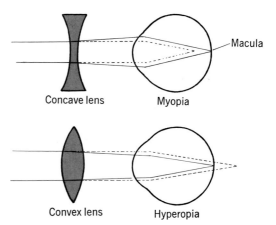

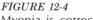

FIGURE 12-4
Myopia is corrected with a concave lens, and hyperopia is corrected with a convex lens.

with this difficulty require glasses when reading or doing other close work.

Retina

GENERAL ORGANIZATION OF THE RETINA

The retina is a mobile portion of the brain, because the retina is a central nervous system structure which moves as the eye moves. In fact, the retina is an extension of the forebrain, which reaches forward from the optic nerve into the eye *1* as the photoreceptive layer (neuroretina) and the pigment epithelium to the ora serrata, *2* as the unpigmented epithelium (ciliary retina) over the ciliary body, and *3* as a pigmented epithelium (iridic retina) over the posterior iris. The *neuroretina* is about the size of a square postage stamp and only slightly thicker. The entire retina is embryologically derived from the two-layered outgrowth of the neural tube, called the optic cup (Fig. 12-5). The outer layer of the cup gives rise to the pigment epithelium of the retina, and the inner layer to the remainder of the retina. The embryonic cavity between the layers—called the optic ventricle—is obliterated during development by the interdigitation

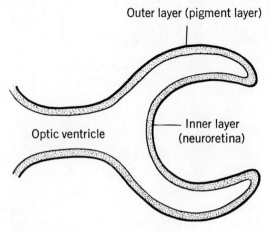

Outer layer (pigment layer)

Inner layer (neuroretina)

Optic ventricle

FIGURE 12-5

The optic cup, an outgrowth of the forebrain, comprises an outer layer and an inner layer.

The outer layer differentiates into the pigment epithelium of the retina. The inner layer differentiates into the neuroretina. Note the optic ventricle, which, in the embryo, is continuous with the ventricular system.

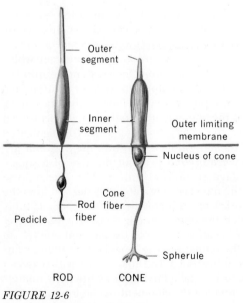

Outer segment

Inner segment

Outer limiting membrane

Nucleus of cone

Cone fiber

Rod fiber

Pedicle

Spherule

ROD   CONE

FIGURE 12-6

A rod and a cone of man.

of extensions of the pigment epithelium with those of the rods and cones.

A cleavage of the retina (*detached retina*) may occur at the interface between the pigment epithelium and neuroretina. It is a common cause of partial blindness. This retinal detachment which "re-creates" the cavity of the optic vesicle, results, in part, because no tight morphologic connection ever develops between the neuroretina and the pigment epithelium except at the ora serrata and the optic disk, where the retina is firmly attached to the choroid layer.

In common with all other vertebrates, man has an inverted retina. In this type of retina, the photoreceptive rods and cones lie in an outer layer and the neuronal cells involved with processing and transmitting neural information to the brain are in the inner layers. In effect, light must pass through all retinal layers (except at the fovea) before reaching the rods and cones (Figs. 12-6 through 12-9). In the fovea the inner layers are spread to the sides, so that light has only to pass through the outer nuclear layer before reaching the photoreceptive elements (Fig. 12-9). The output of the retina is projected via ganglion cells and their axons located in the nerve fiber layer. These fibers converge toward the optic disk to form the optic nerve, which terminates in several processing nuclei of the brain.

CELLS (NEURONS) OF THE RETINA

Layers of the retina Except at the fovea centralis, optic disk, and its peripheral margins near the ora serrata, the neuroretina is conventionally divided into the following layers, from "outer" to "inner" (Figs. 12-8, 12-9).

1 Pigment epithelium

2 Layer of the outer and inner segments of the rods and cones

3 External limiting membrane: junctional complexes (tight junctions) between Müller's cells with rods or cones

4 Outer nuclear layer: cell bodies and fibers of rods and cones

5 Outer plexiform layer: synapses among rods, cones, bipolar cells, and horizontal cells

6 Inner nuclear layer: cell bodies of bipolar cells, horizontal cells, amacrine cells, and Müller's cells

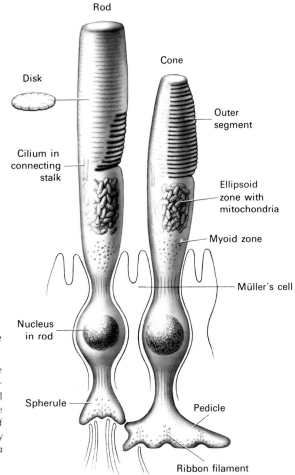

Rod

Cone

Disk

Outer segment

Cilium in connecting stalk

Ellipsoid zone with mitochondria

Myoid zone

Müller's cell

Nucleus in rod

Spherule

Pedicle

Ribbon filament

FIGURE 12-7
Ultrastructure of a cone and a rod.

The new disks of the rods are continually formed by the repeated infolding of the cell membrane at the base of the outer segments. The disks of the cones are not continually replaced. (*Adapted from Young.*)

7 Inner plexiform layer: synapses among bipolar cells, amacrine cells, and ganglion cells

8 Ganglion cell layer: cell bodies of ganglion cells and synapses as in the inner plexiform layer

9 Nerve fiber layer: axons of ganglion cells

10 Inner limiting membrane: junctional complexes of expanded ends of Müller's cells at vitreal surface

The *fovea centralis* is a zone of high density of photoreceptors, in which numerous slender cones and no rods are present. A few cell bodies of the outer nuclear layer are located within the fovea. The other retinal layers and blood vessels are displaced away from the fovea. As a result light rays pass almost directly from the vitreous body without interference to the foveal cones, which are involved with fine visual acuity. The optic disk contains only the axons of the ganglion cells.

Pigment epithelium (Figs. 12-8, 12-9) The cells of the pigment epithelium contain a black melanin pigment called fuscin, which is concentrated in granules. These pigment granules are located mainly in the inner portions of the

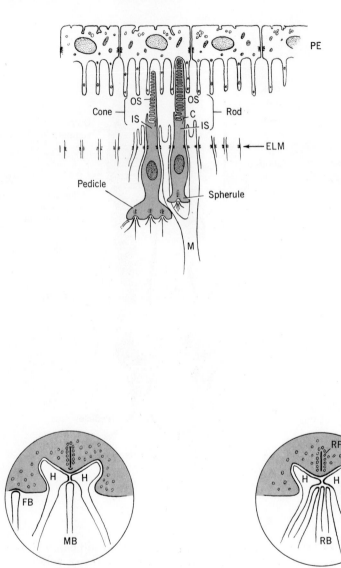

Pedicle

Spherule

FIGURE 12-8
The ultrastructural orga-
nization of a part of the
retina, illustrating the relationship of the rods and
cones to the pigment epi-
thelial cells (PE) and the
processes of Müller's cells
(M).

A cone terminates in a "synaptic" expansion called a pedicle, whereas a rod terminates
as a knoblike "synaptic" ending called a spherule. *Lower
left:* the synaptic contacts of
a pedicle with processes of
midget bipolar cells (MB), flat
bipolar cells (FB), and horizontal cells (H). *Lower right:*
the synaptic contacts of a
spherule with the processes of
rod bipolar cells (RB) and
horizontal cells (H). The
electron-dense line in the
presynaptic terminal is called
a ribbon filament (RF). The
processes of Müller's cells extend outward almost to the
level of the connecting stalks
(C) located between the outer
segments (OS) and inner segments (IS) of the rods and
cones. The external limiting
membrane (ELM) of light microscopy is actually formed by
tight junctions (desmosomes)
at the borders of the apposing
cell membranes of Müller's
cells with those of the rods
and cones (ILM). (*Adapted
from Dowling and Boycott,
1966, by Noback and Laemle,
in* The Primate Brain, *Appleton-Century-Crofts, Inc., New
York, 1970.*)

cells and in their cytoplasmic processes. These
processes interdigitate between the outer segments of the rods and cones. The pigment epithelium absorbs the light rays which were not
successful in activating the photopigments in
the rods and cones. If excess light were not
absorbed, it would backscatter, activate photopigments in other rods and cones, and thus blur

sharp resolution. In addition, these cells provide
metabolic (e.g., active transport of ions) and
functional support for the rods and cones. For
example, the pigment epithelium may be essential to the survival of the photoreceptors, because when it is severely damaged, the adjacent
rods and cones degenerate.

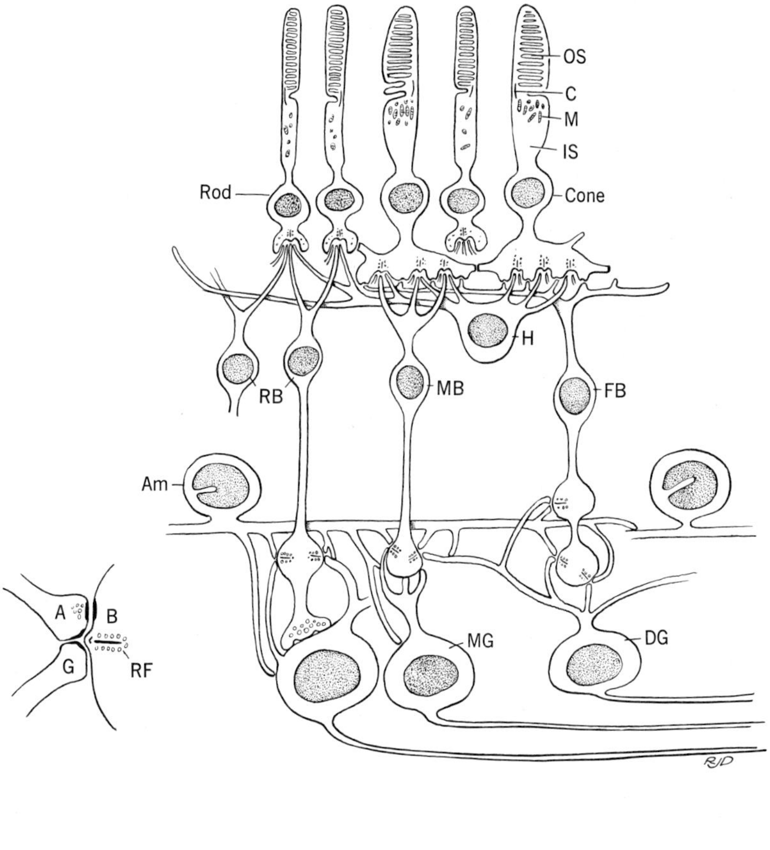

FIGURE 12-9

The ultrastructural orga-
nization of the retina, illustrating the relationship
of the rods, cones, and
intraretinal neurons.

The rod spherules have synaptic contacts with rod bipolar
cells (RB) and horizontal cells
(H). The cone pedicles have
synaptic contacts with midget
bipolar cells (MB), flat bipolar
cells (FB), and horizontal cells
(H). The processes of the
amacrine cells (Am) have synaptic contacts with the three
types of bipolar cells, midget
ganglion cells (MG), and
diffuse ganglion cells (DG).
Insert at lower left: synaptic
contacts between an amacrine
cell terminal (A), ganglion cell
process (G), and a bipolar cell
process (B); this is called a
dyad synaptic complex. The
ganglion cells give rise to
axons of the optic nerve,
chiasm, and tract. Note mitochondria (M) within the inner
segments (IS), cilia within
connecting stalks (C), and the
disks of the outer segments
(OS) of the photoreceptors.
RF, ribbon filament. (*Adapted
from Dowling and Boycott,
1966, by Noback and Laemle,
in* The Primate Brain, *Appleton-Century-Crofts, Inc., New
York, 1970.*)

Rods and cones: the photoreceptors (Figs. 12-6
through 12-9) The rods (rod cells) and cones
(cone cells) are elongated photoreceptors which
are polarized and segmented into subregions
with different functional roles. The *rods* are
slender; in the central part of the retina the rods
are about 2 μm in diameter, whereas in the more
peripheral regions they are about 4 to 5 μm in
diameter. The *cones* vary from those in the fovea
centralis, with a diameter of 1.5 μm, to those in
regions peripheral to the central part, with diameters of about 5 to 8 μm. Each photoreceptor
consists of an outer segment, a connecting

structure (connecting stalk), an inner segment,
a fiber with a cell body, and a synaptic base
(Figs. 12-6, 12-7).

The *outer segment* of a rod is a slender cylindric structure, and that of a cone has a relatively
short conical or tapered shape (Fig. 12-7). Each
outer segment is a stack of hundreds of flattened membranous disks (sacks), which are oriented at right angles to the long axis of the cell.
All the disks of a cone retain their continuity
with the cell membrane. Although some portions of the disks of a rod retain a similar continuity, most of the rod disks have no attach-

ment to the cell membrane. The lamellar membranes of the rod and cone disks are about 50 Å thick, which is roughly the diameter of a rhodopsin molecule (a visual pigment).

The narrow connecting stalk between the outer and inner segments is a cytoplasmic bridge enclosing a *cilium* (Fig. 12-7). The latter extends from a complex basal body in the apex of the inner segment into the outer segment. In fact, each outer segment is considered to be a modified shaft of specialized cilium.

The *inner segment* is divided into an outer portion, called the *ellipsoid zone*, and an inner portion, called the *myoid zone*. The outer portion is filled with mitochondria, and the inner portion contains the Golgi complex and an extensive endoplasmic reticulum. The cytoplasmic organelles of this latter segment—the metabolic center of the cell—are the synthesizers of new proteins, including photoreceptor proteins. After being synthesized, they are conveyed through the connecting structure to the base of the outer segment, where the double-membrane disks of the outer segments are formed (Fig. 12-7). The new disks of the rods are continually being formed at the level of the connecting structure by the successive infoldings of the cell membrane. The visual pigment molecules are incorporated, regularly oriented, and precisely aligned within the membranes. The disks are displaced in a choroid direction as newly formed disks are added. The disks lose their attachment to the cell membrane and become closed membrane sacks. Eventually the disks reach the tip of the outer segment, where they are cast off and incorporated within the pigment cells for disposal. In the case of the cones, the newly synthesized proteins from the inner segment diffuse throughout the outer segment and become incorporated in all disks of the cone.

The *visual pigments* of the rods and cones are constructed on a similar pattern. They are composed of a specific type of protein—called an *opsin*—which is bound to a chromatophore with a special configuration—called *retinaldehyde* (vitamin A aldehyde, retinal, retinene).

Rhodopsin is the photopigment of the rods in man; it has a maximum scotopic sensitivity of about 500 nm. The cones of man contain three photopigments, each cone containing one pigment, with their peak maximum absorptions at approximately 435 nm (blue), 535 nm (green), and 565 nm (red). The cones are called *blue cones, green cones,* and *red cones.* The cone pigments include *cyanolabe* (blue-sensitive pigment), *chlorolabe* (green-sensitive pigment), and *erythrolabe* (red-sensitive pigment). These three cone pigments act as the basis for color discrimination. All four photopigments possess the 11-*cis* retinaldehyde as the chromatophore and are united to four different opsins. The light-trapping efficiency of the outer segment is made optimal by the orientation of the chromatophores of the photopigment molecule in the plane of the disk. The rods and cones are oriented axially to the incident illumination. It is within this segment that the transduction and genesis of the generator (receptor) potential takes place.

The axonlike fiber is a cytoplasmic extension which includes a cell body with the nucleus of the cell. Each fiber terminates in a specialized synaptic body, which is in complex synaptic contact with the nerve fibers of bipolar and horizontal cells. The body of a cone is called a *pedicle*, or *end foot*, because its synaptic surface has a flat base; that of a rod is called a *spherule*, or *end bulb*, because it is small and rounded (Figs. 12-6, 12-8).

Neurons and their synaptic connections The human retina contains several types of cells: photoreceptive cells, bipolar cells or neurons, interneurons, and ganglion cells or neurons (Figs. 12-8, 12-9). It contains one type of glial cell, called Müller's cells. The photoreceptive cells are the rods and cones. The bipolar cells may be classified into three types: rod (mop) bipolar cells, with moplike tuft endings observed in the light microscope; midget bipolar cells; and flat bipolar cells (Dowling and Boycott). The interneurons include the horizontal cell and the amacrine cell (anaxonic neuron, cell without an axon). The two types of ganglion cells are the midget ganglion cell and the diffuse ganglion cell.

The cell bodies of the retinal cells are found

in the three nuclear layers. Those of the rods and cones are in the outer nuclear layer; those of the horizontal, bipolar, and amacrine cells are in the inner nuclear layer; and those of the ganglion cells are in the ganglion cell layer (Fig. 12-9). The main bulk of the synapses are located in two synaptic regions called the plexiform layer and the ganglion cell layer. Synaptic interactions occur among the photoreceptors, horizontal cells, and bipolar cells in the outer plexiform layer. Similar activities take place among the bipolar cells, amacrine cells, and ganglion cells in the inner plexiform layer and ganglion cell layer.

In a general way, the sequence of receptor cells to bipolar cells to ganglion cells conveys neural influences in an axial (vertical) direction within the retina and then to the brain via the axons of the ganglion cells. The horizontal cells and the amacrine cells, with their wide horizontal spread within the plexiform layers, may act to mediate lateral interactions within the retina. The nerve fibers of these cells may be capable of both receiving and transmitting stimuli; it is not possible, as yet, to determine whether each process is a dendrite or an axon.

Müller's cells (Fig. 12-8) These specialized neuroglial cells of the retina are more like astrocytes. Their radially oriented processes fill the interstices among the neurons of the retina, including portions of the rods and cones. In a sense these cells envelop these retinal neurons. In addition to their supportive and insulator rods, Müller's cells are a reservoir for glycogen—a source of energy.

Synaptic organization of the cone pedicles and rod spherules (Figs. 12-8, 12-9) The flat base of each pedicle has from several to as many as 25 invaginations. The region of each invagination represents a synaptic complex composed of a precise arrangement of processes (Fig. 12-9). The lateral elements are the processes of horizontal cells; the central elements are the processes of one or more bipolar cells. These synaptic complexes are called *ribbon synapses*, because, in addition to presynaptic vesicles, a dense ribbon or bar is located in the presynaptic pedicle of a cone. Ribbon synapses are organized to function as feedback loops. The base of each pedicle

has individual superficial synaptic contacts with the dendrites of several bipolar cells.

Each spherule has from one to several ribbon synapses. Within each invagination are the central processes of one or more bipolar cells and the lateral processes of several horizontal cells. In addition, contacts between pedicles, between spherules, and between spherules and pedicles are present.

Bipolar cells (Fig. 12-9) The three types of bipolar cell make the following synaptic connections. Each *rod bipolar cell* is involved with *1* ribbon synapses with from several to many rods and horizontal cells within the outer plexiform layer, and *2* axosomatic, axodendritic, and ribbon synapses with diffuse ganglion cells and amacrine cells within the inner plexiform layer and ganglion cell layer. In general, each *midget bipolar cell* (located in the fovea centralis) has several ribbon synapses in the pedicle of but one cone. In turn, each midget cell makes numerous axodendritic and ribbon synapses with amacrine cells and one midget ganglion cell, and, possibly, with some diffuse ganglion cells. Each *flat bipolar cell* makes synaptic contacts with the bases of many cones within the outer plexiform layer, and axodendritic and ribbon synapses with diffuse ganglion and amacrine cells within the inner plexiform layer.

Ganglion cells, horizontal cells, and amacrine cells (Fig. 12-9) Ganglion cells receive their input from bipolar cells and amacrine cells, and project their output to the midbrain and lateral geniculate body. Some of the synaptic contacts include the regular synapses with presynaptic vesicles and the ribbon synapses with the ribbon filament located in the terminals of bipolar cells.

Each *midget ganglion cell* makes several synaptic contacts with but one midget bipolar cell and several amacrine cells. Each *diffuse ganglion cell* makes synaptic contact with many of the three types of bipolar cells and amacrine cells.

The processes of the *horizontal cells of the outer plexiform layer* and those of the *amacrine cells of the inner plexiform layer* are oriented parallel to the retinal surface and at right angles to the axis of receptor cells to bipolar cells to ganglion cells.

ARTERIAL SUPPLY OF THE RETINA

The retinal cells are dependent upon an un-interrupted, never-ending vascular supply for the maintenance and renewal of their cellular components. Recall that the rods, cones, and other retinal cells are never replaced during a lifetime. The inner layers of the retina contain a capillary plexus, but the outer layers, including that of the rods and cones, are avascular. The fovea centralis is also devoid of blood vessels.

The vascular supply to the eye is derived from the ophthalmic artery. The blood is distributed from this artery via two almost completely inde-pendent systems: the retinal system and the ciliary system. The retinal system is derived from the central retinal artery, which enters the eye through the middle of the optic nerve at the optic disk. This retinal vascular plexus, which is distributed to the inner retina, lacks sphincters. The ciliary system supplies the uveal tract. From the highly vascularized choroid layer, nutriments and oxygen pass to the outer layers of the retina.

GENERAL ORGANIZATION OF THE RETINA

The spatial relations and synaptic connectivity of the neurons of the retina are such that many functionally organized patterns of neurons are possible. In a general way, these cells are geo-metrically oriented in two planes: one perpen-dicular to the curve of the retina, and the other parallel to the curve of the retina. The sequence of rods and cones to bipolar cells to ganglion cells forms *columns* of cells or *signal path-ways* oriented in an axial direction to the reti-nal curve. The horizontal cells of the outer plexi-form layer and the amacrine cells of the inner plexiform layer are oriented parallel to the reti-nal curve; these cells permit interactions among the cells of the "columns." In addition, the "sig-nal pathways" of the retina are organized for convergence; the approximately 120 million rods and 7 million cones process their influences within these "columns" and then project their

output to the brain via only 1 million ganglion cells. Thus there are but 1 million channels of output from the retina. Each ganglion cell is the funnel through which certain rods, cones, and bipolar cells may exert their influences following stimuli from a circumscribed region in the field of vision.

Receptor field, response field, and center-surround Each bipolar cell and ganglion cell of the retina, neuron of the lateral geniculate body, and pyramidal cell of the visual cortex is wired into a pathway through which it may be influ-enced by a certain group of photoreceptors. In turn, each photoreceptor or group of photo-receptors is stimulated by light coming from some definable site in the field of vision, i.e., each of these cells has its own "eye view" of the environment. This eye view of a cell is a site in the field of vision, which will stimulate the cell either with excitatory or inhibitory stimuli. This site is called the *receptor field* or *response field* of that cell (Fig. 12-10).

The *receptor field* of each ganglion cell is organized into two zones (Fig. 12-10): a *small circular zone, called the center, surrounded by a concentric zone, called the annular surround (or periphery)*. The center may be likened to the hole in a doughnut, and the surround to the doughnut. On the basis of functional responses to light in the environment, each response field (receptor field) of a ganglion cell is organized into a *center-surround (circular-concentric) configuration*.

Two general types of receptor fields are found in the light-adapted eye: receptor fields with an on-center and an off-surround (excita-tory-center, inhibitory-surround), and receptor fields with an off-center and an on-surround (inhibitory-center, excitatory-surround). The on-center, off-surround receptor field of a gan-glion cell consists of the center, which fires vigorously when the illumination comes on (or "signs off"), and of a surround which gives a reverse response to a similar stimulus. The off-center, on-surround zones of the receptor field respond in the opposite ways. In both types, the two zones are functionally antagonistic, with the surround antagonistic to the center and the center antagonistic to the surround. One zone may modulate, inhibit, or reduce the activity of the other zone. These influences are exerted by one zone upon the other and are graded according to the intensity of the stimulation.

The concept of central excitation and surround inhibition (or central inhibition and surround excitation) is a basic processing activity in the sensory systems. It is an exquisite mechanism for enhancing contrast and sharpening borders (see the discussion of mutual inhibition, further on in this chapter, under "Functional Aspects of Vision"). This explains the observation that an on-center responds *1* more vigorously if the environmental light is directed on photoreceptors which exclusively influence the on-center, and *2* less vigorously if the same intensity of environmental light is directed on the photoreceptors over the entire on-center and off-surround. As a result of the interactions between center and surround, each retinal ganglion cell relays signals concerning the contrast between the intensity of the illumination in the center as compared with that in the surround. A small intermediate zone, called an on-off field, is recognized in the interface between the center and the surround. In a sense, each neuroretina is a mosaic of about 1 million ganglion cells which relay about 1 million center-surround receptor field transformations via their axons to the lateral geniculate body of the thalamus.

The anatomic basis for the center-surround receptive field has been proposed (Dowling and Boycott). The direct sequence of photoreceptive cells to bipolar cells to one ganglion cell is the basic linkage resulting in an anatomic substrate of the center of a receptive field (Fig. 12-9). The indirect sequence of photoreceptive cells to bipolar cells to amacrine cells to the same ganglion cell is the basic linkage of the surround of that receptive field (Fig. 12-9). The summation of the on-center excitatory activity with the off-surround inhibiting activity is resolved by the ganglion cell. The spread of the dendritic tree of the ganglion cells within the outer plexiform layer corresponds closely with the area of the centers of the receptive fields.

The concept of the receptor field of a ganglion cell applies to color vision responses in the retina. The center of the receptor field would respond maximally to a narrow portion of the visual spectrum (e.g., it may be spectrally sensitive to red wavelengths), whereas the antagonistic surround would respond maximally to

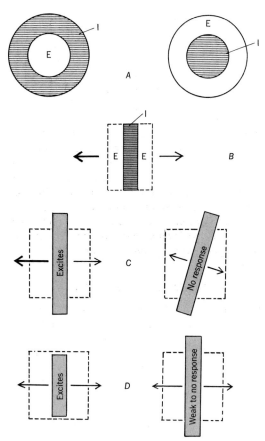

FIGURE 12-10
Receptive fields of neurons of the visual pathway.

A The center-surround receptive fields may have an excitatory center (E) with an inhibitory surround (I) or an inhibitory center (I) with an excitatory surround (E). These annular fields are featured by the retinal ganglion cells, neurons of the lateral geniculate body, and some cells of area 17.
B The simple receptive field of a neuron of area 17 has linearly oriented excitatory areas parallel to an inhibitory area.
C The complex receptive field of neurons of areas 17, 18, and 19 is featured by a moving excitatory slit of light; precise orientation of the slit is critical, but length of slit is not.
D The hypercomplex receptive field of neurons of areas 17, 18, and 19 is featured by a moving excitatory slit of light; precise orientation and length of the slit are critical. Arrows indicate direction in which the slit of light moves to obtain response.

another narrow portion of the spectrum (e.g., it may be spectrally sensitive to green wavelengths). The linkage of red cones to bipolar cells to a ganglion cell comprises the red center, while the linkage of green cones to bipolar cells to amacrine cells to a ganglion cell comprises the green surround to the red center. In theory, the receptive fields include fields with *1* a red center with either a green or blue surround, *2* a green center with either a red or blue surround, and *3* a blue center with either a red or green surround. Because these cells and their linkages are color-coded and exhibit a differential sensitivity to different wavelengths of light, they are called *spectrally opponent cells,* and the theory is the *spectrally opponent concept.*

FUNCTIONAL ASPECTS OF THE RETINA

Rods and cones The quantity of radiant energy and the wavelengths are the two physical factors of light essential to the visual process. The quantity of the radiant energy in light that falls upon a unit area of the retina in a defined unit of time is subjectively interpreted in some degree of brightness. Analogously, a photometer measures light intensity. The various wavelengths are, in man, the basis of color discrimination. The colors of the spectrum are the subjective interpretation of certain wavelengths. The cones and rods of the retina are the photoreceptor cells which are responsive to the amount of radiant energy and to the wavelengths. Those light rays which do not react with the photopigments are absorbed by the pigment in the pigment epithelium of the retina and in the choroid layer.

The functional activities of the photoreceptive rods and cones are divided into *1* transduction, and *2* the genesis of the generator potential. *Transduction* consists of the photochemical reactions which take place in the membranous disks in the outer segments of the rods and cones. In vision, the only action of light is to isomerize the chromatophore retinaldehyde from the 11-*cis* to the all-*trans* configuration (Wald). After this step has been triggered, the remaining chemical steps can take place in

total darkness. One quantum of light supplies the stimulus energy which initiates the reaction in one molecule of visual pigment. The extraordinary sensitivity of the dark-adapted visual system of man is demonstrated by the perception of visual sensation from but 5 to 10 quanta of light. The visual threshold of the dark-adapted human eye is attained when a flash of light composed of 25 to 75 quanta of light at 500 nm enters the retina. Of these, about 5 to 15 quanta are absorbed only by the photopigment (rhodopsin) in the rods. After being bleached by the light, the molecules of the visual photopigments are regenerated quickly, at the rate of thousands of molecules per second. This reconstitution involves the reisomerization of the retinaldehyde to the 11-*cis* form, which is immediately reattached to opsin.

Rods are the sensors for the subjective perception of black, grays, and white. They respond to all radiations in the visual spectrum and even to radiations in the ultraviolet band. Unlike cones, rods do not react selectively to different wavelengths. Man is not normally aware of the visual experience of ultraviolet rays, because these wavelengths are absorbed by the lens. Ultraviolet light can activate the photopigments of the rods in a patient whose lens has been removed for cataracts. Such a person, called an aphakic, can see in an environment "illuminated" exclusively by ultraviolet light. Rhodopsin (visual purple) is the photopigment initiating the train of events leading to black and white vision.

Color vision depends upon *1* the receptor activity of three types of cones, and *2* the processing within the central nervous system. Much is known about the first process and relatively little about the second. In some way, the chemical steps triggered by the light waves in the photopigments are responsible for the *genesis of the receptor* (*generator*) *potential in the rods and cones.* The resulting potentials influence changes in the plasma membranes of the synaptic bodies of rods and cones. Presumably, the presynaptic membranes of the ribbon synapses and other synapses associated with the synaptic bodies are depolarized. In turn, neurotransmitters are released from the photoreceptors to stimulate the postsynaptic membranes of the bipolar cells and the horizontal cells. The *ribbon synapse* is considered to be a feedback circuit. The rods, cones, horizontal cells, bipolar cells, and amacrine cells respond to stimulation with slow, graded potentials. These cells exhibit varying degrees of depolarization and hyperpolarization. They do not have all-or-none action potentials.

Duplicity theory of vision The duplicity theory of vision assumes that the retina is a mosaic composed of two fine-grain emulsions: the rods comprise the black and white emulsion, sensitive to low light intensities, and the cones comprise the color emulsion, sensitive to high light intensities. The rods are specialized for dim-light (twilight or night) vision in which low-threshold sensitivity is at a premium. The cones are specialized for color vision and the registering of fine detail. Because cones have a high threshold, they require bright illumination (daylight vision) to be effective receptors. In a way, the retina is a remarkable photographic plate. It is analogous to a composite black-and-white film and a color film. The black-and-white film has the fast emulsion effective in twilight, and the color film has the slow emulsion effective only in broad daylight.

The modern variation of the duplicity theory does not place so much emphasis on the dichotomy of function between rods and cones; it stresses rather the interplay among the rods, cones, and other neurons of the retina.

Receptor fields of the retina There are roughly 120 million rods, 7 million cones in the retina of each eye, and upward of 1 million ganglion cell nerve fibers to form each optic nerve. The difference between the number of receptors (rods and cones) and the number of ganglion cells is indicative of the convergence operating in the retina.

The rod-free *fovea* contains about 4,000 cones and an equal number of bipolar cells and ganglion cells. In essence the functional unit of one cone, one bipolar neuron, and one ganglion neuron forms a "private-line system" that projects through the optic nerve to the brain. Some interaction occurs among these units. Each receptor field in the fovea is narrow. The *receptor field of a bipolar cell* (or of a ganglion cell) is the retinal area from which it is possible to evoke an impulse from stimulation by light. The *receptor field of a foveal ganglion cell* is that of one private-line cone unit (2 μm wide, subtend-

ing an angle of only a few minutes of an arc at the cornea). The cones in this region are narrow (2 μm wide). As a result, the fovea is the region of maximal discriminative capacity. In fact, the part of an object seen most sharply is that portion which falls on the fovea.

Proceeding from the fovea toward the rest of the retina, the relative number of rods increases until only rods are present in the periphery of the retina. The nonfoveal retina is composed of receptor fields consisting of many rods converging on one bipolar cell with, in turn, many bipolar cells converging on one ganglion cell; and of receptor fields consisting of many rods and cones converging on one bipolar cell and, in turn, many bipolar cells converging on one ganglion cell. As many as 200 rods converge on one bipolar cell and as many as 600 rods converge to influence (through interneurons) one ganglion cell in the peripheral retina. A receptor field in the peripheral retina may be as large as 1 mm in diameter; this corresponds to an arc of 3° in the 160° visual field.

These nonfoveal receptor fields with multiple receptors (rods and cones) are designed to integrate and pool the stimuli from a "relatively" wide area. Hence this portion of the retina has lower discriminatory power but operates at low thresholds. It is specialized to operate in very dim light. In fact, at night one can identify an object with more certainty by not looking directly at it. In this way the object is focused on the nonfoveal retina, instead of on the fovea. When the object is focused on the nonfoveal retina at night the rods are permitted to function maximally with their party-line systems.

Ganglion cell systems *Four types of ganglion cell systems (sets or fibers)* have been described according to the manner in which their discharge is initiated. Some ganglion cells commence to discharge impulses when the light stimulus is *on* and continue to discharge a series of impulses throughout the duration of the photoimpingement on the retina. The firing rate of these units increases under light stimulation. These ganglion cells belong to the *on* system. Other ganglion cells discharge impulses only at the termination of photoimpingement; they belong to the *off* system. Other ganglion cells discharge impulses at the beginning and again at the termination of photoimpingement; they belong to the *on-off* system. Other ganglion cells exhibit a spontaneous steady discharge with no light stimulus acting. The discharge in this *steady-background* system occurs even after the eye has been dark-adapted (kept in the dark) for several hours. Normally the retina is, in fact, discharging at all times, whether it is being photopically stimulated or not. Shadows as well as light can increase retinal activity. In a sense the discharges via the optic nerve are expressed in a frequency modulation (FM) code, with an increase and decrease in the rate of discharge.

The ganglion cell subserving a receptive field yielding an *on* response is surrounded by a concentric band of ganglion cells subserving a receptive field yielding *on-off* responses, which in turn is surrounded by another concentric band yielding *off* responses. The reverse occurs with an *off*-response field surrounded by an *on-off* response band, which is surrounded, in turn, by an *on*-response band. An *on* field can inhibit an *off* field, and an *off* field can inhibit an *on* field. In all likelihood the horizontal neurons of the retina are involved in these inhibitory effects. The main function of these units and their interplay seems to be the response to the contrast in the illumination among the regions of the units. The interactions between elements of these systems are indicative of the complex dynamic nature of the retinal neuronal activity. The *on* sets, *off* sets, and *on-off* sets can also be identified in the lateral geniculate body and the primary visual cortex of the optic pathways.

Functional aspects of vision

SEARCHING MOVEMENTS

The eyes are never still. *Searching movements* are continuously taking place in the pursuit of moving objects. When the object moves, the eye moves. The basic activity is actually a survival legacy from our animal forebears who searched the environment for enemies, food, and shelter.

Perpetual, quick, small oscillations are indicative of the high-frequency scanning essential to maintain a visual image. Actually it is impossible to hold the eyes absolutely still. When an image projected on the retina is held absolutely stationary (which can only be done experimentally), the image fades, its coloration diminishes, and its contours dissolve away.

CONTOUR SHARPENING AND BRIGHTNESS CONTRAST (LATERAL INHIBITION)

In the phenomena of perception called contour sharpening and brightness contrast, our subjective sensations are the result of altered comparisons and contrast. For example, a bulb of a certain brightness will appear brighter subjectively when in a poorly lighted room than in a well-lighted room. The interactions among neurons are significant in distorting and exaggerating our image of the environment to maintain and to enhance boundaries. The retina utilizes such interactions to sacrifice less significant detail, to emphasize more significant detail, and to bias the representation of the patterns of the objects seen. More specifically, the *eye enhances information about the borders and contours and this information is transmitted to the brain at the expense of other details.* An artist conveys effects by exaggerating the depth of black at the edge of a shadow and lightening the whiter edge at the border between dark and light. This phenomenon is normally performed by our visual system. For example, place a white sheet of paper on a blackboard; at the junctional edge of the paper and the board, the paper appears whiter and the blackboard blacker. This effect is perceived but does not really exist. The phenomenon is referred to as "contour sharpening" or "simultaneous brightness contrast." It is utilized effectively by the cartoonist.

Contour sharpening is an expression of lateral (mutual) inhibition. Lateral or cross connections that are inhibitory in their action exist among the neurons of the retina (Figs. 13-1 and 13-2). The horizontal neurons and amacrine cells (cells oriented parallel to the retinal curve) are important structural substrates for these actions; these cells may inhibit nearby neurons associated with different channels and signal pathways. The lateral inhibition is greater on nearby receptor units than on distant units. Widely separated units have minimal reciprocal inhibitory effects on each other. In effect the efficacy of any receptor unit is modified by the inhibitory influences of neighboring receptor units or by their lack.

The contrast effect in shadows occurs commonly in everyday experience. A careful visual examination of the shadow cast on a white paper on the shaded side of a box (Fig. 12-11) demonstrates the consequences of lateral inhibition. Recordings by a photometer indicate that each portion of the shadow in the figure reflects essentially the same intensity of light. Thus, if the visual system "sees" the shadow as it really is, then the subjective sensation should be of a relatively uniform dark shadow. However, this is not what is observed. Viewed from the proper perspective, the area of the shadow near the box is actually seen to be relatively lighter than the darker band along the edge of the shadow adjacent to the unshaded white paper. The differences perceived in the shadow are explained as follows:

1 The lighter area of the shadow appears lighter because the neurons stimulated by the shadow area near the box are minimally inhibited (*mutual inhibition*) by influences from the neurons stimulated by the dark side of the box. The result is that the excitatory influences from these neurons are capable of exerting optimal effects in the cerebral cortex.

2 The darker band along the edge of the shadow appears darker because the neurons stimulated by the shadow are maximally inhibited by influences from the neurons stimulated by the unshaded bright white paper. Hence the excitatory influences from the relatively dark band are inhibited sufficiently to yield the subjective experience of appearing darker.

It is obvious that the retina is not like a simple camera film merely registering an image and relaying it to the brain. The retina is actually a movable (since the eyes move) "little" brain that processes stimuli, selects detail, distorts it, and transmits coded information via the optic nerve to the brain. The retina produces neither a photocopy of nature nor a replica. Mutual inhibition contributes to this end by heightening contrast and discriminating against diffuse light. Information about borders and contours is transmitted at the sacrifice of other details. In a way

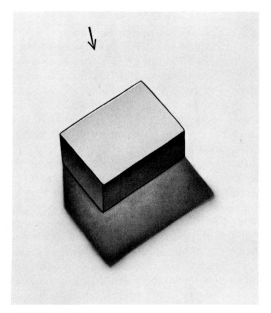

FIGURE 12-11
The phenomenon of *contrast inhibition* explains why certain areas appear lighter or darker than they really are.

The shadow adjacent to the box appears lighter than it really is because inhibition from the dark side of the box upon the shadow is minimal. The area of the shadow adjacent to the white unshaded area appears darker than it really is because inhibition from the light area is maximal. Arrow indicates direction from which light is coming.

we create our own personal image of our environment.

ADAPTATION

The human eye can adapt over a tremendous span of light intensities; it can visually discriminate over a luminance range of about 10 billion to 1. In essence, *adaptation* is an expression of the visual system's attempt to achieve equilibrium with the intensity of environmental light. For example, the completely dark-adapted eye can be stimulated by as much as 1/10,000 less light energy than the light-adapted eye (i.e., the dark-adapted eye is 10,000 times more sensitive to light). Examples of this sensitivity are the change in ability to see during the first half-hour in a darkened motion picture theater and the intense subjective brightness of light upon opening one's eyes after sleeping. The eye which is exposed to good illumination for a time is said to be light-adapted, whereas the eye which has been in darkness for a spell is said to be dark-adapted.

Psychophysical analyses indicate that most of the change in light adaptation is completed within one-tenth of a second, even though it may take as long as a half-hour to become completely dark-adapted. The adjustments to the changes in illumination occur automatically. Several phenomena have been advanced to account for adaptation. The action of the iris and the degree of bleaching of the photopigments may be, at the most, minimally involved. The rapid phase of adaptation is likely to be the result of neural processing in the retina and possibly other optic centers. The constriction and dilation of the pupil may contribute. However, the change in the diameters from a minimally constricted pupil (2 mm) to a maximally dilated pupil (8 mm) represents an areal change of only 16 times. Recent studies suggest that adaptation is not related to the degree of bleached photopigment in the rods and cones.

The dark-adapted eye utilizes the pathways involving rods primarily. These sensitive photoreceptors are not sensitive to the longer wavelengths at the red end of the spectrum, because rhodopsin does not absorb red light. If one wears red goggles when in daylight, the eyes can become dark-adapted. Hence a night fighter pilot or a radiologist can attain and retain his dark-adapted vision by wearing red goggles in the daylight. One can see because the red light stimulates the red cones. When entering the dark environment, dark adaptation is quickly attained by removing the red goggles.

The ability to become dark-adapted is reduced by anoxia. Reduced oxygen levels in the blood constitute one reason why dark adaptation takes longer to achieve at high altitudes.

VISUAL ACUITY

The visual acuity of the eye is a measure of the sharpness with which detail can be distinguished or resolved. In effect, the maximal acuity is the smallest distance by which two lines or two dots can be appreciated without appearing as one line or one dot. When visual acuity is low, fine details are blurred, and outlines and contours become indistinct. Visual acuity can be influenced by such environmental factors as illumination and degree of contrast in detail. In practice, acuity can be measured by the angle of resolution—the angle formed at the retina by the light from any two points in space. The minimal visual angle is slightly less than 1 min.

The "signal pathways" convey information initiated by the rods and cones. They are organized to transmit influences which result in varying degrees of visual acuity. The fovea centralis of the macula is the region of the retina associated with the greatest degree of visual acuity. The cells associated with this zone and its neuronal connections are arranged to ensure this acuity. The fovea centralis consists of a large number of slender cones (no rods) and an outer plexiform layer. The other retinal layers influenced by the foveal cones are displaced radially away from the fovea. Hence light passes almost directly from the vitreous body to these photoreceptors. The cones are linked by a *"private-line" system* of a cone to a midget bipolar cell to a midget ganglion cell to lateral geniculate body to visual cortex. The communication among these separate channels is minimal and is functionally organized to maintain the identity of each channel. Thus the anatomic basis for visual acuity comprises many separate channels, each conveying its distinct bit of fine-grain datum from a receptive field monitored by one cone and relayed centrally by one ganglion cell.

The degree of visual acuity diminishes the farther away the receptive field of a ganglion cell is from the fovea. In these regions, the receptive field is composed of many photoreceptors to a lesser number of rods and flat bipolar cells to one diffuse ganglion cell. Regions associated with lesser visual acuity are regions in which a greater number of photoreceptors is associated with the receptor field of one ganglion cell. In these regions the grain is coarser. Another factor contributing to lesser acuity in these regions is the fact that each photoreceptor cell (rod in areas of least acuity) is associated with fields of many ganglion cells.

Clinically, visual acuity is stated in terms of the size of letters a subject with normal vision can see at 20 ft away as compared with the size seen by the tested subject. In the *Snellen eye charts* used for testing vision, visual acuity is stated as a ratio of 20 over another number. The 20 is the number of feet selected (6 m in Europe) as the distance that the normal eye can see a letter subtending an angle of 1 min. The denominator represents the distance in feet that the observer can identify the same letter. Thus, if a subject can see letters of the standard size that he should be able to see at 20 ft, he has 20/20 vision. If the subject can see only letters that he should be able to read at 100 ft (while standing 20 ft away), he has 20/100 vision. A subject has 20/15 vision if he can distinguish letters at 15 ft that a person with normal vision can see at 20 ft.

COLOR VISION

The visual system reacts to specific wavelengths of light, and, in turn, this information is processed into the subjective experience of color. The entire visual pathway system is involved. The perception of yellow light from the simultaneous flashing of red light into one eye and of green light into the other eye is explained as a consequence of cortical processing. Only a limited number of vertebrates (diurnal animals) have color sense. Many primates, a few other mammals, birds, several groups of fish, and some reptiles can distinguish color. Apparently color vision has evolved independently several times during the phylogeny of the vertebrates.

Colors are characterized by hue or tone, brightness, and saturation or purity. The *hue* or *tone* of a color is a measure of the wavelength perceived. Red, yellow, blue, and green are different hues. *Brightness* is the subjective sensation that is determined by the amount of black in the color—the more black, the less brightness. In effect, the more black in the color, the more light is absorbed and the less light is reflected. The *saturation* or *purity* of a color is the subjec-

tive sensation that is determined by the amount of white in the color. White alters the hue because it is composed of colors. Thus, the less white in the color, the more saturated or pure is the given hue. Pure colors are pastel colors.

In the duplicity theory, cones are the color receptors, and rods are the black-and-white receptors. The *Young-Helmholtz* theory of color vision (or one of its variations) states that specific cones are receptors for specific hues. The trichromatic theory is substantiated by the observations that there is one color receptor for red, one for green, and one for blue.

PURKINJE EFFECT

The *Purkinje effect* was named after the investigator who noted that light blue flowers are bluer at dawn or twilight than at midday. At dusk, red flowers appear black. An artist realizes that color values vary depending on the quantity and quality of light. Our eyes are more sensitive to reds and blues in dim light than in brighter light. The dark-adapted eye is most sensitive to green; the light-adapted eye is most sensitive to yellow. This Purkinje shift in the sensitivity of our eyes to color at different light intensities is probably related to the shift in the sensitivity of the different pigments of the retinal photoreceptors at the different light intensities. The Purkinje effect is analogous to the variations of color values that are obtained when color films are overexposed, underexposed, or "correctly" exposed.

COLOR BLINDNESS

Color blindness is a sex-linked characteristic present to some degree in 8 percent of males and 1.5 percent of females. All classifications are based on subjective defects in perception. Color perception is a behavioral response, not a physiologic one. Many aspects of color blindness are explained on the basis of the amount of photopigments in the blue cones, green cones, and red cones.

Individuals with three-color vision are called

trichromats; there are those with *1* normal color vision, *2* weak red vision (*protanomaly*), *3* weak green vision (*deuteranomaly*), and *4* weak blue vision. Persons in the latter three groups are called anomalous trichromats and are not color blind. The weakness to a color is due to reduction in amount of pigment, not to neural processing. In protanopia, the concentration of the red photopigment, erythrolabe, is reduced; while in deuteranopia, the concentration of the green photopigment, chlorolabe, is reduced.

Subjects with two-color vision are called *dichromats;* there are those who cannot perceive *1* red (*protanopia*), *2* green (*deuteranopia*), and *3* blue (*tritanopia*). In each of these three major classes of dichromats, one of the photopigments is absent and the other two are present in normal amounts. Protanopes lack erythrolabe, deuteranopes lack chlorolabe, and tritanopes lack cyanolabe. Protanopes are insensitive to red and cannot see at all in the red end of the spectrum. Deuteranopes can see red as brightly as a person with normal color vision does, but find it is the same color as green. Individuals who lack either red or green photopigments are said to be *"red-green" color blind.*

Dichromats and tritanopes are said to be color blind; trichromats (except those with normal vision) have a "color weakness." *Tritanopes* and individuals with no color vision (*monochromats*) are rare. The latter see the environment in shades of light and dark; some experience pain during light stimulation.

The reason why more males are color blind than females is that the red gene and the green gene are present, as a recessive trait, on the one and only X chromosome present in a male. Approximately one male out of 50 lacks a red gene, and one out of 16 lacks a green gene; hence 2 percent of men are protanopes and 6 percent are deuteranopes. Because a female has two X chromosomes, female dichromats (with red-green color blindness) occur in only one out of 250 women. The gene for blue is present on an autosome.

AFTERIMAGES

A visual stimulus invariably yields a visual sensation that lags, sometimes imperceptibly, behind the stimulus, but then disappears. Under proper conditions the sensation can persist as an image for as long as several minutes after the stimulus has been removed. Such "afterimages" are either complementary (i.e., negative) or positive.

The *negative afterimage* is produced by gazing at an illuminated object for 10 sec or more, and then gazing at a blank sheet of white paper. The afterimage on the white paper consists of images complementary to the original. Black objects will appear as white images, yellow as blue, blue as yellow, green as red, and red as green. The complementary color in the afterimage disappears after about 15 sec. The afterimage can be prolonged if the eyes are closed for a few seconds. On reopening the eyes, the complementary afterimage is seen again. This phenomenon is presumed to be related to the fatigue or insensitivity of some part of the visual system (possibly in the retina) from the initial strong stimulation. The color effects indicate that linkage factors do exist in color vision.

The *positive afterimage* results after viewing an illuminated object intently for 2 or 3 sec and then closing the eyes. This afterimage resembles the original object in form and color. Colors are true but faded, and bright objects persist as bright images. Positive afterimages are difficult to produce and seldom last more than 10 sec. These effects are presumed to be the result of the persistence of the stimulatory effect of the bright light, possibly through the photochemical activity in the rods and cones.

The visual pathways

The pathways from the eye are involved in two important functional roles: *1* the act of seeing, and *2* the numerous reflex activities which either are important to the visual process (such as accommodation) or are a consequence of the visual process (such as ducking on seeing a blow coming).

The bounded space of the environment seen by one eye (*monocular vision*) while that eye is fixed upon a stationary or fixation point is known as the field of vision of that eye. The *visual field* of a normal eye outlines an irregular oval; from the fixation point the perimeter of the oval extends roughly 60° nasally (medially), 60° upward, 70° downward, and 90° temporally (laterally).

Normally we see with both eyes, i.e., we have a binocular field of vision formed by the almost complete overlapping monocular fields of both eyes. Without changing the fixation of the eyes, the most lateral peripheral areas of the visual fields are seen by one eye only—this is the *monocular* field or crescent (Fig. 12-13). The accurate mapping of the visual fields of each eye can be determined with a perimeter or mapping screen by a process known as *perimetry.* By this method, the patient's fields can be charted, and sites of functional field defects outlined. With the subject gazing with one eye at a central spot directly in front of the eye (with the other eye covered), a small spot of light is moved back and forth across the field of vision. The subject indicates when he can see the spot of light or when he cannot see it. These indications are recorded on the chart. In such an examination the blind spot of the retina is located approximately 15° lateral to the central point of vision.

The projection of the field of vision upon the retina is inverted and reversed with respect to the object because of the lens (Fig. 12-13). We do not perceive objects upside down or reversed (right-left reversal), because the mind makes the essential adjustments in some unknown way. The right half of the field of vision of an eye is projected to the left half of the retina (left hemiretina) and the left visual field to the right hemiretina, while the upper half of the field of vision is projected to the lower half of the retina (lower hemiretina) and the lower visual field to the upper hemiretina. The field of vision of an eye or the retina may be divided into quadrants by two lines; a line in the horizontal meridian and a line in the vertical meridian intersecting in the middle of the macula (the fixation point). Thus the upper temporal quadrant of the field of vision is projected to the

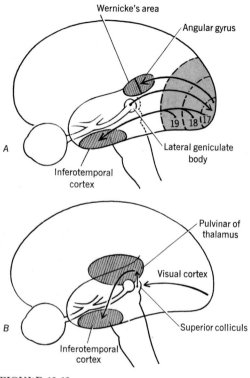

FIGURE 12-12
The two visual pathways.

A The geniculostriate system and *B* the tectal system. The functional significance of Wernicke's area and the angular gyrus is discussed in Chap. 16.

lower nasal quadrant of the retina, while the lower nasal quadrant of the field of vision is projected to the upper temporal quadrant of the retina. The nasal half of the field of vision of each eye is smaller than the temporal half, because of the shadow of the nose.

The retina may be divided another way. The region of the *macula* is the *macular retina;* this region of most acute sight is called the *central area* of vision. Surrounding the macula is the *paracentral (paramacular or pericentral) retina* or area of vision. This is, in turn, surrounded by the *peripheral retinal area of vision,* the region of least acute vision (Figs. 12-13, 12-14).

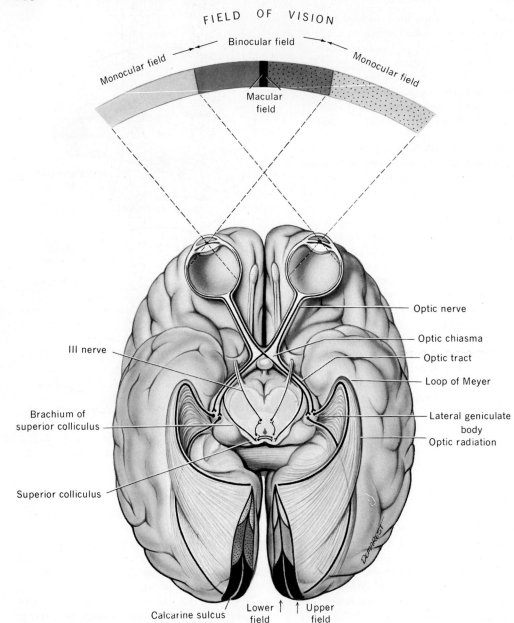

FIELD OF VISION

Binocular field

Monocular field

Monocular field

Macular field

Optic nerve

Optic chiasma

Optic tract

III nerve

Loop of Meyer

Brachium of superior colliculus

Lateral geniculate body

Optic radiation

Superior colliculus

Calcarine sulcus

Lower field ↑ ↑ Upper field

FIGURE 12-13

The visual pathways from the retina to the lateral geniculate bodies and to the primary visual cortex on either side of the calcarine sulcus.

The right visual field is projected to the left primary visual cortex (left visual field to right primary visual cortex). The macular field projects to the posterior aspect of the primary visual cortex (solid black). The rest of the binocular field projects to the visual cortex just rostral to the "macular visual cortex." The monocular field projects to the most rostral portion of the primary visual cortex. The upper half of the visual field projects to the primary visual cortex below the calcarine sulcus. The lower half of the visual field projects to the primary visual cortex above the calcarine sulcus.

Relation of visual fields to the organization of the visual pathways Normal vision is mainly *binocular*, with the temporal hemiretina of one eye "seeing" the same half of the field of vision as the nasal hemiretina of the other eye. When the two hemiretinas do not view precisely the same portions of the visual fields, *double vision (diplopia)* occurs. The visual pathways are organized so that corresponding sites of the images of objects in the real world, which are mapped upon the retina, are matched and fused in the visual cortex in order to obtain binocular vision. To accomplish this, the retinofugal fibers from the nasal hemiretina decussate and terminate in the contralateral lateral geniculate body, while those from the temporal hemiretina do not decussate and terminate in the ipsilateral lateral geniculate body. Thus at the geniculate level the corresponding areas of the two hemiretinas have been projected to the same geniculate body but to different laminae. The fusion of the images from the two hemiretinas into one image occurs at the next level—the visual cortex. To accomplish this transformation the geniculostriate projections to the striate cortex are organized so that corresponding foci terminate with small groups of neurons organized into functional columns. The precision of this connectivity is the means by which the pathways from the two hemiretinas can reinforce one another.

PATHWAYS FROM THE EYE

It is through the axons of the ganglion neurons of the retina that the output of the eyes is conveyed centrally. These axons pass through the optic nerves, optic chiasm, and optic tracts in a retinotopic organization to either the lateral geniculate body of the thalamus or to the tectum of the midbrain. At the present time at least two visual pathways are thought to be involved with visual perception. These are the geniculostriate system and the tectal system (Fig. 12-12).

The *geniculostriate system, or first visual system,* comprises the sequence of retina, to lateral geniculate body, to striate cortex (area 17). In this system the highest processing levels include the primary visual cortex (area 17), association visual cortex (areas 18 and 19), and the inferotemporal cortex (portions of the middle and inferior temporal gyri).

The *tectal system, or second visual system,* is difficult to define precisely at the present time. It may comprise the sequence of retina to superior colliculus, to the pulvinar of the thalamus, to the inferotemporal cortex. The tectum, the major visual integrating center in nonmammals, has presumably retained some older phylogenetic roles and modified others. In addition, the mammalian superior colliculus is actually a cortex—it is a laminated nucleus with a cortical type of neuronal organization, which has direct and indirect neural connections with the cerebral cortex.

Other pathways from the retina include those involved with various reflexes and the pineal gland. The superior colliculus and pretectum are important nuclear structures intercalated in the pupillary reflex, accommodation, and conjugate movements of the eye. The accessory optic system, involving several small nuclei in the midbrain tegmentum, has a significant role in the function of the pineal gland (refer to Chap. 11).

RETINOGENICULOSTRIATE PATHWAY (RETINA TO PRIMARY VISUAL CORTEX)

The axons of the ganglion cells of the retina converge to the head of the optic nerve (blind spot, optic disk). After passing through the lamina cribrosa of the sclera at the head, the axons emerge, become myelinated, and form the optic nerve. *These fibers from the temporal hemiretina course via the optic nerve, optic chiasm, and ipsilateral optic tract before terminating in the ipsilateral lateral geniculate body* (Fig. 12-14). *The fibers from the nasal hemiretina course in the optic nerve, decussate in the optic chiasm, and pass via the contralateral optic tract before terminating in the lateral geniculate body.* Most of the fibers (about 70 to 80 percent) in the optic tracts terminate in the lateral geniculate bodies; the remainder terminate in the midbrain, mainly in the superior colliculi. Although there is some intermingling of the fibers, they are retinotopically localized in their course from the retina to their termination within the six laminae of the lateral geniculate body (Fig. 12-14). The fibers from each temporal hemiretina synapse with neurons in laminae 2, 3, and 5, and those from each nasal hemiretina synapse with

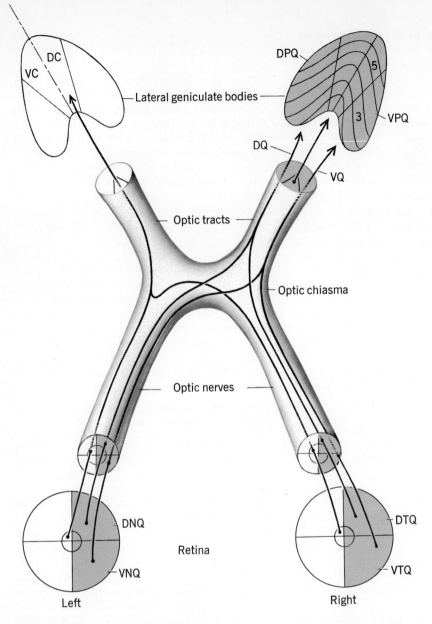

FIGURE 12-14
The course of the ganglion cell fibers from the retina to their terminations within the lateral geniculate bodies.

The crossed fibers from the nasal hemiretina (dorsal nasal quadrant, DNQ, and ventral nasal quadrant, VNQ) terminate in laminae 1, 4, and 6 of the lateral geniculate body (LGB). The uncrossed fibers from the temporal hemiretina (dorsal temporal quadrant, DTQ, and ventral temporal quadrant, VTQ) terminate in laminae 2, 3, and 5 of the LGB. The fibers of the dorsal nonmacular quadrants of the retina pass through the medial parts of the optic tracts (DQ) to the medial aspect of the LGB (DPQ). The fibers of the ventral nonmacular quadrants of the retina pass through the lateral part of the optic tracts (VQ) to the lateral aspect of the LGB (VPQ). The fibers from the macular region project to the wedge-shaped *sector* of the LGB; those fibers from the dorsal macula terminate in the medial part of the *sector* (DC); and those fibers from the ventral macula terminate in the lateral part of the *sector* (VC). (*Adapted from Hoyt and Luis, 1962, by Noback and Laemle, in* The Primate Brain, *Appleton-Century-Crofts, Inc., New York, 1970.*)

neurons in laminae 1, 4, and 6 of the lateral geniculate body.

Each *optic nerve* is composed of about 1 million axons with the fibers organized into about 800 to 1,200 fascicles, each invested by a pial sheath. Actually the optic nerve is not a cranial nerve, but rather it is a tract because its myelin is formed by oligodendroglia (not Schwann cells), and its axons are those of second-order neurons. The bipolar cells of the retina are the first-order neurons. In general, most macular fibers pass through the central region of each optic nerve until they reach the chiasm, where the decussating fibers and the nondecussating fibers ascend and gradually pass into the superior aspect of the optic tracts (Fig. 12-14). These fibers from the macula project to a wedge-shaped sector in the upper posterior two-thirds of the lateral geniculate body, mainly in the small-celled laminae 3, 4, 5, and 6 and only slightly in the large-celled laminae 1 and 2.

The nonmacular fibers from the upper and lower temporal quadrants (those with uncrossed central projections) maintain their superior-inferior temporal positions within the nerve and chiasm; in the chiasm these fibers undergo an inward 90° rotation until *1* the fibers of the upper quadrant shift from their dorsolateral location in the optic nerve to a medial and inferior location in the optic tract, and *2* the fibers of the lower quadrant shift from their ventrolateral location in the optic nerve to their lateral and inferior location in the optic tract.

The nonmacular fibers from the upper and lower nasal quadrants (with crossed central projections) maintain their superior-inferior positions within the nerve and chiasm, until they decussate through the chiasm. The fibers of the lower nasal quadrant shift from their inferior medial location in the optic nerve to the ventrolateral aspect of the contralateral optic tract, while those of the upper nasal quadrant shift from their superior medial location in the optic nerve to the medial aspect of the optic tract.

In general, fibers from corresponding points in the two retinas course together in the optic tract. The fibers from the upper nonmacular quadrants of the retina project to the medial aspect of the lateral geniculate body, and those from the lower nonmacular quadrants project to the lateral aspect of the lateral geniculate body (Fig. 12-14). Some of the fibers from the inferior nasal retinal quadrant loop slightly (Wilbrand's loop) into the contralateral optic nerve before reentering the chiasm.

The retina has precise point-to-point connections with the lateral geniculate body, which is also called the dorsal lateral geniculate body. In man, a small ventral lateral geniculate body, also called the pregeniculate body, is present. The lateral geniculate body consists of six laminae, numbered from 1 to 6. The two ventral laminae (or magnocellular layers), numbers 1 and 2, contain large cell bodies; the four dorsal laminae (or parvocellular layers), numbers 3 to 6, contain small cell bodies. The contralateral projection from the optic tract terminates in layers 1, 4, and 6, and the ipsilateral projection in layers 2, 3, and 5. More precisely, each fiber in the optic tract projecting to the lateral geniculate body synapses with five to six adjacent neurons within a lamina. Some overlapping occurs, with each ganglion cell projecting to the lateral geniculate body synapsing with several geniculate neurons (*divergence*), and with geniculate neurons receiving input from several retinal ganglion cells (*convergence*). Each geniculate cell is monocular, in that it receives input from only one eye. All in all, the number of fibers in the optic tract terminating in the lateral geniculate body is about the same as the number of fibers projecting from the lateral geniculate body to the primary visual cortex.

Lateral geniculate body The receptive field of each neuron of the lateral geniculate body is similar to that of a retinal ganglion cell (Fig. 12-10). The cell's eye view of the visual field is that of a center-surround. On the basis of responses evoked following the stimulation of the retina with monochromatic light, two basic types of neurons are indicated: broad-band cells (spectrally nonopponent cells), and spectrally opponent cells. The *broad-band cells* of the lateral geniculate body respond to all wavelengths and white light. The *spectrally opponent cells* are differentially sensitive to light of different wavelengths. These latter cells are presumed to be concerned with color vision. They are color coded. Five subclasses of color-receptive fields have been described. They include those with   *1* red on-center, green off-surround; *2* red off-center, green on-surround; *3* green on-center, red off-center; *4* green off-center, red on-surround; and *5* blue on-center, green off-surround.

Complex interactions and processing probably occur within the lateral geniculate body among the retinogeniculate endings, corticogeniculate endings, and intrageniculate neurons. However, the precise functional role of the lateral geniculate body in the visual system is not known. One certainty is that each neuron of the lateral geniculate body receives direct input from the retina and, in turn, projects directly to the striate cortex (area 17). The body may act *1* to discard certain influences, *2* to modify the input by compressing it into fewer channels, and *3* to modify the code by recoding.

The only output from the lateral geniculate body to the cerebral cortex is via the geniculocalcarine tract to the striate cortex.

Geniculocalcarine tract   The *geniculocalcarine tract (optic radiation)* is the retinotopically organized pathway from the lateral geniculate body to the primary visual cortex (striate cortex). After it leaves the geniculate body, this tract passes through the caudal aspect of the internal capsule (retrolenticular portion mainly), swings laterally and occipitally as the optic radiation lateral to the atrium and posterior horn of the lateral ventricle, and finally swings medially to terminate in laminae 3 and 4 of the primary visual cortex (area 17). The fibers carrying information from the macula are located in the center of the optic radiation and terminate in the most occipital part of the visual cortex (Fig. 12-13). The fibers carrying information from the upper hemiretinas are located in the upper half of the optic radiation and terminate in the visual cortex above the calcarine sulcus. The fibers carrying information from the lower hemiretinas are located in the lower half of the optic radiation and terminate in the visual cortex below the calcarine sulcus. The lamina of fibers that loop into the temporal lobe before heading occipitally with the rest of the optic radiation is known as the *loop of Meyer* (Fig. 12-13). It

conveys impulses originating from the lower peripheral retina (nasal side of the opposite eye, temporal side of the eye on the same side). As a result, interruption of this loop in the right temporal lobe impairs peripheral vision in the upper quadrant of the left field of vision of both eyes.

VISUAL CORTEX

The visual cortex is conventionally divided into the *primary visual cortex* (*visual area I, striate cortex, area 17*), the *secondary visual area* (*visual area II, area 18, parastriate cortex*), and *visual area III* (*area 19, peristriate cortex*). Areas 18 and 19 are often called the visual association cortex or prestriate cortex.

The primary visual cortex is subdivided into three regions according to the original source of its input from the retina. The *macular (central) fibers* pass from the geniculate body directly through the intermediate part of the optic radiation to the most occipital third of the striate cortex on both sides of the calcarine sulcus. The *paracentral (paramacular) fibers* pass from the geniculate body through the optic radiation just above and below the macular fibers to terminate in the middle third of the striate cortex on both sides of the calcarine sulcus. The *fibers from the peripheral (pericentral) retinal areas* pass to the rostral third of the striate cortex. This most rostral area of the striate cortex is associated with monocular vision; its input is derived from the area of the field of vision which is directed to only one eye. The rest of the primary visual cortex is involved with binocular vision. Note that the small macular area of the retina has a large cortical representation; this is associated with the sharp visual acuity monitored by the macula. The peripheral retinal area, a region registering minimal visual acuity, is represented by a small cortical area.

Each point in the fields of vision is represented only once in the striate cortex, with the neighboring points of the visual field located in neighboring points in the striate cortex. In brief, the points in the visual fields are retinotopically mapped onto the primary visual cortex in a precise and orderly manner.

Of significance is the precise point-to-point retinotopic representation in which the impulses generated by the activity in a small receptor field of the retina are projected to a small discrete group of cells of the lateral geniculate body and inturn to a discrete cortical column. These pathways from the eye to the striate cortex preserve the separate identity of small functional units (center-surround units) of each retina and of one retina from the other. Estimates indicate that one foveal cone influences 100 or more cortical neurons in area 17. Some geniculocortical fibers may directly communicate with up to 5,000 cortical neurons. The fibers of the optic radiation terminate and synapse with neurons in laminae 3 and 4 of the primary visual cortex (Fig. 16-5). The act of fusion of the visual fields from both eyes commences in the laminae other than lamina 4 in the striate cortex. These other five laminae are the site of the initial integration of the information from corresponding points in both eyes. This localized precision and specificity of the optic pathways is neurophysiologically expressed as follows: One specific neuron in the striate cortex can be driven by the neural activity generated by a small spot of light on a specific site of the retina. This same neuron can also be driven by the activity generated by a spot of light focused on, and only on, the equivalent site in the other eye. Apparently neurons in laminae 2, 3, 5, and 6 of the striate cortex are stimulated by both eyes, suggesting that this is an expression of the *act of binocular fusion.*

The neurons of the primary visual cortex are grouped into thousands of columns, which extend from the pial surface through the entire thickness of the cerebral cortex to the white matter perpendicular to the surface. These columns are physiologically defined; they need not have a regular columnar shape. These columnar segments are arranged and oriented as compartments in a beehive comb. Each column receives fibers from a small group of lateral geniculate neurons via the optic radiation. Within each column some neurons (approximately 15 percent of them) are stimulated from influences from one eye, either the ipsilateral or the contralateral eye. The other neurons of the column are driven by both eyes, with some neurons being driven equally from both eyes and other neurons being driven more from one eye than from the other. *Most of the cells in lamina 4 are driven by one eye only,* with some responding to stimuli from the ipsilateral eye and others

to the contralateral eye. *The cells in laminae 2, 3, 5, and 6 are driven binocularly.* In general, the contralateral eye is the most effective in firing the striate neurons—this is the phylogenetically older input.

The primary visual cortex has connections with other regions of the cortex, mainly with areas 18 and 19 (Figs. 12-12, 16-1, 16-2) of the ipsilateral hemisphere. Areas 18 and 19 have direct corticocortical connections through the corpus callosum with areas 18 and 19 of the contralateral hemisphere. Area 17 has no direct connections through the corpus callosum with area 17 of the contralateral hemisphere. In man, the inferotemporal area probably receives its main visual input from the geniculostriate pathway through connections with areas 18 and 19. The inferotemporal area may receive significant input from the superior colliculus via a relay in the pulvinar (Fig. 12-12).

The various cortical areas involved with the visual system have important connections with subcortical centers. Corticofugal fibers to the midbrain comprise the corticotectal fibers to the superior colliculus and the corticoreticular fibers to the midbrain tegmentum. The corticotectal fibers course in the internal sagittal stratum. This stratum is a sheet of fibers located medial to the geniculocalcarine fibers, which comprise the external sagittal stratum. The influences conveyed by these fibers are integrated *1* in such reflexes as accommodation and extraocular movements, and *2* in the tectal system. The corticoreticular fibers are integrated into activities of the midbrain reticular formation. Corticofugal fibers from the visual cortex terminate in such thalamic nuclei as the pulvinar, lateral geniculate body, and lateral dorsal nucleus of the thalamus.

Neurons of the visual cortex The neurons in the binocular regions of the striate cortex (area 17) are responsive to one of four types of receptive field. On the basis of their responses these cells are called *center-surround cells, simple cells, complex cells,* and *hypercomplex cells.* The *center-surround cells* have response features which are basically similar to those found in the ganglion cells of the retina and lateral geniculate neurons.

Simple cells respond optimally to stimulation obtained from straight lines, bars, or edges having a precise orientation and position in space (Fig. 12-10). This critically positioned bar is composed of two bands located side by side; one band, an excitatory one, is separated by a straight edge from the other, an inhibitory one. Strong and brisk activity in simple cortical cells is evoked by moving stimuli passing through the excitatory receptive region. In general, each simple cell will respond to stimuli from either eye, but these cells have a preference for influences from one eye over the other.

Complex cells respond optimally to stimulation obtained from moving straight lines, bars, or edges, each having a precise orientation but a variable position in space (Fig. 12-10). These cells have a definite orientational preference associated with a larger receptive field than a simple cell. The antagonism between the excitatory band and the inhibitory band of the field is not as prominent and the specificity of the position of the stimulus in space is not as critical as for the simple cells.

Hypercomplex cells are detectors of angled and straight lines, bars, or edges, which move through the field of vision (Fig. 12-10). Again the orientation and length are critical. The position of these line segments or corners can vary over a large range.

In summary, center-surround neurons and simple cells are located in area 17, while complex and hypercomplex cells are found in areas 17, 18, and 19.

These cells are presumed to be organized hierarchically. In the sequence from retina to visual cortex, differences are observed in the sensitivity of the neurons to various stimuli; most of the neurons in the central area of the retina and the lateral geniculate body respond to both form and color stimuli, while many neurons in the striate cortex are sensitive either to form or to color, with only a few responding to both form and color.

The center-surround cortical cells are located only in lamina 4 of area 17 (Chap. 16). Each of these neurons is responsive to stimulation from one eye only—either from the contralateral or the ipsilateral eye. Each of these cortical cells has direct connections via the optic radiation from the lateral geniculate body. Some center-surround cells receive their input from the geniculate laminae that have connections with the ipsilateral eye, and the other center-surround cells receive their input from the geniculate laminae that have connections with the contralateral eye; i.e., *these center-surround cortical cells are monocularly driven. The neurons in the other laminae of area 17 are binocularly driven,* in that they are, in varying degrees, responsive to the stimulation from both eyes. This activity is a corollary of the concept that *the act of fusion of the input from corresponding sites of both retinas first occurs in the simple cells of area 17.*

The visual cortex has been conceived to be organized in small columns extending from the pial surface of the cortex to the white matter (Fig. 16-5). Each column is composed of thousands of neurons, which are characterized by physiologic criteria. The columns in the striate cortex are composed of simple cells, complex cells, and hypercomplex cells, while those in areas 18 and 19 contain only complex and hypercomplex cells. Many neurons in the association visual cortex are not classified as complex or as hypercomplex cells. All neurons in a column, whether simple, complex, or hypercomplex, have similar receptive field orientation (Fig. 12-10). According to one theory, several cortical neurons with center-surround receptive fields interact with simple neurons. In turn a complex of simple cells interacts and supplies input to a complex cell, while the activity of a complex of complex cells results in supplying the basic input for the response patterns of hypercomplex cells. Thus many simple cells with similar patterns of orientation are said to synapse with a single complex cell; the latter generalizes a particular contour orientation. Some complex cells are conceived to exert excitatory and others inhibitory influences upon hypercomplex cells. In this way the hypercomplex cells are rendered responsive only to oriented contours of a defined length. Through sequences of serial processing, many orders of hypercomplex cells respond to stimuli from corners, angles, and more complex geometric patterns (Hubel and Wiesel).

The inferotemporal cortex (area 20, Fig. 12-12) may further process visual information from the geniculostriate system. Trigger features evoking responses in some cortical neurons of this area are those with highly specific meaning of visual reality to a monkey. The "shadow" of an extended "monkey's hand" evokes maximal activity, whereas bands or circles yield mild to no responses. Bilateral ablation of area 20 in a monkey impairs visual learning (Gross).

Role of superior colliculus in act of seeing

The *superior colliculus* has several roles in *1* the reflex control and regulation of many movements of the eyes and head (noted below), and *2* certain aspects of vision. This subcortical tectal center has a significant function in attention and perception associated with vision. A lesion limited to the superior colliculus modifies visual activity (this lesion does not involve the direct pathways from the eyes to the visual cortex). A monkey (or cat or dog) with one superior colliculus removed does not pay attention to stimuli from the contralateral visual field. Actually the animal is not blind to contralateral stimuli. It is overresponsive to the visual stimuli from the ipsilateral visual fields; in addition, it continually turns its head to the ipsilateral side. In summary, the *superior colliculus is more than a reflex center, it is an integrative center subserving visual perception.*

Higher functional expressions of the visual system The visual system has roles in both the unconscious and conscious spheres. According to some recent findings, the *concept of "two visual systems"*—i.e., the *geniculostriate system* and the *tectal system*—has been utilized to account for many of the physiologic expressions of the entire visual system (Fig. 12-12). The relative functional contributions of the two systems are incompletely understood. The phylogenetically newer geniculostriate system may mask certain expressions of the phylogenetically older tectal system. An essential primary difference between the two systems may be that the tectal

system answers the question, "Where is it?" in terms of visuomotor responses, and the geniculostriate system answers the question, "What is it?" in the form of learned and conscious responses (Schneider). The activities of the two systems are integrated through interconnections; they are not independent. Visual information is conveyed via the separate channels of these systems to the visual areas of the cerebral cortex where the perception at the conscious level is completed and unified.

Interaction between the geniculostriate system and the tectal system apparently occurs between the cortex and subcortical centers. For example, functional evidence indicates that the direction-selective collicular neurons of the superior colliculus are dependent for their characteristic neurophysiologic activity upon input derived from the direction-selective complex cells (with large receptive fields) of the striate cortex (Palmer et al.).

The tectal system is the phylogenetically older system. In nonmammalian vertebrates, the tectum has the dual roles of acting as visual reflex or visuomotor center and as the crucial center in visual perception. In mammals the visuomotor role is retained with some modification while the perceptive role is only partially retained. The perceptive function of the tectal system has been functionally altered in mammals by the neural connections with the inferotemporal cortex and by the phylogenetically new geniculostriate system. The visuomotor responses can be evoked rapidly through the tectal system, even before the subject is subjectively aware of the stimulus. A common experience is to jerk one's head and eyes and to jump away automatically from an object which suddenly intrudes from the side into the field of vision. The awareness of the object comes after the movements have been initiated. The stimuli responsible for these responses are conveyed largely via the tectoreticular, tectobulbar, and tectospinal fibers. In addition, the tectum may have a role in visual recognition in man. For example, a human patient with complete hemianopia was able to perceive small moving objects in the blind half of the eye, whereas he did not notice a stationary object even after a head movement (Denny-Brown). Rhesus monkeys with the striate cortex bilaterally ablated are able to localize moving objects. Lesions in the superior colliculus in certain mammals are known to produce deficits in pattern vision. The "Where is it?" question is answered by this system through the regulation of orienting movements. These are the acts of adjusting the relation of one's head, body, or body part to the external environment (e.g., movements of eyes or head in response to a new object in the field of vision). Stated otherwise, the tectal system is involved with those movements which orient the body in space and hold objects in the visual field invariant to the eyes through eye and head movements.

The perception mediated via the tectal system may occur bilaterally within each cerebral hemisphere. Apparently the automatic orienting movements are normal in patients with a transected corpus callosum. This system is unified within each cerebral hemisphere.

The functional roles of the visual cortex 17, 18, and 19 of the occipital lobe and inferotemporal cortex of the temporal lobe are discussed in Chap. 16.

Vertical meridian between the visual fields One-half of the common visual field seen by both eyes is projected from two hemiretinas (the nasal hemiretina of one eye and the temporal hemiretina of the other eye) to the visual cortex of one cerebral hemisphere. The other half of the common visual field is projected in a similar way to the visual cortex of the other cerebral hemisphere. Several possible mechanisms have been advanced to explain how the vertical meridians between the visual fields of the two sets of hemiretinas are joined and become continuous. The avoidance of a discontinuity of the vertical meridian may result, in part, because the ganglion cells at, and near, the junctional zone may project fibers bilaterally to both geniculate bodies. Another possibility is that the tectal system may correlate information received from the junctional zone through the posterior commissure before relaying influences via the pulvi-

nar to the inferotemporal cortex. Apparently the tectal system remains functionally unified in human subjects with split brains following sectioning of the corpus callosum. Interconnections between areas 18 and 19 of both cortices through the corpus callosum may contribute to ensuring this continuity.

The visual reflexes

Stimulation of the visual system evokes a number of reflex actions of critical significance to vision. Several of these reflexes will be outlined.

PUPILLARY CONSTRICTION: THE LIGHT REFLEX AND THE CONSENSUAL LIGHT REFLEX

When the eyes are exposed to bright light, the pupils contract, thereby reducing the intensity of the light reaching the retina. This *involuntary light reflex* (Fig. 12-15) is a reflex response to the direct stimulation by light. The involved pathways are as follows: the retinal ganglion cell axons course via the optic nerve, optic chiasma (some fibers decussate), optic tract, and brachium of the superior colliculus (bypassing the lateral geniculate body) to terminate in the pretectum. Interneurons project to the contralateral pretectum through the posterior commissure. Interneurons interact with other interneurons (some probably in the interstitial nucleus), which, in turn, synapse with preganglionic neurons of the oculomotor nerve. These preganglionic neurons project via the third cranial nerve and synapse in the ciliary ganglion (just behind the eye) with postganglionic neurons which innervate the constrictor muscle of the iris in the eye.

When only one eye is exposed to bright light, the pupils of both eyes will constrict. The crossing of some fibers in the optic chiasma and the interconnections across the midline by interneurons of the bilateral pretectum account for this consensual reflex. The reflex resulting in the constriction of the stimulated eye is known as the *direct light reflex*, while the reflex resulting in the constriction of the nonstimulated eye is known as the *consensual light reflex*. The constriction of the pupil in the stimulated eye is more vigorous than in the nonstimulated eye.

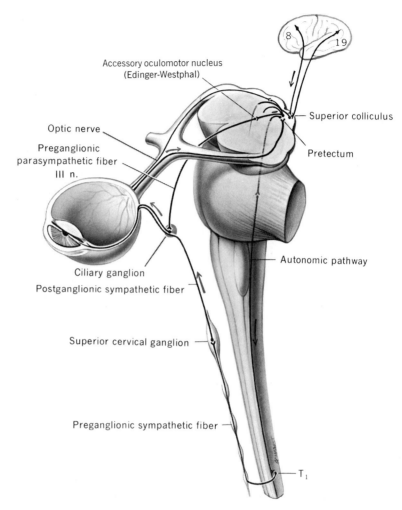

Accessory oculomotor nucleus
(Edinger-Westphal)

Optic nerve

Preganglionic
parasympathetic fiber
III n.

Superior colliculus

Pretectum

Autonomic pathway

Ciliary ganglion

Postganglionic sympathetic fiber

Superior cervical ganglion

Preganglionic sympathetic fiber

T₁

FIGURE 12-15
The light reflex pathways
(pupillary reflex) and the
accommodation pathway.

The light reflex pathways
relay *1* through the midbrain pretectum and the parasympathetic outflow of the
oculomotor nerve (pupillary
constriction), and *2* through
the sympathetic pathways of
the brainstem, upper thoracic
level, and ascending cervical
paravertebral sympathetic
trunk (pupillary dilatation).
Accommodation is mediated
via a pathway which includes
corticocollicular fibers from
the cerebral cortex (occipital
lobe, area 19, and frontal eye
fields, area 8), superior colliculus, and parasympathetic
outflow through the oculomotor nerve. (*After Krieg.*)

PUPILLARY DILATATION

When the eye is exposed to dim light, the pupil
dilates (Fig. 12-15). Optic pathways act through
the reticular formation and descending sympathetic pathways (in the dorsolateral tegmentum
of the brainstem and in the white matter in the
anterior half of the cervical spinal cord) to stimulate the preganglionic neurons of the sympathetic intermediolateral cell column of the C8
and T1 spinal levels. The preganglionic fibers
ascend in the sympathetic chain and synapse in
the superior cervical ganglion (upper part of the

neck) with postganglionic neurons, which, in
turn, travel adjacent to blood vessels to innervate the dilator muscle of the iris (Chap. 6).
Interruption of these fibers may result in Horner's syndrome (Chap. 5).

ACCOMMODATION

The process by which the refractory power of
the lens is changed is known as *accommodation.*
*This reflex action is mediated via the cerebral
cortex* (Fig. 12-15). One can voluntarily focus on
a nearby object or a faraway object. The path-

ways include the optic pathways from the eye to the cerebral cortex; in turn, a projection back from cortical area 19 (and from frontal eye field area 8) via the optic radiation through the brachium of the superior colliculus terminates in the nucleus of the superior colliculus (interneurons interconnect these bilateral nuclei). Through a chain of several interneurons these collicular nuclei are connected to the preganglionic neurons in the accessory motor nucleus of cranial nerve III. These parasympathetic preganglionic neurons project via the third cranial nerve and synapse in the ciliary ganglion with preganglionic neurons, which, in turn, innervate the ciliary muscles in the ciliary body. Pupillary constriction and convergence of the eye accompany accommodation to near vision.

DEPTH PERCEPTION

Depth and distance are judged and perceived in a number of ways. Except for stereopsis, which is a correlate of binocular vision, these qualities can be appreciated to a degree by cues which stimulate only one eye. Shadows, contours, curves, and angles subtended by objects of sizes familiar to the observer are constantly used. To an observer who is in motion, a significant source of information is obtained from the relative movements of near and distant objects from the effect of motion parallax. For example, to the eye of a moving individual, the changing relations of objects at different distances constantly shift. The conscious awareness associated with the focusing of the lens during accommodation is said to contribute to depth perception.

The most precise and accurate means for localizing objects in space utilizes the images seen simultaneously by both eyes. This visual aptitude is called *stereopsis* or *solid vision*. The location of objects in the third dimension by vision is possible, in part, because of the differential selective activity of neurons in the visual cortex, which respond to input from both eyes (Blakemore and Pettigrew). Stereopsis is based upon *1* the fact that the visual cortex on one side receives input from the contralateral nasal

hemiretina and the ipsilateral temporal hemiretina, and *2* the presence of an interhemispheric link through the corpus callosum. Apparently the sole basis of stereopsis is the *horizontal disparity* between the two hemiretinal images. This appears to be related to the fact that the eyes are separated from each other in a horizontal plane through the head, and that the visual pathways from the two eyes are organized both structurally and functionally to maintain a slight disparity. The horizontal disparities between the two hemiretinas viewing the same visual field obtain the cues of depth; in turn, the processing in the neurons of the visual pathway leads to depth perception. Apparently the visual system does not make use of *vertical disparities*. Because of, as yet, undetermined anomalies of binocular vision, stereopsis is not expressed in about 2 percent of the population.

The horizontal disparity is related to the following neural correlates. The pathway from each nasal hemiretina projects dominant, and more precisely localized, influences to the simple and complex cells of the visual cortex, while the pathway from each temporal hemiretina projects less effective and less precisely localized influences to the visual cortex. Stated otherwise, the phylogenetically old crossed pathway conveys more effective projections to the visual cortex than does the phylogenetically new uncrossed pathway. These differences in input from the same half of the visual field via these two pathways from the two eyes create disparities in the neurons of the visual cortex; these horizontal disparities, which vary widely from cell to cell, have a significant role in the ability of these binocularly driven neurons to register distances in space. In effect, different neurons are stimulated optimally by objects located at different distances. The cortical columns in the visual cortex are organized as processing stations, which make use of disparity information for discriminating the relative distances of objects from the eyes. Experimental evidence indicates that about 85 percent of the neurons in visual cortex area 17 are driven by influences from both eyes and that the remainder are driven by either the contralateral or the ipsilateral eye. It is the binocularly driven neurons that register disparity. The disparity range is about 2° in the region of the area centralis and about 6° for those neurons receiving input from the visual field 10° away from the midline (Blakemore).

EYE MOVEMENTS

To obtain true binocular vision the same points in the field of vision common to the two eyes must be focused upon corresponding loci in the two retinas. Optimal visual acuity is attained when the fixation point (center of the visual target) in the field of vision is focused as two images, one on the macula of each retina. The movements of the eyes are exquisitely coordinated to match these corresponding loci. The simultaneous movement of both eyes in the same direction is called a *conjugate movement.* With one exception (convergence), normal eye movements are conjugate. Convergence of the eyes, such as occurs during close-up vision (when the maculae are directed to one fixation point), is a *disconjugate movement.* The system regulating these movements, known as the *oculomotor system,* comprises several central pathways and the lower motor neurons (final common pathway) of cranial nerves III, IV, and VI innervating the extraocular muscles. Each of the three sets of extraocular muscles—medial and lateral recti, superior and inferior recti, and superior and inferior oblique muscles—is reciprocally innervated so that the contraction of one muscle of each pair is synergistically synchronized with the relaxation of the other muscle, in order to direct the gaze to any position (Fig. 7-5). This delicately balanced muscle system is under continuous tension.

The oculomotor system comprises four subsystems (Robinson):

1 The *saccadic system* regulates saccadic movements, which the eyes use to acquire new visual targets in the environment. When searching, the eyes move in sequences of short rapid jerks called saccades. Saccadic movements are the flicks of the eyes as they shift from one stationary point to another when reading or viewing a picture. These flicks are so fast that vision is momentarily impaired—a 10° human saccade lasts 45 milliseconds. Saccades may be initiated spontaneously or in response to a visual stimulus. They usually occur when the observer and the object are stationary.

2 The *smooth pursuit system* controls the automatic eye movements which pursue a moving object. In contrast to the saccades during searching, the movements of the eyes when following are smooth. The smooth pursuit system attempts to match eye velocity to target velocity as the eye tracks the moving target in its course through the environment. The saccadic system operates with this pursuit system to correct an error between the target and the macula. Apparently the purpose of pursuit is to allow the visual system to hold the moving object in a stationary position on the retina in order to gain time to perceive the object. The cerebral cortex (areas 17, 18, and 19) and the superior colliculi are integrated into the central pathways involved with the pursuit system—a system which requires visual stimulation for its essentially automatic response. Electrical stimulation of areas 18 and 19—called the occipital eye fields—produces conjugate eye movements to the opposite side. The neurons in the visual cortex and superior colliculus, which are known to respond to direction and velocity of image movements, are probably integrated in the smooth pursuit movements.

3 The *vestibular system* monitors the orientation of the head in space from the information obtained from the receptors in the vestibular sense organs of the inner ear. In response the head and the eyes move in space "to compensate and maintain the visual axis stable in the environment." This is analogous to a shipboard-mounted radar system, where the tracking device (radar system or eye) is mounted on a moving platform (ship or head); the tracking device operates efficiently when it is automatically stabilized relative to the movement of the platform. In this activity, the vestibular system monitors and evaluates the motion of the head and then, via influences relayed in the medial longitudinal fasciculus, stimulates the extraocular muscles to move the eyes to compensate for the head movements.

4 The *vergence system* is involved with the control of the degree of convergence of the visual axes in its role of maintaining the target image on each macula when the target moves in depth through the field of vision. This is the only system that moves the eyes in opposite directions at one time. The vergence system operates during the shift from one fixation point (X) at one depth to another fixation point (Y) at a different depth. In this shift the eyes follow the sequence of *a* a saccade from point X to a site in which the two visual axes straddle point Y, and *b* a small vergence movement until the visual axes of both eyes are directed to Y. This system is probably influenced via cortical areas 19 and 22, where the information of the slight difference viewed by the corresponding retinal foci is relayed.

Volitional movements of the eye The voluntary fixation mechanism is the means by which we move our eyes voluntarily to locate an object upon which we wish to focus our attention. The *frontal eye field in area 8* (posterior portion of the middle frontal gyrus) is the cortical center that influences voluntary eye movements mediated through cranial nerves III, IV, and VI. If this area, called the *voluntary eye field*, is bilaterally damaged, a patient either will be unable volitionally to move the eyes or will have extreme difficulty in doing so; he is still able to scan a line on the printed page and to fix on and follow a moving object, probably because area 19 is intact. The patient is unable to "unlock" his eyes from one fixation point and shift them to a second point. The movement to the second point may occur if the subject blinks his eyes or covers his eyes for a short period of time.

Automatic eye movements and fixation of the eye Our eyes can, without any volitional effort, scan a line on the printed page or follow a moving object. The neuronal center and pathways involved with locking the eyes upon an object once it has been located is known as the *involuntary fixation mechanism*. These automatic movements include reflex pathways from retina to primary visual cortex to association visual cortex and then via corticotectal fibers to the superior colliculus, from which connections are made with the nuclei of cranial nerves III, IV, and VI. The occipital eye fields in area 19 have a role in controlling the mechanism which

may result in the eyes becoming "locked" upon an object. When areas 19 are damaged bilaterally, the patient is unable automatically to follow objects steadily across the visual field or to scan the line on a printed page.

Accommodation-convergence reaction Immediately after shifting one's attention from a distant gaze to a nearby object (near-point), three ocular adjustments occur. The eyes converge with the contraction of both medial rectus muscles so that the maculae of both eyes are directed to the object to be observed. *Accommodation* for near-sight vision follows, with the rounding up of the lens. Some further sharpening of the image occurs with constriction of the pupils. The convergence may be, in part, the consequence of influences from the frontal eye fields in area 8 which are conveyed via corticobulbar fibers to the superior colliculus and from there, via interneurons, to the nucleus of the oculomotor nerve. The pupillary constriction may result from influences conveyed from the occipital visual association cortex via corticotectal fibers to the superior colliculus, which, in turn, stimulates through interneurons, the neurons of the accessory oculomotor nucleus (nucleus of Edinger-Westphal).

The so-called *Argyll-Robertson pupil* may occur in syphilis of the central nervous system. In this syndrome, the pupil is small in dim light and does not constrict further when the eye is exposed to bright light. This same pupil will respond by constricting further during the accommodation-convergence reaction. The precise explanation for this differential effect of pupillary constriction is unresolved. The usual stated cause for this dissociation of the pupillary reflex is a lesion in the pretectum.

Lesions of the optic pathways and related phenomena

The impairment of a small area of the retina results in a *scotoma* (*blind spot*) in the field viewed by that eye. The optic disk is a natural blind spot, for it contains no rods and cones. A partial defect at a site anywhere along the visual pathway may result in a scotoma.

The complete interruption of the optic nerve

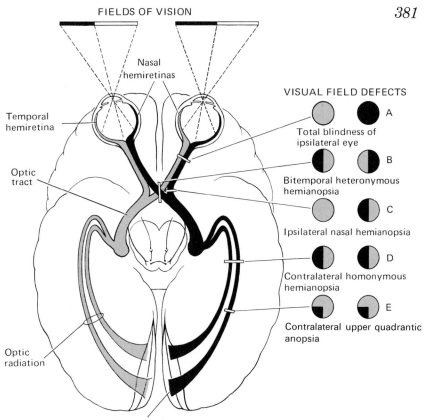

Nasal hemiretinas

Temporal hemiretina

Optic tract

Optic radiation

Lower field

VISUAL FIELD DEFECTS

A

Total blindness of ipsilateral eye

B

Bitemporal heteronymous hemianopsia

C

Ipsilateral nasal hemianopsia

D

Contralateral homonymous hemianopsia

E

Contralateral upper quadrantic anopsia

FIGURE 12-16
Some common lesions at various levels within the visual pathways.

The corresponding *visual field defects* are represented on the right side.

results in permanent blindness in one eye—called *monocular blindness* (Fig. 12-16*A*). However, the blind eye can still accommodate and show the consensual light reflex because the normal eye activates the intact reflex arcs through the pretectum and superior colliculus and oculomotor nerve to the blind eye. A fixed dilated pupil may be a sign of pressure on the oculomotor nerve.

A midline lesion of the optic chiasm (as from pressure from a tumor of the hypophysis) may interrupt the decussating retinofugal fibers (Fig. 12-16*B*). The result is loss of reception in the nasal hemiretina of each eye, accompanied by loss of vision in the temporal half of the visual field of each eye, called *bitemporal hemianopia* (*hemianopsia*). Such a defect is *heteronymous*; this means that portions of both retinas which view different areas of the fields of vision are in-

volved. Interruption of the nondecussating fibers on both sides of the optic chiasm produces a *binasal hemianopia*, i.e., loss of reception in the temporal hemiretina of each eye; this is accompanied by loss of vision in the nasal half of the visual field of each eye (Fig. 12-16*C*). In the early stages of its growth, a hypophyseal tumor expands upward to interrupt the lowermost decussating fibers of the optic chiasm first; in this situation impairment of vision occurs in both upper temporal quadrants (fields) initially, because of impairment of fibers from the lower nasal retinal quadrant of each eye. If diagnosed correctly at this stage, the chances are favorable that surgical removal of the tumor can save the vision of the patient. A hypophyseal tumor, in addition to interrupting the decussating fibers in the optic chiasm, may damage the anterior hypothalamus. This may result in a persistent *hyperpyrexia* (hyperthermia, elevated body temperature) and diabetes insipidus.

The complete interruption of the optic tract or the lateral geniculate body or the optic radiation or the entire primary visual cortex on one (right) side results in a *left contralateral homonymous hemianopia*, or blindness in the field of vision on the side opposite the lesion. *Homonymous* refers to corresponding regions of both retinas, hence to a single visual field. A thrombus of the posterior cerebral artery may result in destruction of the visual cortex, except possibly for that for the macular area; in this condition, central (macular) vision is spared (preserved bilaterally). In some cases of homonymous hemianopia, macular sparing is said to occur after lesions of the optic radiation near or within the visual cortex. This form of macular sparing may be more apparent than actual. This is because the subject with a hemianopia sees with the normal half of the macula and then automatically shifts the eye with a saccade to view the field previously in the blind area. It is possible to differentiate whether the homonymous hemianopia is caused by a lesion in the optic tract or by a lesion in the optic radiation or visual cortex by testing whether the stimulation of the blinded half of one retina can elicit the pupillary light reflex. This reflex should be evoked if its arc through the optic tract to the pretectum is intact. Light is directed into the blinded half of one retina; if the pupillary reflex can be elicited, the lesion is located beyond the lateral geniculate body, but if the pupillary reflex is absent, the lesion is probably located in the optic tract.

Partial lesions of the visual pathways produce partial defects in the fields of vision. A *lower quadrantic homonymous anopsia* results from a contralateral lesion in the upper (superior) half of the optic radiation or the entire primary visual cortex (area 17) above the calcarine sulcus. This field defect occurs because the pathways from the upper temporal quadrant of the ipsilateral retina and the upper nasal quadrant of the contralateral retina are interrupted. A lesion of the loop of Meyer will produce a *contralateral upper quadrantic anopsia* because pathways from the lower temporal quadrant of the ipsilateral retina and the lower nasal quadrant of the contralateral retina are interrupted (Fig. 12-16E).

Although the fibers of the visual pathways from corresponding regions of the retina terminate in a precisely organized pattern upon the neurons of the visual cortex, these fibers are not necessarily adjacent to each other within the optic tract and optic radiation. As a result lesions of a portion of the primary visual cortex result in a homonymous field defect in which the field defect of one eye is exactly superimposed upon that of the other eye; the loss is *congruous*. A lesion within the optic tract or optic radiation results in a field defect in which the fields from each eye are not exactly superimposed—the loss is said to be *incongruous*. Field defects in the optic radiation produce a more congruous loss than those in the optic tract.

A blow or an injury that damages the choroid layer of the eye may result in *sympathetic ophthalmia*. In this condition not only may sight be impaired in the affected eye, but the other eye may gradually lose its sight. In some patients the injured eye must be removed to preserve the sight in the normal eye. Apparently, the cause is that the body responds to certain substances released from the injured choroid layer by regarding them as foreign materials. The consequence is an immunologic activity which results in the destruction of both eyes.

True albinos shun light and have difficulty seeing because melanin pigment is absent in the iris, choroid, and retinal pigment layer of their eyes. In these individuals the light passes through the retina, and light which is normally absorbed by the melanin pigment is reflected as scattered light. Hence a discrete spot of light excites more receptors over a wider area than it usually does. In addition, the unpigmented iris permits diffuse light to enter the vitreous body and stimulate many photoreceptors. As a consequence, the visual acuity of albinos is rarely better than 20/100 to 20/200.

Brindley, G. S.: *Physiology of the Retina and Visual Pathway.* Edward Arnold (Publishers), Ltd., London, 1970.

Davson, H.: *Physiology of the Eye.* Academic Press, Inc., New York, 1972.

—— (ed.): *The Eye.* Academic Press, Inc., New York, 1969, 1970.

Doty, R. W., and N. Negrão: Forebrain commissures and vision. Ablation of visual areas in the central nervous system, in R. Jung (ed.), *Handbook of Sensory Physiology,* vol. VII, part 3. Springer-Verlag, Heidelberg, 1973.

Dowling, J. E., and B. B. Boycott: Organization of the primate retina: electron microscopy. Proc. Roy. Soc. Lond. (Biol.), 166:80–111, 1966.

—— and F. S. Werblin: Synaptic organization of the vertebrate retina. Vision Res., Suppl., 11:1–15, 1971.

Duke-Elder, S., and K. C. Wybar: In S. Duke-Elder (ed.), *The Anatomy of the Visual System. System of Ophthalmology.* The C. V. Mosby Company, St. Louis, 1961.

Fine, B. S., and M. Yanoff: *Ocular Histology:* A Text and Atlas. Harper & Row, New York, 1972.

Fuortes, M. G. F. (ed.): Physiology of photoreceptor organs, in *Handbook of Sensory Physiology,* vol. VII, part 2. Springer-Verlag, Heidelberg, 1972.

Gross, Charles G.: Visual functions of infero-temporal cortex, in R. Jung (ed.), *Handbook of Sensory Physiology,* vol. 7, part 3. Springer-Verlag, Heidelberg, 1972.

Hogan, M. J., J. A. Alvarado, and J. E. Weddell: *Histology of the Human Eye.* W. B. Saunders Company, Philadelphia, 1971.

Hoyt, W., and O. Luis: Visual fiber anatomy in the infrageniculate pathway of the primate. Arch. Ophthalmol., 68:94–106, 1962.

Hubel, D. H., and T. N. Wiesel: Receptive fields and functional architecture of monkey striate cortex. J. Physiol., 195:215–243, 1968.

—— and ——: Anatomical demonstration of columns in the monkey striate cortex. Nature, 221:747–750, 1969.

Mishkin, M.: Cortical visual areas and their interactions, in A. G. Karczmar and J. C. Eccles (eds.), *Brain and Human Behavior,* pp. 187–208. Springer-Verlag, Berlin and New York, 1972.

Noback, C. R., and L. K. Laemle: Structural and functional aspects of the visual pathways of primates, in C. Noback and W. Montagna (eds.), *The Primate Brain,* pp. 55–82. Appleton-Century-Crofts, Inc., New York, 1970.

Palmer, L. A., A. C. Rosenquist, and J. M. Sprague: Corticotectal systems in the cat: their structure and function, in T. L. Frigyesi, E. Rinvik, and M. D. Yahr (eds.), *Corticothalamic Projections and Sensorimotor Activities.* Raven Press, New York, 1972.

Pettigrew, J. D.: The neurophysiology of binocular vision. Sci. Am., 227:84–96, 1972.

Rattliff, F.: *Mach Bands: Quantitative Studies on Neural Networks in the Retina.* Holden-Day, Inc., Publisher, San Francisco, 1965.

Robinson, D. A.: Eye movement control in primates. Science, 161:1219–1224, 1968.

Schneider, G. E.: Two visual systems. Science, 163:895–902, 1969.

Straatsma, B. R., M. O. Hall, R. A. Allen, and F. Crescitelli: *The Retina: Morphology, Function and Clinical Characteristics.* University of California Press, Berkeley and Los Angeles, 1969.

Wald, G.: The receptors of human color vision. Science, 145:1007–1016, 1964.

Young, R. W.: Visual cells. Sci. Am., 223:80–91, 1970.

CHAPTER **13**
THE SENSORY SYSTEMS
AND THE THALAMUS

The internal and external environments of the organism are the sources of the stimuli that trigger the sensors in the body to initiate the transmissions of coded input to the central nervous system. This input is subsequently processed in the nuclear stations of the nervous system. Much of this information is utilized at subconscious levels in a variety of reflex activities. Some of this input may eventually lead to the formulation of a representation of the environments by the mind. In this way, each individual creates his own world, a world that is not a stereotyped duplication of nature. This copy is a biased, rather than a faithful, reproduction. In fact, an animal is actually aware only of its own senses and their effects on the nervous system. For example, the physical movements of molecules in the air are vibrations, not sounds. The concert pianist generates air vibrations, not music as such. It is the ear and the brain that transform the vibrations into sounds and music. The air vibrations are transformed by the ear into the coded messages of nerve impulses. These messages are transmitted and processed in the auditory pathways and the higher brain centers, where the air vibrations are subjectively heard and interpreted as sounds.

Coding and processing in the nervous system

SENSORY ENDINGS AND ENVIRONMENTAL ENERGIES

The sensory endings are the sources of information for the nervous system. These sensors are stimulated by a limited spectrum of the multi-

tude of specific energies which impinge upon us. We cannot directly sense cosmic rays, radiowaves, ultrasonic waves, and many other environmental energies, but we can sense "light" waves, "sound" waves, contact, and certain chemicals, among other forms of energy.

Information about the outer world is differentially sensed by an organism, because the threshold levels of its sensory receptors are different. This is used to advantage. For example, if the eyes were stimulated by all the radiations emanating from the sky at night, the sky would appear as an intensely "lighted" expanse. With the eyes sensitive to only a narrow band of radiation the stars are visible against the dark background of space.

In addition, man and other organisms can sense similar stimuli as different perceptions. For example, the retina is sensitive to energies perceived as light in the range of 4×10^{14} to 8×10^{14} vibrations per second, while the skin is sensitive to radiant heat ranging from 3×10^{14} to 8×10^{14} vibrations per second. Note the overlap; i.e., some vibration frequencies are both seen and felt. A gradation of mechanically induced vibrations from 1 to about 20,000 cycles per second, transmitted through various media, can be sensed by man. The lowest frequencies are felt as touch. The frequencies up to 1,500 cycles per second are perceived as vibrations (tested with the base of a tuning fork on a joint). The range of vibrations of from 30 to over 20,000 cycles per second are sensed as sound. Again note the overlap.

Each sensory receptor responds when adequately stimulated, quite specifically and regardless of the stimulus. For example, retinal stimulation results in the perception of light, whether the source of stimulation consists of "light" waves, electric shocks, or a blow on the eye. A specific energy which is capable of stimulating different types of receptors will evoke the perception of a different sensation from each sensor. For example, when electric stimulation is applied to taste buds, taste may be sensed; when applied to the spiral organ of Corti of the inner ear, a sound may be sensed; or when applied to the retina, light may be sensed.

RECEPTOR MEMBRANE, TRANSDUCTION, AND RECEPTOR POTENTIAL

The subjective sensation felt by the organism is not due to any known uniqueness in the basic neurophysiology of the neurons, but is rather a function of the regions of the brain stimulated. Apparently all neurons are fundamentally similar; they all seem to exhibit similar neurophysiologic properties. Sensory neurons may differ only in that the various neurons are stimulated by different specific energies. However, these differences end at the receptor membrane of the neuron. The sequence of neurophysiologic events exhibited by a sensory neuron, commencing with its stimulation, includes the transduction, formation, and conduction of the code to the synaptic effector site. The code may exert a role in generating a new code in the postsynaptic neuron.

Transduction is the process of converting the signal of the environmental energy into the receptor (generator) potential at the nerve ending (Chap. 3). The receptor potential is graded in some proportion to the intensity of the stimulus. In a sense the receptor membrane corresponds to amplitude modulation (AM). The receptor can be enhanced by both spatial summation and temporal summation. The simultaneous stimulation of many of the arborizing endings of one nerve fiber can summate spatially to create a receptor potential of sufficient magnitude to trigger an action potential (Chap. 3), whereas an increase in the frequency of stimulation of a nerve ending can summate temporally to increase the magnitude of the receptor potential.

CODING IN THE NERVOUS SYSTEM

At the present time only a start has been made in the identification and evaluation of the codes employed by the nervous system to transmit information. Only a few aspects of coding are indicated in this account.

Each stimulus, which may be eventually comprehended as a modality, is a composite of several components. Presumably each of these components evokes several codes and even subcodes which are transmitted to the nuclear processing centers in the central nervous system. These components include intensity (a quantitative function), duration (a temporal function), location of stimulus either within or outside the organism, frequency (number of stimuli per unit time), and the dimensions of shape and motion.

The generator potentials evoked by a stimulus in a nerve receptor trigger an all-or-none action potential (digital pulse, spike) at the nodal point in a neuron (Chap. 3). The spike transmitted along the conductile segment (axon channel) is an expression of a code. The frequency of the spike (or of the interval between spikes) forms a basis for coding information; it may be utilized for evaluating gradations in the intensity of a given modality. The more intense the stimulus, the greater the number of impulses transmitted per unit time to the central nervous system. The number of fibers stimulated is also significant. According to the pattern theory (Chap. 5), information as to the quality of a modality is transmitted via combinations of nerve fibers. This information is conveyed in these various axon channels as a spectrum of velocities ranging from the slow speeds in unmyelinated fibers to the fast speeds of heavily myelinated fibers. The pulse signals traveling in the various temporal patterns and velocities in a number of axon channels are organized into the coded data to which a nucleus is "listening" and from which a nucleus abstracts and processes information before transmitting its output code to other nuclei.

TRANSFER OF INFORMATION FROM ONE NEURON TO ANOTHER

The transfer of coded information from one neuron to another occurs at the synapses by the secretion of neurotransmitter substances through each presynaptic membrane into the synaptic cleft where the secretion can influence the postsynaptic membrane of the receptive segment of the neuron. A new code-carrying signal is generated in the postsynaptic neuron. In effect, *each synapse performs a transformation function.*

PROCESSING IN THE NERVOUS SYSTEM

The ascending (and descending) pathways function both as processors and as transmitters of coded information. *The processing within the nuclear stations of the pathways is information-linked not energy-linked.* For example, as noted above, stimulation of the optic system evokes sensations related to visions, regardless of whether the stimulus is light, an electrical shock, or blow on the eye. One critical unsolved problem is: How are the signals selected in the presence of noise? Comparators and information generators may be present in the nervous system. The novelty of the stimulus and the degree of the deviation from random background activity in the nervous system may contribute.

Because a neuron may have numerous synaptic connections with many other neurons (divergence) and each neuron may be stimulated by many other neurons (convergence), the possibilities for interactions among neurons are great. The interactions of the impulses generated in neurons produce excitatory postsynaptic potentials (EPSPs) and inhibitory postsynaptic potentials (IPSPs) which are resolved in each of the neurons of the ascending pathways. One EPSP alone is not able to stimulate a neuron sufficiently to trigger an action potential; hence the importance of algebraic summation of the EPSPs and IPSPs on the receptive membrane of a neuron (Chap. 3).

A pathway does not merely comprise a series of "relay" stations receiving input and relaying output like a bucket brigade. The relay or nuclear stations are the sites which alter the characteristics of the transmitted code. For example, the number of neuron channels delivering input into a nucleus, as the result of a stimulus, does not necessarily equal the number of neuron channels discharging output from the nucleus. Actually in each nucleus reassessments are made and new codes are generated.

The influences arriving via these multiple axonal channels to a nuclear processing station are biased, enhanced, or dampened within the nucleus. In effect the nucleus acts as an editor. *Feed-forward and feedback inhibitory circuits* and descending centrifugal fibers from higher centers have a significant role in this editing. Inhibitory interneurons are essential elements within these pathways.

1 A feed-forward inhibitory circuit is characterized by having one or more inhibitory interneurons within the circuit; these interneurons convey influences in a forward direction toward the more distal levels of the pathway. In such a circuit, the axons of the excitatory neurons have some axon collaterals which excite one or more inhibitory neurons. In turn, these neurons exert inhibitory influences upon other neurons in a forward direction. Feed-forward inhibitory circuits are illustrated in Figs. 5-20, 5-23, and 13-2. The afferent fiber from the neuromuscular spindle receptors within a muscle excites, among others, an inhibitory interneuron which exerts inhibitory influences upon the alpha motor neuron innervating a voluntary muscle (Figs. 5-20, 5-23). Neuron C excites interneuron F, which excites inhibitory neuron I_4 to inhibit neuron E postsynaptically (Fig. 13-2).

2 A feedback inhibitory circuit is characterized by having one or more inhibitory interneurons which convey inhibitory influences back (feedback) to the original output neuron. A feedback inhibitory control circuit performs its role through both presynaptic and postsynaptic inhibition (Chap. 3). Feedback inhibitory circuits utilizing postsynaptic inhibition are illustrated in Figs. 3-13 and 13-2. The axon collateral of the lower motor neuron excites the inhibitory interneuron (Renshaw cell), which feeds back to inhibit the lower motor neuron (Fig. 3-13). The axon collateral of neuron D excites interneuron I_3, which feeds back to inhibit output neuron D (Fig. 13-2). Feedback inhibitory circuits utilizing presynaptic inhibition are illustrated in Figs. 13-1 and 13-2. The axon collaterals of neurons C and D excite inhibitory neurons, which feed back to inhibit neurons A and B by presynaptic inhibition (Fig. 13-1). Recall that presynaptic

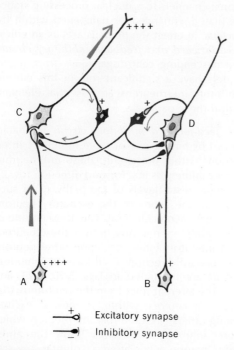

+ ─○) Excitatory synapse

● Inhibitory synapse

FIGURE 13-1
Neural processing utilizing presynaptic inhibition.

The strong input from neuron A and weak input from neuron B can stimulate discharge in neurons C and D, respectively. This same discharge traveling along recurrent collateral branches of C and D excites "inhibitory neurons" which feed back inhibitory stimuli to the presynaptic terminals of A and B. The stimuli are sufficient to prevent D from firing but insufficient to prevent C from firing.

inhibition is exerted via an interneuron which excites (Chap. 3). The axon collateral of neuron E excites interneuron I, which feeds back to inhibit neuron E by presynaptic inhibition (Fig. 13-2).

3 The descending centrifugal fibers from higher centers (e.g., corticonuclear fibers, Chap. 16) to the nuclei of the ascending pathways incorporate inhibitory interneurons. This is illustrated in Fig. 13-2. The descending fibers of neuron G

excite inhibitory neuron I_2, which inhibits neuron D postsynaptically.

These inhibitory circuits exert their effects in the nuclei of both the ascending reticular and the ascending lemniscal systems. The modulating influences act to suppress some of the input channels, possibly those which are transmitting noise. The effectively inhibited channels surround excitatory foci which serve to stimulate the output channels; these output channels transmit the signals with less noise. For example, the inhibitory ring of *off* sets surrounding an excitatory focus of an *on* set, as found in the visual pathways, illustrates the interaction of inhibitory activity in nuclear processing. A negative feedback inhibitory circuit tends to prevent those neurons with relatively weak excitatory input from firing (filters out the noise); it may modify but not prevent those neurons with relatively strong facilitatory input from firing (contain the coded signals). This is an example of lateral (mutual, afferent contrast, Chap. 12) inhibition, which has an important role in sharpening, focusing, and contrasting effects. Some information being transmitted in a coded pattern is lost at synaptic relays. Within the nervous system inhibition produces hyperpolarization of the postsynaptic neurons (Chap. 3). The critical significance of inhibition is that it lowers the background activity so that the message can come through. Inhibition acts "to clear the addresses of the computer." *In a sense, the signals are strengthened and the noise is suppressed.*

Many sensory endings are under the influence of efferent neurons. Certain neurons, each with its cell body in the central nervous system, project axons to sensory receptors (feedback from a nucleus). These efferent cells may facilitate or inhibit, thereby making sensory endings more or less receptive. Although this view is not fully documented as yet, it is likely that the degree of receptivity of most if not all peripheral sensors is modified by efferent neurons. The gamma efferent fibers to the neuromuscular spindles and the cochlear efferent fibers to the spiral organ of Corti are two examples of such efferent neurons. The gamma efferent fibers stimulate the intrafusal muscles of the neuromuscular spindle receptor to contract, thereby enhancing the firing rate of the neuromuscular spindle. This is significant in the stretch reflex because it ensures a continuous flow of infor-

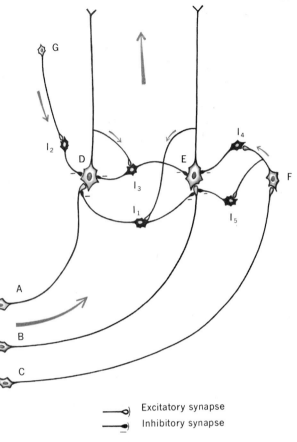

FIGURE 13-2
Neural processing utilizing presynaptic
and postsynaptic inhibition.

Normally neurons *A* and *B* can excite neurons
D and *E* to fire. However, inhibitory influences
can modify the receptivity of neurons *D* and
E. The recurrent collateral branch from neuron
E can excite interneuron I_1, which exerts presynaptic inhibitory influences on the terminal
ending of neurons *A* and *B*. The recurrent
collateral branch from neuron *D* can stimulate
interneuron I_3, which exerts postsynaptic inhibitory influences on neurons *D* and *E*. The
descending efferent neuron *G* (corticonuclear
fiber) can stimulate interneuron I_2, which exerts postsynaptic inhibitory influences on neuron *D*. Excitatory stimuli from neuron *C* can
exert through interneurons *F*, I_4, and I_5 presynaptic inhibitory influences on the terminal
ending of neuron *B* and postsynaptic inhibitory influences on neuron *E*.

mation from the receptor to the spinal cord
(Chaps. 5, 14). The cochlear efferent fibers to the
hair cells in the cochlea inhibit the flow of input
from the ear to the brain (Chap. 10). The
"biasing" of the input data commences at the
receptor level and occurs in the nuclei of the
central nervous system; this implies that even
the receptors are not precise indicators of the
modalities they register.

ADAPTATION

Adaptation (Chap. 3) has a significant role in the
way information from the sensors is employed.
An organism utilizes the slowly adapting receptors as a source of background (tonic) information about the environment, and the fast-
adapting receptors as a source of information

about changes (phasic) in the environment.

*The slowly (or non-) adapting endings con-
tinue to discharge at a steady frequency of digital pulses as long as the stimulus is maintained
unchanged,* because, for some unknown reason,
the generator potential is sustained at a level
sufficient to fire action potentials. The slowly
adapting neuromuscular spindles provide the
background data for tonic muscular action.
Pressure receptors in the skin, thermoreceptors,
pain receptors, the spiral organ of Corti, and the
retina are among the endings which continue
to respond up to several minutes (a long time
for the nervous system) to the continuous
bombardment of stimuli.

*When stimulated, a fast-adapting ending fires
a burst of digital pulses.* With continued unchanged stimulation, the endings soon cease to

fire or drastically lower their firing rate, because the generator potential is insufficient to trigger the generation of more action potentials. The Pacinian corpuscles adapt in about 5 milliseconds. These fast-adapting endings, including touch endings, joint receptors, and endings around hair follicles, provide the phasic data about changes in the environment. They are mainly mechanoreceptors. In a sense, after these endings serve their immediate role, the slate is wiped clean in preparation for sensing a change in the intensity of the stimulus.

Roles of the ascending reticular and ascending lemniscal systems

The input to the nervous system has a role in *1* determining the level of alertness (general awareness) of an organism, *2* supplying information for unconscious reflex mechanisms, and *3* providing the data essential for the conscious appreciation of the sensory modalities. The level of alertness of the organism is mediated primarily through the ascending reticular system, while the pathways significant to the appreciation of the sensory modalities are those mediated through the lemniscal system. The delineation of the ascending pathways into these two systems, characterized by various structural and functional criteria (Chap. 8), is a useful conceptual schema, but is not absolute. These systems are not independent but interact with each other.

RETICULAR SYSTEM

The ascending reticular (nonspecific) system is the complex afferent system with widespread connections throughout the nervous system (Chap. 8). It provides the structural and functional substrates which operate to influence, modulate, and regulate the state of the organism in the sleep-wake cycle as overtly expressed by its attentiveness and its degree of arousal. This system receives its input from a wide variety of sources, via spinoreticular pathways, antero-

lateral column–spinal lemniscus pathway, trigeminal pathways, lateral brainstem reticular formation, auditory pathways, optic pathways, and olfactory pathways (Fig. 8-15). This input is ultimately integrated in the functional expression of the reticular system, which may intensify and dampen the effect of stimuli. A neuron of the reticular system is subject to the influence of stimuli from many sites of the body (e.g., skin, joints, retina, spiral organ of Corti, and viscera). In this respect, the reticular system is composed of complex units, each responding to stimuli of many modalities. The sensory inputs from the visual system and olfactory system are not sufficient to support even transient wakefulness. The further addition of sensory input from the face (via the trigeminal nerve) to the ascending reticular pathways makes it possible to maintain the arousal state.

The protopathic sensation of pain, temperature, and erotic sensibilities with their significant input to the brainstem reticular formation are powerful activators of the ascending reticular system. In addition to their effects on the sleep-wake cycle, these influences contribute through connections with the descending reticular pathways (Figs. 5-17, 8-15, and 8-16) in evoking such responses as the wincing, grimacing, and biting associated with intense pain; as the facial expressions and visceral activities associated with sexual excitement; and as the somatic and visceral activities associated with exposure to temperature changes.

The reticular system furnishes the background activity for the performance of the lemniscal system. The presentation of a new stimulus to an animal evokes an alerting response which is accompanied by an action orientating the organism to the stimulus (searching movement). These expressions of the reticular system are requisite for the more efficient use of the input transmitted through the lemniscal system. The reticular system is geared primarily to make the animal aware of the stimulus being received, not to deliver and report the specific modality. Even in deep anesthesia, the lemniscal systems (specific afferent stimuli) convey neural signals to the cerebral cortex; this information is unrecognized by the organism because anesthesia suppresses the expression of the ascending reticular system. As a result, the awareness of the lemniscal-transmitted information is lost.

For example, in an animal anesthetized with a barbiturate sedative, the lemniscal pathways continue to conduct nerve impulses in a relatively normal manner to the cortex but the ascending reticular pathway does not conduct impulses. The latter is electrically silent.

The reticular system within the brainstem and hypothalamus is important in the tonic activation of the cerebral cortex. This is objectively expressed in the maintenance of a state of wakefulness (or sleep) for sustained periods of time. On the other hand, the thalamic reticular nuclei are critical in the phasic activation of the cerebral cortex. This latter drive is expressed in the responses to changes in the intensity of sensory input by the immediate shifts in the attentiveness of an organism.

The major ascending pathway of the reticular system is the indirect spinothalamic pathway (paleospinothalamic pathway, Fig. 5-15, Chap. 5). This pathway receives additional inputs within the brainstem reticular formation (Chap. 8) from the cranial nerves and from collateral branches of such ascending pathways as the neospinothalamic tract. The central tegmental tract is the main ascending route from the brainstem reticular formation to the hypothalamus and thalamus (Fig. 8-12). This nonsomatotopically organized system contains the multineuronal paleospinothalamic pain pathway which conveys diffuse, poorly localized pain. These pain sensations are felt after a long latency following the stimulation; they may persist for a long time after the withdrawal of the stimulation.

LEMNISCAL SYSTEM

The lemniscal system conveys and processes the neural information associated with the specific modalities (Chap. 8). The four major ascending lemniscal pathways are *1* pain, temperature, and light-touch pathways (Figs. 5-13 and 5-17); *2* touch and deep-sensibility pathways (Fig. 5-16); *3* auditory pathways (Fig. 10-8); and *4* visual pathways (Fig. 12-13). After the attention of the organism has been focused by the activity of the reticular system, the lemniscal system operates by accurately locating, assessing, and organizing the specific sensory input. The lemniscal pathways are high-fidelity systems in which peripheral sensors have a precise func-

tional representation in the nuclei and cerebral cortex projection area of a pathway. The processing within each system of pathways endows it with a tremendous capacity for sensory discrimination. These pathways project primarily to the ventral posterior thalamic nucleus and geniculate bodies and then to the cortex.

The nuclei of the lemniscal pathways in the spinal cord and brainstem are involved with the initial processing of neural information before it is transmitted rostrally to the higher centers. The nuclei of the thalamus (and possibly of the midbrain) are sites where the conscious awareness of certain senses occurs, viz., crude touch, pain, general temperature sense, and even sounds. The highest stations in the cerebral cortex in conjunction with some mesencephalic and thalamic nuclei are the centers involved in the conscious appreciation of discriminatory general senses, vision, and audition.

Some ascending lemniscal pathway systems, commencing from the periphery, are composed of a relay of three neurons (each with a long axon) extending from the receptors of the body and to the cerebral cortex.

The first neuron (first-order), with its receptor ending in the body and its terminal ending in a nucleus of the central nervous system, has its cell body located in the sensory ganglia (spinal ganglion of spinal nerve and cranial ganglion of cranial nerve).

The second neuron (second-order) has its cell body in a nucleus of the central nervous system (on the same side as the first-order neuron). Each of these second-order neurons has a long axon which decussates to the contralateral side, ascends in a lemniscal tract (some axons ascend on the same side), and terminates in the thalamus.

The third neuron of the sequence (third-order) has its cell body in the thalamus and projects its axon to the cerebral cortex.

Interneurons in the nuclei of these lemniscal pathways have a role in processing the information conveyed via these three-neuron relay systems. Several other pathways are included with the specific systems; the specific relay thalamic nuclei (noted below) are major processing centers in these specific pathways. One of these pathway complexes is the dentatothalamocortical system (Chap. 9).

A neuron (or group of neurons arranged as a column or point) of the lemniscal pathways is subject to the influences of stimuli from a small peripheral area (spot or point) as, for example, in the skin, joint, retina, or spiral organ of Corti. Each neuron of this system may be involved in a point-to-point (column-to-column) relay, and it responds to only one modality; such a neuron is modality-specific. In brief, the lemniscal systems are composed of many point-to-point relay units with "secure," tight synaptic connectivity of presynaptic neurons with postsynaptic neurons. This tight coupling is insensitive to anesthetics; conduction and transmission via these systems are normal when subjects are under anesthesia. This is one factor basic to fine discrimination; point-to-point relays tend to maintain the integrity of each bit of information.

PAIN AND TEMPERATURE PATHWAYS

The lemniscal pathways conveying the protopathic modalities of pain and temperature are the direct spinothalamic tract (Fig. 5-13) and the anterior trigeminothalamic tract (Fig. 8-15). These phylogenetically new tracts, which are well developed in many mammals, are also called neospinothalamic and neotrigeminothalamic tracts. The former is also called the anterolateral–spinal lemniscal pathway, because it is located in the anterolateral portion of the lateral column of the spinal cord and is a lemniscal tract composed of fibers originating in the spinal cord. The trigeminothalamic tracts are often called the trigeminal lemniscus. The anterior spinothalamic tract conveying light touch is included in the anterolateral–spinal lemniscal pathway.

The disagreeable subjective aspects of pain are important as a message that warns the organism of a harmful event. The fundamental reaction is the flexor withdrawal reflex (Fig. 5-23). The intensity of the subjective feeling of pain is not necessarily proportional to the intensity of the stimulus; a mild stimulus may evoke in-

tense pain, and an intense stimulus may evoke mild pain. The rare individuals who do not possess a sense of pain are handicapped because they may sustain serious injury before realizing it. Pain is a conceptualized perceptual modality.

The direct pain and temperature pathway is composed of a sequence of three neurons from the periphery to the cerebral cortex.

A neuron of the first order, with its cell body in a spinal ganglion, extends from a peripheral receptor, through a spinal nerve, to the spinal cord, where its axon terminates and synapses in the posterior horn.

A neuron of the second order, with its cell body within the gray matter of the spinal cord, has an axon which crosses over to the opposite side, ascends in the somatotopically organized lateral spinothalamic tract, and terminates and synapses in the ventral posterolateral, parafascicular nuclei and posterior region of the thalamus. A small proportion of the fibers of the neospinothalamic tract project to the ipsilateral ventral posterolateral nucleus of the thalamus, perhaps because of fibers which do not decussate in the spinal cord or to fibers which, after having crossed in the spinal cord, redecussate in the lower brainstem or posterior commissure.

A neuron of the third order in the thalamus projects its axon through the posterior limb of the internal capsule to the cortex of the postcentral gyrus.

The pain and temperature pathway from the head is conveyed via the sequence of *1* a neuron of the first order with its cell body in the trigeminal ganglion, *2* a neuron of the second order with its cell body in the spinal nucleus of the trigeminal nerve, and *3* a neuron of the third order with its cell body in the ventral posteromedial nucleus of the thalamus (Chap. 5). These three-neuron pathways convey the sharply localized pain that is felt immediately following the stimulus (short latency) and lasting throughout the duration of the provoking stimulus.

Many factors are involved in the perception of this complex modality called pain. Athletes sustain severe punishment of which they are hardly aware. Acutely wounded soldiers often deny feeling pain from extensive wounds, yet normally these same men complain of a venous puncture with a hypodermic needle. The degree of pain perception is influenced by anticipation and anxiety (placebo effect). The fact that the intensity of pain is not proportional to the stimulus suggests that pain is a function of the whole individual, including his fears, drives, and state of mind. The culture affects the perception of pain. For example, the suppression of pain by an adult male is, in part, a response to our cultural values; it is expected that a man will "grin and bear it."

Pain is called a thalamic sense because it is probably brought to consciousness in the thalamus. This idea is consistent with the concept that many primitive modalities are thalamic senses. It is possible that pain may also be perceived at the collicular level, if one assumes that the spinotectal fibers (which accompany the spinothalamic pathway) convey pain. The cerebral cortex is involved with pain perception, particularly in the emotional, interpretive, and psychic spheres. The different roles of the thalamus and the cerebral cortex in pain can be illustrated by several examples. Following a prefrontal lobotomy (Chap. 16), a patient is aware of pain but its distressing quality is reduced or eliminated. Injuries or stimulation of the cerebral cortex are not significantly painful, whereas damage or stimulation within the thalamus evokes a nonlocalized intense pain.

The direct and indirect descending (centrifugal) neural pathways from higher to lower centers are involved in the suppression, intensification, or modification of pain perception through their effect on the nuclei of the ascending pathways. These pathways are important in determining the quality and intensity of the ultimate perceptive experience.

TOUCH–DEEP SENSIBILITY PATHWAYS (POSTERIOR COLUMN–MEDIAL LEMNISCAL PATHWAY))

The main pathway conveying the mechanoreceptive modalities of touch-pressure, including two-point discrimination, position sense, and kinesis, is the posterior column-medial lemniscal pathway (Fig. 5-16). This pathway is composed of a sequence of three neurons from the periphery to the cerebral cortex, each synapsing directly with the next one in the sequence. Interneurons in the nucleus gracilis, nucleus cuneatus, and thalamic nucleus are essential to the processing within each nucleus.

A neuron of the first order, with its cell body in a spinal ganglion, extends from a peripheral receptor through a spinal nerve and the dorsal columns of the spinal cord (fasciculus gracilis and fasciculus cuneatus) to the lower medulla, where it terminates and synapses directly with the neurons of the second order located in the nucleus gracilis or nucleus cuneatus.

A neuron of the second order decussates in the lower medulla as the internal arcuate fibers and ascends in the contralateral medial lemniscus until it terminates and synapses directly with the neurons of the third order located in the ventral posterolateral nucleus of the thalamus.

A neuron of the third order projects through the posterior limb of the internal capsule to the cortex of the postcentral gyrus.

The posterior column–medial lemniscal pathway, with its direct projections to the ventral posterolateral thalamic nucleus, is a phylogenetically new pathway (comparable to the neospinothalamic pathway). The contralateral rostral projections of the nucleus gracilis to the midbrain reticular formation, magnocellular portion of the medial geniculate body, and posterior thalamus may represent a phylogenetically old multineuronal pathway from the posterior columns to the thalamus and cerebral cortex (comparable to the paleospinothalamic pathways).

The touch–deep sensibility modalities from the head are conveyed via the sequence of *1* a neuron of the first order with its cell body in the trigeminal ganglion of the fifth cranial nerve, *2* a neuron of the second order with its cell body in the principal sensory nucleus of the fifth nerve, and *3* a neuron of the third order with its cell body in the ventral posteromedial nucleus of the thalamus (Fig. 8-16). Some neurons of the second order decussate and terminate in the contralateral thalamus, whereas other neurons do not decussate and terminate in the ipsilateral thalamus (Chap. 8).

The modality of light touch is also conveyed via the anterior spinothalamic tract, which is located near the spinothalamic tract in the lower brainstem and near the medial lemniscus in the upper brainstem.

AUDITORY AND OPTIC PATHWAYS

The lemniscal pathways of the special somatic senses of audition and vision have basic features in common with the lemniscal pathways of the general senses. A thalamic nucleus is intercalated into each of these lemniscal pathways— the medial geniculate body in the auditory pathway (Chap. 10) and the lateral geniculate body in the optic pathway (Chap. 12). Each of these nuclei receives a contralateral projection from the appropriate sense organ. Unlike the lemniscal pathways of the general senses, the auditory pathway has a significant ipsilateral projection to the medial geniculate body, and the optic pathway has a massive ipsilateral projection to the lateral geniculate body.

GENERAL STATEMENT ON THE ASCENDING SYSTEMS

Each pathway system should be considered as a whole. The entire tract is significant, because normal conscious perception is dependent on the functional integrity of the entire pathway. Each nucleus is not a simple relay locus but a processing station contributing to the ultimate sensory, perceptive, and mnemonic realization. The nuclei with their many interneurons are the sites where convergence, divergence, lateral inhibition, centrifugal efferent influences, and other neural expressions are utilized to "distinguish" and enhance differences and to "note" similarities.

Each lemniscal and special sensory pathway (except taste) is probably a composite of many precise point-to-point "relay" units. Each of these component relays commences in a small zone of peripheral receptors and continues through small groups of neurons in each of the nuclei up to the cerebral cortex. For example, two-point discrimination is appreciated in part because the integrity of each of the relay units is maintained from periphery to primary somesthetic cortex. The stimulation of a touch spot evokes a response in only a few neurons in the postcentral gyrus. This security of transmission

from point to point is important in maintaining the separation and distinction between two spots. This activity in the cortex illustrates the concept that the threshold of the receptors of a spot is the threshold of the relay unit. This precise point projection is maintained by at least two neural mechanisms: *1* Each small group of neurons in each nucleus is surrounded by a zone of inhibition. This is an expression of (lateral) mutual inhibition (Chap. 11). *2* The descending centrifugal fibers from higher centers contribute a flow of feedback influences (Chap. 10) which can inhibit noise and other information. The nuclei of the ascending system receive stimuli through synapses from neurons with cell bodies in nuclei located at higher levels.

Thalamus

GENERAL ROLES OF THE THALAMUS

The (dorsal) thalamus is the complex of nuclear processing stations that are coordinators and regulators of the functional activity of the cerebral cortex. Most of the direct input to the cerebral cortex is derived from the thalamus. In turn, the thalamus receives much of its input via direct and indirect connections from the cerebral cortex. Many thalamic nuclei have reciprocal connections with the cerebral cortex; however, these cortical connections are not the substrate for reverberating circuits.

The thalamus serves four basic roles.

1 Role in the sensory systems: All sensory pathways, except those of the olfactory system, have direct projections to certain thalamic nuclei, which, in turn, convey through their axons influences to restricted sectors of the sensory cerebral cortex. In addition, large sectors of the sensory cerebral cortex have connections with many thalamic nuclei. The conscious awareness of the crude aspects of the sensations pain, touch, pressure, and temperature are probably realized in the thalamus.

2 Role in motor systems: The thalamus has a crucial role in projecting critical influences to the cortex involved with somatic motor activities (motor and premotor cortex). Actually, it is intercalated between a number of subcortical structures and the cerebral cortex. The two neuronal circuits which are significant in this regard are the pathway of the cerebellum to the thalamus to the cortex (Chap. 9), and the feedback circuit of cortex to corpus striatum to thalamus to cortex (Chap. 14).

3 Role in general background neural activity: The thalamus has an essential role in processing through its connections those neural influences which are basic, for example, to the rhythms of the cerebral cortex (as expressed in the electroencephalogram—EEG) and in the phases of the sleep-wake cycle. These activities are fundamental physiologic and behavioral expressions of the activities of the nonspecific thalamic nuclei and the entire ascending reticular system.

4 Role in affect and the highest expressions of the cerebral cortex: The thalamus is involved in some subtle way with affect and many of the expressive aspects of emotion and behavior through its connections with the limbic lobe (Chap. 15) and the prefrontal cortex (Chap. 16). Reciprocal and related circuits act to integrate the thalamus and the association areas of the cerebral cortex, which contain the structural substrates critical to the "highest-ordered" cortical activities, including thought, symbolisms of communication, and creativity.

NUCLEAR GROUPS OF THE THALAMUS

The thalamus is roughly divided into the *anterior nuclear group, lateral nuclear group,* and *medial nuclear group* by a plate of neural tissue called the internal medullary lamina (Table 13-1 and Figs. 13-3, 13-4). The anterior nuclear group is flanked between the two arms of the rostral bifurcation of this lamina. Within the internal medullary lamina is the *intralaminar nuclear group.* On the rostral and lateral surface of the thalamus adjacent to the internal capsule is the external medullary lamina, within which is the *thalamic reticular nucleus.* A narrow lamina on the medial surface of the thalamus, lining the third ventricle, contains several small nuclei called the *midline nuclear group.* The lateral nuclear group is divided into a *ventral tier* and a *dorsal tier.* The *metathalamic group* is the caudal extension of the ventral tier of the lateral nuclear group.

TABLE 13-1
Thalamic nuclei

Nonspecific nuclei

Intralaminar nuclear group
  Centromedian nucleus (CM)
  Parafascicular nucleus (PF)
  Paracentral nucleus
  Central lateral nucleus (CL)
  Central median nucleus
Thalamic reticular nucleus (RN)
Midline nuclear group
  Parataenial nucleus
  Paraventricular nucleus
  Reuniens nucleus
  Rhomboid nucleus

Specific cortical relay nuclei

Anterior nuclear group
  Anteroventral nucleus (AV)
  Anteromedial nucleus (AM)
  Anterodorsal nucleus (AD)
Lateral nuclear group (ventral tier)
  Ventral anterior nucleus (VA)
    Principal part (VApc)
    Magnocellular part (VAmc)
  Ventral lateral nucleus (VL)

Specific cortical relay nuclei (cont.)

    Oral part (VLo)
    Caudal part (VLc)
    Medial part (VLm)
  Ventral posterior nucleus (VP)
    Ventral posterior lateral nucleus (VPL)
    Ventral posterior medial nucleus (VPM)
Metathalamic group
  Nucleus of lateral geniculate body (LGB)
    Dorsal part
    Ventral part (pregeniculate)
  Nucleus of medial geniculate body (MG)
    Parvocellular part (MGpc)
    Magnocellular part (MGmc)

Specific association nuclei

Lateral nuclear group (dorsal tier)
  Lateral dorsal nucleus (LD)
  Lateral posterior nucleus (LP)
  Pulvinar or posterior nucleus (P)
Medial nuclear group
  Dorsomedial (medial) nucleus (DM)
    Parvocellular part
    Magnocellular part

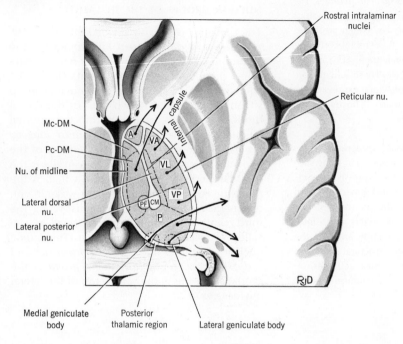

Mc-DM

Pc-DM

Nu. of midline

Lateral dorsal
nu.

Lateral posterior
nu.

Medial geniculate
body

Posterior
thalamic region

Lateral geniculate body

Rostral intralaminar
nuclei

Reticular nu.

FIGURE 13-3
The major thalamic nuclei in a, composite of several horizontal sections through the thalamus.

The arrows indicate the general location of the cortical projections within the internal capsule. A, anterior nuclear group; CM, centromedian nu.; P, pulvinar; PF, parafascicular nu.; VA, ventral anterior nu.; VL, ventral lateral nu.; VP, ventral posterior nu.

The intralaminar nuclear group has the following anatomic relations. The large centromedian nucleus (CM) is located in the middle third of the thalamus between the medial nuclear group and the ventral posterior nucleus of the lateral nuclear group. The smaller parafascicular nucleus (PF) is found medial to the CM and adjacent to the fasciculus retroflexus (habenulopeduncular tract). Rostral to these nuclei are the other intralaminar nuclei; the central lateral and central median nuclei are located caudal to the paracentral nucleus. The former group is referred to as the centromedian-parafascicular nuclear complex (large in man) and the latter as the rostral intralaminar group (small in man).

The *anterior nuclear group* is divided into the anterolateral, anteromedial, and anterodorsal nuclei. The anteroventral nucleus is large.

The *nuclei of the ventral tier* of the lateral nuclear group are arranged in a rostrocaudal order as the ventral anterior nucleus, ventral lateral nucleus, and ventral posterior nucleus. The ventral posterior nucleus is subdivided into the medially located *ventral posteromedial*

(arcuate, semilunar) nucleus and the laterally located *ventral posterolateral nucleus*. The metathalamic group (metathalamus) comprises the nuclei of the medial and lateral geniculate bodies.

The *nuclei of the dorsal tier* are arranged in a rostrocaudal order as the lateral dorsal nucleus, lateral posterior nucleus, and pulvinar. The large pulvinar has been subdivided into the medial, inferior, and lateral nuclei.

The medial nuclear group is divided into a medially located magnocellular part and a laterally located parvocellular part.

Because the dendrites and axons of many neurons of adjacent thalamic nuclei overlap and interdigitate, the precise delineation of each thalamic nucleus may not be critical considering our present-day knowledge of the precise function of each nucleus.

SOME THALAMIC NUCLEI ACCORDING TO OTHER TERMINOLOGIES

The description and anatomic delineation of the thalamic nuclei are imprecise because of the indistinct cytoarchitectural boundaries between

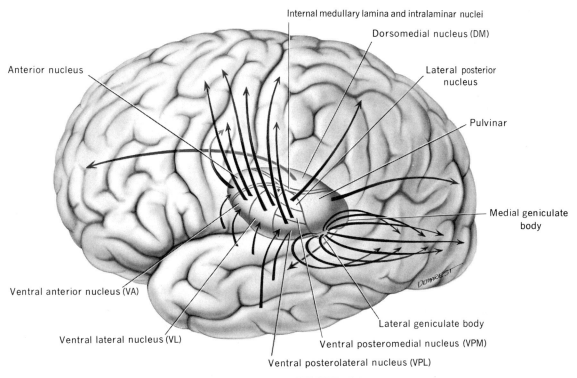

Internal medullary lamina and intralaminar nuclei

Dorsomedial nucleus (DM)

Lateral posterior nucleus

Pulvinar

Anterior nucleus

Medial geniculate body

Ventral anterior nucleus (VA)

Ventral lateral nucleus (VL)

Lateral geniculate body

Ventral posteromedial nucleus (VPM)

Ventral posterolateral nucleus (VPL)

FIGURE 13-4
The thalamus and its major nuclei and cortical projections. * Lateral dorsal nucleus.

the "named nuclei." Accordingly other nuclear groupings have been proposed, especially with regard to the ventral tier of the lateral nuclear group.

The term *ventrobasal complex* is defined on the basis of physiologic criteria. It is the nuclear complex whose cells respond to the stimulation of somatic sensory receptors, particularly those modalities conveyed by the medial lemniscus. In general the ventrobasal complex corresponds to the ventral posterolateral and ventral posteromedial nuclei. The cells of the ventrobasal complex are excited predominantly by mechanical stimulation, including pressure, touch, vibration, and joint movement. Stimuli associated with thermal sense and possibly pain (nociceptive modality) may activate cells of the ventrobasal complex.

The ventral tier of the lateral nuclear group, exclusive of the metathalamus, has been subdivided into six nuclei by Hassler. In the following list, these six nuclei are noted, along with the probable equivalent portion of the ventral tier:

1 lateropolaris (LPO) is equivalent to the VA

2 ventralis oralis anterior (VOA) is equivalent to the anterior basal region of the VL

3 ventralis oralis posterior (VOP) is equivalent to the posterior basal region of the VL

4 dorsalis oralis (DO) is equivalent to the dorsal region of VL

5 ventralis intermedius (VIM) is equivalent to the rostral region of VP

6 ventralis caudalis (VC) is equivalent to the remainder of VP.

SPECIFIC NUCLEI AND NONSPECIFIC NUCLEI

In the most widely used classification, the thalamic nuclei are grouped as *1 specific cortical relay nuclei* (specific thalamic nuclei), *2 spe-*

cific association nuclei (association thalamic nuclei), and *3 nonspecific nuclei* (Table 13-1).

Specific nuclei A specific nucleus is one which projects to localized regions of the cerebral cortex. These nuclei can be demonstrated *1* anatomically by the retrograde degeneration of the cell bodies of the thalamocortical fibers following the removal (ablation) of the cerebral cortex, and *2* physiologically by stimulating the cells within the nuclei and recording the discharge of the thalamocortical projections within the cerebral cortex. The specific nuclei are often called *"cortically dependent" nuclei,* because their cell bodies exhibit the retrograde degeneration response after the destruction of their axon terminals by the cortical ablation. Some cell bodies with axons terminating in the cortex do not exhibit the retrograde degeneration response; they remain normal because their axons have *sustaining axon collateral branches;* these branches project either to several widely dispersed cortical regions or to other thalamic nuclei.

The *specific cortical relay nuclei* are arranged into three groups on the basis of the major sources of their inputs and the objects of their outputs:

1 The *sensory relay nuclei* include the ventral posteromedial (VPM) nucleus, ventral posterolateral (VPL) nucleus, and the nuclei of the medial and lateral geniculate nuclei. These nuclei receive their major inputs from the ascending sensory pathways and project their output to the primary and secondary somesthetic, primary visual, and primary auditory cortices.

2 The *"motor" relay nuclei* include the ventral anterior (VA) and ventral lateral (VL) nuclei. They receive their major inputs from the cerebellum, basal ganglia, and substantia nigra and project their outputs to the motor and premotor cortex.

3 The "limbic" relay nuclei include the nuclei of the anterior nuclear group and the lateral dorsal nucleus. They receive input from the basal diencephalic regions and project to sectors of the limbic cortex.

The *specific association nuclei* have profuse connections with other diencephalic nuclei with the association areas of the cortex. They receive no input or possibly a slight input from the ascending pathways. The lateral nuclear group has connections with the association cortical areas of the temporal, parietal, and occipital lobes, while the medial nuclear group has connections with the prefrontal cortex.

Nonspecific nuclei The nonspecific nuclei are considered to be rostral extensions of the brainstem reticular formation. The *magnocellular part of the ventral anterior (VAmc) nucleus* is also considered to be a nonspecific nucleus. These nuclei receive their major input from descending fibers from the cortex and from ascending fibers of the brainstem reticular formation. They seem to have numerous reciprocal connections with some other nonspecific nuclei and specific nuclei of the thalamus. The intralaminar nuclei project prominently to the neostriatum. Although the intralaminar nuclei exert powerful effects over the cerebral cortex, the projections to the cortex seem to be limited to a pathway from some nonspecific nuclei to the orbitofrontal cortex. The reticular nucleus has extensive connections with thalamic nuclei and a caudal projection to the midbrain reticular formation. The nonspecific thalamic projection system is known as the *Generalized Thalamocortical Projection System.* After ablation of the cortex, the cell bodies of the nonspecific nuclei do not undergo retrograde degeneration changes.

Duality A duality exists within the thalamocortical systems. The *specific thalamic nuclei* and their projections are primarily organized as precise conveyors and processors of information utilized in the sensory sphere (e.g., touch, sight) and in the motor sphere (e.g., a movement). The *nonspecific thalamic nuclei* and their projections are organized primarily as signal systems subserving an energizing function over wide sectors of the thalamus and cerebral cortex. The powerful internuclear activity within the thalamus modulates, regulates, and modifies thalamocortical activity. The interactions between the thalamic specific nuclei and thalamic nonspecific nuclei are extensive. Much of the internuclear processing is exerted through intense excitatory and inhibitory synaptic activity between the interneurons and neurons of the specific and nonspecific nuclei.

The *intralaminar nuclear group* receives *1* ascending input from the brainstem reticular formation, spinothalamic and associated fibers, and the cerebellum, and *2* influences from the cerebral cortex and basal ganglia. The *centromedian nucleus* receives input from area 4 (motor cortex) of the cerebral cortex and the globus pallidus, and projects output to the putamen. The *parafascicular nucleus* receives input from area 6 (premotor cortex), and projects output to the caudate nuclei. These intralaminar nuclei probably interact with the magnocellular part of the ventral anterior nucleus (VAmc), which is a reticular nucleus with projections to the orbitofrontal cortex. Interconnections between intralaminar nuclei and the specific thalamic nuclei are extensive and significant to the functional roles of the thalamus. The spinoreticulothalamic pathways terminate in all intralaminar nuclei. The lateral spinothalamic tract terminates, in part, in the parafascicular nucleus and the rostral intralaminar group.

In general, the basic connections of the nonspecific nuclei are 1 reciprocal interconnections with the specific nuclei, 2 ascending afferent input from the brainstem reticular formation, 3 descending input from the cortex, and 4 output to the orbitofrontal cortex.

The *thalamic reticular nucleus* is a thin lamina of cells flanking the rostral and lateral aspect of the thalamus. The input to this nucleus is derived from the reticular formation and the cerebral cortex. The output from this nucleus is directed to the specific and nonspecific thalamic nuclei and caudally to the midbrain reticular formation. Rostrally directed projections are not demonstrable. The thalamic reticular nucleus is presumed to have a critical role in the integration of intrathalamic activities. It is suggested that this nucleus may be related to the synchronized low-frequency high-amplitude rhythms associated with light sleep and with drowsiness (Chap. 16).

The *midline nuclear group* consists of small nuclei located in the periventricular gray, including the interthalamic adhesion. Their connections with the hypothalamus suggest that they are involved with visceral activities.

SPECIFIC THALAMIC NUCLEI

Anterior nuclear group The *anterior nuclear group* is intercalated between the mamillary body of the hypothalamus and the cortical areas 23, 24, and 32 of the cingulate gyrus. The input to this group is conveyed from the mamillary body via fibers of the mamillothalamic tract and from the hippocampus via fibers of the fornix (Fig. 15-4). The medial mamillary nucleus projects to the large anteroventral (AV) and the small anteromedial (AM) nuclei, and the lateral mamillary nucleus projects to the small anterodorsal nucleus (AD) of the group. Some fibers from the anterior nuclear group project to the mamillary body via the mamillothalamic tract. Reciprocal influences are conveyed between this nuclear group and the cingulate gyrus via thalamocortical and corticothalamic fibers which pass through the anterior limb of the internal capsule. The anterior nuclear group is a processing and relay station in the "Papez circuit" of the limbic system (Chap. 15). Stimulation or ablation of this nucleus results in changes in blood pressure and other expressions of the autonomic nervous system. A cat with a lesion in this nuclear complex is more difficult to excite to anger; it has an elevated threshold for rage. The lateral dorsal nucleus (LD) of the lateral nuclear group may be a posterior extension of the anterior nuclear group.

Lateral nuclear group (ventral tier) The *ventral anterior nucleus* (VA) has a dual role as a specific thalamic nucleus and as a nonspecific thalamic nucleus of the reticular system. Input is derived from the globus pallidus (fibers pass via the ansa lenticularis and lenticular fasciculus to the principal part of VA), from the pars reticularis of the substantia nigra (fibers terminate in the magnocellular part of the VA nucleus—VAmc), and from the brainstem, intralaminar nuclei, nuclei of the midline, and collateral branches of descending fibers from the premotor area of the cerebral cortex. VA may receive some input from the cerebellum. The major role of the VA in the regulation of somatic motor activity is effected, at least in part, by complex circuits involving the intralaminar nuclei and basal ganglia, which feed back influences to the VA, VL, and CM (Chap. 14). In turn, this processed information is projected to area 6 (the premotor cortex, Chap. 16). The VA is a significant link in the reticular system; its effect upon the elicitation of the recruiting response (noted above under "Nonspecific Nuclei") is thought to be exerted by *1* the projection from magnocellular parts of the VA to the orbitofrontal cortex, and *2* by activation of the nonspecific thalamic nuclei. The VAmc and its projection to the orbitofrontal cortex may act as the "trigger zone" for the recruiting response and the synchronous electrocortical activity over wide areas of the neocortex (Chap. 16).

The *ventral lateral nucleus* (VL) is an integral nucleus in the feedback circuits from the cerebellum and basal ganglia to the motor cortex (precentral gyrus, area 4). The feedback circuits include *1* cerebral cortex to cerebellum to VL to motor cortex (Chap. 9), and *2* cerebral cortex to basal ganglia to VL to motor cortex (Chap. 14). Through the projection to the motor cortex, the *VL exerts its role as the main gateway to and prime mover of the motor pathways.* It receives its main input from the contralateral cerebellar hemisphere (primarily via the dentatothalamic tract and partly from the nucleus interpositus) and the ipsilateral red nucleus via the dentatorubrothalamic tract. Other input comes from the ipsilateral medial segment of the globus pallidus via the thalamic fasciculus and from the substantia nigra. The VL has somatotopically organized reciprocal connections with the precentral and supplementary motor cortex: the medial region of the VL with the face area, the intermediate region with the upper extremity and body area, and the lateral region with lower extremity area of area 4. The input and output are distributed differentially within the VL. *In general, VLo (oral part) receives input from the cerebellum and some from the globus pallidus, and VLm (medial part) receives input from the globus pallidus and substantia nigra.* VLo and VLc (caudal part) have reciprocal connections with the motor cortex. The neural processing within the VL of the various inputs, including that from the reticular nuclei, results

in the production of the powerful influences exerted by the VL upon motor activity. Thus there appears to be a blending of the afferent input from the basal ganglia and the cerebellum by the overlap of their fiber terminals in VLo. The motor cortex is the source of the fibers of the corticobulbar, corticospinal, corticoreticular, and corticorubral tracts. Surgical lesions in the VL may ameliorate the tremors and rigidity on the contralateral side of patients with Parkinson's disease.

The *ventral posterior nucleus* (VP) *is the primary somatic processing relay nucleus for the general sensory and gustatory pathways.* The VP nucleus comprises two large nuclei: the ventral posterolateral (VPL) and the ventral posteromedial (VPM). Most of the neurons of the VP respond to one of the following stimulus modalities: tactile sense (e.g., light pressure or bending of hair), mechanical distortion of deep structures (position sense or joint movements), or intense mechanical distortion, often associated with pain. Each neuron is place-specific (from a precise locus on the body) and modality-specific. Whether or not pain cells or thermal cells are located in the VP has not been resolved.

The *VPL nucleus* is the nucleus of termination of the lateral spinothalamic tract (pain and thermal sense from the body), medial lemniscus (touch, deep sensibility, and vibratory sense from the body), anterior spinothalamic tract (light touch from the body), and spinocervicothalamic tract (tactile and kinesthetic sense). These ascending pathways terminate somatotopically within the VPL. One schema indicates that the thoracic and lumbar regions are represented dorsally and the distal parts of the limbs ventrally in the VPL; in addition, sacral segments are represented laterally and cervical segments medially in it. Another schema indicates that the pathways from the lower extremity terminate in the posterolateral part, those from the body segments in the intermediate location, and those from the upper extremity in the anteromedial part of the VPL. The sensory homunculus is a distorted image of the body proportional to the innervation density; those parts of the body (e.g., the hand) with great tactile sensitivity occupy a greater volume of the nucleus than those with relatively minimal sensitivity (e.g., the back).

The *VPM nucleus* is the nucleus of termination of the fibers of the crossed anterior trigeminal tract from the principal and spinal trigeminal nuclei and the uncrossed posterior trigeminal tract from the principal trigeminal nucleus. The modalities are topographically localized within the VPM; taste is projected to the medial portion of the nucleus (referred to as the parvocellular part, VPMpc), tactile sense to the lateral portion, and temperature to the intermediate portion. The tactile sense from the face and oral cavity is conveyed via crossed and uncrossed fibers to the VPM.

The VP nucleus has precise point-to-point projections to the primary somesthetic cortex (postcentral gyrus, areas 3, 1, and 2). This is consistent with the somatotopic organization of this cortical area and with the modality-specific cortical neurons. Lateral VPL projects to the dorsal sectors of the gyrus, intermediate portions of the VP to the midsector of the gyrus, and the VPM to the lower sector of the gyrus. Although cortical areas 3, 1, and 2 receive projections from the VP, most of the fibers terminate in area 3. In addition, the VP probably has some connections with somatic sensory area II. As in the other ascending systems, descending influences from the postcentral gyrus are projected to the VP.

Metathalamus The nucleus of the lateral geniculate body (LGB) is the thalamic relay nucleus of the visual pathway. Each LGB *1* receives input from both eyes via the retinofugal fibers of the optic tract and from the primary visual cortex (area 17) via corticogeniculate fibers of the optic radiation, and *2* projects output to the visual cortex via the geniculocalcarine tract (optic radiation). Intrathalamic connections are made with the pulvinar and other nuclei of the lateral thalamic groups.

The nucleus of the *medial geniculate body* is divided into the dorsally located parvocellular part (MGpc) and the ventrally located magnocellular part (MGmc, posterior thalamic region or zone). The MGpc is the thalamic relay nucleus of the auditory pathway and of the vestibular system. A vestibular pathway from the vestibular receptors in the membranous labyrinth to the MGpc has been proposed, but its course is unknown. Vestibular influences are thought to be projected from the MGpc to the face region of the primary somatic sensory cortex. In this sector of the cortex there are cells which respond to vestibular influences. This system may have a role in our sense of orientation of the head in space. These cells also respond to kinesthetic stimuli in joints.

Each MGpc *1* receives input from the spiral organs of Corti of both ears via the ascending fibers of the brachium of the inferior colliculus and from the primary auditory cortex (area 41) via descending fibers of the auditory radiation, and *2* projects output to the primary auditory cortex (superior temporal gyrus, transverse gyri of Heschl, area 41) via the auditory radiation (geniculotemporal fibers). Intrathalamic connections are made with the pulvinar and other nuclei of the lateral thalamic groups.

A region caudal to the VP including the magnocellular (medial) portion of the medial geniculate body is called the *posterior thalamic region (zone)*. It is a significant processing and relay nucleus in the general sensory pathways with a critical role in the perception of painful and noxious stimuli. Bilaterally derived influences from the ipsilateral and contralateral sides of the body are conveyed to the posterior thalamic region via the spinothalamic tract, ascending reticular pathway, and some fibers from the other ascending pathways. In effect, *this complex receives polysensory input* from the visual, auditory, vestibular, and somatosensory systems. Its cells are not modality-specific. Rather they respond to a variety of inputs from tactile, vibratory, and auditory sources. This posterior thalamic region has direct connections with the secondary somatic sensory area (somatic area II) of the cortex.

Lateral nuclear group (dorsal tier) The *dorsal tier of the lateral nuclear group* consists, in a rostrocaudal direction, of the lateral dorsal nucleus (LD), the lateral posterior nucleus (LP), and the massive pulvinar. The *lateral dorsal nucleus* is now considered to be a caudal extension of the anterior nuclear group. In common with the latter, the LD has its primary connections with the cingulate gyrus. Reciprocal connections with the cortex of the precuneus have been reported. Information concerning input to LD is wanting. The *lateral posterior nucleus*, located dorsal to the VP, blends into the pulvinar. The input to the LP is apparently derived primarily from the VP and adjacent thalamic nuclei. Its reciprocal connections with the superior parietal lobule (areas 5 and 7) suggest that the LP has a role in processing information of the general somatic sensory system.

The *pulvinar*, the largest of all the thalamic nuclei, receives subcortical input from other thalamic nuclei, including the nuclei of the medial and lateral geniculate bodies and the intralaminar nuclei. Some input from the visual system may come via projections from the superior colliculus. Direct fiber connections from the optic tract or geniculate bodies are apparently lacking. This is interesting because the pulvinar has numerous reciprocal connections with the association cortex of the posterior parietal, occipital, and posterior temporal lobes, areas with a significant role in higher sensory processing. The pulvinar is regarded as a polysensory nucleus, receiving input from the visual, auditory, and somatic sensory systems. The three nuclei within the pulvinar have specific connections with the cortex: its *medial nucleus* interconnects with the cortex of the posterior parietal lobe, its *inferior nucleus* interconnects with the occipital cortex in the peristriate cortex (area 18 and possibly 19), and its *lateral nucleus* interconnects with the cortex of the posterior temporal lobe. The lateral posterior nucleus and the pulvinar are complex processing stations involved with the normal functioning of the association cortex, which subserves the highest levels of somesthetic, auditory, and visual integration (Chap. 16). No functional or behavioral changes in the sensory sphere have been observed in animals or human beings with lesions in the pulvinar. Reduction in the degree of spasticity as indicated by decrease in hypertonus and clonus in certain spastic patients has been reported.

Medial nuclear group The massive *dorsomedial nucleus* (*DM, medial*), located between the internal medullary lamina and the third ventricle, is divided into a *magnocellular* (*large-cell*) part and a larger, *parvocellular* (*small-cell*) part. This nucleus has extensive intrathalamic connections with the intralaminar nuclei, nuclei of the midline, and the nuclei of the lateral thalamic group. The medially located magnocellular part of the DM has connections primarily with subcortical structures, while the laterally located parvocellular portion is linked with the prefrontal cortex (areas 9, 10, 11, and 12—all rostral to areas 6 and 32). Via fibers in the inferior thalamic peduncle, the magnocellular part has connections (some of which are reciprocal) with the amygdaloid body, lateral hypothalamus, basal olfactory centers, and temporal and caudal orbitofrontal neocortex. The parvocellular part has massive topically organized reciprocal connections with the prefrontal cortex.

The integration and elaboration of this input and its relation with the hypothalamus (Chap. 11) and the prefrontal cortex (Chap. 16) may help to explain why this elaborate nucleus is involved with the affect of an individual rather than with specific sensory activities. The affective tone is expressed as euphoria or as mild depression, as a feeling of well-being or ill-being, or as a pleasant response or an unpleasant response to environmental stimuli. The hypothalamus, as the highest center of the autonomic nervous system, has the expressive role, whereas the prefrontal cortex is a higher elaborator of affect. The ablation of the DM has been used therapeutically, as has prefrontal lobotomy, in certain psychosurgical procedures (Chap. 16). Destruction of the DM in cats produces an animal that has a lower threshold for rage, is easily irritated, and is less adept at solving problems.

THALAMIC PEDUNCLES

The thalamocortical and corticothalamic fibers between the thalamus and cerebral cortex course through the limbs of the internal capsule (Fig. 16-10 and Chap. 16) as the so-called *thalamic peduncles* or *thalamic radiation*. Many of these fibers reciprocally interconnect the thalamus and cortex. The *anterior* (*frontal*) *peduncle* comprises the fibers in the anterior limb of the internal capsule which connect the DM with the prefrontal cortex and the anterior thalamic nuclear group with the cingulate cortex. The *middle* (*superior* or *centroparietal*) *peduncle* comprises fibers in the genu and posterior limb of the internal capsule which connect the VP with the postcentral gyrus, the VL with the precentral gyrus (area 4), the VA with the premotor cortex (area 6), and the dorsal tier thalamic nuclei with the association cortex of the parietal lobe. The *posterior* (*occipital*) *peduncle* comprises fibers in the posterior limb proper and the retrolenticular portion which connect the lateral geniculate body with the visual cortex (area 17) and the dorsal tier thalamic nuclei with the association cortex of the occipital lobe. The *inferior (temporal) peduncle* comprises fibers in the sublenticular portion of the internal capsule which connect the medial geniculate body with the auditory cortex (a few fibers may connect the pulvinar and the association cortex of the temporal lobe).

SOME FUNCTIONAL ASPECTS OF THE THALAMUS

The thalamus is interconnected with the ipsilateral cerebral cortex and with subcortical nuclear complexes, e.g., the hypothalamus and basal ganglia. The ipsilateral thalamus does not have direct connections with any structures on the contralateral side of the brain. Any functional projection of thalamic activity to the opposite half of the brain must take place at other levels through the indirect connections of commissures and decussating pathways.

The thalamus has a significant role in two other types of sensation, viz., affective and discriminative. The "affective" domain of sensory appreciation is apparently mediated through the thalamic reticular system, dorsomedial nucleus, and anterior thalamic nucleus. The affect of an individual relates to his emotional tone and somewhat to the phase of the sleep-wake cycle. Well-being, malaise, and a state of contentment are expressions of affect. The degree of agreeableness or disagreeableness of any stimulus depends on the state of an individual. The same objective degree of pain, temperature, or touch can evoke a remarkable variety of subjective degrees of reactivities. This variety is an expression of affective sensory mechanisms. Discriminative sensation is an aspect of sensation mediated through the thalamic specific nuclei. Such sensations include the "objective" appreciation of sensory stimuli from the general somatic and visceral sensors and the special sensors of vision, audition, and taste. The thalamus has a significant role in the generation of many rhythms, including brain waves (see further on in this chapter, "Rhythms in the Nervous System").

The thalamus has a significant role in the conscious appreciation of sensation. The more general aspects of many sensations (pain, crude touch, vibratory sense, crude temperature discrimination, and possibly general sound detec-tion) are brought to the conscious level in the thalamus. The finer sensory discriminations (those of the somesthetic, visual, auditory, and gustatory senses), which are elevated to the conscious sphere in the cerebral cortex, require the input of the information processed in thalamic nuclei for their final resolution. In brief, the conscious appreciation of sensory input takes place at both thalamic and cortical levels.

INTEGRATIVE AND SYNCHRONIZING ROLES OF THE THALAMUS

Many of the major pathways interact with one another at many levels of the nervous system, including the cerebral cortex, basal ganglia, diencephalon, and brainstem. This integrative activity is essential to the concept that the pathway systems are interdependent. According to this concept, the thalamus is crucial because *1* many of its nuclei are the final processing stations of systems which project to the cerebral cortex, and *2* the thalamic reticular system apparently acts as a monitor, a modulator, and a modifier of the activity of the thalamic nuclei of the specific system. Through these connections, the thalamus exerts the essential regulatory drive upon the cerebral cortex. This thalamic drive is projected to pools of cortical neurons; these influences are directed through the stellate neurons of the cortex either to subpools of dendrites (axodendritic synapses) or to subpools of somas (axosomatic synapses). Numerous pieces of neurophysiologic evidence support the concept that the thalamus is the key generator of much of the synchronized activity of the nervous system.

The genesis of this recruitment activity is thought to take place in pacemaker cells in the intralaminar nuclei with natural rhythms of between 6 to 12 per second. The stimulation of 8 to 10 per second brings these neurons in synchrony with their pacemaker frequency. This synchrony of the neurons within the thalamic nuclei is brought about by inhibitory circuits. The stimulated cells discharge through axon collaterals to inhibitory interneurons (Figs. 13-1 and 13-2), which, through their connections, hyperpolarize many other cells within the thalamus for about a 100-millisecond interval. Then these cells are stimulated, while in the same phase, to fire together in synchrony. In turn, these synchronized cells, through their axon collaterals and inhibitory interneurons, hyperpolarize many more cells. This recruitment of more cells continues until the rhythm is established.

The thalamus is essential to such expressions of synchrony as *1* the rhythmic brain wave activity evidenced in the electroencephalogram (Chap. 16), and *2* the phasic and tonic movements mediated by the motor pathways. *The thalamus, through the VL, is considered to be a "prime mover" of the motor pathways. The nonspecific thalamic reticular system has a major role in the synchronizing effects of the thalamus;* it exerts this role through precise neuroanatomic connections and neurophysiologic inhibitory and excitatory influences on the specific thalamic nuclei. The various brain wave rhythms are apparently set by the thalamic reticular system (see further on, "Rhythms in the Nervous System"). The phasic and tonic movements are largely the products of the influences of the thalamic reticular system upon specific thalamic nuclei and thus upon specific systems. These modulatory effects are exerted through *1* the cerebellothalamo- (ventral lateral nucleus) cortical pathway, and *2* the basal ganglia-thalamo- (ventral anterior nucleus) cortical pathway. Through these integrative and synchronizing activities, the thalamus exerts a major effect upon the motor expressions through the cerebral cortex and its projection pathways, including the corticospinal, corticostriate, and corticoreticular tracts, among others (Chaps. 14, 16).

Repetitive electrical stimulation (6 to 12 per second) of the nonspecific thalamic nuclei evokes responses with long latency in the cerebral cortex by recruitment through multineuronal chains from these nuclei to the cortex. Neural influences from these nuclei are presumably relayed to the VA thalamic nucleus and then from the VA to the orbitofrontal cortex. This cortical area probably serves as a trigger zone for activating the entire cortex.

This cortical recruitment response is a type of electroencephalogram (EEG) which is in some way analogous to the normal arousal EEG response (Chap. 16). It is called a recruitment response because the activity increases in a step-by-step manner as more and more neurons are recruited in the course of this cortical response initiated by the repetitive thalamic stimulation. No cortical response is obtained from a single stimulus. With a continuous repetitive stimulation the cortical responses increase to a maximum, then decrease, then increase (wax and wane). The phenomena of recruitment, waxing and waning, long latency, and diffuse cortical activity to repetitive stimulation at this frequency are attributable to the multineuronal chain (which favors neuronal interaction) through other thalamic nuclei terminating in numerous axodendritic synapses of the pyramidal cortical neurons. The many inhibitory postsynaptic potentials and excitatory postsynaptic potentials on the cortical cells are the bioelectric responses responsible for much cortical activity recorded by neurophysiologists and electroencephalographers (EEG, Chap. 16). Destruction of intralaminar nuclei is said to result in temporary somnolence, lethargy, and minimal reactivity to noxious stimuli. Many of the nuclei of the midline have strong connections with the hypothalamus; these nuclei apparently do not influence the cortex. The nucleus centrum medianum has a direct connection with the caudate nucleus and putamen which is integrated in the activity of the somatic motor system (Chap. 14).

Low-frequency electrical stimulation of certain specific thalamic nuclei (e.g., the nuclei of the ventral tier) evokes short-latency responses restricted to the primary cortical projection areas. These recorded potentials on the surface of the cortex are known as *augmenting responses* (cf. waxing and waning of the recruiting responses). The influences involved in these responses are conveyed from the specific thalamic nuclei via fibers which are projected to the middle third of the shaft of the apical dendrites of pyramidal cells (Fig. 16-5). These terminals make effective connections because they are relatively close to the nodal sites that fire these cortical neurons. In addition, the augmenting responses are diphasic; they increase in magnitude during the initial four or five repetitive stimulations of the specific nuclei.

A change in an individual's reaction to pain can occur following a prefrontal lobotomy or thalamotomy (lesion of the dorsomedial and intralaminar nuclei, or possibly of the pulvinar). Following such surgery, the subject perceives pain but he is not unduly disturbed once the fear and dread of the pain and anxiety about it are gone. This operation is often helpful in alleviating the intractable pain associated with metastatic cancer.

A thrombosis of a branch of the posterior choroidal or posterior cerebral arteries in man may produce the *thalamic syndrome.* A transitory contralateral hemianalgesia may be an immediate consequence. Soon painful sensations appear upon the application of noxious stimulation. Later pain is provoked by pressure, touch, and vibration. In time a state of spontaneous, constant or paroxysmal pain on the affected (opposite) side is evoked without the application of any external stimulus. In this syndrome, the threshold for pain, temperature, and tactile sensations is usually raised on the opposite side of the body from the lesion. In addition mild stimuli may evoke disagreeable sensations. Stimuli may produce exaggerated and perverted sensations on the affected side of the body. The feelings elicited from a pinprick may be an intolerable burning and agonizing pain. Heat, ice, cold, and pressure of one's clothes can be exceedingly uncomfortable. Even the sound of melodious music may produce unpleasant sensations on the affected side. Intractable pain, which does not respond to analgesics, may be a consequence. Affect qualities such as swelling, pulling, compression, and numbness are exaggerated during emotional stress.

These highly overactive sensory responses are probably the result of alterations in frequencies and patterns of input to the thalamus, irritation of injured neurons, and changes in the quality of the output to the cerebral cortex. In addition the release (phenomenon) from some cortical influences upon the thalamus may be contributory. Emotional control is modified, as exhibited by forced laughter and sobbing. Mild stimuli may provoke an overresponse with agreeable and pleasant feeling tones. The application of a warm object to the hand may be pleasurable.

Lesions of the ventral posterior nucleus and nuclei of the medial and lateral geniculate bodies produce deficits in the modalities subserved by the pathways associated with these specific nuclei.

The conscious appreciation of crude general sensations occurs in the thalamus. One clinical indication of this phenomenon is that, following lesions of the thalamocortical projections, the sensations of pain and crude touch and some thermal sense are retained.

Lesions in the VLo result in the reduction of muscle tone and rigidity in Parkinson's disease. The probable explanation for the reduced rigidity is that the lesion isolates the processed input of the muscle stretch receptor within the cerebellum, preventing it from being projected to the motor cortex (area 4).

Rhythms in the nervous system

Oscillatory activities as expressed in the rhythms of the electroencephalogram (Chap. 16), in the jerky movements of the eye (Chap. 12), in the tremors of cerebellar dysfunction (Chap. 9), and in the respiratory cycles are the products of the functional organization of the neurons resulting from the gaited discharge of nerve cells. The spatial distribution and the timing of the activity at the excitatory and inhibitory synapses of a group of neurons are essential to the phasic discharge of this group of neurons. Some of the neurophysiologic activities suggested as being contributory to these rhythms include an "autorhythmicity" of pacemaker neurons, hyperpolarization of the receptive membranes of neurons, presynaptic inhibition, postsynaptic inhibition, disinhibition, facilitation, and closed self-reexciting neuronal circuits.

Pacemaker neurons exhibiting an "autorhythmicity" may contribute to the genesis of such gaiting; however, the experimental documentation for this concept in mammals is inadequate at present. Some neurons are known to become hyperpolarized by a retrograde spread from the initial segment (trigger point) which has just generated an axon potential in the conductile segment. The simultaneous hyperpolarization of the receptive segment of each neuron (dendrites and cell body) of a group places all neurons in the same state of activity. In this hyperpolarized state, each neuron is in the same phase, a probable prerequisite for a rhythm.

Closed self-reexciting chains of neurons have a significant role in generating rhythmic waves. These circuits are feedback loops in which are linked interneurons exerting presynaptic and postsynaptic inhibitory influences. The cortically projecting thalamic neurons, which are associated with brain wave activity, are integrated into these feedback circuits as follows (Figs. 13-1 and 13-2). An axon collateral branch of the cortically projecting thalamic fiber synapses with one or more interneurons, which, in turn, may have axosomatic and axodendritic synaptic connections with several cortically projecting thalamic neurons, or may have axoaxonic synapses with axons terminating on these thalamic neurons. Functionally this is a negative feedback circuit, with the axon collateral branches exciting the interneurons, which, in turn, inhibit the thalamocortical neurons through postsynaptic inhibition (axosomatic and axodendritic synapses) and presynaptic inhibition (axoaxonic synapse). This recurrent inhibitory circuit (functioning mainly through postsynaptic inhibition in the thalamus) tends to suppress the thalamocortical projecting neurons; these neurons are now in phase; all are dampened. These momentarily inactive (for 100 milliseconds or so), cortically projecting neurons now do not feed back information via the feedback circuit to generate new IPSPs on the thalamocortical neurons; hence these previously inhibited cells are now released from inhibitory influences and are phased to receive facilitatory influences to resume the next cycle of the rhythm. The 10-per-second alpha rhythm (Chap. 16) of the electroencephalogram may be generated by such a system. In brief, inhibition has a crucial role in gaiting the rhythms of the nervous system.

The interrupted flow patterns of the plays of a football game offer a crude analogy to this concept of the generation of rhythms. Each play, from huddle to grounding of the ball, is analogous to the activity commencing preliminary to inhibition of the neurons and ending with the completion of the synchronized discharge of the group of neurons. The interval between two plays is the time for the operation of the negative feedback to the referee and players. The synchronously discharging neurons are the players, and the interneurons of the feedback circuit are the referee and the quarterback. The whistle of the referee and the call of the quarterback alert and coordinate the players to line up in the set position. The final signal of the quarterback is the key which releases the inhibition and supplies the excitation triggering the synchronous discharge of each player to perform his assignment. At the termination of the play negative feedback relay commences.

Bibliography

Carmel, P. W.: Efferent projections of the ventral anterior nucleus of the thalamus in the monkey. Am. J. Anat., 128:159–184, 1970.

Carpenter, M. B.: Ventral tier thalamic nuclei, in D. Williams (ed.), *Modern Trends in Neurology*, vol. 4, pp. 1–20. Butterworth & Co. (Publishers), Ltd., London, 1967.

Ebbesson, S. O. E., J. A. Jane, and D. M. Schroeder: A general overview of major interspecific variations in thalamic organization. Brain Behav. Evol., 6:92–131, 1972.

Geldard, F. A.: *The Human Senses*, 2d ed. John Wiley & Sons, Inc., New York, 1972.

Gerard, P. W., and J. W. Duyff (eds.): *Information Processing in the Nervous System*, Proceedings of the International Union of Physiological Sciences. Excerpta Medica Foundation, Amsterdam, 1964.

Graybiel, A. M.: Some fiber pathways related to the posterior thalamic region in the cat. Brain Behav. Evol., 6:424–452, 1972.

Harmon, L. D., and E. R. Lewis: Neural modeling. Physiol. Rev., 46:513–592, 1966.

Hess, W. R.: *Diencephalon: Autonomic and Extrapyramidal Functions.* William Heinemann, Ltd., London, 1954.

Mehler, W. R.: The posterior thalamic region in man. Confin. Neurol., 27:18–29, 1966.

Petras, J. M.: Connections of the parietal lobe. J. Psychiat. Res., 8:189–201, 1971.

Purpura, D. P., and M. D. Yahr (eds.): *The Thalamus.* Columbia University Press, New York, 1966.

Riss, W., K. Koizumi, and C. M. Brooks (eds.): Basic thalamic structure and function. Brain Behav. Evol., 6:1–560, 1972.

Rosenblith, W. A. (ed.): *Sensory Communication Symposium on Principles of Sensory Communications.* The M.I.T. Press, Cambridge, Mass., and John Wiley & Sons, Inc., New York, 1961.

CHAPTER **14**
THE SOMATIC MOTOR SYSTEMS
AND THE BASAL GANGLIA

NERVOUS SYSTEM AS AN EFFECTOR

The nervous system may be thought of as a complex assemblage of neural circuits functioning primarily to regulate the activity of the effectors of the body—its muscles and glands. It is only by stimulating muscles to contract (or to relax) and glands to secrete that the nervous system can overtly express itself. The somatic nervous system has the specific role of regulating the activity of striated (voluntary) muscles, while the autonomic (visceral) nervous system (Chap. 6) has the role of influencing the heart, nonstriated (involuntary) muscles, and glandular cells.

Postures are the body poses that are basic to the complex somatic motor activities. Each of the postures is maintained through an elaborate series of reflexes and reactions which utilize continuously acting feedback circuits operating through several segmental levels of control. The smooth flow of striated muscle activities from one posture to another posture is a movement. In this context, postures are the framework for all movements, whether crude, stereotyped, skilled, or volitional. The evaluation of these concepts is the subject of this chapter.

SEGMENTAL LEVELS FOR THE REGULATION AND CONTROL OF SOMATIC MOTOR ACTIVITY

Input from the peripheral sensors is essential for the nervous system to function as an efficient effector. Most of the vast amount of incoming sensory data is integrated and processed in many neuronal pools of the central nervous system before the resulting influences are transmitted via the somatic motor pathways. These influences from the various levels of the brain and spinal cord are funneled to the pools of motor neurons directly innervating the striated muscles. In addition, the motor pools receive a continuous flow of input directly from peripheral sensors (especially neuromuscular spindles).

The control of muscular activities may be thought of as being regulated from successive segmental levels of the spinal cord and brain. The intrinsic neural patterns in the spinal cord levels are the circuits which are basic for coordinated motor activity (Chap. 5). In the lower brainstem is located the vestibular level, which has a significant role in static reactions, labyrinthine accelerating reactions, and tonic head, neck, and eye movements (Chap. 9). At the pontocerebellar level is located the integrative complex crucial to the synergistic regulation of muscular coordination (Chap. 10). From the processing centers in the midbrain tectum are projected influences from the auditory and optic systems to the other levels. The basal ganglia located at the cerebral level are integrated in the control of automatic movements, while the cerebral cortex is the location of centers involved with volitional movements.

The motor pathways from the brain actually make relatively few direct synaptic connections with alpha and gamma motor neurons of the spinal cord. In fact, descending influences are directed primarily to the spinal interneurons, which, in turn, synapse with the alpha and gamma motor neurons. Stated otherwise, these spinal interneurons are intercalated between the descending pathways from the brain and the lower motor neurons.

FACILITATORY AND INHIBITORY CENTERS

The motor pathways contain many neuronal centers (pools) which are called facilitatory and inhibitory centers. Each of these pools can simultaneously facilitate and inhibit the motor pools essential to an action. For example, the center which evokes the extension of a limb facilitates the motor neurons innervating the extensor muscles and inhibits the motor neurons innervating the flexor muscles. By convention, *a facilitatory center (nucleus or pathway) is one that facilitates extensor reflexes and inhibits flexor reflexes, while an inhibitory center (nucleus, pool, or pathway) is one that inhibits extensor reflexes and facilitates flexor reflexes.* This reciprocal activity on antagonistic muscle groups is essential to integrated action.

It is important to note that the center is defined by the evoked response following its stimulation. This has several implications, because of the interaction among the various centers. For example, a *facilitatory center may, in fact, be the source of inhibitory influences, because it may actually inhibit an inhibitory center (disinhibition) and thereby evoke (facilitate) a response. In the same way an inhibitory center may also facilitate when it stimulates by inhibiting an inhibitory center.* Many areas, neuronal pools, and centers in the brain can modify the activity of the spinal motor neurons. The cortex of the anterior limbic lobe, septal nuclei, caudate nucleus, and globus pallidus exert inhibitory influences on the extensor reflexes. The epithalamus exerts facilitatory influences. The cerebral motor cortex, hypothalamus, brainstem tegmentum, and cerebellum have some areas which exert facilitatory influences, and other areas which exert inhibitory influences.

The interactions of the stimuli from the descending motor pathways with those from the peripheral sensors are crucial to normal muscle activity. The significance can be gauged in the case where all the sensory spinal roots from the upper extremity are transected—in effect, preventing the motor neurons to the limb from receiving sensory data from the limb. The limb after deafferentation, with its motor neurons intact, exhibits a flaccid paralysis; however, the stimulation of the motor cortex can induce movements in it.

In the vertebrates, all peripheral somatic efferent (lower motor) neurons are excitatory nerves; when these peripheral nerves are stimulated, the voluntary muscles they innervate contract. There are no peripheral inhibitory somatic efferent nerves. However, in the autonomic nervous system there are inhibitory visceral peripheral nerves that innervate involuntary muscles. These nerves inhibit the activity of the cardiac muscles and the smooth muscles of the many visceral organs, including those of the vascular system and digestive system. Inhibition of the activity of the voluntary muscles is exerted exclusively through the inhibitory activity of the central nervous system (central inhibition). In brief, inhibition is a property of certain neurons of the central nervous system and peripheral autonomic nervous system but not of the neurons of the peripheral somatic efferent system.

The regulation of posture

Posture, or the attitude of the body, is the product of automatic muscle activity which counters the action of gravity. The various attitudes are not under volitional regulation because they are assumed without conscious effort. Posture is fundamental, for every movement begins from and ends in a posture. A movement may be considered as a change in posture; and a posture, as the point of change in a movement. In addition, all movements are actually reflexes modified by influences from the brain.

Gravity and the proprioceptive receptors are basic to the maintenance of posture. The erect posture is an antigravity response dependent on muscle activity stimulated by the proprioceptors. These antigravity responses are countered by antagonistic muscle groups, so that a balance of tone is maintained between the agonist and the antagonist muscle groups. All muscles are under some continuous tension which is maintained by streams of asynchronous volleys; these volleys are continually being fed to the muscle groups to maintain muscle tonus.

In man, the antigravity muscles include the

back muscles, posterior neck muscles (which hold the head up), jaw muscles, extensors of the lower extremity (for erect stance), and flexors of the upper extremity (which hold the arms up). The asynchronous discharge from the peripheral sensors is the source of stimulation for the smooth contractions which sustain a static antigravity posture.

The regulation of posture is dependent primarily on the stimuli from muscle and vestibular proprioceptors, their integration in the central nervous system, and their influence on the lower motor neurons. The visual system has a lesser role. The information from muscle receptors is utilized at the spinal level in the spinal reflexes. Much information is transmitted to supraspinal levels, even to the cerebral cortex. The descending pathways from the brain transmit facilitatory and inhibitory influences which have their effects on the spinal reflexes (Chap. 8). A reflex act may be operationally defined as an activity which originates in the peripheral nervous system and is relayed through the central nervous system before stimulating (or inhibiting) lower motor neurons. The significance of reflex activity in the regulation of posture is discussed below.

EXTENSOR REFLEXES—THE BASIC POSTURAL REFLEXES

The monosynaptic extensor (stretch) reflex (myotatic reflex, stretch extensor reflex) is basic to the maintenance of upright posture, because it is the main source of stimulation to the antigravity muscles. The arc formed by this two-neuron monosynaptic reflex includes the neuromuscular spindle receptor, the sensory neuron with its annulospiral endings in the spindle, and the alpha motor neuron (Chap. 5). This simple circuit with short latency forms a direct connection from the bag region of the spindle to an extensor muscle (Fig. 5-21). Because this arc involves only one synapse (and thus no interneurons), its effects are not diffuse. Furthermore, afterdischarge is lacking, the response lasting only as long as the stimulus.

When the back muscles and the extensor muscles of the lower extremity commence to relax, the standing individual begins to sag from the effects of gravity. These muscles and their spindles are now stretched until the spindle bags stimulate the afferent neurons to increase their firing rates. In turn, this excites the antigravity muscles to contract until the spindles are passively shortened. Then the firing rates of the spindles decrease until the muscles begin to sag, and the feedback cycle is resumed. The main function of the neuromuscular spindle is to exercise a significant role in the subconscious control of muscle contraction, both during steady contraction (posture) and during movement.

The stretch reflex cannot be maintained exclusively by the passive stretching and shortening of the spindles. The stimulation of the gamma efferent neurons by the motor pathways from the brain is also essential. The gamma fibers stimulate the intrafusal muscle fibers of the spindle to contract and thereby stretch the bag region of the spindle (Figs. 2-18 and 5-21). The stretched bag activates the stretch reflex.

Passive stretch has more effect than gamma fiber stimulation upon spindle activity (Chap. 5). In the maintenance of posture, muscle stretch is paramount to the generation of tone in the antigravity muscles. It is effective in overcoming the continual tendency of the legs to collapse under gravity. The gamma efferent neurons have a facilitatory role in the stretch reflex.

Polysynaptic extensor reflexes also have a significant role in motor activities. In the crossed extensor reflex, the flexion of one leg is coordinated with the extension of the contralateral leg (as in walking). This arc consists of receptors initiating flexion, sensory neuron, spinal interneurons crossing to the contralateral side, and alpha motor neuron to the contralateral extensor muscles. In the polysynaptic extensor thrust reflex, the extremity extends in response to moderate pressure on the sole of the foot. This arc consists of pressure receptors, sensory neuron, spinal interneuron, and alpha motor neuron to the ipsilateral extensor muscles.

FLEXOR REFLEXES—THE BASIC PROTECTIVE REFLEXES

The flexor reflex is primarily a withdrawal reflex protecting the organism from the effects of a noxious stimulus (Chap. 5). It acts in concert with the extensor reflex through reciprocal connections. The reflex arc of at least a three-neuron disynaptic reflex includes, in order, *1* one of several afferent neurons associated with cutaneous receptors (free nerve endings and touch-pressure receptors) and muscle receptors (flower spray endings of the muscle spindle), *2* an interneuron or more than one in the spinal cord, and *3* alpha motor neurons (Fig. 5-23). This reflex can be equated with diffusion of action, especially when many interneurons are intercalated. The polysynapticity of this reflex may result in afterdischarge (contraction outlasting the stimulus) and in a mass action response.

The disynaptic flexor reflex (stretch flexor reflex) originates in flower spray endings of the muscle spindle receptors in either flexor or extensor muscles. The polysynaptic flexor reflexes (flexor twitch) include the nociceptive (flexion withdrawal) reflex and the scratch reflex. Several interneurons are present in these reflexes. In the nociceptive reflex, the pain receptor endings in the skin initiate a reflex, ending with the withdrawal from a noxious stimulus. In the scratch reflex, the "irritation" of sensory receptors in the skin stimulates the reflex activity.

A monosynaptic flexor reflex (pluck reflex) is expressed by the jaw jerk. The reflex arc consists of annulospiral endings of the muscle spindle receptors in the flexor muscles (closed jaw), sensory neuron with a cell body in the mesencephalic nucleus of the fifth nerve (Chaps. 7, 8), and a lower motor neuron in the motor nucleus of the fifth cranial nerve.

The role of the Golgi tendon ending is expressed in a three-neuron, disynaptic reflex arc which transmits inhibitory influences to the alpha motor neuron (Fig. 5-22). This acts to inhibit the generation of extreme tension in the contracting muscle (Chap. 5).

STATIC REFLEXES (POSTURAL REACTIONS OR ATTITUDINAL REFLEXES)

Local static reaction *The local static reactions are the ipsilateral segmental reflexes directed to the support of the body.* The positive supporting action is the product of the simultaneous contraction of the antagonistic extensor muscles and flexor muscles (of the lower extremity in man) to form pillar-like posts. This support enables us to stand erect. The integration of the reciprocally acting extensor reflex and flexor reflex for the contraction of opposing muscle groups is a reaction to *1* gravitational pull, *2* muscle stretch from the sagging body, and *3* neuromuscular spindle stimulation.

The role of the cutaneous exteroceptive endings in the generation of this static reaction is illustrated by the "magnet reaction." When the extensor side (sole or palm) of the free flexed limb comes in contact with a surface, the cutaneous receptors are stimulated. As the surface is slowly withdrawn, the limb attempts to maintain contact by flowing with the touched surface (magnet reaction) until the limb is fully extended. At this point the pillar attitude is assumed and maintained by proprioceptive stimuli if the surface provides an active resistance. The "magnet reaction" is more readily demonstrated experimentally.

For the maintenance of the postural reactions, the descending influences on the gamma motor neurons are more important than those on the alpha motor neurons. The functional role of the gamma motor neurons is to stimulate the neuromuscular spindles and thus maintain the sensitivity of the spindles so that they fire asynchronous volleys to sustain a smooth contraction. In posture, the stabilization of the stretch reflex is paramount.

Segmental static reactions *The segmental static reactions are the bilateral segmental reflexes as expressed in the bipedal walking gait* (with compensatory upper limb movements) in man and the quadrupedal gait in many mammals. These coordinate movements arise from the effect of the movements of one extremity upon the contralateral extremity. The crossed extensor reflex and the spinal intersegmental reflexes (Fig. 5-11 and Chap. 5) are basic to these static reactions. The interactions of the movements of the lower limb on the upper limb are dependent on complex circuits and reciprocally innervated muscle groups. The rhythmic and automatic sequences during walking (which commence with flexion of the right hind limb, extension of the contralateral hind limb, extension of the right forelimb, and flexion of the contralateral fore-limb) are mediated through intrinsic circuits within the spinal cord (Fig. 5-11).

In certain experimental transected preparations, the crossed extensor reflex is obtained if a noxious stimulus (e.g., pinching a foot which cannot be felt) is presented. If the noxious stimulus is prolonged, the reflex activity grades into the rhythmic stepping movements called mark-time movements. As Charles S. Sherrington remarked, "The irritated foot is withdrawn from harm and the other legs run away."

General static reactions The general static reactions are postural reflexes initiated by spindle receptors in the neck muscles and proprioceptors in the utricle and saccule of the inner ear (Chaps. 5 and 10). The postural attitudes assumed are related to the actual position of the head in space.

The tonic neck reflexes are instrumental in influencing the extensor tonus of the extremities through multineuronal circuits with long recruiting latencies. The following attitudes illustrate general static reactions.

1 Imagine a cat preparing to jump up on a table. The contraction of the back neck muscles elevates the head so that the cat looks up. The attitude which is reflexly assumed is that of forelimbs extended to raise the forebody and hind limbs flexed to lower the hindquarters in preparation for the jump.

2 Imagine a cat with its head down preparing to jump off a table. The tonic neck reflexes are instrumental in initiating the flexion of the forelimb and the extension of the hind limbs.

3 A cat that turns its head to the right to catch a glimpse of a mouse assumes the following attitude prior to taking off. The tonic neck reflexes initiate the influences resulting in his right limbs' being reflexly extended and his left limbs' being flexed for the takeoff.

The tonic neck reflex initiates certain reflex actions. For example, the driver of a car may steer to the left when a distraction suddenly appears on the right. The reflex of quickly rotating the head to the right may cause an accident because the right upper extremity may reflexly extend and the left upper extremity may flex. The steering wheel turns and the car veers to the left, the driver having assumed a "Statue of Liberty pose," with face to the right, left upper extremity flexed, and right upper extremity extended and raised.

The precise role of the utricle and saccule of the vestibular labyrinth (Chap. 10) in normal activity is difficult to assess. In general the labyrinthine righting reaction is the result of stimuli from the utricle and saccule acting on the neck muscles to keep the head in a position consistent with gravity regardless of the position of the body. This reflex is expressed by a blindfolded cat held in the air with its legs up and its back to the ground (see "The Vestibular System," in Chap. 10). When the cat is dropped, its head twists to the position assumed when the cat is in a normal posture on the ground; the rest of the body twists as the animal rights itself and lands upright. This reflex is not highly developed in man.

LABYRINTHINE ACCELERATING REACTIONS (KINETIC REFLEXES, STATOKINETIC REFLEXES, OR ACCELERATOR REFLEXES)

These reactions are a consequence of a change in the rate of movement (acceleration and deceleration). The response may be to linear (progressive) acceleration (movement in a straight line) or to angular (rotatory) acceleration (movement at an angle). The utricle and saccule contain the sensors for responses to linear acceleration, while the semicircular canals contain the sensors for angular acceleration (Chap. 10).

Responses to linear acceleration are demonstrable in a blindfolded cat held with head down and supported by the pelvis. When such a cat is suddenly lowered, the forelimbs are extended and the toes spread. This is the reaction a cat assumes when it is about to land after a jump from a height.

Angular acceleration of the head evokes responses in the muscles of the eyes, neck, limbs, and trunk. Nystagmus is the reaction expressed by the eyes; the accompanying body and limb responses to maintain balance and stance are the reactions of the body and limb muscles. Neuroanatomic and neurophysiologic aspects are discussed under "The Vestibular System" in Chap. 10.

Nystagmus and the accompanying movements are basically the attempt of the organism to locate a fixed point for the eyes to focus on. The fast component is the nystagmus phase, or searching for the fixed point; the slow component is the phase of holding the fixed point in the view of the eyes. In the situation of watching telephone poles from a car window, the slow component of the eye movements occurs at the interval while the eyes are focused on a pole.

POSTURAL REACTIONS DEPENDENT ON THE CEREBRUM AND THE CEREBELLUM

The precise positioning (placing) of the feet on the ground beneath the body is essential for normal stance. The normal animal uses several sensory cues to effect the *placing reactions.* Visual, exteroceptive, and proprioceptive stimuli resulting from the sight, contact, position, or movement of the supporting surface contribute to these reactions.

The corrective movements of the extremities to secure a more stable standing posture are known as *hopping reactions.* When an animal held and left standing on one leg is moved forward, backward, or sideward, the dragged limb in contact with the supporting surface will hop in the direction of the movement so that the limb is directly under the body in a supporting posture (assuming the role of a rigid pillar). The hopping reaction is probably the result of stimulation from muscle stretch.

Both the placing reaction and the hopping reaction are dependent on the cerebral cortex and the cerebellar cortex.

REGULATION OF POSTURAL TONUS AS AN AUTOMATIC CONTROL SYSTEM

The interactions leading to the stabilization of the tonic muscular contractions in the postural reflexes utilize the principle of a closed-loop control system with negative feedback (Chap. 3). In this servomechanism, the negative feedback (a fraction of muscle tension acts as a stimulus for feeding back impulses generated by the neuromuscular spindles and Golgi tendon organs; the impulses are transmitted via the sensory nerves to the neuronal pools in the spinal cord) serves to maintain the predetermined goal (tonic muscular contractions) of the control system. This performance (goal) is accomplished through a sequence of self-correcting adjustments which are a consequence of the feedback of the prior performances (tonic muscle contractions) of the system to a control box (neuronal pool in the spinal cord). The feedback is negative because the corrections are in the opposite direction (reduced muscle tonus) to the positive divergence (increased muscle tonus) from the predetermined goal (tonus necessary to maintain posture). Constant surveying, utilizing feedback, is evidenced by the continuous sequences of tiny adjustment movements of muscle groups. The control box in the spinal cord directs the maintenance of the muscle tonus through the alpha motor neurons. The tonus fluctuates about the predetermined tonus set by the activity of the neuronal pools in the spinal cord. The entire system is goal seeking in the attempt to match the predetermined tonus. The intensity of the tonic contractions can be altered (this is comparable to changing the preset temperature in the thermostat) by the descending influences transmitted via the motor pathways from the brain. These descending influences account for the difference in the intensities of the tonic contractions in the upper extremity between holding a 1-lb weight and holding a 10-lb weight. The increase (or decrease) in the excitatory state of the neuronal pool stimulates the gamma motor neurons to increase (or decrease) the firing rate of the neuromuscular spindle; in turn, this increases (or decreases) the degree of muscle tone.

The sequence of events in the regulation of posture may be summarized as follows: the upper motor neurons can influence the state of excitability of the neuronal pools in the spinal cord (the control box); this acts to determine the degree (intensity) of muscle tonus. A comparison is made in the neuronal pool between the feedback from the muscle receptors and the state of excitability. After this action, an error-correcting signal is generated in the form of postsynaptic potentials which lead to an increase (or decrease) in the firing rate of the alpha motor neurons. The change in the contractions of the muscle and the subsequent changes in the sensitivity of the muscle receptors are fed back to the neuronal pool for another comparison. This negative feedback loop is important to the maintenance of posture.

ALTERATIONS IN THE OPERATION OF CONTROL SYSTEM

Three sensory systems have significant roles in influencing our orientation in space: the general proprioceptive system with sensors in the muscles, the special proprioceptive system with sensors in the labyrinth of the ear, and the visual system. The proprioceptive systems monitor certain relations between the body and gravity, and the movements of the body. The exteroceptive visual system senses the relation of the organism to the external environment.

Any two of these three systems are sufficient for the efficient operation of the control system that regulates normal posture. The paucity of input from one system may be compensated for by the other systems. For example, in tabes dorsalis (Chap. 5) the impairment of the input from the general proprioceptive sensors results in an unsteady gait unless compensated for by influences from the visual system. In this situation the visual system substitutes for the normal feedback system.

Spasticity is a consequence of injury to the upper motor neuron pathways (Chap. 5). The deprivation of these descending influences coupled with some local changes (collateral nerve sprouting and denervation sensitivity, Chap. 5) in the spinal cord has altered the level of the control box (spinal cord neuronal pools). The spasticity is a consequence of the profound uninhibited facilitatory effect that a slight stretch of the neuromuscular spindle has on the activity of the neuronal pools.

Another example of altered control over the feedback system is the clasp-knife reflex. The break, which follows after the resistance, occurs at the time when the Golgi tendon organs fire and get the upper hand (Chap. 5).

RESPONSES IN EXPERIMENTAL ANIMALS

Many of the significant observations pertinent to understanding the role of the nervous system in motor activities have been made on experi-

mental animals. Such experimental preparations include *1* the "spinal animal," i.e., one with its spinal cord transected (Chap. 5), *2* the decerebrate animal, with its brainstem transected at a low midbrain level, *3* the "midbrain animal," with its brainstem transected at a high midbrain level, *4* the "thalamic animal," with its cerebrum transected at a "high" thalamic level, and *5* the decorticate animal, with its cerebral cortex ablated.

Decerebrate animal The decerebrate animal has an intact hindbrain and a spinal cord which is deprived of the influences from the cerebrum and midbrain. If food is placed in the animal's mouth it is moistened by the flow of saliva, chewed, and swallowed. Coughing and sneezing are evoked by the irritation of the mucosal lining of the trachea and bronchial tubes of the lungs. Blinking of the eyelids and flow of tears follow corneal stimulation. These reflexes are a consequence of intact circuits involving cranial nerves and the lower brainstem. The animal is cool because hypothalamic control is absent. The state of intense hypertonus, especially of the extensor muscles, is called *decerebrate rigidity*. When placed on its feet, the animal can stand and support its weight because the facilitatory influences on the stretch reflexes are strong. If the animal is placed on its side, it remains motionless. The vestibular reflexes associated with posture are active; when the animal's head is held down by a handler, the forelimbs become flexed and the hindlimbs become extended (simulating the jumping-down posture). With the animal's head bent up, the forelimbs become extended and the hindlimbs become flexed (simulating the jumping-up posture).

"Midbrain animal" The "midbrain animal" is able to stand and display righting reflexes. It does not exhibit decerebrate rigidity. The animal performs the righting reflexes and recovers its normal posture if displaced from it. It keeps its head in the normal horizontal position and its eyes parallel to the ground (this head-righting response is a vestibular *labyrinthine-righting reflex* initiated by endings in the utricle and saccule, Chap. 10). The attempt is made to bring

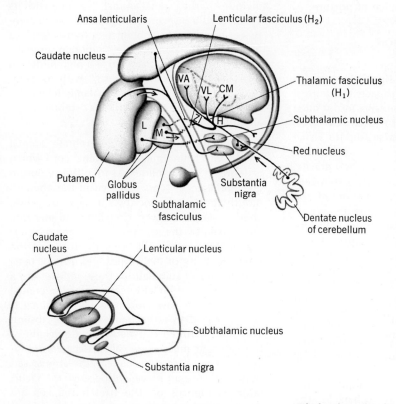

FIGURE 14-1
Lower: The location of the basal ganglia with reference to the lateral ventricle.
Upper: The fields of Forel and some efferent projections of basal ganglia and cerebellum.

The pallidofugal fibers pass through three bundles: ansa lenticularis, lenticular fasciculus (H_2), and subthalamic fasciculus. The former two bundles and the cerebellar projections join in the H field of Forel (prerubral field) and continue as the thalamic fasciculus (H_1) to various thalamic nuclei. CM, centromedian nucleus; H, the H field of Forel; L and M, lateral and medial segments of the globus pallidus; VA, ventral anterior thalamic nucleus; VL, ventral lateral thalamic nucleus; ZI, zona incerta.

the neck and the body into the relationship with each other and with the head that is present in the normal posture of the animal. The *neck-righting reflexes*, through which head position influences the position of the body, and the *body-righting reflex*, through which body position influences the position of the neck, are active. The labyrinthine-righting reflexes, neck-righting reflexes, and body-righting reflexes are reactions operating to maintain the normal positional relations of head to neck (or neck to head) and neck to body (or body to neck). These reflexes are dependent on the uneven stimulation of the bilateral labyrinths and on the unequal stimulation of the pressure receptors in the body. The organism adjusts until the stimulation from one side is balanced by the stimulation from the other side. The *optic-righting reflexes* are not elicited because they are dependent on the cerebral cortex.

"Thalamic animal" The "thalamic animal" exhibits all the reflex activity of the "midbrain animal." Because the hypothalamus is active, this animal has a normal body temperature. Behavioral patterns are complex. Trivial stimuli evoke sham rages, viz., dilated pupils, growling, hissing, and hair standing on end.

Decorticate animal The chronic decorticate animal moves about in an essentially normal manner. Its sleep-wake cycle alternates regularly. It has no sense of smell but apparently feels pain (because its thalamus is intact). When irritated, the animal will growl, bark, or hiss. If food is placed in contact with the mouth, the animal eats in a normal fashion. The decorticate animal has lost all learned behavior, viz., it does not answer to its name and cannot be trained. A decorticate dog or monkey is not totally blind for he is apparently able to distinguish light from dark.

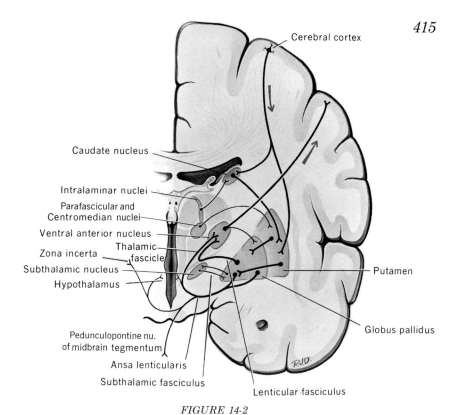

Cerebral cortex

Caudate nucleus

Intralaminar nuclei

Parafascicular and
Centromedian nuclei

Ventral anterior nucleus

Zona incerta — Thalamic fascicle

Subthalamic nucleus

Hypothalamus

Pedunculopontine nu.
of midbrain tegmentum

Ansa lenticularis

Subthalamic fasciculus

Lenticular fasciculus

Putamen

Globus pallidus

FIGURE 14-2
Some major interconnections of the basal ganglia, thalamus, and cerebral cortex.

Concept of pyramidal and extrapyramidal systems

By convention, each somatic motor "tract" is classified as belonging to one of two motor systems, pyramidal or extrapyramidal. The pyramidal system includes the corticospinal and the corticobulbar tracts. All other motor systems and the basal ganglia (Fig. 14-1) influencing the lower motor neurons are collectively grouped into the extrapyramidal system; thus the name *extrapyramidal system* is a term of exclusion. (Many investigators insist that the term *extrapyramidal* should be discarded; however, it is commonly used.)

PYRAMIDAL SYSTEM

The corticobulbar tract is a direct tract extending from the cerebral cortex to the brainstem tegmentum, where it innervates, through interneurons, the motor nuclei of the cranial nerves and nuclei in the reticular formation. Because of its

terminations in the brainstem reticular formation, the corticobulbar tract has been called a corticoreticular tract. The corticospinal tract is the only direct tract from the cerebral cortex to the spinal cord (Fig. 5-24). This phylogenetically new tract is found in mammals. Along its course collateral branches project successively to the putamen, substantia nigra, nucleus ruber, and brainstem reticular nuclei (Figs. 14-2, 14-3). The pyramidal tracts are necessary for skilled voluntary movements. They act as the major pathway through which the individual selects the prime mover of an activity; and they have a role in coordinating the resulting action. The contraction of individual muscles is largely a function of the pyramidal system. Through its collateral branches to the putamen and the nuclei in the brainstem, the pyramidal system influences the extrapyramidal system. Hence its effect on the spinal cord may be expressed, in part, through

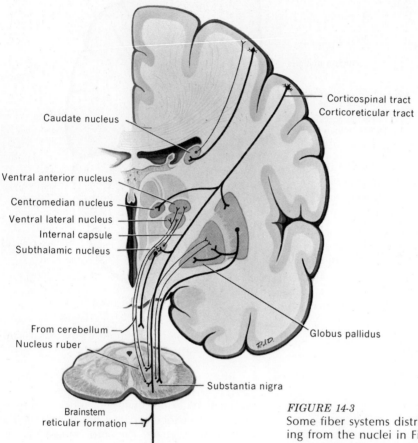

Caudate nucleus

Corticospinal tract
Corticoreticular tract

Ventral anterior nucleus

Centromedian nucleus

Ventral lateral nucleus

Internal capsule

Subthalamic nucleus

From cerebellum
Nucleus ruber

Globus pallidus

Substantia nigra

Brainstem
reticular formation

FIGURE 14-3

Some fiber systems distributing to and projecting from the nuclei in Fig. 14-1.

Collateral branches from the corticospinal and corticoreticular tracts project to the centromedian nucleus, putamen, subthalamic nucleus, and nucleus ruber. The cerebral cortex and neostriatum have reciprocal connections.

the reticulospinal tracts of the extrapyramidal system. The corticobulbar tract may influence the extrapyramidal system through its terminal connections in the brainstem reticular formation.

The extrapyramidal tract functions as the activator and coordinator of postural adjustments and of automatic movements. This system is basic to motor activity. Some extrapyramidal circuits can influence the pyramidal system (see "Circuitry," further on in this chapter). The pyramidal tract may influence the activity of the extrapyramidal system, and on the other hand,

the extrapyramidal may influence the activity of the pyramidal tract. In addition, the pyramidal system may influence the ascending pathway systems through its connections with the nucleus gracilis, nucleus cuneatus, dorsal (Clarke's) nucleus, and trigeminal nuclei of the brainstem (Chap. 13).

The sectioning of the pyramids of the medulla interrupts the corticospinal tracts. A monkey with such a lesion has a paresis, with some hypotonus and no clonus. Gross voluntary movements of the limbs are coordinated, well controlled, and apparently normal. Voluntary finer movements, especially those of the hands and feet, are impaired.

EXTRAPYRAMIDAL SYSTEM

The *extrapyramidal system* is composed of a continuous lattice of neural systems including nuclei, feedback circuits, and descending pathways. In general, the extrapyramidal system includes, among other structures and circuits, the cerebral cortex, the basal ganglia, some thalamic nuclei (e.g., VA, VL, and intralaminar nuclei), nuclei of the ventral thalamus (subthalamic nucleus), nuclei of the midbrain (red nucleus and substantia nigra), nuclei of the pons and medulla (nuclei of the reticular formation), some feedback loops, and a number of tracts and pathways, including the corticorubrospinal and corticoreticulospinal pathways. The cerebellum and its pathways are often included.

This phylogenetically old system, which has its ancient roots in the nonmammalian vertebrates, is involved in stereotyped motor activity of a postural and reflex nature. These well-coordinated basic motor expressions are regarded as primitive motor reactions. The extrapyramidal system projects descending streams of influence which supply the neuronal pools of the spinal cord with continual subliminal stimulation; this acts (by facilitation) to keep the spinal reflex arcs in a "ready" state. In addition, the extrapyramidal system provides a background reference which the pyramidal system

utilizes for expressing its activities. Many pathway circuits of the extrapyramidal system are organized to feed back to the cerebral cortex.

BASAL GANGLIA, RELATED CENTERS, CIRCUITS, AND FUNCTION OF THE EXTRAPYRAMIDAL SYSTEM

Basal ganglia and related centers   The nuclear complexes usually classified as basal ganglia comprise the amygdaloid body, corpus striatum, and claustrum (Table 14-1). The subthalamic nucleus, substantia nigra, and red nucleus are sometimes included. The amygdaloid body, a nuclear group associated with the limbic system, is not considered to be a basal ganglion by some authors.

The corpus striatum is subdivided into the paleostriatum and the neostriatum (striatum). The paleostriatum is also called the globus pallidus or pallidum; the neostriatum is divided into the putamen (60 percent of the striatum by volume) and the caudate nucleus. The amygdaloid body (archistriatum), neostriatum, and claustrum are telencephalic structures, while the globus pallidus and subthalamic nucleus are diencephalic derivatives. During development the fibers of the internal capsule insinuate themselves so as to divide some regions of the diencephalon and telencephalon; the result is that the internal capsule separates the subthalamus from the globus pallidus and divides the neostriatum into the caudate nucleus and putamen. The globus pallidus and putamen, both

TABLE 14-1
Basal ganglia and related centers

Archistriatum (amygdaloid body, amygdala, amygdaloid nucleus)

Corpus striatum
- Paleostriatum (globus pallidus, pallidum)
  - Medial segment
  - Lateral segment
- Neostriatum (striatum)
  - Putamen
  - Caudate nucleus

Lentiform (lenticular) nucleus

Claustrum
Subthalamic nucleus*
Substantia nigra*
Red nucleus*

*Sometimes included.

located lateral to the internal capsule, are together called the lentiform (lenticular) nucleus. The globus pallidus is subdivided into a medial (inner or internal) segment and a lateral (outer or external) segment (Fig. 14-1). The subthalamus is considered to be the rostral continuation of the midbrain tegmentum into the diencephalon. The red nucleus (nucleus ruber) is a major midbrain tegmental nucleus (Chap. 8). The substantia nigra is a large pigmented nucleus located in the midbrain (Fig. 8-14).

BASIC PRINCIPLES

Functional The general role of the basal ganglia is to serve as processing stations linking the cerebral cortex to certain thalamic nuclei; in turn, the latter project to the cerebral cortex. This is indicated by circuitry which conveys influences from widespread areas of the cortex to the neostriatum to globus pallidus to thalamus. The specific functional roles of the basal ganglia are not, as yet, resolved. According to one concept, the basal ganglia are nuclei where many influences, including those from visual, labyrinthine, and proprioceptive sources, are integrated in activities which involve the initiation and direction of voluntary movements and motor responses. This is based upon some of the symptoms observed in patients with damage to the basal ganglia. Such patients have difficulty in initiating willed movements, and defects in some of the attributes that contribute to normal motor activities. According to another concept, the basal ganglia, although they do influence somatic motor activity, are not basically motor in function. This is indicated, in part, by their efferent projections; the basal ganglia do not have direct connections with nuclei or cortical regions which give rise to the motor pathways projecting directly to the spinal cord.

A most important suggested role for the corpus striatum is that it acts as a nuclear processing linkage between the association cortex (involved in some way with the mnemonic system) and that system of the brain involved with handling this sensory experience properly for meaningful responses. The following statement by Mettler expresses this role: "Without the striatum the animal is quite unable to relate itself to its environment at a satisfactory level of self-maintenance. Without its cortex it is unable to relate itself accurately to its environment but it can still do it. The cat . . . is able to get along reasonably well without much cortex, but if you add a sizable striatal deficit to this, the animal looks at you with vacuous eyes and . . . will walk out of a third story window with complete unconcern."

Circuitry Two subcortical structures are central to the circuits influencing the motor and premotor cortex. They are the corpus striatum and the cerebellum. Two key loops involved with the corpus striatum are *1* wide areas of cerebral cortex to corpus striatum to VA and VL of the thalamus to motor and premotor areas of the cerebral cortex (Fig. 14-4), and *2* corpus striatum to intralaminar nuclei of the thalamus to corpus striatum (Fig. 14-4). Two key circuits involved with the cerebellum include *1* wide areas of cerebral cortex to pontine nuclei to cerebellum to the VA and VL of the thalamus to motor and premotor cortex (Fig. 14-6), and *2* cerebellum to intralaminar nuclei of thalamus (Fig. 14-6 and Chap. 9).

These circuits and loops apparently have a significant role, supplying input to the motor and premotor areas of the cerebral cortex which give rise to such important motor pathways as the corticospinal, corticorubrospinal, and corticoreticulospinal tracts. Note that there are structures which are common to both the cerebellar and striatal systems. These are *1* wide areas of the cerebral cortex (source of input), *2* VA and VL of the thalamus, *3* intralaminar nuclei, and *4* motor and premotor areas of the cerebral cortex (site of output). This does not imply that the neurons in these structures are all common to both systems. However, many of the neurons are probably functionally integrated into both systems.

Connections and circuits

The cerebral cortex, basal ganglia, and related nuclei are organized into complex linkages of interconnections, feedback circuits, and de-

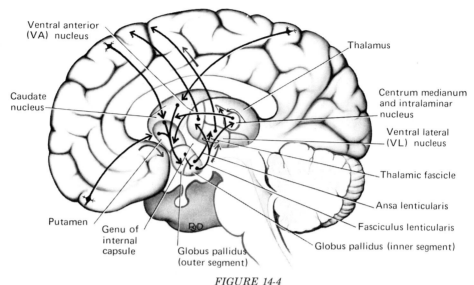

Ventral anterior
(VA) nucleus

Thalamus

Caudate
nucleus

Centrum medianum
and intralaminar
nucleus

Ventral lateral
(VL) nucleus

Thalamic fascicle

Ansa lenticularis

Fasciculus lenticularis

Putamen
Genu of
internal
capsule

Globus pallidus (inner segment)

Globus pallidus
(outer segment)

FIGURE 14-4
Some of the major interconnections of the "extrapyramidal system" involving the cerebral cortex, basal ganglia, thalamus, and brainstem. (Arrows indicate major direction of projections.)

scending pathways. The following schemata outline some of the major proposed circuits of the extrapyramidal motor system (Figs. 14-4 through 14-6).

CIRCUIT 1

Cerebral cortex → striatum → globus pallidus → thalamus → cerebral cortex (Fig. 14-4).

Nearly all regions of the cerebral cortex project corticostriate fibers in a topographically organized arrangement to the ipsilateral striatum (both caudate nucleus and putamen). Additionally, fibers from the sensorimotor cortex (pre- and postcentral gyri) may project to the contralateral striatum; they cross the midline in the corpus callosum. There are no fibers which interconnect the caudate nucleus with the putamen. In turn, fibers from the striatum terminate topographically in both segments of the globus pallidus. Fibers from the lateral segment of the globus pallidus terminate in both the medial segment of the globus pallidus and the subthalamic nucleus. From the medial pallidal segment fibers course via the *ansa lenticularis* (loops under the internal capsule) and *fasciculus lenticularis* (penetrates through internal capsule); these fascicles join to form the *thalamic fascic-*

ulus before terminating in the VA, VL, and centrum medianum (CM) nuclei of the thalamus. The VA and VL nuclei project somatotopically to the premotor cortex (areas 6 and 8) and to the motor cortex (area 4), respectively.

Other connections of the nuclear centers of this circuit add to the complexity. The CM nucleus (which receives input from the globus pallidus) and other intralaminar thalamic nuclei project to the striatum: the CM projects to the putamen, and other intralaminar nuclei project to the caudate nucleus. In a sense the CM is incorporated in a closed circuit relaying back to the striatum. In addition, the globus pallidus projects pallidotegmental fibers to the pedunculopontine tegmental nucleus (Fig. 8-9) and other brainstem reticular nuclei.

CIRCUIT 2 (Fig. 14-5)

This circuit involves the substantia nigra. It comprises the following sequences: *1* Cerebral cortex to the striatum to the substantia nigra.

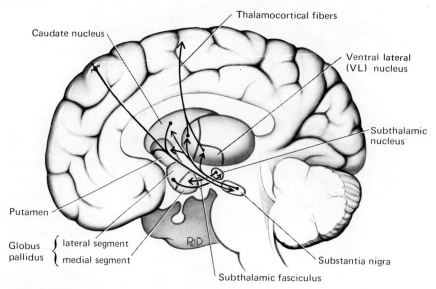

FIGURE 14-5
Some of the major circuits of the "extrapyramidal system."

The nigrostriatal (substantia nigra to striatum) fibers compose the dopamine neuronal pathway. Arrows indicate major direction of projections.

The striatonigral fibers project to both the pars compacta and pars reticularis of the substantia nigra. *2* The projections from the substantia nigra are directed rostrally via *a* nigrostriatal fibers to the striatum, or *b* nigrothalamic fibers to the VA and VL thalamic nuclei, which project to the motor and premotor cortical areas. Direct corticonigral fibers probably do not exist.

The substantia nigra is divided into the anteriorly located pars reticularis (adjacent to the crus cerebri) and the posteriorly located pars compacta. The *pars reticularis* is rich in iron and lacking in melanin pigment. The *pars compacta* contains neurons rich in dopamine (a catecholamine) and melanin. Reciprocal topographic projections apparently are the main interconnections *1* between the pars reticularis and the VA and VL thalamic nuclei, and *2* between the pars compacta and the striatum. The striatonigral connections are primarily between the rostral portion of the substantia nigra and the caudate nucleus, and between the caudal two-thirds of the substantia nigra and the putamen. The substantia nigra does not project caudally. The nigral efferent projections to the VA and VL thalamic nuclei terminate in different regions of these thalamic nuclei than those projections from the globus pallidus (no overlap). The nigrostriatal fibers compose the *dopamine neuronal system;* the substantia nigra, nigrostriatal fibers, and striatum are rich in dopamine, which may be an active neurotransmitter substance (see discussion of paralysis agitans, below).

CIRCUIT 3

The *subthalamic nucleus* is integrated in the above circuitry (Figs. 14-1, 14-5). Fibers from the lateral segment of the globus pallidus terminate in the subthalamus, which, in turn, projects back to the medial segment of the globus pallidus.

CIRCUIT 4

Another circuit influences the extrapyramidal system. Its sequence includes the cerebral

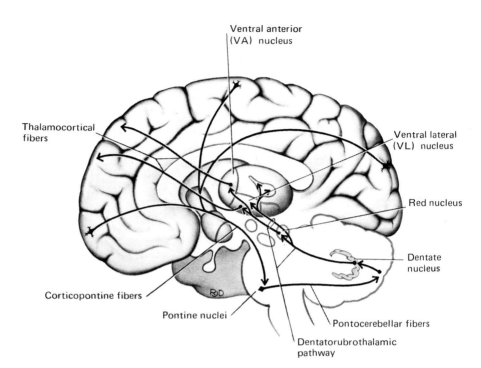

Ventral anterior
(VA) nucleus

Thalamocortical
fibers

Ventral lateral
(VL) nucleus

Red nucleus

Dentate
nucleus

Corticopontine fibers

Pontine nuclei

Pontocerebellar fibers

Dentatorubrothalamic
pathway

FIGURE 14-6
Some major circuits of the "extrapyramidal system." (Arrows indicate major direction of projections.)

cortex → ipsilateral pontine nuclei (corticopontine fibers) → contralateral cerebellar cortex (pontocerebellar fibers) → dentate nucleus of the cerebellum → contralateral VL, VA, and intralaminar thalamic nuclei (dentatothalamic fibers) → cerebral cortex (areas 4, 6, and 8) (Figs. 9-4, 14-6).

There is an overlapping of the dentatothalamic fibers from the cerebellum and pallidothalamic fibers from the globus pallidus in the VL thalamic nucleus. Some influences from the cerebellum to the thalamus are also conveyed via the dentatorubrothalamic pathway (see Chap. 9).

CIRCUIT 5

The extrapyramidal subcortical influences upon the cerebral cortex are, in turn, projected from the cerebral cortex to the brainstem and spinal cord motor nuclei via several descending pathways (Figs. 8-19, 8-20). These include the pyramidal pathways (corticospinal and cortico-

bulbar tracts), corticorubrospinal pathway, corticoreticular pathway, and corticoreticulospinal pathway (medial and lateral reticulospinal tracts).

The pyramidal system can serve as both a source of input and a pathway for the output of the extrapyramidal system (Fig. 14-2). The influences from the pyramidal system are transmitted through collateral branches to the putamen, centrum medianum, subthalamic nucleus, substantia nigra, red nucleus, and brainstem reticular formation. Through part of the feedback loop of cerebral cortex to basal ganglia to thalamus to cerebral cortex, the influences from the basal ganglia to the cerebral cortex can eventually be relayed through the pyramidal tract and the corticobulbar and corticoreticular tracts.

PALLIDOFUGAL FIBERS AND THE H FIELDS OF FOREL (Fig. 14-1)

The output from the globus pallidus is conveyed via pallidofugal fibers which are organized in three bundles of fibers. These bundles, arranged in a rostrocaudal sequence, are the ansa lenticularis, the lenticular fasciculus (H_2 of Forel), and the subthalamic fasciculus.

The *ansa lenticularis* arises from the ventral portion of the medial segment of the globus pallidus, loops ventromedially around the internal capsule near the crus cerebri, curves to pass upward and caudally, and then joins the fibers of the lenticular fasciculus at the H field of Forel (prerubral field) of the subthalamus.

The *lenticular fasciculus* arises from the dorsal portion of the medial segment of the globus pallidus, penetrates as the comb bundle (because it resembles the teeth of a comb) through the posterior limb of the internal capsule (rostral to the subthalamic nucleus), and then courses medially and caudally between the subthalamic nucleus (located ventrally) and the gray matter called the zona incerta (located dorsally). The lenticular fasciculus then joins the ansa lenticularis in the H field of Forel; the fibers of the fasciculus and ansa recurve and project rostrally just dorsal to the zona incerta as the thalamic fasciculus (H_1 field of Forel).

The *zona incerta* is the rostral extension of the midbrain reticular formation into the ventral thalamus. It is located within the subthalamus between the subthalamic nucleus and the thalamic fasciculus. The thalamic fasciculus is a key bundle. Its fibers convey influences from the cerebellum and globus pallidus to the thalamic nuclei (VA and VL); these nuclei project their output to the motor and premotor cortex.

The *subthalamic fasciculus* consists of fibers passing through the internal capsule as a comb bundle. It consists of pallidosubthalamic fibers passing from the lateral segment of the globus pallidus to the subthalamic nucleus and of subthalamopallidal fibers passing from the subthalamic nucleus to the medial segment of the globus pallidus. Another pallidal projection,

consisting of the pallidotegmental fibers, leaves the H field and descends to the pedunculopontine reticular nucleus of the midbrain.

PHYSIOLOGY

The extrapyramidal system has a significant role in the regulation of stereotype movements. In man and primates, this system is capable of stimulating the performance of complex volitional motor acts, for, as previously noted, such activities are exhibited even when the corticospinal tracts are interrupted in the pyramids of the medulla.

The precise role of each nucleus of the extrapyramidal system is not known. The complex connectivity implies that each nucleus expresses its role through facilitatory or inhibitory influences (or both) on several other nuclei and systems. Release phenomena may be expressed when some inhibitory influences are suppressed. Such emotionally triggered gestures such as yawning, stretching, and tics may be related to the connections of the basal ganglia with the hypothalamus and the descending reticular system.

Skilled and voluntary movements

All normal movements are to a greater or lesser degree skilled. Even "crude" reflexes are the product of exquisite neural integration. The most skilled acts may range from the contraction (and relaxation) of a few muscles for the execution of each brush stroke by a van Gogh to the continuous muscle flow of an Olympic gymnast. These highest skills may include *1* the unilateral control of finger movements, as in writing and playing a piano, and *2* the bilateral control of word formation by the vocal cords, throat, mouth, tongue, and lips. Inhibition is as significant to skilled movements as is excitation. The inhibition of nonessential movements and of antagonist muscles is essential to each skilled act.

A voluntary movement is a focal act of which the executor is consciously aware. The acquisition of the ability to perform these actions takes time. Learning to walk, to write, or to play a musical instrument occurs only after a number of complex motor patterns have been mastered.

Persistent efforts and repeated trials are required before such movements are gradually integrated into automatic patterns and into voluntarily controlled actions. The automatic aspect of each movement is subcortically regulated, while the volitional aspect is largely controlled by the cerebral cortex. A voluntary act may be operationally defined as an activity produced by a stimulation originating within the central nervous system. The term "voluntarily controlled act" is not wholly accurate; although the doer is consciously controlling the act, he is not aware of the means to attain the end. *The focus of a voluntary movement is called the focal act; this expresses the fact that one concentrates on performing one movement at a time.* Trying to perform many acts simultaneously is difficult if not impossible. In executing a voluntary act many movements accompany the focal act. For example, a typist is conscious of the control of her fingers, but unaware of a whole complex of supporting movements. The latter include the slight adjustment movements of the hand, forearm, and arm, the stabilizing muscle contractions of the shoulder, the maintenance of the posture of the body, and the head and eye patterns as the lines on a page are followed.

The corticospinal tracts are essential substrates to volitional actions. These tracts, which are largest in man, have a crucial role in the manipulative skills and the independent movement of man's extremities, particularly of the fingers.

EFFECTS OF STIMULATION AND ABLATION OF BASAL GANGLIA

In general, stimulation of the neostriatum evokes different effects than does stimulation of the paleostriatum. Apparently the neostriatum exerts inhibitory influences on somatic motor activity (specifically, the inhibition of spontaneous activity, of a motion in progress, or of deep tendon reflexes). Stimulation of the globus pallidus produces a minimum of effects, such as increased muscle tonus. This hypertonus occurs after a long latency, and it outlasts the stimulus. A prolonged stimulus can produce a tremor. Effects evoked by stimulation of the pallidum occur on the contralateral side.

The unilateral ablation of the globus pallidus or of the putamen produces slight, if any, objec- *tive signs of malfunction. The bilateral ablation of either structure gives evidence of the release phenomenon.* The bilateral ablation of the putamen produces a hyperactive animal that wanders about continuously, with a disregard of its environment. For example, the animal will walk into a wall and continue to push against the obstruction (forced progression), or it will walk across a table and continue until it falls off the edge (labyrinth disregard). In addition, behavioral changes in affect are exhibited. A cat shows no fear and may even purr when confronted by a hostile dog. In contrast, the bilateral ablation of the globus pallidus produces a hypoactive animal, exhibiting hypotonus and somnolence. Such an animal seldom moves about. If placed in a bizarre enforced posture, it can retain the posture for an extended period of time. For example, a monkey with bilateral ablation of the globus pallidus makes little or no effort to assume a natural posture if the upper extremity is placed behind the neck with the hand touching the opposite shoulder and if a lower extremity is lifted until the foot rests against the back of the neck. The hypoactivity has a resemblance to that in Parkinson's disease. However, these animals do not exhibit any tremor or rigidity.

Violent flinging ballistic movements, especially in the contralateral upper extremity, are exhibited in men and monkeys with discrete lesions in portions of the subthalamic nucleus (the syndrome is called *ballism* in man). This hyperactivity is another manifestation of a release phenomenon producing an abnormal movement.

Functional and clinical considerations

The extrapyramidal system is functionally organized into an exquisitely "tuned" complex of interconnected nuclei. The role of the basal ganglia and associated nuclei is to modulate motor activities through circuits which directly and indirectly feed back to the cerebral cortex. In turn, the cortex projects its influences to the brainstem and spinal levels through the descending pathways upon the alpha and gamma motor neurons. The malfunction of various nuclear complexes results in an imbalance in the interactions within the complex circuitry of the extrapyramidal system. This is a plausible explanation for the variety and assortment of symptoms and signs noted in the clinically observed disorders in the control of posture and movements when the harmonious interactions are altered within this system. Posture is modified by an increase in muscle tone to a similar degree in the agonists and antagonists of a muscle group without an accompanying increase in reflex activity; this is called *rigidity*. The abnormal involuntary movements, called *dyskinesias*, may be rhythmic or arrhythmic, generally without paralysis of the muscles. The motor disorders resulting from the improper functioning of the extrapyramidal system, the basal ganglia, and associated nuclei include paralysis agitans (Parkinson's disease), athetosis, choreas, and ballism.

Paralysis agitans (Parkinson's disease) is characterized by rigidity and tremor. The rigidity is essentially the same in all muscles; it is accompanied by poverty of movements but with normal deep tendon reflex activity. As a limb is passively forced through flexor or extensor movements, the muscular resistance alternately increases and decreases to give a cogwheel effect. The patient exhibits resistance to passive movements in all directions. From a standing position, the patient has difficulty in starting to take his initial steps. The subject also has the same problem in arresting the movement. The rigidity is the disabling symptom. During forward locomotion, short, shuffling steps are taken. The masked face has a fixed expression accompanied by no overt spontaneous emotional response. The tremor with its regular frequency and amplitude occurs while the subject is at rest; it is lost or reduced during a movement and is aggravated by emotional tension. Degenerative changes in the globus pallidus and substantia nigra are present in Parkinsonian patients; in addition there is a marked reduction to absence of dopamine in the substantia nigra and striatum. Surgical lesions in the globus pal-

lidus or ventral lateral thalamic nucleus may reduce or abolish the tremor and rigidity. *L-dopa* in low doses may ameliorate the rigidity and in high doses may decrease the tremor. L-dopa is a common precursor of melanin and dopamine. The symptoms of Parkinsonism are probably due to the removal of the inhibitory influences which are normally exerted upon the globus pallidus.

The movements of *athetosis* are slow and are exaggerated by voluntary movement. Spasticity is characteristic. The slow, writhing character of the involuntary movement of the extremities appears wormlike. The alternating adduction and abduction of the shoulder joint are accompanied by flexion and extension of the wrist and fingers. Usually the wrist is flexed, and the fingers hyperextended. Grimaces of the face may occur during the limb movements. This dyskinesia may be due to a lesion in the striatum, mainly in the putamen, following the trauma of a birth injury. Such injury suggests that the striatum has an inhibitory role.

Torsion dystonia is a form of dyskinesia in which the athetoid movements are expressed largely by sustained contractions of the axial musculature. This results in an abnormal degree of fixity of postural configurations with severe torsion of the neck, shoulder girdle, and pelvic girdle. In contrast, athetosis is primarily expressed by spasticity of the musculature of the extremities.

Choreas (dances) are characterized by jerky, irregular, brisk, rapid, purposeless, continuous flow of different movements of the limbs accompanied by involuntary twitchings of the face. These movements are expressed primarily by the distal segments of the extremities. Muscles are hypotonic. In advanced cases, the patient is almost always in motion when awake. There is no reduction in muscle power. *Huntington's chorea* is a hereditary form, which becomes progressively worse with age after its initial appearance, often in the late thirties. Damage to the striatum and the cerebral cortex are presumed to be causal.

Ballism ("throwing") is characterized by violent, abnormal, flail-like movements originating mainly from the activity of the proximal appendicular muscles of the shoulder and pelvis. The movements cease during sleep. There is a marked reduction of muscle tone. These symptoms are exhibited unilaterally with a lesion in the contralateral subthalamic nucleus.

Symptoms associated with the malfunctioning of the basal ganglia are usually observed bilaterally. However, those symptoms on one side result from lesions in the contralateral basal ganglia; this is a consequence of the circuits by which the basal ganglia project to the ipsilateral cerebral cortex, which, in turn, relays its influences via the corticofugal pathways to the contralateral side (see the comments on ballism, above). The abnormal movements resulting from lesions in the basal ganglia circuitry are an expression of release phenomena in which the inhibitory influences on such structures as the globus pallidus or ventral lateral nucleus of the thalamus are lost or reduced. Surgical lesions of these "released structures" (globus pallidus and the VL nucleus) are known to ameliorate the symptoms in many patients. In this context, the loss of dopamine, noted in patients with Parkinsonism, is presumed to account for the reduction or loss of inhibitory influences upon the striatum.

It is not possible to state that any clinically observed "basal ganglia disease" is due to the damage of a certain nuclear structure or part of a structure. At autopsy, patients with these diseases are found to have extensive lesions of many regions, including many structures other than the basal ganglia. These observations contribute to the enigma concerning the precise role(s) of the basal ganglia. In addition, with the exception of ballism, none of the basal ganglia diseases has been reproduced by the experimental ablation of parts of the basal ganglia. Symptoms of ballism can be produced by an experimentally produced lesion in the subthalamic nucleus. It must be remembered that the symptoms observed in an organism with a lesion of a certain structure do not necessarily tell us

what the normal functional role of the damaged structure is; rather the symptoms express the functional activity of the nervous system in the absence of the normal functioning of the damaged structure.

Bibliography

Denny-Brown, D.: *The Basal Ganglia and Their Relation to Disorders of Movement.* Oxford University Press, London, 1962.

————: *The Cerebral Control of Movement.* Charles C Thomas, Publisher, Springfield, Ill., 1966.

Evarts, E. V.: Brain mechanisms in movement. Sci. Am., 229:96–103, 1973.

Frigyesi, T. L., E. Rinvik, and M. D. Yahr (eds.): *Corticothalamic Projections and Sensorimotor Activities.* Raven Press, Hewlett, New York, 1972.

Granit, R.: *The Basis of Motor Control.* Academic Press, Inc., New York, 1970.

Haymaker, W.: *Bing's Local Diagnosis in Neurological Diseases,* 15th ed. The C. V. Mosby Company, St. Louis, 1968.

Martin, J. P.: *The Basal Ganglia and Posture.* Lippincott Company, Philadelphia, 1967.

Mettler, F. A.: Muscular tone and movement: their cerebral control in primates, in S. Ehrenpreis and O. C. Solnitzky (eds.). Neurosci. Res., 1:176–250, 1968.

Roberts, T. D. M.: *Neurophysiology of Postural Mechanisms.* Plenum Publishing Corporation, New York, 1967.

Szabo, J.: Projections from the body of the caudate nucleus in the rhesus monkey. Exp. Neurol., 27:1–15, 1970.

Yahr, M. D., and D. P. Purpura (eds.): *Neurophysiological Basis of Normal and Abnormal Motor Activities.* Raven Press, Hewlett, N.Y., 1967.

CHAPTER **15**
THE OLFACTORY SYSTEM
AND THE LIMBIC SYSTEM

The olfactory system

SENSE OF SMELL

The sense of smell is a modality with a long phylogenetic history. This chemical sense was important even in the most primitive of fish, hundreds of millions of years ago. It remains as a dominant sensation in many living vertebrates; many contemporary animals live largely in a world of odors. Olfaction is critical to the survival of many animals and species, e.g., in hunting for food, in finding a mate, in recognizing friends, and in warning against enemies. An animal often identifies another by the odor it generates. Vertebrates with a well-developed sense of smell are known as *"macrosmatic,"* and those with a poorly developed sense of smell are known as *"microsmatic."* Even in microsmatic man, olfaction is a complex sense. Odors generate complex associations of ideas and images and personal interpretations modified by past experiences. Aromas of fresh-mown hay, of a chemical laboratory, or of a fish market conjure up more than smells. The blind and deaf Helen Keller was able to describe a garden and other objects because of her acute sense of smell. Tea sniffers, wine tasters, and perfumers develop their sense of smell until it becomes finely discriminative.

The olfactory system is more than just a perceiver of odors; it is an activator and a sensitizer of other neural systems—those which are substrates for emotional behavior patterns. The aromas emanating from many foods evoke salivation and lip smacking, the characteristic scent from a doe stirs responses in a buck deer in rut, and the olfactory sense can produce aggressive reactions in a dog. Even man's reactions to odors are instinctive.

Odors are describable only in subjective terms; there are no basic odors comparable to the primary colors or the notes of a scale. This explains the hazards inherent in predicting the smell of mixtures. The fragrance of flowers and the aroma of roast coffee are the product of complex interactions of literally scores of volatile chemicals.

The olfactory system can be activated by mere traces of excitants in the atmosphere. In man, the sense of smell can be a more sensitive detector of certain chemicals than the most efficient chemical analytic techniques. Many odors are sensed immediately by smell in such minute concentrations that the most sophisticated chemical methods either cannot detect them or can identify them only after procedures requiring many days of analyses.

Odorous chemicals must be volatile, water-soluble, and lipid-soluble. Although volatility is important for odor detection, the degree of volatility is not necessarily proportional to the intensity of smell. For example, highly volatile water has no odor, whereas poorly volatile musk is a powerful odorant used as a base in perfumes. Estimates indicate that 1 Gm of muscone would retain its odoriferous capacity after a million years with a loss of only 1 percent of its weight. These three qualities are essential, otherwise the odoriferous particles would not reach the nose, dissolve in the aqueous secretion coat of the olfactory region, and penetrate the final lipid barrier of the olfactory receptor cell. The water solubility need be only infinitesimal. Nonvaporizing and lipid-insoluble chemicals do not produce odors. In addition, odorif-

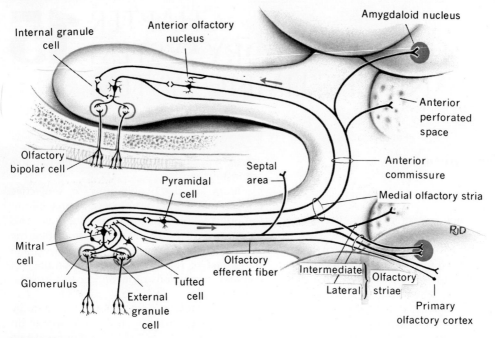

FIGURE 15-1
The olfactory pathways.

The anterior olfactory nucleus is located in the posterior olfactory bulb and along the olfactory tract and striae.

An impaired sense of smell, as experienced during a cold, is reflected in the bland taste of food; the aroma of food has an important role for the gourmet.

erous chemicals are usually organic substances with molecular configurations that stimulate the olfactory receptor cells. These olfactory sensors will adapt rather quickly to a continuous stimulus. This explains why an unchanging odor may soon become unnoticed.

Sensitivity to odors may depend on obscure factors. For example, women can detect a certain steroid compound excreted in the urine by its odor. After an ovariectomy this ability is lost. However, this compound can be smelled by an ovariectomized woman given female sex hormones.

The loss of the sense of smell does not have great significance in man, as indicated by the fact there is no common expression for loss of smell (anosmia) as there is for the loss of sight (blindness) or for the loss of hearing (deafness).

OLFACTORY PATHWAY

The olfactory receptor cells in man are located in a small 2.5-sq-cm epithelial patch of the olfactory mucosa high up in each nostril; we sniff to help direct air to this olfactory mucosa. The more than 10 million receptor cells in man are bipolar neurons, each of which is surrounded by sustentacular cells. The short dendrite of each neuron (the cell body within this layer) is directed peripherally and terminates as a tuft of six to eight olfactory hairs (filaments or streamers) which are slightly motile cilia. These cilia form a feltwork that is embedded in the odor-absorbing secretion coating the mucosa (Fig. 15-1). The receptor sites where the *odorant-receptor interaction* takes place are probably located on the cilia and/or the microvilli on the free surfaces of these bipolar receptor neurons. The initial segment may be located on the cell body where the action potential commences. The axons project from the olfactory mucosa, forming the fascicles of the olfactory nerve which pass through the cribriform plate. These unmyelinated fibers are among the smallest and slowest-conducting fibers of the nervous system. They average about 0.2 μm in diameter. Groups of these unmyelinated axons are collectively enclosed in one sleeve of a neurolemma cell (Fig. 2-13); hence axons are in direct contact with one another (separated by 100-Å spaces). Cross-talk between these axons is theoretically possible. The receptor potentials are generated in the dendrites as a reaction to the odoriferous molecules acting at the olfactory hairs. The resulting action potentials are then transmitted via the axons to the olfactory bulb within the cranial cavity. Each bipolar cell acts in a dual role as an olfactory chemoreceptor cell and as the first-order olfactory neuron; each is a chemical detector, a transducer of a stimulus, and the transmitter of the nerve impulse. Each *sustentacular cell* has about 1,000 microvilli on its free surface. These microvilli and the numerous organelles within these cells are indicative of the presumed secretory nature of these cells; the sustentacular cells are probably not just supporting cells.

The receptor neurons and sustentacular cells undergo a constant regeneration. These new cells are apparently derived from small basal cells of the olfactory mucosal epithelium. Estimates indicate that there is an annual decrease of about 1 percent in the number of receptor neurons throughout life.

The *olfactory bulb* is the primary center in the central nervous system for the olfactory system (Fig. 15-1). The key structures of the bulb are the *glomeruli*. Each glomerulus is the complex synaptic "ball" where the terminal arborization of the axon of the receptor bipolar cell synapses with the dendritic arborization of the mitral cells (which resemble a bishop's miter in shape) and of the tufted cells of the olfactory bulb. The axon of a bipolar cell does not branch until it enters a glomerulus.

Figures on the cell populations of the olfactory mucosa and olfactory bulb are available only for the rabbit, but they give some indication of the interacting units of this system. There are approximately 50 million receptor bipolar cells per nostril, and 45,000 mitral cells, 150,000 tufted cells, and 2,000 glomeruli in each olfactory bulb. The interactions within the bulb result in a significant amount of neural processing. Approximately 25,000 bipolar cells converge upon each glomerulus. This is indicative of the tremendous spatial summation (facilitation) occurring in the neurons of the olfactory bulb. Each mitral cell further summates, because its dendrites synapse in several glomeruli. Thus there is convergence of neural influences from several glomeruli to each mitral cell. In turn, recurrent axon collateral branches from the mitral cells synapse with interneurons which feed back to the glomeruli.

The *mitral cells* project axonal branches to the pyramidal cells in the anterior olfactory nucleus and project other branches through the olfactory tract and olfactory striae to the primary olfactory cortex, amygdaloid body, anterior perforated substance, and septal area. The anterior olfactory nucleus is composed of cells in the posterior part of the olfactory bulb, of cells scattered along the olfactory tract and olfactory striae, and of a few cells in the olfactory cortex and anterior perforated substance. The pyramidal cells of the anterior olfactory nucleus project recurrent axon collateral branches which synapse with internal granule cells and tufted cells, and main axons which, after passing through the anterior commissure, synapse with internal granule cells in the contralateral olfactory bulb. Tufted cells receive input from several glomeruli and from recurrent collateral branches of the pyramidal cells of the anterior olfactory nucleus and, in turn, project axons to other glomeruli. External granule cells interconnect the neurons within a glomerulus with the neurons in other glomeruli. Internal granule cells receive input from recurrent collateral branches of the pyramidal cells of the anterior olfactory nucleus and from pyramidal cells of the contralateral anterior olfactory bulb and, in turn, project axons to the dendrites of the mitral cells.

The axons of the mitral cells project via the olfactory tract and the olfactory striae to the primary olfactory cortex. The medial olfactory stria terminates largely in the cortex and nuclei of the septal region, while the lateral olfactory terminates mainly in the prepiriform cortex (uncus region—area 28) and in the amygdaloid body. These striae and the intermediate olfactory stria, when present, also end in the anterior perforated substance (olfactory tubercle). The *primary olfactory cortex* comprises the cortex of the uncus and adjacent areas: this includes the rostral portions of the parahippocampal gyrus, periamygdaloid cortex (overlying the amygdaloid body), and the prepiriform cortex in the rostral uncus. The course of olfactory impulses beyond these areas is not clear.

Little is known about the neural mechanisms by which odors are sensed and distinguished, and their intensities determined. The glomeruli have been implicated as being critical sites of this activity. The discharges from the olfactory epithelium and the feedback stimuli are integrated so that patterns of glomerular activity are expressed in the discharges of the mitral cells to the olfactory cortex. Each glomerulus sorts and integrates its input before relaying stimuli to the cortex.

Alone among the senses, *olfaction has no primary projection to the thalamus.* Because of this, the olfactory bulb has been considered to be an analogue of the thalamus. The primary olfactory cortex includes such cortical regions as the prepiriform area (rostral part of the uncus), the anterior perforated substance (sometimes called the "olfactory tubercle"), and the septal area. The olfactory bulb may project many fibers to the corticomedial nuclei of the amygdaloid body but none to the hippocampal formation or postuncal cortex (area 36). This primary olfactory cortex has connections with such structures as the hypothalamus and reticular system (via the dorsal longitudinal fasciculus), amygdaloid body, and possibly through interconnections to the thalamus and to most of the limbic lobe. In addition, direct olfactory influences are conveyed to the hypothalamus via the medial forebrain bundle to the lateral hypothalamus.

The term *rhinencephalon,* or "smell brain," is used in various ways. In its most restricted

sense, the rhinencephalon is limited to the olfactory nerves, olfactory bulbs, olfactory tracts, and to those neural structures receiving direct connections from the olfactory bulbs. The latter include the anterior perforated substance, prepiriform cortex, septal area, and corticomedial nuclei of the amygdaloid body. In the broadest definitions the rhinencephalon also includes the limbic cortex. The term *allocortex* is used synonymously with *rhinencephalic cortex.* The broad definition includes, at least in theory, all neural structures influenced by the sense of smell. Elimination of the term *rhinencephalon* has been suggested; after all, the terms "visual brain" and "auditory brain" are not used.

In theory, the *olfactory bulb is the crude indicator of smell* (as the thalamus produces crude awareness of pain) and the primary olfactory cortex and its associative cortex are the processors of finer odor discrimination. Electric recordings obtained from the olfactory bulbs of man suggest that the quality of an odor is coded, at least in part, in the frequency patterns. The detection of an odor, following an adequate signal strength, is characterized by greater amplitude patterns. The complex neuronal interconnections operate to intensify, enhance, and suppress the neural processing within the olfactory pathways. This includes the activities of the feedback circuits, reciprocal dendrodendritic synapses (Chap. 2), and the olfactory efferent (corticofugal) fibers from the olfactory cortex to the olfactory bulb (Fig. 15-1).

The limbic system

FUNCTIONAL ROLE

Many of the neuroanatomic substrates underlying the behavioral and emotional expressions of animals reside in the limbic system, otherwise known as the "visceral brain." This system is integral to those activities essential to the self-preservation of the organism, e.g., feeding, fight, and flight; and those essential to the preservation of the species, e.g., mating, procreation, and care of offspring. The limbic system is influenced by all sensory systems, including the olfactory, optic, auditory, and general exteroceptive and interoceptive systems. *The main outlet for its activity is via the pathways from the hypothalamus to the brainstem and spinal cord (largely via the autonomic nervous system), and the pathways to the hypophysis (endocrine gland)*. The somatic motor system also serves as an outlet for the expression of the activities of the limbic system. Autonomic and somatic motor responses and feelings of a variety of sensations can be evoked by electrically stimulating structures belonging to the limbic system. Depending upon the structure stimulated and the nature of the stimulation, there are differences in the quality of the responses evoked.

1 *Somatic motor responses* evoked by limbic stimulation include *a* those associated with food acquisition and ingestion such as sniffing, licking, chewing, and swallowing movements; *b* those associated with behavioral patterns of activity such as grooming and goal-seeking searching movements; and *c* those associated with attack and defense such as snarling, clawing, and various posturing movements.

2 *Autonomic responses* include changes in the rate of the heartbeat, in blood pressure, in the motility and secretory activity of the gastrointestinal tract, and in the level of many hormones in the blood. Many hormonal effects of the autonomic nervous system are mediated via the hypothalamus and hypophysis (Chap. 11).

3 *Sensory modalities* evoked include the olfactory sensations (often sensed as an unpleasant quality), feelings of vertigo, and visceral sensations such as those felt within the abdomen. Other "sensory" responses evoked are emotional feelings noted later on in this chapter, under "'Pleasure Centers' and 'Punishing Centers.'"

ANATOMY

The precise identification of all the structural elements associated with the limbic system is not possible at the present state of our knowledge. This is so because it is difficult to establish morphologic correlates with the subtle physiologic and behavioral criteria by which the limbic system is characterized. The following are generally considered to be *core structures of the limbic system:*

1 the olfactory pathway comprising the olfactory nerve, olfactory bulb, anterior olfactory nucleus, olfactory tract, olfactory striae, and primary olfactory cortex

2 the amygdaloid body and its efferent projections via the stria terminalis and ventral amygdalofugal fibers

3 the hippocampus and its efferent projections comprising the alveus, fimbria of the fornix, and fornix

4 the limbic lobe (Figs. 1-4, 15-2)

5 the hypothalamus.

Other nuclei and pathways associated with the limbic system are included later on in this chapter.

The *hippocampus* consists of the pes hippocampus, alveus, and fimbria (Fig. 1-24). The alveus and the fimbria are fibers forming a thin lamina over the hippocampus; they continue as the bundle of fibers called the fornix, the successive parts of which are its crus, body, and columns (Fig. 1-24). The term "hippocampal formation" is obsolete. The *commissure of the fornix* (formerly called the *hippocampal commissure*) consists of fibers crossing from the body of one fornix to the other. These fibers interconnect the two hippocampi.

The *limbic lobe* is a ring of cortex around the ventricular system of the cerebrum. It includes the septal area, cingulate gyrus, isthmus, indusium griseum, fasciolar gyrus, parahippocampal gyrus, subiculum (entorhinal cortex), uncus, and the primary olfactory cortex (Figs. 1-4, 15-2). The cortex of the limbic lobe is phylogenetically older than the neocortex; it is called the allocortex (Chap. 16).

The *septal (subcallosal) area* consists of the paraterminal body (subcallosal gyrus) and the parolfactory area of the orbitofrontal cortex (Fig. 15-2). The *septal region* is composed of the septum pellucidum, septal nuclei, and septal area. The *septum pellucidum* is a lamina of glial cells and some nerve fibers; at its base in the vicinity of the column of the fornix are located clusters of nuclei, called the septal nuclei (Fig. 15-3). The *indusium griseum* (associated with medial and lateral longitudinal striae) is a thin layer of gray matter on the upper surface of the corpus callosum (Fig. 15-4); it continues around the splenium of the corpus callosum and becomes continuous rostrally with the paraterminal body and occipitally with the fasciolar gyrus (Fig. 15-3). The *fasciolar gyrus* is the transitional area between the indusium griseum and the dentate gyrus. The *isthmus,* located on the

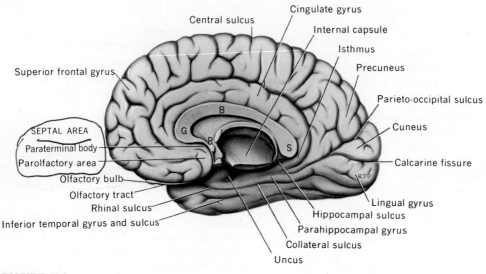

FIGURE 15-2
Median surface of the cerebral hemisphere.

The internal capsule and the limbic lobe are exposed by the removal of the entire brainstem and cerebellum. The limbic lobe consists of the septal area, cingulate gyrus, isthmus, parahippocampal gyrus, and uncus. The corpus callosum is subdivided into a rostrum (R), genu (G), body (B), and splenium (S).

occipital side of the fasciolar gyrus, is the transitional area between the cingulate gyrus and the hippocampus. The medial and lateral longitudinal striae consist of fibers within the indusium griseum which interconnect the hippocampus with the septal area. The *subicular area* (subiculum) is a transitional band of cortex, located between the hippocampus (archicortex) and the neocortex of the parahippocampal gyrus (Fig. 1-4). The *prepiriform cortex* is a cortical area adjacent to the lateral olfactory stria on the rostral portion of the uncus. The *piriform lobe* (cortex) is the cortex of the uncus (includes prepiriform cortex). The septal area, along with preoptic hypothalamus and the hypothalamus, has been called the septopreopticohypothalamic component of the reticular formation (Chaps. 8 and 11).

The limbic structures of the telencephalon, just noted, are connected by pathways with the neocortex, diencephalon, and mesencephalon. The structures in the latter regions of the brain are considered to contain other morphologic substrates of the limbic system (Chap. 11). *1* The neocortex along the margin of the limbic lobe is interconnected with the limbic lobe; it particularly includes the neocortex of the orbitofrontal, medial temporal, and central lobe (insular) gyri. Even the prefrontal cortex may be considered to be a neocortical representation of the limbic system. *2* The major thalamic nuclei integrated into the limbic system include the medial dorsal nucleus (DM) and the anterior ventral nucleus of the anterior nuclear group. *3* Other important diencephalic structures comprise the fibers of the stria medullaris thalami and habenula of the epithalamus, and many nuclei of the hypothalamus. *4* The mesencephalic components of the limbic system are the interpeduncular nucleus, median midbrain reticular formation, dorsal and ventral tegmental nuclei of Gudden, superior central nucleus (brainstem raphe nucleus), and periaqueductal gray matter.

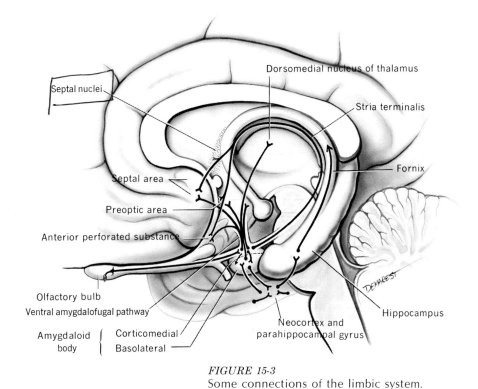

Septal nuclei

Dorsomedial nucleus of thalamus

Stria terminalis

Fornix

Septal area

Preoptic area

Anterior perforated substance

Olfactory bulb

Ventral amygdalofugal pathway

Amygdaloid body { Corticomedial / Basolateral

Neocortex and parahippocampal gyrus

Hippocampus

FIGURE 15-3
Some connections of the limbic system.

GENERAL CIRCUITRY OF THE LIMBIC SYSTEM

The complexities of the neuroanatomy of the limbic system (Figs. 15-3 through 15-5) may be schematized into *1* the pathways within the limbic lobe and its immediate nuclear stations, including the hippocampal formation, amygdaloid body, and septal area; *2* the pathways interconnecting this complex with the diencephalon, including *a* epithalamus (habenular nuclei), *b* thalamus (anterior thalamic nuclear complex, dorsomedial nucleus, and the intralaminar nuclei), *c* hypothalamus; and *3* the pathways interconnecting the diencephalon with the midbrain tegmentum, raphe nuclei, and the interpeduncular nucleus. The ramifications of the input to and output from these circuits add to their intricacy. The major efferent projections from the hypothalamus are elements incorporated into the reciprocal connections with the limbic forebrain and midbrain structures.

Amygdaloid body, hippocampal formation, and other connections of the limbus The amygdaloid body and hippocampal formation are among the most prominent of the processing stations of the limbic system. Their pathways of input and output are outlined first (Figs. 15-3 and 15-4).

The amygdaloid body is divisible into two groups of nuclei: corticomedial amygdaloid and basolateral amygdaloid. The corticomedial group receives its major input from the olfactory bulb (via the lateral olfactory tract) and has interconnections with the contralateral amygdaloid body and the ipsilateral basolateral nuclear group. This corticomedial group projects its output chiefly via the stria terminalis (which parallels the arc of the fornix) to the septal region and the preoptic area of the hypothalamus of the same and opposite side (crossing over in the anterior commissure). The

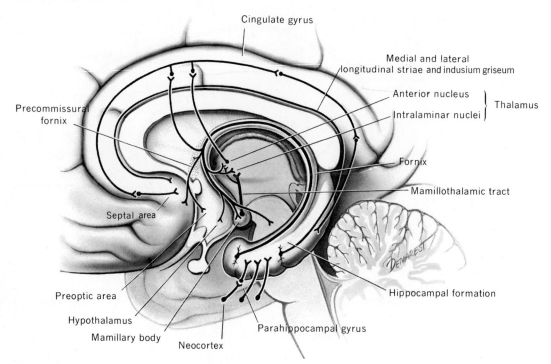

FIGURE 15-4
Some connections of the limbic system.

The "Papez circuit": hippocampus via fornix → mamillary body via mamillothalamic tract → anterior nuclear group of thalamus → cingulate gyrus → hippocampus.

basolateral group has many reciprocal interconnections with the cortex of the parahippocampal gyrus. This latter has important connections with the neocortex of the temporal pole, and through neuron chains rostrally to the cortex of the frontal lobe and caudally to the cingulate gyrus—in effect, with much of the limbic lobe. Other connections of this group are through the hippocampal formation.

The output from the amygdaloid body utilizes two major pathways: the stria terminalis and the ventral amygdalofugal fibers. The latter is the larger. The amygdaloid body projects to the hypothalamus (lateral, ventral, and preoptic regions), dorsomedial thalamic nucleus, septal region, and anterior perforated substance.

The hippocampus is interconnected with many regions (Fig. 15-4). In a general way the input to this complex comes via *1* multineuronal chains from the adjacent temporal lobe neocortex, which, in turn, receives its input from many association areas of the neocortex, *2* the fornix from the septal region (septohippocampal fibers), *3* the fornix and commissure of the fornix from the hippocampus of the opposite side, and *4* the longitudinal striae from the septal region. In brief, this archicortex integrates multidimensional information which subserves the emotional state.

The outflow from the hippocampus is transmitted mainly, if not exclusively, via the axons of pyramidal cells that form the fornix. Some axons project commissural fibers via the commissure of the fornix and the contralateral fornix to the hippocampus of the opposite side. The precommissural fornix (which passes rostral to the anterior commissure) contains fibers pro-

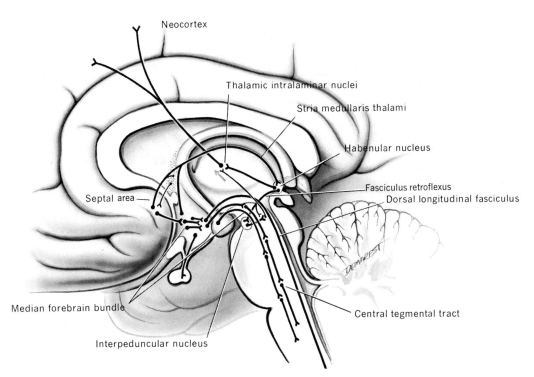

Neocortex

Thalamic intralaminar nuclei

Stria medullaris thalami

Habenular nucleus

Septal area

Fasciculus retroflexus
Dorsal longitudinal fasciculus

Median forebrain bundle

Central tegmental tract

Interpeduncular nucleus

FIGURE 15-5
Some connections of the limbic system.

The median forebrain bundle is a multineuronal pathway extending from the septal area through the lateral hypothalamus to the brainstem tegmentum. Note the pathway system comprising the sequence of septal area and preoptic area → habenular nucleus → midbrain tegmentum and interpeduncular nucleus. The latter projects to the midbrain tegmentum.

jecting to the septal region, preoptic nuclei, and cingulate gyrus. The 1,200,000 fibers of the column of the postcommissural fornix project to the mamillary body, anterior intralaminar nuclei, anterior nuclear group of the thalamus, lateral hypothalamic nucleus, and the rostral central gray of the midbrain. The hippocampus and dentate gyrus are interconnected with the paraterminal body (subcallosal gyrus) via the medial and lateral longitudinal striae. These striae are located within the vestigial convolution called the indusium griseum (Figs. 1-4, 15-4).

The cingulate cortex has diffuse projections. Many of its pyramidal cells have axons which bifurcate into two long axonal branches, each branch projecting to a different region (Fig. 15-4). The cingulate cortex has connections via the cingulum to other areas of the cingulate gyrus (Chap. 16), via the uncinate fasciculus with the temporal lobe (Chap. 16), via the ipsilateral internal capsule to the corpus striatum, via the corpus callosum to the contralateral cingulate gyrus and corpus striatum, and via perforant

fibers (fibers perforating through the corpus callosum) through the septum pellucidum and fornix to other limbic nuclei.

The hippocampus and its associated gray matter have connections through the fornix with the septal area and the preoptic region. In addition, afferent fibers from the septal area via the fornix project to the hippocampus. The amygdaloid body projects via the stria terminalis to the septal region.

Connections of the limbic lobe with the diencephalon The hippocampus projects fibers via the fornix to the anterior thalamic nuclear complex, the intralaminar thalamic nuclei and lateral dorsal nucleus of the thalamus, the lateral hypothalamus, and the mamillary bodies (Fig. 15-4). The amygdaloid body projects fibers via the stria terminalis to the preoptic region, the hypothalamus, and the dorsomedial thalamic nucleus.

Pathways from the septal region and the preoptic portion of the hypothalamus (common terminus for some input from the hippocampus and the amygdaloid body) project via *1* the stria medullaris thalami bundle to the habenular nuclei of the epithalamus, and *2* the median forebrain bundle to the lateral hypothalamus and the tegmentum of the midbrain. The median forebrain bundle is an intricate complex of short multisynaptic chains of neurons extending from the septal region to the midbrain; many hypothalamic nuclei are intercalated within this bundle (Fig. 15-5). These nuclei include the preoptic, anterior hypothalamic, and lateral hypothalamic nuclei.

Connections of the diencephalon with the midbrain The hypothalamus has three pathways which interconnect with the midbrain (Chap. 11). *1* The *median forebrain bundle* is a complex of reciprocal connections between many hypothalamic nuclei and the midbrain tegmentum. The *tegmental nuclei* include the median midbrain reticular formation and such brainstem raphe nuclei as the dorsal and ventral tegmental nuclei of Gudden and the superior central nucleus (Figs. 8-9, 11-4, and 11-5). *2* The mamillary body projects to the midbrain tegmentum via the *mamillotegmental tract*, and *3* via the *dorsal longitudinal fasciculus* of the periventricular gray (Chap. 11). In addition, the mamillary body projects to the anterior thalamic nuclear group via the *mamillothalamic tract* (Fig. 11-5).

The habenular nucleus of the epithalamus is the nucleus of origin of the *fasciculus retroflexus* (habenulopeduncular tract); this tract has connections with the midbrain tegmentum and the interpeduncular nucleus. The latter projects

to the midbrain tegmentum. The habenular nucleus also projects to the nucleus centrum medianum, one of the thalamic reticular nuclei.

Overall view of the limbic pathways The full significance of the limbic interconnections is unknown. However, several aspects of these pathways illustrate the interactions, with probable functional correlates (Figs. 15-3 through 15-5).

The midbrain and thalamic reticular nuclei receive inputs from several limbic pathways. The multiple projections to *1* the midbrain tegmentum from the habenular nucleus and from the hypothalamus (Fig. 15-5), and *2* the thalamic intralaminar nuclei from the hippocampal formation exert influences that undoubtedly affect the activities of the reticular system (Chap. 8).

The influences on the hypothalamus, which is the major center regulating the autonomic nervous system, play a major role in the autonomic reactions which are associated with emotional and behavioral patterns.

The interactions of the limbic lobe cortex with the neocortex underline the postulated functional division which associates emotional processes with the limbic cortex, and intellectual processes with the neocortex. The limbic lobe is a link between emotional and cognitive mechanisms.

In theory, feedback circuits which interact within the limbic system and with other structures of the nervous system have been suggested. For example, there is the postulated circuit of hippocampal formation through the fornix to the mamillary body through mamillothalamic tract to anterior thalamic nucleus through internal capsule to cingulate gyrus through multisynaptic chains in the allocortex back to the hippocampal formation. This "reverberating circuit" was suggested by James W. Papez in 1937, in his classic theory, as the basis for the central mechanism for emotion underlying the psychic expression of the neocortical areas (Fig. 15-4). This was the milestone that initiated research leading to the modern concepts of the function of the limbic system. Other circuits with numerous nodal sites for accepting input and discharging output are available for the complex interactions essential to the subtle displays of behavioral patterns. These circuits are a complex of direct feedback circuitry involved in homeostatic control systems. The major pathway for the outflow of influences from the neocortex to subcortical levels is the internal capsule (Chap. 16). In a comparable sense, the major pathway for outflow from the limbic lobe to subcerebral levels is the median forebrain bundle (limbic lobe to hypothalamus to brainstem tegmentum). Another route of outflow is the habenulopeduncular tract. The output from these pathways may exert effects through *1* the hypophysis (hypophyseal–pituitary fibers, and the hypophyseal portal vein (Fig. 11-2), *2* the descending autonomic pathways, and *3* the hypothalamotegmental pathways, central tegmental tract, and the reticulospinal pathways to the spinal cord.

Terminology An understanding of the terminology associated with emotion and behavior is basic to this discussion. Subjective terms should be distinguished from objective terms. *Feeling tone* and *affect* describe the subjective feeling state of an individual. When affect is prolonged in time, a mood sets in. *Emotion* generally refers to affect or a mood when it is accompanied by an active expression. The expression may be mediated through the autonomic nervous system (e.g., heart palpitations) or the somatic nervous system (e.g., fidgeting). In this context emotion combines subjective feelings (such as an empty feeling, pleasantness, unpleasantness, depression, elation, alertness, and contentment) with objective signs. *True rage* combines intense antagonistic subjective feelings (anger) with pronounced objective activity (the snarling or clawing of a cat). A *sham rage* (*pseudoaffective reflex*) is a rage without the subjective side but with the objective signs. An animal without a cortex may exhibit a sham rage because it presumably has no subjective feelings. *Behavior* is a constellation of expressions of an animal noted by an observer. Subjective signs are not observed, only inferred. Observed behavior includes the schooling of fish, the nesting of birds, and the stalking by lions. *Agonistic behavior* and *agonistic responses* refer to the behavior manifested by animals in an attack and defense contest during fight or flight. *Motivation* is the drive that urges the

animal to activity; it is reduced after the goal is reached, e.g., hunger is reduced following a meal. Several aspects of the relation of emotion and the limbic lobe will be outlined below.

EMOTIONAL BEHAVIOR AND PUTATIVE NEUROTRANSMITTERS

The limbic system has an essential role in processing input which influences the activity of the autonomic and somatic motor systems. These influences act to suppress or to enhance those expressions of the organism which we interpret as emotional behavior. Some of the input to telencephalic limbic structures is conveyed via ascending pathways from the nuclei of the midbrain and lower brainstem reticular formation. These include the adrenergic and serotoninergic pathways described in Chap. 8 (Figs. 8-12 and 8-13). These pathways release norepinephrine and serotonin, which are putative neurotransmitters in many structures of the limbic system. These putative neurotransmitters are presumed to have a critical role in influencing emotional behavior. The tranquilizing and mood-elevating drugs probably exert their effects through action upon these pathway systems. Most of the mood-elevating drugs are known to be central antagonists of the catecholamines and serotonin.

Klüver-Bucy syndrome Monkeys with the anterior temporal lobe ablated bilaterally (Klüver-Bucy syndrome) exhibit a constellation of emotional expressions. In the Klüver-Bucy syndrome the visual and other sensory systems are disconnected from the limbic lobe. This loss of the amygdaloid body, uncus, anterior pole of the temporal lobe, parts of the hippocampal formation, and the parahippocampus alters the animal's behavioral patterns. The animal is able to see and to locate objects visually, but it is unable to recognize objects by sight. (This visual agnosia in human beings with comparable damage is characterized by the loss of recognition of friends and places.) Animals in this condition probably have auditory and tactile agnosias, but these are difficult to determine. Such animals exhibit strong oral tendencies, expressed by a compulsiveness to examine objects with the mouth and lips. An object, once seen, is contacted, placed in the mouth, bitten, and often gently chewed. Unless edible, each object is immediately dropped. This overreacting animal is said to be stimulus-bound, as he has an irresistible impulse to touch every object in sight. Behavioral changes are profound and dramatic, for the animal is apparently released ("release phenomenon") from expressing fear. Wild or aggressive monkeys become tame and docile. The marked absence of emotional responses, such as anger or fear, is accompanied by the loss of the usually associated facial expressions and vocal protests. Monkeys that were formerly fearful of a mouse or a snake will pick up a live mouse or snake and handle it without fear. Dietary habits are altered; monkeys will eat fish and other food not usually eaten. Food is often consumed in excess. Hypersexual behavior is marked, with many manifestations of autosexual, homosexual, and heterosexual activities. Unilateral temporal lobe ablation does not produce such behavioral patterns, although it does make animals tamer.

Amygdaloid body   Electrical stimulation of the amygdaloid body and the immediate region in the unanesthesized monkey produces a number of behavioral actions. Activities associated with nutrition are elicited, including sniffing, licking, biting, swallowing, and retching movements. Monkeys exhibit agonistic behavior patterns. The peaceful monkey becomes a furious and aggressive animal that attacks and bullies. Once the stimulus is turned off, the peaceful monkey reappears. The stimulated cat is transformed into a ball of fury, with pupils dilated, claws extended, and back hair on end. Any approaching object is attacked. After the stimulus is turned off, the cat becomes a friendly, purring animal. Cats so stimulated can exhibit emotional behavior. If the amygdaloid body is stimulated in one of two cats, a fight ensues between the two animals. After this activity is repeated several times, the cats retain their newly acquired an-

tagonism and will fight even without such stimulation. They are now emotionally driven.

An opposite response may be elicited. A stimulated cat may even express friendly behavioral patterns; it will sniff and lick, and nuzzle and rub other cats. In addition, such stimulation can inhibit a hungry and thirsty cat from eating and drinking and even prevent the hungry cat from sniffing food.

The increase in the secretion of digestive juices in the alimentary canal after repeated acute stimulations of the amygdaloid body may be followed by the appearance of erosions similar to peptic ulcers in the stomachs of monkeys and cats. The possibility of psychic excitation in the production of peptic ulcers in man is implied.

Human beings with bilateral temporal lobe damage exhibit visual agnosia, as seen in their lack of recognition of people and objects. They become docile and hypersexual. Nymphomania in the female and satyrism in the male are manifested. The behavior change may not be apparent to the casual observer, for the patient may be outwardly unchanged, with normal powers of reason and understanding. Stimulation of the amygdaloid body in man produces the feeling tones of fear, anxiety, and rage.

Limbic lobe and neocortex   Psychomotor epileptic seizures originating in the temporal lobe of man illustrate the interplay and interaction that may occur between the limbic lobe and the neocortex. In a seizure, the patient may experience difficulty in speech (showing the influence of the neocortex) and may be in a confused state (showing the effect of the limbic lobe).

LIMBIC SYSTEM AND GOAL-DIRECTED BEHAVIOR

The limbic system may act as a link between the sensorium and motivated activity. This linkage is probably an essential substrate in influencing the motor systems in goal-directed behavior. Some ingenious experimental studies with monkeys indicate that the amygdaloid body has a functional role in the motivational aspect of many motor responses (Doty). Monkeys with an ablated amygdaloid body can be demonstrated to have their mnemonic systems in normal working order. These animals react to visual stimuli; they are able to recognize objects and events in their environment. However, they do not respond behaviorally to these same visual stimuli; they exhibit a loss in their emotional expressions and in their ability to evaluate their environment. In summary, there is a definite loss in motivational behavior when mnemonic information is disconnected from the amygdaloid body; the latter may act as an intermediary between the neocortex and the parts of the limbic system.

Memory The limbic lobe, especially the amygdaloid body and hippocampal formation, has been implicated in the memory for recent events. The neural mechanisms subserving the fleeting memory traces which are forgotten after a few minutes to several days are not known. The role of the hippocampus and the amygdaloid body in this phenomenon has been indicated by experimental work on animals and by human patients. Individuals with bilateral lesions of the amygdaloid body–hippocampal region of the temporal lobes retain memory of events prior to the surgical operation (long-term memory). Subsequent to the operation they may forget any information obtained ten or so minutes previously. These patients carry on normal conversations but cannot recall their content shortly thereafter. They are unable to commit anything to memory. If given a message to convey to another person, some patients can carry out this task only within a 5- or 10-min period after getting the instructions. After that, the message is forgotten. Lesions are found in the hippocampus in some cases of senile dementia. Patients with hippocampal lesions in the dominant hemisphere may have mild disturbances of memory. This may be related to *Korsakoff's syndrome,* in which there is loss of recent memory and sense of time along with intellectual impairment. These patients have a tendency to fabricate and to become easily confused. For example, the subject forgets the question just asked and may reply with irrelevant answers (called compensatory confabulation).

The hippocampus is probably not the locale for the actual storage of the memory trace; rather it may be thought of as being involved in the decision to tape and to store information

for future recall. Information storage is thought to be a function of the entire brain or of many regions throughout the brain.

The neurons of the hippocampus are relatively more likely to be induced into convulsant activity, which can spread to other structures of the limbic system. In general, this activity tends to remain localized within limbic structures. This is an expression of the observation that hippocampal seizures generally do not become generalized epileptic seizures accompanied by loss of consciousness. It also accounts for the many bizarre changes in behavior observed in some patients during psychomotor attacks.

Stimulation of limbic lobe Stimulation of the hippocampus results in respiratory and cardiovascular changes and in a generalized arousal response. Such sexual activities as grooming and erection can be elicited. In this capacity, the hippocampus acts as a supplemental motor area by inducing such expressive somatic movements as facial grimaces, shoulder shrugging, and hand movements that are considered normal behavioral gestures. After the bilateral removal of the hippocampus, monkeys appear normal and feed themselves but are lethargic, apathetic, and slow to anger. They lack emotional tone.

Electric stimulation of the cingulate gyrus, the septal cortex, and other areas of the limbic lobe may evoke responses indicative of activity of the autonomic nervous system. Some responses include changes in the tone of the blood vascular system, in the activity of the digestive system, and in respiratory rhythms. These actions have even been observed in man.

Aggressiveness can be inhibited or decreased in either monkeys or cats by electrical stimulation of the septal area or the caudate nucleus. The "boss" monkey in a colony of monkeys dominates the other members so that their behavior reflects their underdog position. The stimulation of the septal region of the "boss" monkey with implanted electrodes reduces the aggressive behavior of this dominant monkey. If this stimulation of the "boss" monkey is prolonged, the other monkeys sense this change. They lose their fear of the former bully and will take new liberties, such as securing a larger share of food or invading his territory. The former situation returns after the stimulation ceases. The aggressive monkey that attacks and bites becomes gentle when its caudate nucleus is electrically stimulated. This nonaggressive, easily handled, relaxed animal returns to its former self immediately after stimulation ceases.

"Pleasure centers" and "punishing centers"
The stimulation by implanted electrodes of certain regions of the limbic system of cats, dogs, dolphins, monkeys, apes, and man drives the animal to seek further stimulation. The animal will trip the lever over and over again and thus continually restimulate itself—*an expression of positive reinforcement on self-stimulation.* Such nodal sites have been named *pleasure centers* or *rewarding centers.* The stimulation of some regions excites the animal to avoid further stimulation—*an expression of negative reinforcement on self-stimulation.* Such sites have been named *punishing centers* or *aversion centers.* A "pleasure center" may be located a fraction of a millimeter from a "punishing center."

The general approach to locating these areas is to implant electrodes in the brain and to permit the animal to stimulate itself with small shocks by pressing a bar lever. Each press of the lever evokes a shock. With electrodes in the "pleasure centers" animals will press the lever thousands of times per hour (as many as 11,000 times per hour in some regions), hour after hour until physically exhausted. If an animal is permitted to indulge in this bar-pressing self-stimulating performance each day for an hour or so, the daily self-stimulation will be intensely performed for months on end with no indication of satiety. Such animals would rather press the lever than eat if hungry, or drink if thirsty. They will brave painful shocks to their feet to continue the self-stimulation ritual. This activity is in the nature of a positive feedback phenomenon. The several human beings whose septal areas were stimulated had feelings of pleasure or a "brightening of their attitude." They giggled, talked more, and expressed themselves

more freely when the current was on. The stimulation changed their mood and made them "feel good." These so-called "pleasure centers" have been located within most of the limbic system, septal region, cingulate cortex, hippocampal formation, amygdaloid body, hypothalamic preoptic area, anterior nuclei of the thalamus, medial forebrain bundle, and midbrain tegmentum.

Shocks from electrodes within the "punishing centers" evoke behavioral patterns to which animals are averse. Monkeys grimace, quiver, and shake. They bite and tear objects with their mouths, their eyes dilate, and their hair stands on end. If stimulated for hours, the monkey becomes irritable, refuses to eat, and may become ill. These effects can be eliminated by stimulating a "pleasure center." If an animal is conditioned to expect a shock to a "punishing center" after a certain cue and it finds out that the shock can be avoided by some action such as pressing a lever, it becomes motivated to nullify the stimulus. Avoidance responses to the stimulation of these "aversion centers" are exhibited by rats and cats as well as by monkeys. The midbrain tegmentum and certain areas of the thalamus and hypothalamus are the sites of these "punishing centers." In man, the response evoked is one of fear or terror.

Expressions of limbic system function The effects of the electric stimulation or the ablation of various regions of the limbic system are diverse and intricate. In effect, these regions are nodal sites that activate or inhibit many other functional complexes of the nervous system. Electric shocks to the area (or the ablation of a region) disturb, alter, and bias the dynamics of the preexisting physiologic and psychologic patterns. The effects are multifaceted—utilizing both the somatic nervous system and the autonomic nervous system. The responses can be expressed both subjectively and objectively, because the stimuli may modify the behavioral patterns, including moods and emotional states.

Uncinate fits are generally the consequence of involvement (by tumor or other disease process) of the uncus region and amygdaloid body. The immediate area is associated with the olfactory system and possibly with the gustatory system. A patient with a lesion in this area may have an olfactory aura; the hallucination usually consists of the smelling of a nonexistent disagreeable odor. Associated with this olfactory illusion is a difficult-to-describe fear of the unreality of the environment.

PREFRONTAL CORTEX AS A LIMBIC STRUCTURE

The prefrontal cortex may be a major neocortical representative of the limbic system (Nauta). This interpretation is based on morphologic and behavioral criteria. The prefrontal cortex has multiple reciprocal connections with many core structures of the limbic system, including the cortex of the limbic lobe and the hypothalamus. The frontohypothalamic interconnection is the only known direct route from the neocortex to the hypothalamus. Functionally the prefrontal cortex may serve as a critical link between other regions of the cerebral cortex and the limbic system. This linkage is presumed to act as a channel through which the prefrontal cortex monitors and modulates limbic mechanisms and thereby influences the organism's affective and motivational states (Chap. 16).

Bibliography

Beidler, L. M.: Olfaction, in *Handbook of Sensory Physiology*, vol. IV, part 1, pp. 1–517. Springer-Verlag, Berlin and New York, 1971.

Clemente, C. D., and M. H. Chase: Neurological substrates of aggressive behavior. Ann. Rev. Physiol., 35:329–356, 1973.

Grossman, S. P.: *Essentials of Physiological Psychology.* John Wiley & Sons, Inc., New York, 1973.

Hockman, C. H. (ed.): *Limbic System Mechanisms and Autonomic Function.* Charles C Thomas, Publisher, Springfield, Ill., 1972.

Klüver, H.: "The temporal lobe syndrome" produced by bilateral ablations, in E. E. Wolstenholm and C. M. O'Connor (eds.), *Neurological Basis of Behaviour,* pp. 175–182. Churchill, London, 1958.

Magoun, H. W.: *The Waking Brain,* 2d ed. Charles C Thomas, Publisher, Springfield, Ill., 1969.

Moulton, D. G., and L. M. Beidler: Structure and function in the peripheral olfactory system. Physiol. Rev., 47:1–52, 1967.

Raisman, G., W. M. Cowan, and T. P. S. Powell: An experimental analysis of the efferent projections of the hippocampus. Brain, 89:83–108, 1966.

Sprague, J. M.: The effects of chronic brain stem lesions on wakefulness, sleep and behavior. Res. Publ. Assoc. Nerv. Ment. Dis., 45:148–194, 1967.

Stensaas, L. J.: The development of hippocampal and dorsolateral pallial regions of the cerebral hemisphere in fetal rabbits. J. Comp. Neurol., 132:93–108, 1968.

Valenstein, E. S.: *Brain Stimulation and Motivation.* Scott, Foresman and Company, Chicago, 1973.

Valverde, F.: *Studies on the Piriform Lobe.* Harvard University Press, Cambridge, Mass., 1965.

CHAPTER 16
THE CEREBRAL CORTEX

The cerebral cortex is the gray mantle of the cerebrum, composed of about 10 to 15 billion neurons and 50 billion glial cells (Figs. 16-1 through 16-4). Its intricate networks are essential to our intellectual faculties and to the other higher neural expressions. This matrix has been likened to "an enchanted loom where millions of flashing shuttles weave a dissolving pattern" (Charles S. Sherrington).

The cerebral cortex covers about $2\frac{1}{2}$ sq ft of surface area. In thickness it varies from 4 mm in the precentral gyrus (motor cortex) to 1.5 mm in the primary visual cortex near the calcarine sulcus. Its total weight of 600 Gm—about 1 lb, or roughly 40 percent of the total brain weight —is estimated to be divisible into about 180 Gm of neurons, including their processes, and 420 Gm of glial cells and blood vessels.

The cortex of man achieves its maximal weight by the eighth year of life. No reliable data even suggest a relation between cortical weight (normal ranges) and intelligence.

Organization of the cortex

GROSS ORGANIZATION

The cerebral cortex has been parceled into a number of areas, depending on which structural and functional criteria are emphasized by an author. Even the validity of many of the criteria is questioned.

On the basis of phylogenetic, ontogenetic, and functional criteria, the *cerebral cortex* (*pallium*) is subdivided into *archicortex (archipallium)*, *paleocortex (paleopallium)*, and *neocortex (neopallium)*. The archicortex and paleocortex attain relatively large proportions early in mammalian evolution and during early development. The neocortex, although indicated in rep-

tiles, is actually an "organ" of mammals. The paleocortex has a significant role in olfaction (Chap. 15). The archicortex is integrated into the neural mechanisms associated with emotional and affective behavior.

The neocortex constitutes the bulk of the cortex (90 percent) in man. Other names for it, besides *neopallium*, are *homogenetic cortex*, *isocortex*, and *dorsal area*. This cortex has a six-layered laminated cytoarchitectural pattern (discussed below).

ALLOCORTEX

The paleocortex and archicortex are collectively known as the *heterogenetic cortex* or *allocortex* (Chap. 15). This ancient cortex either is nonlaminated or, if laminated, has fewer than six cytoarchitectural layers. Although the allocortex has a phylogenetically ancient history, many portions of it have become highly evolved in man and the higher primates.

The archicortex is subdivided into hippocampus, dentate gyrus, and subiculum. The hippocampus forms the floor of the temporal horn of the lateral ventricle; the subiculum is a transitional area adjacent to the neocortex; and the dentate gyrus is wedged in between the hippocampus and the subiculum. The hippocampal formation consists of the hippocampus, dentate gyrus, and possibly the subiculum. The hippocampus is the ridge in the floor of the temporal horn of the lateral ventricle. It comprises *1* the pes hippocampi, which is the rostral extension; *2* the alveus hippocampi, which is a thin layer of white matter covering the ventricular surface of the hippocampus; and *3* the fimbria hippocampi (fimbria of the fornix), which is composed of many efferent and afferent fibers projecting from and to the mamillary body (Fig. 1-24).

The *paleocortex* (essentially equivalent to the

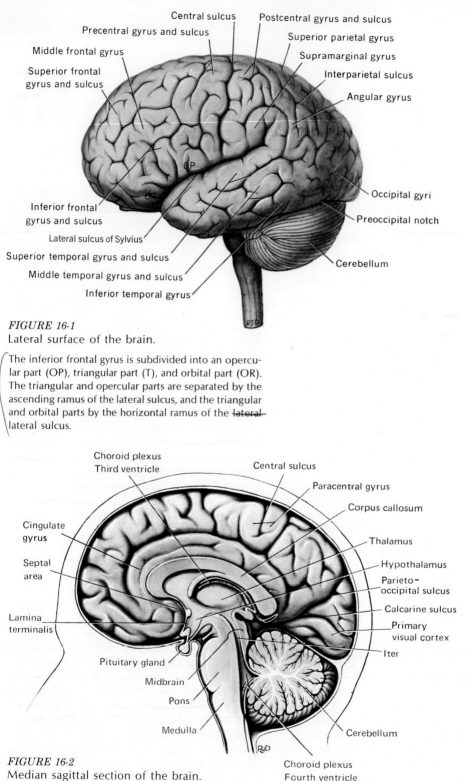

Central sulcus
Precentral gyrus and sulcus
Postcentral gyrus and sulcus
Middle frontal gyrus
Superior parietal gyrus
Superior frontal gyrus and sulcus
Supramarginal gyrus
Interparietal sulcus
Angular gyrus
Occipital gyri
Preoccipital notch
Inferior frontal gyrus and sulcus
Lateral sulcus of Sylvius
Superior temporal gyrus and sulcus
Middle temporal gyrus and sulcus
Inferior temporal gyrus
Cerebellum

FIGURE 16-1
Lateral surface of the brain.

The inferior frontal gyrus is subdivided into an opercular part (OP), triangular part (T), and orbital part (OR). The triangular and opercular parts are separated by the ascending ramus of the lateral sulcus, and the triangular and orbital parts by the horizontal ramus of the ~~lateral~~ lateral sulcus.

Choroid plexus
Third ventricle
Central sulcus
Paracentral gyrus
Corpus callosum
Cingulate gyrus
Thalamus
Septal area
Hypothalamus
Parieto-occipital sulcus
Lamina terminalis
Calcarine sulcus
Primary visual cortex
Iter
Pituitary gland
Midbrain
Pons
Medulla
Cerebellum

FIGURE 16-2
Median sagittal section of the brain.

Choroid plexus
Fourth ventricle

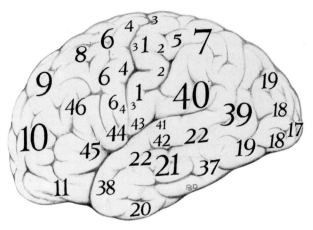

piriform area) is relatively and absolutely larger in man than in other primates. It generally includes the uncus, parahippocampal gyrus medial to the rhinal sulcus, prepiriform cortex, anterior perforated substance, and some small adjacent areas of cortical tissue (Figs. 1-4, 15-2). The mesocortex (mesallocortex, juxtallocortex) includes the cortex of the cingulate gyrus.

Neocortex

GENERAL ORGANIZATION

On the basis of cytoarchitectural criteria, the cortex has been parceled into 20 areas (Campbell), 47 areas (Brodmann), 109 areas (von Economo), and over 200 areas (Vogt). The numbered areas of Brodmann are commonly used (Figs. 16-3, 16-4). These subdivisions are useful for discussion purposes, but their precise functional roles are not fully resolved. Many of these areas are readily distinguished by microscopic criteria, but many others are based on subtle criteria. In a general way, the "motor" or "expressive cortex" is mainly located rostral to the central sulcus; the "sensory or receptive cortex" is mainly located occipital to the central sulcus.

The frontal lobe comprises the motor cortex (precentral gyrus, area 4), premotor cortex, prefrontal cortex, supplementary motor cortex, and

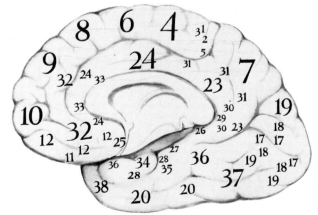

446

Broca's speech area; the parietal lobe consists of a general somatic sensory cortex (postcentral gyrus, areas 1, 2, and 3), second sensory cortex (including part of area 4), and an association area; the occipital lobe consists of a primary visual cortex (area 17) and an association area; and the temporal lobe consists of a primary auditory cortex (area 41) and an association area (areas 42 and 22). The association cortical areas of the parietal, temporal, and occipital lobes are concerned with the "higher integrative functions" of the general senses, vision, and audition. A wide area of the anterior temporal lobe association cortex has been called the "interpretive cortex." The association areas receive input from the adjacent primary and secondary sensory areas and are interconnected by reciprocal connections with several thalamic nuclei. The processing of the more elemental forms of the sensory input takes place within these association areas and the dorsal tier of the thalamic nuclei.

MICROSCOPIC ANATOMY OF THE NEOCORTEX

Horizontal organization The neocortex is laminated into six horizontal sheets. These conventionally recognized six laminae (Figs. 16-5 and 16-6), beginning at the cortical surface, are *1* plexiform layer, or molecular layer of nerve fibers oriented tangential to the cortical surface, *2* external granular layer, or layers of small pyramidal cells, *3* layer of medium-sized and large pyramidal cells, or external pyramidal layer, *4* internal granular layer, or layer of small stellate and pyramidal cells, *5* inner or deep layer of large pyramidal cells, and *6* spindle cell layer, layer of fusiform cells, or multiform layer.

The neocortex with each of the six laminae clearly evident is known as the "homotypic cortex" (generalized six-layered type), whereas the neocortex with the six laminae present but not clearly demarcated is known as the "heterotypic cortex." The heterotypic cortex with a scant number of granule neurons (discussed below) is called the "agranular cortex," while that with numerous granule (stellate) neurons is called the "granular cortex" ("koniocortex"). The pri-

mary visual cortex (area 17) is a heterotypic granular cortex; the primary auditory cortex (areas 41, 42) and the primary somesthetic cortex (areas 1, 2, and 3) are homotypic granular cortices; and the primary motor cortex (area 4) is a homotypic agranular cortex. The heterotypic cortex is the more common neocortical pattern. Other cytoarchitectural schemas have been described.

Neocortical neurons Five basic neuronal types may be considered representative of the more than 60 cortical cell types that have been described. The pyramidal neurons and the stellate (granular) neurons are the most common. There are approximately 5.5 billion *pyramidal cells* and 4.5 billion *stellate cells*. The other three basic

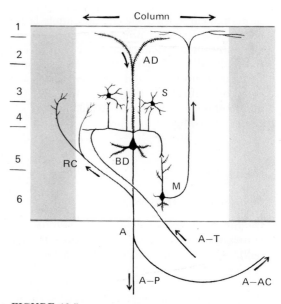

FIGURE 16-5
Schema of the vertical columnar organization of the cerebral cortex.

The basic types of cortical neurons are indicated. A, axon of a pyramidal neuron; A-AC, axon of association or commissural fiber; AD, apical dendrite of a pyramidal neuron; A-P, axon of projection fiber; A-T, axon of neuron in a specific thalamic nucleus; BD, basilar dendrites of a pyramidal neuron; M, Martinotti cell; RC, recurrent collateral branch; S, stellate cell (granule, Golgi type II cell). Each pyramidal neuron may be an association neuron, commissural neuron, or projection neuron, but not all three. Arabic numerals indicate the six horizontal laminae of the neocortex.

SURFACE OF CEREBRAL CORTEX

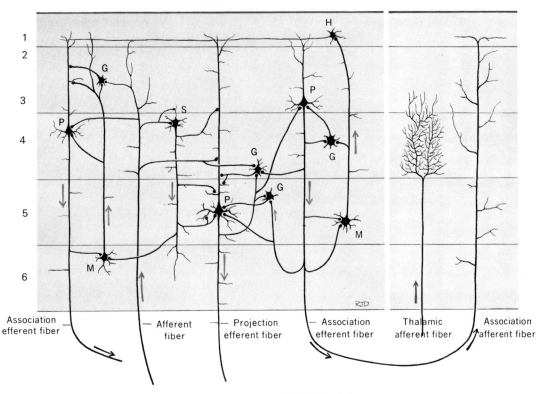

1
2
3
4
5
6

Association
efferent fiber — Afferent
fiber — Projection
efferent fiber — Association
efferent fiber — Thalamic
afferent fiber — Association
afferent fiber

FIGURE 16-6
Some intracortical circuits of the neocortex.

neocortical cell types are the *horizontal cells of Cajal, cells of Martinotti,* and *polymorph (multiform) cells.*

Each *pyramidal cell* has a pyramid-shaped cell body with its apex directed toward the cortical surface (Figs. 16-5 through 16-8). The apex is continuous as the apical dendrite that terminates as several branches in the molecular layer. Short collateral branches extend horizontally from the apical dendrite. Several horizontally directed dendrites, known as "basilar dendrites," extend from the cell body. The branches of all dendrites have numerous spines, which increase the surface area of the neuron. The cell bodies (ranging from 10 to over 50 μm in diameter) of pyramidal cells are found in all cortical laminae, except the molecular layer. The giant pyramidal cells, called Betz cells, are found in layer 5 of cortical area 4. The relative amount of synaptic activity on the dendrites as compared with that on the cell body of a pyramidal cell

Afferent fibers to the cortex include the thalamocortical, commissural, and association fibers. Some stellate cells (S) have long axons which extend vertically to the deeper cortical layers. The Martinotti cells (M) have long axons which extend vertically to the superficial cortical layers. Other stellate cells (granule cells, G) have short axons which terminate in their immediate vicinity. Pyramidal cells (P) have long axons which, before emerging from the cortex, send recurrent and transverse collateral branches to terminate within the cortex. The horizontal cells of Cajal (H) are located in lamina 1. (*Adapted from Lorente de Nó.*)

can be gauged from the estimate that 90 percent of the dendritic–cell body surface area of each pyramidal cell is located on the dendrites.

The axon of a pyramidal cell extends from the base of the cell body into the subcortical white matter. Before leaving the gray matter, all axons

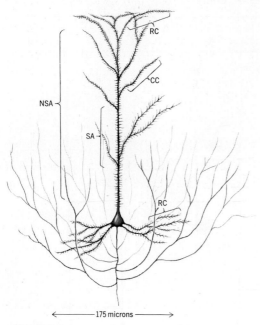

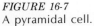

FIGURE 16-7
A pyramidal cell.

Note the source of the input to the various regions of the dendritic arborization. The afferents from the specific afferent thalamic nuclei (SA) terminate on the central third of the apical shafts of cells with cell bodies in lamina V. The afferents of corpus callosal fibers (CC) are distributed to oblique branches of apical dendrites. The axon recurrent collaterals (RC) of other pyramidal cells are distributed on the tips of apical arches and basilar dendrites. The nonspecific afferents (NSA) terminate widely on the apical dendrites. (*Adapted from Scheibel, Scheibel, and Globus.*)

have one or more branches, called "axon collateral branches," which project back (recurrent axon collaterals) or extend horizontally (horizontal axon collaterals) into the gray matter as intracortical association fibers (Fig. 16-5). These collaterals synapse in the immediate vicinity with stellate neurons. The main axon projects into the subcortical white matter. These axons project as *1* association fibers to other cortical areas in the same hemisphere; *2* commissural

fibers to the same cortical areas in the opposite hemisphere; or *3* projection fibers to subcortical gray matter of the cerebral hemispheres (corpus striatum), the diencephalon (thalamus), the brainstem, and the spinal cord.

There are many varieties of pyramidal cells, including the fusiform cells of layer 6. Ontogenetically, the pyramidal cells tend to mature in the following sequence: *1* the apical dendrites differentiate slightly before the basilar dendrites, and *2* the axodendritic synapses develop somewhat before the axosomatic synapses.

Each *stellate cell* (granule cell, Golgi type II cell, star-shaped cell) has a star-shaped cell body with short, extensively branched dendrites and with a short axon that arborizes in the immediate area. These intracortical cells are found in all cortical laminae (Fig. 16-6). Numerous varieties of stellate cells exist.

The *cells of Martinotti* are multipolar neurons with short branched dendrites (Fig. 16-6). Each cell has a myelinated axon that extends to the molecular layer. Horizontal collateral branches of this intracortical neuron extend into the various laminae. These association cells of Martinotti may be considered as modified stellate cells.

The *horizontal cells of Cajal* are small neurons of the molecular layer. These association cells have dendrites and axons that are parallel in direction to the cortical surface. These neurons, which are present in young but rarely in adult animals, are the only cortical neurons oriented entirely in the horizontal plane.

Many neurons may be modified types of pyramidal cells; the cell bodies of these neurons have a wide variety of shapes and contours, hence *polymorph, multiform, and fusiform neurons.* They are more commonly found in the sixth cortical layer. The dendrites of these neurons extend into the more superficial cortical layers, and the axons project into the white matter.

Vertical or columnar organization Microelectrode studies of the primary somesthetic cortex (areas 3, 1, and 2) of the cat lead to the concept that the elementary organization of the cortex is a "column" of neurons (from one to several neurons thick) oriented vertically to the cortical surface (Fig. 16-6). Many vertical cylinders of

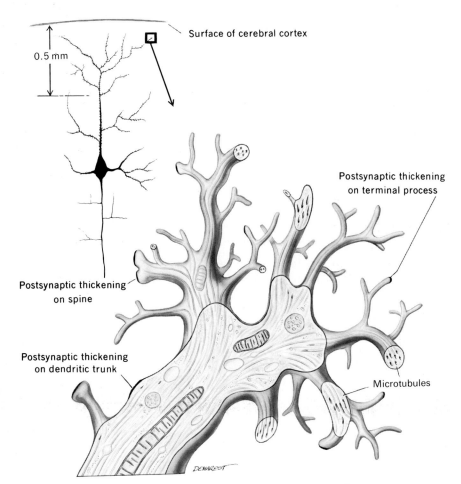

Surface of cerebral cortex

0.5 mm

Postsynaptic thickening
on terminal process

Postsynaptic thickening
on spine

Postsynaptic thickening
on dendritic trunk

Microtubules

DEMAREST

FIGURE 16-8
Terminal processes of a small dendritic branch
of a pyramidal neuron of the neocortex as reconstructed from electron micrographs.

The thickenings of the subsynaptic membrane are indicated *1* on the dendritic trunk, *2* on a dendritic
spine, and *3* on a terminal process. A major portion
of the total dendritic surface does not contain postsynaptic thickenings. (*Pappas and Purpura*, Exp. Neurol., *Academic Press, Inc., New York, 1961.*)

neurons constitute this cortical area. A specific
cylinder is activated by one and only one of the
following stimuli: *1* movement of groups of
hairs, *2* pressure on the skin, and *3* deformation of the tissues deep to the skin from a specific "spot" of the body. The primary visual cortex (area 17), the primary auditory cortex (areas
41, 42), and the primary motor cortex (area 4)
are also organized as vertical columns of neurons. These vertical columns of neurons are
connected with other areas of the cortex by
association fibers and with subcortical nuclei by
projection fibers. Each electrophysiologically
defined column of neurons may be considered
as the ultimate in cortical parcellation.

The columns are not simple geometric ar-
rangements but complexes of neurons and
neuronal circuits which are more functionally
real than anatomically apparent. They differ in
size. Although an individual column may have

a sharp physiologically defined boundary, it usually overlaps with adjacent columns. Thus a cortical neuron may be located within several columns. These columns are close enough so that one neuron may be located within several columns and that cross-talk probably occurs between two columns.

There is a morphologic basis for the cylindric columns of different sizes. The afferent fibers to the cortex terminate in cylindric spreads. Those from cells in the specific thalamic nuclei arborize in a plexus of about 200 to 500 μm in diameter, while the nonspecific thalamic afferent fibers terminate in spreads up to 3 mm in diameter (Scheibel and Scheibel). The pyramidal cells have dendrites which radiate from the central axis of the cell body and main shaft of the apical dendrite. The horizontal spread of the basilar dendrites and distal branches of the apical dendrites range from 150 to 300 μm (Figs. 16-5, 16-7), although spreads of 500 μm for the apical dendrites and 600 μm for the basilar dendrites have been reported. The axons of the stellate cells, Martinotti cells, and fusiform cells are generally oriented vertically within the cortex. They provide the essential circuitry for a vertical column.

The general organization of the fibers conveying input to and output from the cortex is consistent with the cortical columnar organization. Although the afferent fibers to the cortex form fasciculi which enter the cortical sheet at an angle (Fig. 16-5), each afferent fiber, as noted above, terminates in a cylindric arborization. The efferent fibers emerge from the cortex as fasciculi oriented perpendicular to the neocortex (Fig. 16-5).

Input to the pyramidal neurons (Fig. 16-7)   The afferent projections to the cortex terminate in organized patterns upon the pyramidal cells and other cortical neurons. These inputs are directed differentially to a number of sites of each pyramidal cell (Globus and Scheibel). The following is a general, but incomplete, statement. The specific sensory afferent fibers synapse with the central third of the main shaft of the apical dendrites of pyramidal cells with cell bodies in the fifth cortical layer. Nonspecific afferent inputs from the thalamus and brainstem are exerted over the entire main shaft and some branches of the apical dendrites. The commissural fibers of the corpus callosum terminate upon oblique branches of the shaft of the apical dendrites. The recurrent collateral axonal branches of pyramidal cells are distributed to the outer segments of the basilar and apical dendrites of other pyramidal cells. Although much input to the pyramidal cells is through direct synaptic connections, most of it is conveyed to the cortical interneuron, e.g., stellate cells; they are intercalated between the association, projection, and commissural fibers and the pyramidal cells.

White matter of the cerebrum

The white matter of the cerebrum is composed of association, commissural, and projection fibers.

ASSOCIATION, OR INTRAHEMISPHERIC, FIBERS

The *association fibers* are the axons of pyramidal cells projecting to other cortical areas of the same hemisphere. An innumerable number of short association fibers interconnect adjacent gyri or adjoining sectors within a gyrus. These short association fibers may remain wholly within the cortex (*intracortical*) or may pass through the white matter (*subcortical*). Long association fiber bundles reciprocally interconnect distant cortical areas within the same hemisphere.

The *intracortical association fibers* project their axonal branches (recurrent and transverse collateral branches) for short distances probably restricted to the confines of a cluster of vertical columns. The *subcortical association fibers* form bundles of fibers, called *arcuate or U association fiber bundles*, which pass from a cortical area of one gyrus to an area of an adjacent gyrus. These fibers course in an arc within the white matter deep and transverse to the sulcus between the gyri. Fibers do not pass lengthwise along the long axis of a gyrus. Some fascicles of arcuate fibers may extend deep to two or three sulci before terminating in the cortex.

The *long association fibers* form several

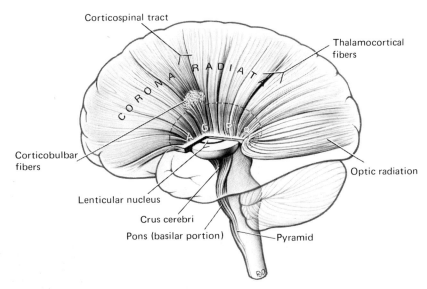

Corticospinal tract

Thalamocortical fibers

Corticobulbar fibers

Optic radiation

Lenticular nucleus

Crus cerebri

Pons (basilar portion)

Pyramid

FIGURE 16-9
Some component fiber tracts of the internal capsule and their cortical projections.

A, anterior limb; G, genu; P, posterior limb; R, retrolenticular portion of the posterior limb.

named intrahemispheric bundles: superior longitudinal fasciculus, arcuate fasciculus, inferior occipitofrontal fasciculus, inferior longitudinal fasciculus, uncinate fasciculus, and vertical occipital fasciculus. The fiber components of each fasciculus are organized precisely. The fibers originating from a limited area project and terminate in definite regions of the cortex. These regions of termination are usually located within cytoarchitecturally delimited zone(s) within a Brodmann area(s); this indicates that each Brodmann area projects fibers in an organized pattern to other Brodmann areas.

The *superior longitudinal fasciculus* interconnects most of the frontal lobe with the parietal and occipital lobes; the main mass of the fasciculus is located just above the insula. The *arcuate fasciculus* is an extension of the superior longitudinal fasciculus which arcs around the insula and extends into the temporal lobe. The *inferior occipitofrontal fasciculus* interconnects the inferior part of the frontal lobe with the temporal and occipital lobes; the main mass of the bundle passes beneath the lenticular nucleus and insula. The *uncinate fasciculus* is a compact arc of fibers which interconnects the cortex of the basal frontal lobe with the cortex of the temporal pole. The *inferior longitudinal fasciculus* is a fiber bundle extending from the temporal lobe to the occipital lobe. Both the

uncinate fasciculus and the inferior longitudinal fasciculus can be considered to be portions of the inferior occipitofrontal fasciculus. The *vertical occipital fasciculus* consists of fibers connecting the inferior parietal lobule and adjacent occipital lobe with the caudal portions of the temporal gyri and adjacent occipital cortex.

COMMISSURAL, OR INTERHEMISPHERIC, FIBERS

The commissural fibers are pyramidal cell axons that generally interconnect an area of one hemisphere with its counterpart area of the contralateral hemisphere. They form the corpus callosum, anterior commissure, commissure of the fornix, and habenular commissure.

The corpus callosum is the massive commissure interconnecting most of the neocortical areas of one hemisphere with the other hemisphere (Figs. 15-2, 16-9, and 16-10). The primary visual cortex (area 17), somatosensory cortex

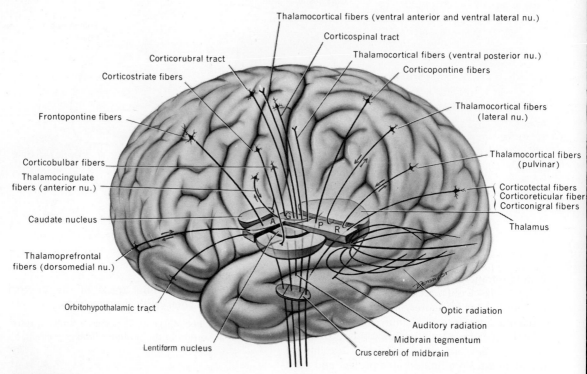

Thalamocortical fibers (ventral anterior and ventral lateral nu.)

Corticospinal tract

Corticorubral tract

Thalamocortical fibers (ventral posterior nu.)

Corticostriate fibers

Corticopontine fibers

Frontopontine fibers

Thalamocortical fibers (lateral nu.)

Corticobulbar fibers

Thalamocortical fibers (pulvinar)

Thalamocingulate fibers (anterior nu.)

Corticotectal fibers
Corticoreticular fiber
Corticonigral fibers

Caudate nucleus

Thalamus

Thalamoprefrontal fibers (dorsomedial nu.)

Orbitohypothalamic tract

Optic radiation

Auditory radiation

Midbrain tegmentum

Lentiform nucleus

Crus cerebri of midbrain

FIGURE 16-10
Some component fiber tracts of the internal capsule and their cortical connections.

Reciprocal projections between a thalamic nucleus and a cortical area are indicated by arrows pointing in two directions. The nuclei refer to nuclei of the thalamus. A, anterior limb; G, genu; P, posterior limb; R, retrolenticular portion of the posterior limb.

(areas 3, 1, and 2), part of the primary auditory cortex (area 41), and the regions of the motor cortex serving the upper and lower extremities (area 4) give rise to and receive few, if any, callosal fibers. The face, pectoral girdle, trunk, and pelvic girdle regions of the motor cortex (area 4) are the sites of the origin and termination of many callosal fibers. The fibers of the corpus callosum originate from pyramidal cells with cell bodies mainly in lamina 3; they terminate in laminae 1 to 4 of the corresponding areas of the contralateral cerebral cortex.

Callosal fibers may have many collateral branches in addition to those terminating in the cortex. This extensive collateralization may include projection fibers, which may terminate in the corpus striatum of either the same or the opposite side. Some projection fibers from the cortex may pass successively through the corpus callosum and internal capsule before terminating in the subcortical centers; these fibers do not have any collateral branches that terminate in the cortex.

The anterior commissure interconnects portions of the paleocortex and neocortex. The paleocortical regions connected by this commissure include the cerebral cortex medial to the rhinal sulcus. In man there are, at the most, only sparse anterior commissural fiber connections between the amygdaloid bodies, olfactory bulbs, and anterior perforated substances of the two sides. A shift occurred during evolution so that in man, the anterior commissure is primarily a neocortical commissure. It interconnects neocortical areas which are not interconnected by the corpus callosum. Thus the anterior commissure is mainly a commissure for the neocortex of the anterior temporal cortex, which includes portions of the superior, middle, and inferior temporal gyri and the inferotemporal visual area of each side.

The *commissure of the fornix* consists of fibers that originate in the hippocampus, pass through the fimbria of the fornix, decussate across the midline (ventral to the splenium of the corpus callosum), pass through the fimbria, and terminate in the contralateral hippocampus. This is a commissure of the archicortex.

The habenular commissure consists of fibers of the stria medullaris thalami crossing to the contralateral habenular nucleus (Fig. 15-4). Some fibers passing through the commissure are said to interconnect the habenular nuclei or the amygdaloid body or the hippocampal formation. This commissure is of unknown significance.

PROJECTION FIBERS

The projection fibers include *1* the descending (corticofugal) pathways which originate in the cortex (axons of pyramidal cells) and project to the nuclei of the basal ganglia, diencephalon, brainstem, and spinal cord; and *2* the ascending (corticopetal) pathways which mainly originate from diencephalic nuclei, project to, and terminate in the cortex (Fig. 16-10). The corticofugal fibers to the basal ganglia, hypothalamus, substantia nigra, red nucleus, and nuclei of the ascending pathways are sometimes referred to as "corticonuclear fibers." These projection fibers are funneled through the fornix, external capsule, and internal capsule. The fornix conveys fibers to and from the hippocampus (Chap. 15). The external capsule is partly made up of fibers projecting to the corpus striatum (corticostriate fibers) and to the brainstem tegmentum (corticotegmental, corticoreticular, or corticobulbar fibers). The internal capsule is the main "highway" for input to and output from the cerebral cortex.

INTERNAL CAPSULE

The internal capsule has the shape of an open Japanese fan (Fig. 1-7). The ribs of the fan parallel the course of the fiber bundles (Figs. 16-9 and 16-10). The handle of the fan is analogous to the crus cerebri of the midbrain; the lower half of the fan, to the internal capsule; the upper half of the fan, to the corona radiata (radiating crown) of the cerebral white matter; and the distal margin of the fan, to the gray matter. The pathways of the internal capsule, their sites of origin, and their sites of termination are outlined below. Many fibers do not extend through all portions of the "fan" (e.g., striate fibers and thalamocortical fibers are not found in the "handle").

The *anterior limb of the internal capsule* contains fibers projecting either to or from the frontal lobe (Figs. 16-9, 16-11). The reciprocal connections include *1* fibers from the prefrontal cortex to the dorsomedial thalamic nucleus, and from the dorsomedial thalamic nucleus to the prefrontal cortex; and *2* fibers from the cingulate gyrus to the anterior thalamic nuclei, and from the anterior thalamic nuclei to the cingulate gyrus (Chap. 15). The frontopontine fibers to the nuclei located in the pons are integrated into the cerebellar systems (Chap. 9). The orbitohypothalamic fibers of the median forebrain bundle (Chap. 15) and some corticostriate fibers (Chap. 14) to the caudate nucleus (subcallosal fasciculus) pass through this limb.

The *genu of the internal capsule* contains the corticobulbar and corticoreticular fibers (Figs. 16-9 through 16-11). The fibers from the frontal eye fields (Chap. 12) synapse in the brainstem tegmentum with interneurons that innervate the motor nuclei of the eye muscles (oculomotor, trochlear, and abducent motor nuclei) in complex patterns so as to influence the conjugate movements of the eyes. Other corticobulbar fibers terminate in the tegmentum on interneurons that innervate the motor nuclei of the trigeminal nerve, facial nerve, and hypoglossal nerve, nucleus ambiguus, and nucleus of the spinal accessory nerve (Chaps. 7 and 8). Some ascending (sensory) thalamic fibers project to the "motor cortex" of the frontal lobe.

The *posterior limb proper (thalamolenticular portion)* is composed of both motor pathways and sensory pathways (Figs. 16-9 through 16-11).

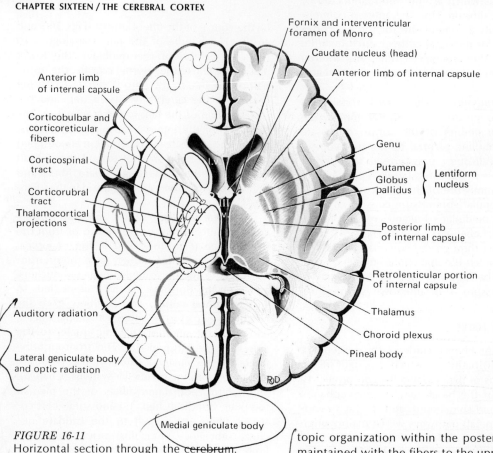

FIGURE 16-11
Horizontal section through the cerebrum.

Note the location of the head of the caudate nucleus, lentiform nucleus, and thalamus relative to the ventricles and the internal capsule. The components of the internal capsule are indicated on the left side. The somatotopic organization of the corticospinal tracts is indicated by: U, upper extremity; T, trunk; L, lower extremity.

Through the rostral half of this limb pass fibers that are associated with the cortex of the posterior aspect of the frontal lobe. These include the major motor output from the cerebral cortex. The corticospinal tract (pyramidal tract) originates primarily from neurons in areas 4 and 6 of the frontal lobe and some portions of the parietal lobe. Its fibers terminate mainly in laminae 4, 5, 6, and 7 of the spinal gray matter; a few fibers terminate in lamina 9. The somato-topic organization within the posterior limb is maintained with the fibers to the upper extremity located rostrally (next to the genu) to those fibers to the trunk and lower extremity, respectively. Through the caudal half of this limb pass many of the pathways from the thalamus (thalamocortical radiation) to the parietal cortex and temporal cortex. The thalamic radiation from the ventral anterior thalamic nucleus and the ventral lateral thalamic nucleus projects to areas 4 and 6 of the frontal lobe (Chap. 14). The radiation from the ventral posterior nucleus projects to the postcentral gyrus (areas 1, 2, and 3). Some corticofugal connections from the postcentral gyrus terminate in the ventral posterior nucleus. Extensive reciprocal connections exist between the lateral thalamic nuclear group and the parietal cortex and temporal cortex.

The retrolenticular and sublenticular portions of the internal capsule comprise the fibers associated with the auditory and visual cortical areas of the temporal and occipital lobes (Figs. 16-9 through 16-11). The auditory radiation originates in the medial geniculate nucleus, and terminates in the transverse temporal gyri of Heschl. Some descending cortical fibers terminate in the medial geniculate body and in the inferior colliculus. The optic radiation originates in the lateral geniculate body and terminates in the primary visual cortex (area 17). Descending fibers from visual association area 18, 19, and 20 terminate in the pulvinar of the thalamus, pretectal region, and superior colliculus (Chap. 12), and in the brainstem reticular formation. The major corticopontine pathways project from extensive cortical areas to the pontine nuclei (Chap. 10); this includes the frontopontine, parietopontine, temporopontine, and occipitopontine tracts.

The precise course of the projection of the thalamic reticular system from the thalamus to the cerebral cortex is debatable. The pathways from the thalamic reticular nuclei are relayed through interneurons whose axons ultimately synapse with the cortical neurons.

Functional circuitry of the cortical neurons

In contrast to the horizontal orientation of the cortical laminae, the functional "units" of the cerebral cortex are actually oriented in "vertical patterns" at right angles to the laminae (see "Microscopic Anatomy of the Neocortex," earlier in this chapter). These vertical "units" are organized into chains of neurons forming loops within other loops of varying complexity. Within the numerous variations of the basic neuronal types in the various regions of the neocortex, there "is a basic constancy in the general organization of the cortical afferents, intracortical neurons and intracortical distribution of the axons. What remains constant is the arrangement of the plexuses of dendritic and axonal branches; i.e., of the synaptic articulations through which nerve impulses are transmitted" (Lorente de Nó).

The following account is an abstraction of a complex organization that is, as yet, incompletely understood.

TWO-NEURON AND THREE-NEURON LOOPS

In theory the simplest loop is a *two-neuron chain;* it is similar to the two-neuron spinal reflex arc. Such a loop would include a neuron with its cell body in the thalamus and a pyramidal neuron with its cell body in the cerebral cortex. The thalamic neuron from a specific thalamic nucleus synapses with a pyramidal cell that projects to a subcortical nucleus (Fig. 16-6). In the analogy with the spinal arc, this thalamic neuron is comparable to a spinal ganglion neuron, and the pyramidal cell is the equivalent of the anterior horn motor cell of the spinal cord.

The pyramidal cell is integrated into another loop. The recurrent axon collateral (and the horizontal collateral) branch of each pyramidal cell feeds back and synapses with one (or more) of the stellate interneurons that, in turn, may synapse with the original pyramidal neuron. This circuit is similar to the spinal cord circuit, with the stellate interneuron playing a role similar to that of the Renshaw interneuron (Chap. 5). The essence of a *three-neuron chain* can be constructed from the sequence of thalamic afferent neuron to interneuron stellate cell to cortical pyramidal cell (Fig. 16-6).

The basic two-neuron and three-neuron loops are the structural base from which other loops can be visualized. The projections from the specific nuclei of the thalamus (Chap. 13) arborize into a profuse terminal plexus, mainly in layer 4 and to a lesser extent in layer 3 of the cortex. The projections from the nonspecific nuclei (ascending reticular system) of the thalamus through, as yet, unknown connections have their terminal arborization in probably all cortical layers but especially in the superficial four layers (Fig. 16-6).

In general, the thalamic projections to the cortex terminate as synaptic connections with the stellate interneurons. In turn, these stellate cells synapse with the pyramidal cells. Direct connections with pyramidal cells are also present. Apparently the specific thalamic nuclei exert their influences largely upon the cell bodies and the adjacent portions of the dendrites (*axosomatic synapses*) of the pyramidal cells.

The nonspecific (reticular) thalamic nuclei exert their influences largely on the apical dendrites and the basilar dendrites (axodendritic synapses) of the pyramidal cells.

INTRACORTICAL LOOPS

Intracortical loops of neurons within the "units" of vertical chains contribute to the complexity (Fig. 16-6). Recurrent collateral branches of pyramidal cells synapse with Martinotti cells in the deep layers of the cortex. The Martinotti cells project to the superficial layers and synapse with stellate interneurons or with pyramidal cells. The long loops utilizing the Martinotti cells are considered to be phylogenetically old. Loops comprised of a pyramidal cell (through a recurrent collateral branch), a stellate interneuron with short axon, and a pyramidal cell are numerous in the cortex of man and higher primates. These short loops are phylogenetically new. The tremendous numbers of these stellate cells with short axons are significant. As Lorente de Nó states, *"Cajal assumed that the large number of cells with short axons was the anatomical expression of the delicacy of function of the brain of man. At present this assumption is almost a statement of fact."*

Some intracortical influences may be exerted laterally, largely through the horizontal cells of Cajal. This activity is minimal. These cells of Cajal are generally absent after neonatal life.

COMPLEX INTRA- AND INTERHEMISPHERIC LOOPS

The "units" of intracortical loops of one cortical area are connected with those of another area through the association pyramidal neurons (intrahemispheric) and the commissural pyramidal neurons (interhemispheric). These interconnections form intrahemispheric and interhemispheric loops. The axons of the pyramidal cells (and some deep stellate cells) comprise the long and short association fibers which have terminal branches in most layers of another area of the cortex (few in layers 1 and 4). Small cortical areas project, through pyramidal association neurons, to the small cortical areas from which they received projections; this forms the basis for reciprocally connected areas. The association neurons have synaptic connections with stellate interneurons and with pyramidal neurons. In addition, the commissural pyramidal cells form interhemispheric loops through their reciprocally connected pathways.

Further complexities are integrated through connections with subcortical nuclei. Many of the pyramidal cells of the cortex project to many thalamic nuclei and basal ganglia. In turn, many of these subcortical nuclei project back to the cerebral cortex, either through "direct feedback loops" between reciprocally interconnected cortical areas (Chap. 13) or through "indirect feedback loops" between the cortex and one or more subcortical nuclei before the projection back to the cortex (Chap. 14).

CYTOARCHITECTURAL FEATURES OF NEOCORTICAL AREAS

The outer layers of the cortex (laminae 1, 2, 3, and 4) are often called the *receptive layers*, because most of the afferent input fibers terminate in these layers. The deeper layers (laminae 5 and 6) are often called the *discharge layer,* because the many pyramidal cells concentrated in these layers are a major source of efferent projection and association fibers (Fig. 16-6). This stratification into receptive and discharge layers is not absolute, for, in effect, each cortical area and each lamina of the sensory, motor or association cortex is both a terminus for input and a source of output.

Nerve fibers which are oriented parallel to the cortical laminae form small bundles called *stripes,* or *bands.* These horizontal stripes are more prominent in some layers than in others: the stripe of Kaes in lamina 2, the inner stripe of Baillarger in lamina 5, and the outer stripe of Baillarger in part of lamina 4. The two stripes of Baillarger form a common stripe called the *line of Gennari* in the primary visual cortex (17). These stripes are visible to the naked eye in some areas. The fibers that comprise them include the basilar dendrites and horizontal axon collaterals of the pyramidal cells, as well as some collateral and terminal branches of afferent fibers.

Neurophysiology of cortex and electroencephalogram

The neurophysiologic activity of the brain induces variations in the electrical potentials that can be recorded with electrodes placed on the surface of the scalp. The record of these voltage shifts is known as an *electroencephalogram* (EEG). The fluctuating potential differences on the unshaven scalp surface usually range between such minute amounts as 50- to 100-millionth of a volt (microvolts). This is about one-tenth of the voltage induced by the heart on the body surface (electrocardiographic potentials of the ECG). From the EEG record of a patient lying quietly in bed in semidarkness, an encephalographer can tell if a patient is awake, asleep, or excited.

The brain waves recorded by the electroencephalogram are largely produced by the electrical activity at the axosomatic synapses, axodendritic synapses, and the all-or-none axon potentials in the cerebral cortex. These scalp surface recordings are the result of the algebraic summation of the excitatory postsynaptic potentials (depolarization), inhibitory postsynaptic potentials (hyperpolarization), and the axon spike (all-or-none) potentials in the cerebral cortex. These activities are, in turn, influenced by the complex interactions derived from such subcortical stations as the specific thalamic nuclei and nonspecific thalamic nuclei, and from other cortical areas. The encephalogram is produced by the amplified electrical activity recorded as movement of a pen on a slowly moving sheet of paper. The EEG of an adult, like a fingerprint, is characteristic for the individual under standard conditions. However, it varies according to the state of the individual, i.e., whether he is alert, startled, drowsy, dreaming, or in deep sleep. The rhythms of children are less stable. The EEG pattern varies from one area to another area and from one person to another person.

The brain waves (rhythms) are described in terms of amplitude (in microvolts, one-millionth

of a volt) and of frequency (number of oscillations or waves per second). When the subject is awake, frequencies of about 10 per second constitute a normal rhythm. This is the alpha rhythm of the EEG. This alpha (α) rhythm is a high-voltage, slow-frequency rhythm (HVS) of 50 microvolts at a frequency of 8 to 14 per second. This rhythm is most prominent in the occipital region when the eyes are closed and is poorest in the frontal region. When an individual is alert, this resting alpha rhythm is replaced by an irregular, reduced-amplitude, rapid oscillation (desynchronization of alpha rhythm or alpha blocking) called the beta (β) pattern. This rhythm is present during states of attention and problem solving. The beta rhythm is a low-voltage, fast-frequency rhythm (LVF) of 5 to 10 microvolts at a frequency of from 15 to 30 per second. This is most prominent in the frontal and parietal regions. The HVS activity is referred to as a "synchronized" EEG pattern, and the LVF activity is called a "desynchronized" EEG or "activation" pattern.

The desynchronization of the alpha rhythm to the beta rhythm results from activation. It can be induced by a set of stimuli that produces sudden arousal. This arousal reaction is probably produced by ascending reticular system activity. Visual stimuli and alerting stimuli desynchronize the alpha rhythm to the beta pattern. Mental concentration can abolish the alpha rhythm. Beta rhythms are present at birth; the alpha rhythms generally are not found until about 9 years of age. The typical adult EEG pattern is usually established at about 17 or 18 years of age.

The complexity of the EEG patterns is largely regulated by subcortical activity (Chap. 13). Although the details of the factors responsible for these cortical rhythms are not fully known, this rhythmicity is dependent on the integrity of the thalamus. In fact, the cortex deprived of thalamic connections exhibits no rhythmic patterns. Rhythms generated in thalamic reticular nuclei project their influences through the unspecific thalamocortical pathways utilizing recruiting activity (Chap. 3). Only after several (8 to 10) electrical stimuli are applied to thalamic reticular nuclei is the maximal effect recorded upon the cortex, apparently largely through axodendritic synapses of the pyramidal cells.

Sleep

Normal consciousness is a state of psychologic awareness of the environment, sensations, and the self. Wakefulness, perception, and cognition are some of the qualities generally associated with consciousness. On the basis of subjective criteria, sleep seems to be quite different from the wakeful state. This is not so, for sleep is essentially an altered expression of consciousness. In one sense, sleep is a state of diminished consciousness in which, as compared to wakefulness, there is a change in the quality of the reactivity of the brain to events in the environment. During sleep mental activity does not cease and the capability to discriminate is retained. Actually the brain is not unaware. For example, even the muted cry of her baby will readily arouse the sleeping mother, whereas repetitive or insignificant, fairly loud sounds may not noticeably affect her sleep at all. Although sleep is essential for our well-being, the basic biologic significance of sleep is, as yet, unresolved.

The brain is often considered to be an organ that wants to sleep. This altered state of consciousness has been conceived as being induced *1* passively through the deprivation of sensory input (passive theory of sleep), or *2* actively through "sleep centers" (active theory of sleep). The two theories are not mutually exclusive.

Before 1950, sleep was thought to be primarily a passive phenomenon associated with a marked decrease in the amount of stimulation. According to this concept, the brain is said to fall asleep when it is not excited. There is some validity to this concept. The nature of the sensory influences conveyed from the periphery to the cerebrum via the ascending reticular pathways (Chap. 8) has profound effects on the sleep-wake cycle. When the cerebrum is de-

prived of this input by large lesions in the midbrain reticular formation, there is a drastic reduction in the sensory input to the cerebrum. Patients and animals with such lesions are behaviorally and electrophysiologically (i.e., as seen in the EEG rhythm) in a permanent sleep state. In these preparations, the cerebrum, although lacking reticular input, presumably receives all the lemniscal input from the brainstem and spinal cord and sensory input from the olfactory and visual systems.

It is now known that sleep is the expression of active phenomena occurring within the brain. The activity of subcortical neuronal pools accounts for the rhythms expressed by the EEG during sleep (Chap. 13). Electrical stimulation of certain "hypnogenic regions" within the thalamus induces sleep; damage to such regions produces permanently awake, insomniac animals. Low-frequency stimulation of a "hypnogenic region" results in a sleeping animal, whereas high-frequency stimulation (about 100 cycles per second) in the same region arouses the sleeping animal to the awakened state. Low-frequency stimulation is comparable to the sleep induced following the rhythmic stimulation of vestibular receptors by the gentle to-and-fro motion of the rocking chair. An active sleep center has been demonstrated to be present in the medulla (Chap. 8).

REM and NREM sleep Sleep is not a unitary but rather a complex, multifaceted phenomenon. On the basis of electroencephalographic (EEG), behavior, and psychologic criteria, two major types of sleep are recognized: rapid eye movement (REM) sleep and nonrapid eye movement (NREM or non-REM) sleep. NREM sleep is divided into four stages. The various types and stages of sleep can be differentiated from one another by differences *1* in the EEG wave patterns, *2* in behavior as expressed by somatic and autonomic activities and by the stimulus intensities required to awaken the sleeping subject, and *3* in psychologic manifestations of dreams and sensations related by an individual after arousal.

REM sleep is characterized by bursts of rapid conjugate eye movements accompanied by fluttering of the eyelids. It is called paradoxic sleep or behavioral sleep because the EEG exhibits a low-voltage fast EEG wave pattern (20 to 30 Hz), which is similar to that found in the aroused or awakened state. During REM sleep, vivid dreaming occurs, the heart rate and blood pressure are elevated, respiration is irregular and increased, and muscle tone is completely abolished. Cerebral blood flow is greater during dream sleep than during the waking state.

NREM or regular sleep is also called slow-wave sleep because the EEG potentials have a high-voltage, slow (1 to 10 Hz) wave pattern activity. During NREM sleep, the heart rate and blood pressure are somewhat reduced, respiratory rate is slow and regular, the pupil is constricted, and the motility and secretory activity of the gastrointestinal tract is normal. The somatic muscles are relaxed. Monosynaptic reflexes are slightly depressed. The antigravity muscles (e.g., neck, back, and extensors of the lower extremities) have less tone than those in the awake subject.

NREM sleep is divided into four stages. Stage 1 is characterized by slow rolling eye movements, regular respiration, drowsiness, decreased heart rate, and 7- to 10-Hz low-voltage EEG wave patterns. Stage 2 is characterized by light sleep from which the subject is readily aroused and by 3- to 7-Hz low-voltage EEG wave patterns with bursts of 12- to 14-Hz sleep spindles. (So-called K complexes occur; they are high-voltage bursts of waves before or after a sleep spindle.) Stage 3 is characterized by moderate-depth sleep, slow heartbeat, reduced blood pressure, constricted pupils, slightly depressed monosynaptic reflexes, and 1- to 2-Hz high-voltage EEG wave patterns with a few sleep spindles. State 4 is characterized by deep sleep, with 1- to 3-Hz high-voltage EEG wave patterns, which is similar to that occurring in a coma.

Sleep has a rhythmicity. A normal night's sleep consists of from 4 to 6 sleep cycles. Each cycle lasts about 1½ hr and consists of an NREM period followed by a REM period. In an average sleep cycle an individual spends a few minutes in the "half-awake, half-asleep" lightest phase of sleep (stage 1) before reaching the "medium" kind of sleep (stage 2). Later the subject passes into the deep-sleep phases (stages 3 and 4) and then gradually eases into REM sleep. Stages 3 and 4 are thought to be the most restorative and recuperative sleep periods. The relative time spent by an average young adult in each of the stages of one cycle may be divided roughly as

follows: 5 percent in stage 1 NREM, 50 percent in stage 2 NREM, 20 percent in stages 3 and 4 NREM, and 25 percent in the REM stage. The REM period of the first cycle is usually the shortest, lasting no more than 5 min (it may even be absent). The later REM periods may last from 30 to 60 min. Most NREM sleep occurs during the first third of a night's sleep, while most REM sleep takes place during the last third of sleep.

ONTOGENY OF SLEEP

The character of sleep changes with age. On the average, premature infants spend about 18 hr per day in active sleep. This is reduced to about 12 to 16 hr in the neonate, to about 8 hr in the adolescent and young adult, and to less than 6 hr in old age. The relative amount of NREM to REM sleep also shifts with age; neonates divide their sleep time equally between REM and NREM sleep, whereas the old subjects spend only an hour in REM sleep. During REM sleep, babies grimace and smile in bursts; their rapid eye movements can be observed under the eyelids. The neonate and young child have a polyphasic sleep-wake pattern in which a sleep period alternates with an awake period. The newborn infant has about seven of these sleep-wake cycles, which alternate fairly regularly during a 24-hr period. By the age of 4 this has been modified into a long night's sleep period supplemented by an afternoon nap. This grades into the monophasic sleep pattern of one sleep period per 24-hr day. It is not certain whether this ontogenetic change from polyphasic to monophasic sleep is induced by learning or is a natural inborn maturation phenomenon.

FUNCTIONAL CONSIDERATIONS OF THE SLEEP CYCLE

REM sleep is the dream stage. When awakened during this stage, four out of five individuals will describe a vivid, active dream colored by much imagery and some fantasies. Powerful inhibitory influences are exerted upon the lower motor neurons during REM sleep; this is a true paralysis, expressed by a marked decrease in the spontaneous and reflex somatic motor activity. The difficulty in making rapid movements (e.g., running) in a dream imagery is presumably the consequence of these inhibitory influences. REM sleep is the deepest state of sleep; it is more difficult to awaken a sleeping individual from REM sleep than from any of the NREM sleep stages.

Dreams with slight, if any, imagery may be experienced during NREM sleep. When awakened from this type of sleep, the aroused individual may describe a dream related to thought processes or experiences associated with mental activity.

Normally, there is a reduction in gastric secretions during sleep. In contrast, patients with chronic duodenal ulcers experience an increase in gastric acid secretion during REM sleep. Individuals afflicted with nocturnal migraine headaches almost always experience these headaches upon waking during or just following REM sleep. Alcohol, tranquilizers, and sleeping pills inhibit the amount of REM sleep.

Somnambulism, enuresis (bedwetting), and frightening nightmare attacks (of the type associated with a suffocating feeling and terror) occur, surprisingly, during NREM sleep stage 4, not during REM sleep. These phenomena are not thought to be manifestations of dreams.

The serotoninergic neurons with cell bodies in the brainstem raphe nuclei (Chap. 8) may have a significant role in the sleep-wake cycle. The destruction of these serotoninergic neurons results in an animal that is almost continuously awake. Animals treated with drugs which elevate the serotonin levels of the brain experience an increase in the duration of the NREM stage and a reduction in the amount of the REM state. Serotonin may be involved with triggering REM sleep. Norepinephrine is believed to mediate REM sleep.

Primary and secondary sensory areas

The areas of the cerebral cortex with the most direct afferent connections with the peripheral sensors are called the primary and secondary sensory areas (Figs. 16-12 through 16-14). The primary somesthetic area is located in the postcentral gyrus (areas 1, 2, and 3); the primary visual area, in the cortex on both sides of the calcarine sulcus (area 17); the primary auditory area, in the transverse gyri of Heschl (areas 41, 42); the primary gustatory area, in the ventral part of the postcentral gyrus (area 43); the "primary vestibular area," probably in the temporal lobe near the primary auditory cortex; and the primary olfactory cortex, in the cortex in the region of the uncus.

The secondary sensory areas are smaller than the primary sensory areas (Fig. 16-13). Whereas ablation of the primary sensory areas results in dramatic deficits in sensory appreciation, the ablation of the secondary areas results in slight, if any, deficits. Information on the secondary sensory areas in man is scant. A secondary somatic sensory area (somatic area II) is located in the cortex just above the lateral sulcus in the precentral and postcentral gyrus; a probable secondary auditory area (auditory area II) is located near the primary auditory area; and a probable secondary visual area (visual area II) is located on the lateral surface somewhere anterior to the primary visual cortex in areas 17 and 18.

Except for the olfactory cortex, the primary sensory area and the secondary sensory area receive their main input from the specific thalamic relay nuclei (ventral posterior nucleus, lateral geniculate body, and medial geniculate body). The primary olfactory cortex receives its input from the olfactory bulb.

Parietal lobe

The parietal lobe has a major role in the higher-level processing of the general sensory modalities and in the integration of neural data from the auditory, visual, and somesthetic cortical areas; it has a lesser role in motor activities.

PRIMARY SOMESTHETIC AREA
(AREAS 1, 2, and 3)

The postcentral gyrus or the primary receptive somesthetic area (areas 1, 2, and 3, primary somatic sensory area, somatic area I, SI) receives

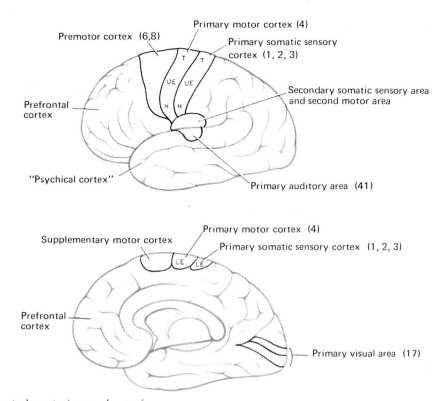

FIGURE 16-12
The location of several functional areas of the cerebral cortex.

The representation of body parts on the primary motor and somatic sensory cortices includes the head (H), upper extremity (UE), trunk (T), and lower extremity (LE). Numbers represent areas of Brodmann.

its input from the ventral posterior nucleus of the thalamus. This primary projection area has a somatotopic localization pattern in the form of a sensory homunculus (Fig. 16-14). The amount of cortical area associated with a body area is proportional to the sensory innervation density of the body area rather than to the size of the area (e.g., lips, tongue, and thumb have a relatively large representation). Area 2 responds to stimuli from the deep tissues of the body, especially to movements of joints; this is significant for the appreciation of movement and position sense. Area 3 responds to cutaneous stimuli. Most of the neurons of the ventral posterior thalamic nucleus project to area 3, and a lesser number to area 1. Most of the axons projecting to area 2 are apparently the collateral branches projecting to areas 3 and 1. The primary somesthetic area is often called a sensorimotor structure. This is so because 80 percent of the electric stimulations of its cortex in the awake human evoke sensations, while the remaining 20 percent evoke motor responses. Some fibers from this area project to such thalamic nuclei as the ventral posterior, ventral lateral, and reticular nuclei.

Some fibers originating in the postcentral gyrus descend via the pyramidal tract before terminating in the nuclei of the ascending pathways (refer to "Corticonuclear Fibers," later on in this chapter). These include the nuclei gracilis and cuneatus of the posterior column–medial lemniscal pathway. It is through these descending fibers that the somesthetic area influences this ascending pathway. This may explain why a monkey, following a lesion of the pyramidal tract, has a deficit in its ability to make certain kinesthetic discriminations.

Taste The primary area for taste is claimed to be located either at the base of the precentral gyrus and postcentral gyrus slightly rostral to the

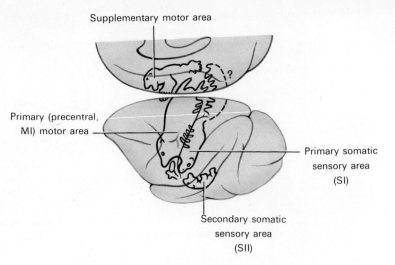

Supplementary motor area

Primary (precentral,
MI) motor area

Primary somatic
sensory area
(SI)

Secondary somatic
sensory area
(SII)

FIGURE 16-13
Some motor and sensory
areas of the monkey cortex,
with somatotopic representation.

The upper portion represents the
medial aspect. (*After Woolsey.*)

somesthetic area or in the immediate adjoining area of the insula (area 43). Stimulation of these areas may produce gustatory hallucinations.

SECONDARY SOMESTHETIC AREA

A secondary somesthetic area is apparently lo-cated at the base of the postcentral gyrus—occupying the same part of the cortex as the second motor area (Fig. 16-13). This area has also been called the secondary somatic sensory area, somatic area II, SII, and supplementary sensory projection area. This area has been located in primates by electrophysiologic techniques and is presumed to be also present in man. The somatotypic patterns in this area are less precise than in the primary somesthetic area (somatic area I). The face, mouth, and throat are appar-ently not represented in the secondary sensory area.

Functional considerations Stimulation of the primary somesthetic area in man evokes sensory effects on the contralateral side of the body. Numbness, absence of sensation, tingling, a feeling of electricity, or a sense of movement may result from focal stimulation. Patients do not inquire whether some object is in contact with the body region where sensation is felt. Actually the sensation is perceived as an unusual rather than a normal experience. Stimulation of

somatic sensory area II may evoke sensations similar to those produced by stimulation of the primary somesthetic area except that the sensa-tion may be felt bilaterally. This phenomenon may be explained by the fact that this sensory area receives input from the posterior thalamic region, which, in turn, receives input from both sides of the body.

Ablation of the postcentral gyrus is followed by loss of the finer and more subtle aspects of sensory awareness. When an object is handled (with the eyes closed) the patient can feel it but cannot appreciate its texture, estimate its weight, or gauge slight changes in its tempera-ture. Difficulty is experienced in appreciating the position of one's body or its parts. The crude aspects of the general sensory modalities are apparently sensed in subcortical nuclei. The conscious recognition of pain, temperature, and gross contact sense are apparently functional correlates of the midbrain tectum and the thala-mus in man. Ablation of somatic sensory area II produces no known deficits. The primary re-ceptive cortex integrates the information re-ceived from subcortical sources, and it is here that the more complex aspects of touch, deep sensibility, pain, and temperature are sensed. These perceptions include the appreciation of the location and position of a body part; the sensing of the movements of the body; the lo-

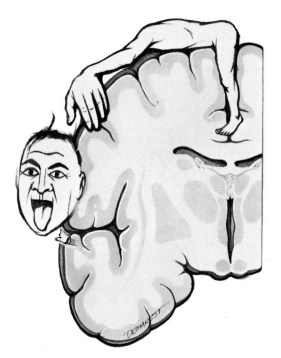

FIGURE 16-14
A motor homunculus on the precentral gyrus.

It shows the somatotopic localization of motor activity (following focal cortical stimulation). The sensory homunculus has a similar configuration.

calization of the source of pain, temperature, and tactile stimuli; and comparison of these sensed modalities with those formerly experienced.

SOMESTHETIC ASSOCIATION AREA

Areas 5, 7, and 40 of the parietal lobe are known as the "somesthetic association area." These areas receive an extensive input from the postcentral gyrus. In addition they have well-developed reciprocal connections (thalamocortical and corticothalamic pathways) with the lateral nuclear group of the thalamus, including the pulvinar (Chap. 13). These areas also make a contribution to the descending pathways through some corticospinal, corticotegmental, and corticopontine fibers. The integration essential to the appreciation of the finer and more discriminative aspects of the somesthetic senses is a functional correlate of the somesthetic asso-

ciation cortex. The expression of this higher-level sensory station is the product of the processing of the information received from the receptive somesthetic cortex and the interaction with the lateral nuclear group of the thalamus.

The parietal associative cortex integrates and correlates impulses associated with the somesthetic modalities and those associated with the auditory, gustatory, and visual senses. The whole complex of associative patterns subserves the knowledge and awareness of the individual of his environment. The conceptualization of qualities and quantities utilizes the basic somesthetic modalities. The qualities of shape, form, roughness, smoothness, size, and texture of an object (stereognosis) can be ascertained from a manual examination and can even be imagined. Quantities that can be deduced include weight, temperature changes, and the degree of pressure sensations. Of great significance is the awareness of body image, of location of body parts, of postural relation of body parts, one to the other, and of one's self. The consciousness of one's physical being is a dimension of the general senses.

Supramarginal gyrus Lesions in area 40, called the supramarginal gyrus, especially on the dominant side, produce deficits in the sphere of higher general sensations—cortical astereognosis and the failure of the so-called *body scheme.* Cortical astereognosis (*tactile agnosia*) is the inability to recognize common objects through cues from the general sensory receptors; it is the failure to appreciate the significance of the sensory stimuli. The agnosia may be in the visual sphere (*visual agnosia*), in the tactile sphere (*tactile agnosia*), or in the auditory sphere (*auditory agnosia*). Agnosia refers to those disturbances in which there is a failure to recognize, to identify, or to discriminate somatic sensory, visual, auditory, smell, or taste information. It is presumed that patients with pure agnosia have no basic deficits within the afferent pathways and in the reception of the primary input at the cerebral cortical level.

When a patient with lesions in the supramarginal gyrus feels a watch with the hand on the side opposite the lesions, he does not recognize the object as a watch. The intact primary cortex is functional because the patient can tell that the watch is smooth, cold, and light in weight, and he may sense the vibrations of the watch movements. Recognition of position sense and fine discrimination are not impaired. However, in this tactile agnosia the patient is unable to integrate the bits of information into the concept of a watch. The recognition of an object through the general senses requires an intact parietal association cortex, whereas the awareness of the various sensory modalities can be brought into the conscious sphere through subcortical centers and the postcentral gyrus cortex.

A large lesion in the superior parietal cortex usually results in the failure to recognize the body scheme. The recognition of self is impaired. For example, a patient with such a lesion may be unaware that his arm on the contralateral side of the lesion is his arm. In some patients the half of the face contralateral to the lesion is denied; that side may not be washed or shaved. Some mild motor effects such as hypotonia may be due to interruption of motor fibers originating from this area of the cortex.

ANGULAR GYRUS (AREA 39) AND WERNICKE'S AREA (AREA 22)

Areas 22 and 39 have rich connections with association fibers from the somesthetic (5 and 7), auditory (41 and 42), and visual (18 and 19) association cortex. These cortical areas subserve such complex expressions as the comprehension of the written word and the ability to conceive the symbols of language. The stimulation of these cortical areas in man evokes no effects. A lesion of area 39 in the dominant hemisphere produces dysfunctions indicative of the significant role this part of the cortex has to communication in man. Words are seen but not recognized (visual agnosia). The comprehension of the written word, whether in script or in type, is lost. This word blindness is expressed as the inability to read (*alexia*) or the inability to copy (*agraphia*). This is a form of *sensory* or *receptive*

aphasia. In sensory aphasia, the patient is unable to comprehend the written or spoken language. This visual receptive aphasia is so severe that words written by the patient himself are not recognized as words. Note that area 39 is adjacent to visual association cortex 18.

Bilateral lesions of the angular gyrus may produce a disorientation of spatial discrimination. The location of objects and the relating of one to another in space are so misjudged that the patient gropes about and often runs into these "seen" objects.

Lesions in *Wernicke's area* of the dominant hemisphere produce defects of an even "higher" order of complexity (Fig. 16-15). The patient loses the ability both to comprehend spoken words (auditory aphasia) and to express himself through them. Auditory agnosia is more complete if the damage to area 22 is bilateral, probably because auditory input to the cortex is bilateral. The intelligent, thinking person with this injury is at a loss to communicate his thoughts because words are unavailable to him. He has lost the tool of verbal expression. In effect he is a mute, although technically all the motor facilities for speech are unimpaired. (Refer to "Cerebral Dominance" and " 'Twin-Brain' Man," later on.)

Occipital lobe

The occipital cortex is composed mainly of the visual cortex. It is subdivided into striate area 17, known as the primary visual cortex, parastriate area 18, and the peristriate area 19. Areas 18 and 19 are called the *visual association area.* A secondary visual area may be located in areas 17 and 18 in man.

The striate cortex receives its input from the lateral geniculate body via the optic radiation and in turn projects its output via associative fibers to the visual association area. The visual association area has reciprocal connections with the pulvinar of the thalamus.

PRIMARY VISUAL AREA (AREA 17)

The primary visual area (area 17, visual area 1) is the primary receptive area for visual stimuli. Its loss in man results in complete blindness, indicating that our subcortical centers are not capable of elevating visual sensations to the conscious level. A patient can "see" with area 17 intact, even with a massive lesion in the association visual area. He may even avoid walking into a table, but he is unable to identify or appreciate the significance of the table through visual cues. Stimulation of this area in the normal man evokes no elaborate hallucinations but rather flashes of lights, shadows, and colors with movements in the contralateral fields of vision.

VISUAL ASSOCIATION AREA
(AREAS 18 AND 19)

Areas 18 and 19 subserve interpretive vision or the recognition of visual stimuli. Area 18 is often designated as visual area II (secondary visual area). Area 19 is often called visual area III. The objects "seen" by the striate cortex are processed and made meaningful in the association area. With lesions of the visual association area, especially on the dominant side, a *visual agnosia or psychic blindness* results. The patient cannot recognize or name an object. He has difficulty in determining its function or appreciating its significance from visual cues.

Electrical stimulation of areas 18 and 19 evokes an imagery similar to that sensed from stimulation of area 17. Restimulation of the same cortical site may produce the same or a different visual sensation. Flashes, stars, streaks of light, whirling disks in color or in black and white are perceived. These visual sensations move about and vary in brightness. Similar images are visualized by patients with irritative lesions in these areas. Stimulation of the anterior temporal lobe produces complex images of scenes and people. (See "Temporal Lobe 'Psychical Cortex,'" further on.)

Temporal lobe

The temporal lobe cortex comprises the neocortex and the allocortex. The neocortex has a major role in the "higher" functions of audition. It is also concerned with the visual sense and the vestibular sense. The anterior temporal pole neocortex is involved in the sphere of behavior, emotion, and personality through its connec-

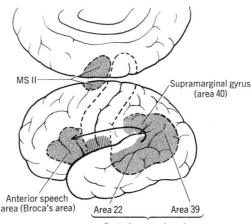

FIGURE 16-15
Location of some of the major functional association areas of the cerebral cortex.

The line and arrow indicate the location of the arcuate association fibers interconnecting the association areas in the parieto-occipital-temporal region with the frontal region. MSII, secondary somatic sensory and motor area. (*After Penfield and Roberts.*)

tions with the frontal and limbic lobes (Chaps. 13, 15), and in the visual and auditory spheres through extensive interconnections with the visual and auditory association areas. The anterior pole of the temporal lobe has been called the *psychical cortex.*

The allocortex is integrated with the olfactory sense and with the limbic system (Chap. 15).

PRIMARY AUDITORY AREA
(AREAS 41 AND 42)

The transverse gyri of Heschl (areas 41 and 42) comprise the primary auditory cortex (auditory area I). A tonotopic pattern is present, with low tones localized laterally and high tones medially (Fig. 10-6). A second auditory area (auditory area II) is probably located medial to the primary reception cortex. This auditory area II, identified in the monkey, has a reverse tonotopic representation and exhibits a higher threshold than the primary cortex. Area 22 of the superior temporal gyrus is the auditory association area.

The cortex of the superior temporal gyrus just rostral to the auditory cortex in man may subserve a conscious phase of the vestibular activity. Stimulation of this cortical area can evoke dizziness and even make the patient feel that he is rotating. This is considered to be the primary vestibular area.

Stimulation of the areas 41, 42, and 22 elicits sensations of sounds described as cricket chirping, bells, humming, buzzing, and whistling. The sounds may be heard as coming from the opposite ear. During stimulation, conversation picked up by the ears cannot be heard. At times, deafness may be subjectively sensed.

A patient can hear with areas 41 and 42 intact with a lesion in area 22 on the dominant side. He has profound difficulty in the interpretation of sounds; the spoken language may be utterly meaningless or extremely difficult to comprehend. He is not deaf, but cannot understand the conversation. This condition is known as *word deafness* and *auditory receptive aphasia*. The patient can speak but he makes many mistakes without realizing it.

Lesion of areas 41 and 42, on one side, results in the inability to locate the source of sound readily from auditory cues, but in only a slight loss of hearing. Subcortical centers and the redundancy in the central auditory pathways are functional and account for the high margin of physiologic safety (Chaps. 10 and 13).

TEMPORAL LOBE ASSOCIATION CORTEX

The posterior cortex of the temporal lobe is an association cortex where integration of the input from auditory, visual, and somesthetic sources occurs. Large lesions of the association cortex on the dominant side result in visual and auditory aphasia. The patient loses his ability to comprehend the written and spoken word and the symbolism associated with language. Agnosia is a consequence. Defect in the memory associated with these senses may occur. A deep lesion may interrupt the portion of the optic radiation which arcs into the temporal lobe (loop of Meyer); this results in a homonymous hemianopsia on the contralateral side (Chap. 12). The nonauditory cortex of the temporal lobe does not have such extensive connections with subcortical nuclei as does the association cortex of the occipital and parietal lobes.

TEMPORAL LOBE "PSYCHICAL CORTEX"

The neocortex of the region in the vicinity of the temporal pole has been called the "psychical cortex," because the responses obtained by stimulation of this area include associations relative to "experiences." Stimulation may elicit the recall of objects seen, or of music heard. Visual and auditory hallucinations may be produced; illusions which are similar to objects felt, seen, or heard in everyday experience. Feelings of fear may arise. The hallucination may be recall of an experience of the recent or distant past. It is a clear reenactment, unencumbered by confusion. A subsequent stimulation may evoke the same memory or a different memory. For example, the elicited experience may be a symphonic melody that is thought to be broadcast over a radio. The patient may, if requested, hum the tune at the tempo in which it is "heard." Later he will recall that he "heard" an orchestra playing the specific composition. The stimulation may evoke the recall of a conversation of a previous year. The patient with temporal lobe tumors may have auditory and visual hallucinations. He may see vivid scenery and friends not present, and he may hear songs not being sung. All these hallucinations can be consistent with experiences of reality because all could have been seen or heard in the past (*déjà vu*). The patient is cognizant of the hallucinations. Fearful feeling may ensue.

MOTOR ACTIVITY AND THE TEMPORAL LOBE

The temporal cortex may influence motor activity. Stimulation of this cortex, in man, may elicit facial movements on the same and opposite sides. In primates, bilateral movements of each of the four extremities can be evoked by stimulation of the temporal lobe on one side.

Insula

The cortex of the insula is somehow involved in both somatic and visceral functions. Its fiber connections are incompletely known. In the somatic sphere, the insula may have a supplementary motor area; stimulation of the insular cortex of a monkey may evoke somatic movements. The insula is apparently associated with visceral sensibility and visceral motor activity. Stimulation and irritation of this cortex (as in certain epileptic seizures) may produce some visceral sensations referable to many visceral organs. The insular cortex may have a role, probably minor, in such expressions as nausea, salivation, alteration in blood pressure and respiratory rhythms, piloerection, desire to urinate and to defecate, and belching.

Cortex and the motor pathways

Many areas of the cerebral cortex have roles in motor activity. These motor regions receive their main direct stimulation from the thalamus and from other cortical areas. The ventral lateral nucleus and the ventral anterior nucleus of the thalamus project powerful input to the cortex, mainly through axosomatic synapses with the pyramidal neurons, whereas the thalamic reticular nuclei exert their influences mainly through axodendritic synapses with the same cortical cells. The numerous association fibers from wide areas of the ipsilateral cortex and many callosal commissural fibers from the contralateral cortex are major sources of input to the motor cortex.

The motor areas project influences via a number of descending pathways to many subcortical nuclei and via association fibers and commissural (corpus callosum) fibers to many other areas of the cerebral cortex. The descending pathways include *1* the corticospinal tract, *2* corticobulbar fibers to cranial nerve motor nuclei, *3* corticoreticular fibers, *4* corticothalamic and corticostriate pathways, *5* corticonuclear fibers to nuclei of the ascending pathways, and *6* corticopontine tracts.

CORTICOSPINAL (PYRAMIDAL) TRACT

The corticospinal tract is composed of the axons of pyramidal cells located in frontal, parietal, occipital, and temporal lobes (Chap. 5). These fibers collect to form the pathway that descends in order through the rostral part of the posterior limb of the internal capsule, cerebral peduncle of the midbrain, pons proper, pyramids of the

medulla, and spinal cord (Fig. 5-24). Approximately two-fifths of the fibers project from the motor and from the premotor cortex (areas 4 and 6), another one-fifth project from the postcentral gyrus (areas 1, 2, and 3), and the remaining two-fifths project from the association cortex of the parietal lobe and possibly from the temporal and occipital lobes. In the precentral gyrus are the 34,000 giant (Betz) pyramidal cells which probably give rise to the small percentage of fast-conduction fibers of the pyramidal tract. Many collateral branches terminate in subcortical nuclei of the brainstem (Chap. 14). Roughly 90 percent of the 1 million fibers of the pyramidal tract cross over in the pyramidal decussation and terminate mainly on spinal cord interneurons, which, in turn, synapse with both alpha and gamma motor neurons (Chap. 5).

CORTICOBULBAR FIBERS TO CRANIAL NERVE MOTOR NUCLEI

The corticobulbar fibers consist of the axons of pyramidal cells located in many neocortical areas. For example, the frontal cortex (area 8), lower aspect of the precentral gyrus (area 4), and occipital association area can influence eye movements. Most of these axons descend through the genu of the internal capsule and terminate mainly on brainstem reticular formation interneurons, which, in turn, synapse with the lower motor neurons of the cranial nerves (Chap. 14). The course of the fiber groups of this pathway in the brainstem varies in different individuals. Bundles of corticobulbar fibers are found in both the basilar and tegmental portions of the brainstem. Because the fibers of this pathway synapse with interneurons in the reticular formation, they may be included with the corticoreticular fibers.

CORTICORETICULAR FIBERS

The corticoreticular fibers arise from pyramidal cells of wide areas of the neocortex, many from areas 4 to 6. These fibers pass through the internal capsule and terminate in the brainstem tegmentum. Many fibers terminate in the red nucleus (corticorubral tract), the tectum (corticotectal tract), and other tegmental nuclei.

This system exerts influences on the reticular nuclei of the pons and medulla, especially on those nuclei projecting to the spinal cord via the reticulospinal tracts (Chap. 5). Other descending fibers exert influences on the ascending reticular activating system (Chap. 8).

CORTICOTHALAMIC PATHWAYS AND CORTICOSTRIATE PATHWAYS

The cortex has connections with many of the subcortical nuclei, especially with certain thalamic nuclei, the corpus striatum, nucleus centrum medianum, subthalamus, substantia nigra, and some nuclei in the brainstem (Chaps. 13 and 14). The primary somesthetic cortex projects fibers to the ventral posterior thalamic nucleus, the primary visual cortex to the lateral geniculate body, the primary auditory cortex to the medial geniculate body, and the primary motor cortex (area 4) to the ventral lateral thalamic nucleus. The reciprocal interconnections of the neocortex with the other thalamic nuclei are discussed in Chap. 13 (Fig. 13-4). The cortex has many reciprocal connections with the thalamic nuclei. They do not form reverberating circuits.

The corticostriate fibers from frontal areas 4, 6, 9, and others have connections with the caudate nucleus, putamen, and substantia nigra. These pathways are integrated in the complex feedback circuitry that includes the globus pallidus and ventral anterior thalamic nucleus (Chap. 14).

CORTICONUCLEAR FIBERS (DESCENDING FIBERS FROM CORTEX TO NUCLEI OF ASCENDING PATHWAYS)

Many corticofugal fibers synapse, either directly or through interneurons, with the nuclei of the ascending pathways. These pathways transmit information that influences the processing occurring within these nuclei (Chaps. 8, 13). Included are the neocortical projections from the primary sensory areas to the ventral posterior thalamic nucleus (general senses), to the lateral geniculate body (vision), and to the medial geniculate body (audition). These descending pathways from the cortex also terminate in *1* the nucleus gracilis, nucleus cuneatus, and ventral posterior thalamic nucleus of the posterior column–medial lemniscus system; *2* the nucleus of the inferior colliculus, medial geniculate body, and other nuclei of the auditory pathways; *3* such brainstem nuclei as the cranial nerve nuclei of the trigeminal nerve; and *4* such spinal cord nuclei as the thoracic (Clarke's) nucleus and the gray matter of the posterior horn (Chaps. 5, 8, and 10). Because these fibers project from the cortex to subcortical nuclei, they are called corticonuclear fibers.

CORTICOPONTINE TRACTS

The corticopontine tracts are pathways which arise from the neocortex of all cerebral lobes, descend in order through the corona radiata, internal capsule, and crus cerebri before terminating within the ipsilateral pontine nuclei. These tracts are integrated into the feedback circuitry of the cerebellum with the cerebral cortex (Chap. 9).

Frontal lobe

The cortex of the frontal lobe is subdivided into several areas, with each subserving one or more roles.

1 The motor areas comprise the cortex of the precentral gyrus and the adjacent cortical areas of the superior, middle, and inferior frontal gyri (cortical areas 4, 6, and 8). They are associated with certain somatic motor activities.

2 The prefrontal cortex includes the cortex rostral to areas 6 and 8. It is somehow functionally integrated in circuits basic to many expressions of emotion and behavior.

3 The orbitofrontal cortex on the inferior surface of the frontal lobe (areas 11 and 12) is apparently the site of the linkage between the ascending reticular pathways and the neocortex (Chap. 15).

4 Broca's speech area is the cortical area of the opercular and triangular parts of the inferior frontal gyrus (areas 44 and 45). It is involved with the formulation of speech.

Primarily on the basis of observations of movements evoked by electrical stimulation of the cerebral cortex, several so-called motor areas have been designated. Ablation of these regions may result in changes in the qualities of the movements. These motor areas include *1* the primary motor area (area 4, MI, "the motor cortex"), which is the cortex of the precentral gyrus; *2* the premotor cortex (areas 6 and 8), located just rostral to the precentral gyrus; *3* the secondary motor area (second motor area, MII), located at the base of the precentral and postcentral gyri adjacent to the lateral sulcus, and coextensive with somatic sensory area II; and *4* the supplementary motor area, which is the portion of area 6 on the medial surface of the superior frontal gyrus rostral to area 4. The supplementary motor area is designated as MII by some authors.

The primary, secondary, and supplementary motor areas are somatotopically organized in caricature figurines. Each figurine is called a *homunculus* (Fig. 16-14). The head and body image represented by the MI homunculus is large as compared with images represented by the MII and supplementary motor homunculi. The MI figurine is oriented "upside down" on area 4, with the head located near the lateral sulcus and the lower extremity in the paracentral lobule (Fig. 16-13). In a general way, motor area MI faces sensory area SI as mirror images, with the line of the central sulcus acting as an interface. The body image of MII in man is presumed to be oriented with the upper body located rostrally and the lower extremity caudally. The homunculus of the supplementary motor cortex is sequentially organized with the head located rostrally and the lower extremity caudally. Although electrical stimulation of each of these areas normally evokes a motor response, such stimulation does, at times, evoke a sensation; hence these motor areas are often called sensorimotor areas.

Association fibers interconnect some of the motor areas with one another and with somesthetic sensory areas. The primary motor area projects topographically to MII, supplementary motor area, premotor area, and somesthetic sensory areas SI and SII. The premotor cortex has connections with MI, MII, and adjacent prefrontal cortex. The supplementary motor area has topographic connections with MI and the pre-

motor cortex. The corticofugal projections from these motor areas to the subcortical nuclei, brainstem, and spinal cord are conveyed via several descending fiber pathways.

In general, the major corticofugal outflow from the motor areas comprises the corticospinal, corticobulbar, and corticorubral fibers from MI and the corticoreticular and corticostriate fibers from all the motor areas. Neural influences to the motor nuclei of the cranial nerves are conveyed from the motor areas via corticobulbar and corticoreticular fibers (Chap. 8). The output of the motor areas to the motor nuclei of the spinal nerves is projected from the primary motor cortex via the corticospinal, corticorubrospinal, and corticoreticulospinal pathways. The other motor areas are presumed to exert their functional roles via their connections with the primary motor cortex and via fibers of the corticoreticulospinal pathway. The corticostriate fibers are integrated into the feedback circuits involving the basal ganglia and thalamus (Chap. 14).

PRIMARY MOTOR AREA (MI)

The primary motor area, often called the "motor cortex," is located in area 4 of the precentral gyrus. Direct topical electrical stimulation of this region evokes movements of the voluntary muscles. A map of this electrically excitable motor cortex produces the configuration of a homunculus indicative of the somatotopical representation of different parts of the body (Fig. 16-14). In addition to its major projection via the pyramidal tract to the spinal cord, cortical area 4 projects to many subcortical nuclei, including the ventral lateral thalamic nucleus, nucleus centrum medianum, subthalamic nucleus, red nucleus, substantia nigra, and many brainstem reticular nuclei. Many of these connections are via collateral branches of the corticospinal fibers. MI receives subcortical input from the ventral lateral thalamic nucleus.

In a general way this homunculus is upside down, with the head region near the lateral sulcus and with the lower extremity on the medial surface in the paracentral lobule. The homunculus reveals that larger proportions of motor cortex are associated with those cortical regions evoking movements of the face, larynx, tongue, and hand as compared with the smaller regions associated with the trunk and lower extremities. The detailed representation of the thumb and fingers is consistent with the paramount importance of manual dexterity in man's primacy. The amount of the motor cortex devoted to specific regions is roughly proportional to the delicacy of control that is possible in each body region.

Stimulation of the motor cortex elicits phasic activity in groups of muscles, rather than from individual muscles per se. Experimentally induced movements include changes in facial expression, swallowing, torsion of the body, rotation of an extremity, and flexion of limbs. Focal stimulation may occasionally produce the contraction of individual muscles, such as an adductor muscle of the thumb. Flexor responses occur more frequently than extensor responses. The specific localized movements are usually expressed on the side of the body opposite the cortical stimulation, although some ipsilateral activity may be elicited. Stimulation of the postcentral gyrus (areas 1, 2, and 3) in man may evoke motor responses when area 4 is intact. The responses are similar to those obtained from stimulating area 4, but weaker.

The ablation of the precentral gyrus in a monkey produces an initial paralysis; a monkey with an ablated precentral gyrus exhibits an immediate severe impairment of voluntary movements, hypotonia, and diminished reflexes on the contralateral side. With the passage of time, the monkey has a good return of function, but with a persistent flaccidity and some impairment of skilled actions. The paresis is accompanied by an almost normal tonus, no major increase in the deep tendon reflexes, and no clonus. The main loss is of the fine voluntary movement, particularly of the fingers and feet. However, the monkey has sufficient manual dexterity to be able to pick up objects by the apposition of the thumb with the index finger. Effects are more pronounced in the distal muscles than in the proximal muscles of a limb.

The abnormal stimulation of the motor cortex may produce patterned convulsions. The *Jacksonian seizure* (*epilepsy*) offers a vivid example of such responses. In a focal seizure, the convulsive movement of a group of muscles may be manifested. The repeated contractions may be restricted to the muscles of the face, an arm, or a leg, taking the form of tonic and clonic movements, such as a twitch of the cheek, finger, or ankle. In the Jacksonian march, the seizure, which may commence with a finger twitch, spreads in an orderly progression from the distal to the proximal muscles of the limb, down the same side of the body, down the lower extremity, across to and up the other lower extremity, up the body to the upper extremity and face, following the order of representation of the homunculus of one side and then the homunculus of the opposite side. Consciousness is lost, unless the seizure is confined to one side. During a seizure, the patient can see and hear but cannot communicate.

PREMOTOR CORTEX

The premotor cortex comprises areas 6 and 8 on the lateral surface of the hemisphere. Area 6 on the medial surface of the frontal lobe is the supplementary motor area. The major subcortical input to area 6 is derived from the ventral anterior nucleus of the thalamus. Electrical stimulation of part of area 6 in man may produce motor responses which are similar to those evoked by stimulating the primary motor cortex. These responses may be elicited through relays via association fibers to the primary motor area and then via the corticospinal, corticobulbar, and corticoreticular pathways to the brainstem and spinal cord.

Stimulation of area 6 on the lateral cerebral surface often produces adversive movements which are different from the precise movements obtained from stimulation of area 4. *Adversive movements* or *orientation movements* are generalized actions, such as turning the head and eyes, twisting movements of the trunk, and general flexion or extension of the limbs. These movements are thought of as directional—the motor reaction to attention. Stimulation of area 8 (just rostral to area 6) results in conjugate movements of the eye to the opposite side. This frontal eye field influences the volitional eye movements. Adversive movements may be elicited by stimulating other regions of the cortex. Stimulation of areas 9 and 10, which projects fibers to the caudate nucleus, inhibits the deep tendon reflexes and movements in progress. Ablation limited to area 6 on the lateral hemispheric surface (avoiding the primary motor and supplementary motor areas) does not produce a monkey with paresis, motor impairment, hypotonia, hypertonia, or grasp reflexes. The ablation of premotor area and primary motor area results in a flaccid paralysis with a slight increase in muscle tone. The explanation for these observations is not known.

SECONDARY MOTOR AREA
(SECOND MOTOR AREA, MII)

The secondary motor area is the small cortical region at the base of the pre- and postcentral gyri (Fig. 16-12); its precise function in motor activity is unknown. Electrical stimulation of this area generally produces sensations rather than motor responses. This greater prominence of sensory phenomena following its stimulation suggests that the role of the MII area in motor activity is minimal. When motor responses are evoked, they are usually elicited on the contralateral side, especially of the more distal segments of the extremities. At times ipsilateral and bilateral responses can also be evoked. The electrical stimulation of this area may elicit in man the desire to make a specific movement. No obvious sensory or motor deficits have been observed in experimental animals with this cortical area ablated. This is probably so because the secondary motor area is functionally overpowered by the primary motor area.

SUPPLEMENTARY MOTOR AREA

The supplementary motor area is found on the medial surface of the superior frontal gyrus (area) rostral to the paracentral lobule (Fig. 16-12). Stimulation of this area outlines a small homunculus with its head located rostrally. The motor responses in man evoked by electrical stimulation are largely bilateral movements of a tonic or postural nature, resulting from the activity of the axial, pectoral girdle, and pelvic girdle musculature. These generalized responses are slow and outlast the stimulation for a short time. They include such posturing movements

as turning the head contralaterally and raising the contralateral upper extremity. The stimulation can also evoke vocalization as well as fine movements of the thumb, fingers, and hand.

These bilateral responses elicited by the stimulation of each supplementary motor area are probably evoked through influences conveyed by the corticospinal and corticoreticulospinal pathways from both sides. These pathways can be activated directly or indirectly by some of the following known connections from each supplementary motor area: *1* direct corticoreticular fibers projecting to the brainstem, *2* association fibers projecting to the primary motor area and premotor cortex of the same side, *3* corpus callosal fibers projecting to the contralateral supplementary motor area, and *4* corticofugal fibers projecting bilaterally to the ventral lateral and intralaminar nuclei of the thalamus (the decussating fibers cross through the anterior commissure). There are no direct projections from the supplementary motor area to the spinal cord.

The bilateral removal of both supplementary motor areas produces an animal exhibiting hypertonus, hyperactive deep tendon reflexes, spasticity, and increased resistance to passive movements of the extremities; there is no paralysis. The ablation of only one supplementary motor area results in a monkey with only minimal symptoms, such as weak but transient grasp reflexes, lasting slowness of movement of the contralateral extremities, and moderate hypotonia of the shoulder musculature. The removal of the contralateral supplementary motor area six or more months later produces an animal exhibiting minimal effects, with no spasticity. Reasons for these phenomena are unknown. However, the simultaneous ablation of the supplementary motor cortex and the motor cortex on the same side produces a monkey that exhibits symptoms of upper motor neuron paralysis accompanied by marked spasticity, without paresis. The ablation of the entire cortex on both frontal lobes in the monkey results in an animal with spastic paralysis symptoms, including clonus and hyperactive deep tendon reflexes. These animals are unable to stand up, walk, or feed themselves.

These observations are similar to those obtained in monkeys and chimpanzees with bilaterally transected pyramids in the medulla (Chap. 8). When all corticospinal tract fibers are interrupted at this site, the animals are characterized by a marked impairment of their motor activities. They can move about and feed themselves. They exhibit slow stereotyped movements accompanied by hypotonus and no clonus.

The motor areas are not absolutely essential to movement. After bilateral ablation of the primary, supplementary, and premotor areas (areas 4 and 6), adult monkeys can walk and right themselves.

PREFRONTAL CORTEX

The prefrontal cortex (areas 9 through 12) is well developed in higher primates, especially in man. This cortex has rich reciprocal connections with the parvocellular part of the dorsomedial nucleus of the thalamus (Chap. 13). Many complex reciprocal projections are made with other neocortical and limbic areas, both of the same and opposite side. Efferent fibers project to the hypothalamus (corticohypothalamic fibers).

The bilateral ablation of areas of the prefrontal cortex or the interruption of the white matter deep to the cortex in both prefrontal lobes (*prefrontal lobotomy, leukotomy*) may produce permanent changes in an individual. The patient may become less excitable and less creative. The relief from anxiety is accompanied by a change in the patient's outlook and disposition. Less altruism toward others and a release from many inhibitions make the patient free to express himself frankly, often without the restraint demanded by society. A neat, precise individual may become indifferent and sloppy in appearance. Surprisingly, this change in personality, including a reduction in the awareness of self, is generally accompanied by no real change in mental processes. Drive, not intelligence, is altered.

Alleviation of suffering from pain may follow a lobotomy. Relief from intractable pain and other effects of a phantom limb is also obtained.

The pain remains, but the patient is unconcerned about it; it can be ignored, for the psychic feeling associated with the intensity of the pain is lost.

The prefrontal lobe may be thought of as a regulator of the depth of feeling of an individual. Basically it is involved not in the perception of sensations, but rather in the "affect" associated with the sensation. The special quality of "feeling tone" or state of mind is apparently the result of the processing of the input from the numerous subcortical and cortical sources. This may form the basis for many of the emotional aspects associated with behavioral responses. The relative pitch of one's being is influenced in this region. The complex responses of an individual from calmness to ecstasy, from gloom to elation, from friendliness to disagreeableness—have their roots in areas 9 to 12. One concept suggests that the prefrontal cortex is the neocortical representation of the limbic system; this view is based on *1* the rich direct and indirect interconnections between this lobe and the limbus, and *2* the similarities of the functional expressions of the prefrontal cortex and the limbic system. The autonomic responses associated with various emotional states are probably mediated through the frontopreoptic tract, frontohypothalamic tract, and fronto-dorsomedian thalamic nuclear hypothalamic pathways (Chap. 13). The hypothalamus exerts its effects on the blood pressure, respiratory rate, and gastrointestinal activity through the autonomic nervous system (Chap. 11).

Functional considerations of the neocortex

The functional role of an ablated area of the cortex should not and cannot be objectively inferred from observations of the residual activity of the organism. The expressions remaining following the ablation of an area may be taken to indicate, in effect, the performance of the nervous system without the influences of this missing region. Additionally it may reveal the prior expression of the rest of the nervous system plus the degree to which the nervous system compensates.

The activity evoked from focal stimulation does not necessarily tell the real function of the area stimulated. The stimulation acts as a nodal site which sets off a complex of other integrated systems with its multiplicity of inhibitory, excitatory, and feedback effects. Each cortical area actually functions in conjunction with many other cortical and subcortical regions. The specific part stimulated is a segment integrated into the complex circuitry of the brain. The cortical influences are exerted not directly on the end organs (muscle cells and glands) but actually through intermediaries of from one to many intercalated nuclear complexes.

MOTOR EXPRESSION OF THE CEREBRAL CORTEX

The part of the cerebral cortex associated with motor expression is influenced by a multitude of afferent stimuli. These sources of input are essential to the activity of the motor areas of the cortex. The influences come from other cortical areas—both contralateral and ipsilateral; from feedback circuits involving the basal ganglia, cerebellum, brainstem, and possibly the spinal cord (spinocortical tract), and from peripheral afferent sources through subcortical nuclei (Chaps. 14 and 15). The motor pathways are really the efferent arms of complex arcs having afferent arms.

The motor systems of the cerebral cortex may be provisionally thought of as operating in the following manner. The pyramidal system is the pathway essential to special actions and skilled and learned movements. It is a phylogenetically new specialized system. The "extrapyramidal systems" are involved with the stereotyped and grosser movements and with the automatic association motions and gestures. This complex is important in the learned skills such as writing and the athletic dexterity exhibited by a baseball pitcher. These are the underlying systems with a long phylogenetic history. The multiplicity of motor areas, whether called primary, supplementary, or second motor areas, provides, at least in part, the substrates for the subtle and wide range of motor expressions. Many of these are associated with the behavior patterns and with the personal motor nuances peculiar to each individual as a personality.

AUTONOMIC NERVOUS SYSTEM AND THE NEOCORTEX

Cortical activity is also expressed through the autonomic nervous system, e.g., those behavior patterns colored by emotion. Intellectual decisions, all cortically derived, are set in an emotional environment. All lobes of the cerebrum contribute primarily through connections with the hypothalamus, limbic system, and midbrain tegmentum (Chap. 15). The autonomic expressions elicited during emotional states can be evoked by the electrical stimulation of the neocortex. Among these responses are cardiovascular effects (vasodilatation, vasoconstriction, and blood pressure changes), digestive influences (salivation, peristalsis, and gastric discomfort), temperature changes, and alterations of pupillary size. These actions have their emotional counterpart in heart palpitations, cold sweat, paleness, and blushing.

ROLE OF THE CORTEX IN "HIGHEST-ORDER" ACTIVITIES

The cortex is essential in the neural processing underlying the loftiest activities of the nervous system. Among these activities are the fullest comprehension of the afferent input, expression through the symbolisms of communication of the unique nuances of each personality, and abstract creativity. Only a few indications of the role of the cortex in these spheres will be made.

The cortex of the parietal lobe, occipital lobe, and temporal lobe is necessary for the comprehension of the afferent input. Defects in these lobes produce individuals with receptive aphasias. These patients receive input from visual, auditory, and somesthetic pathways—can see, hear, and feel. The receptive aphasia is indicated when they are unable to process this information in order to comprehend the written word, the spoken word, or the felt object. Visual aphasia, auditory aphasia (word deafness), and somesthetic aphasia are expressions of malfunction in the highest levels of neural integration in the neocortex.

The ultimate of afferent processing in the

cerebrum of man is seen in the neural activities expressed as abstract and creative thought. These highest expressions may not necessarily be accompanied by any overt motor activity.

The motor aspect of expression through the symbolism of language is in part a function of the frontal lobe. The motor aphasias (motor apraxias) are indications that these regions are essential to the performance of these activities. Broca's speech area (areas 44 and 45 of the inferior frontal gyrus) is a nodal site concerned with ability to produce the spoken word. Lesions of Broca's area, especially of the left dominant hemisphere, may result in motor or expressive aphasia. More often these lesions lead to a transient speech defect. This loss of articulate speech occurs even though there is no demonstrable paralysis of any muscles associated with speech. Complete loss of articulate speech—the ability to say only several words, mispronunciation of common everyday words, or repetition of the same word over and over again—may be a consequence of the total destruction of Broca's speech area. At times these patients may express themselves with better facility when under emotional stress.

The "sensory" association cortex has a role in subtle motor activity. Injury to the somesthetic association cortex (supramarginal gyrus) may result in a sensory apraxia. The patient is capable of performing the various separate movements of a sequence but may not be able to carry out volitionally all the movements of the sequence in their intended or proper order. He knows what and how to execute the sequence but is unable to do it volitionally or on command. He is unable to handle a screwdriver although he can explain its use. He may be able to brush his teeth, comb his hair, and tie his shoes automatically but is unable to perform these tasks when instructed to do so.

CEREBRAL DOMINANCE

Cerebral dominance refers to the fact that the control of certain forms of learned behavior in man is exerted predominantly by one of the two cerebral hemispheres. Handedness, perception of language, performance of speech, and appreciation of spatial relations are, in all but a few individuals, primarily expressions of one or the other hemisphere.

Roughly 90 percent of adults are right handed. In these right-handers the left hemisphere is motor dominant because the cerebral motor center on the left side controls the right hand. In left-handers, the right hemisphere is considered to be dominant for handedness. In about 98 percent of the adults, the comprehension of the spoken and written word as well as the motor control of language (speech) are expressions of the left cerebral hemisphere. Only in about 2 percent of the population are the speech centers (e.g., Broca's areas 44, 45) located in the right hemisphere.

Apparently the lateralization of *speech centers* is not causally related to handedness. About 90 percent of right handers have speech centers in the left hemisphere, while the other 10 percent have speech centers in the right hemisphere. About 65 percent of left handers have speech centers in the left hemisphere, 20 percent in the right hemisphere, and the remaining 15 percent have speech centers bilaterally located in both hemispheres. Naturally ambidextrous subjects have their speech centers located as follows—60 percent in the left hemisphere, 10 percent in the right hemisphere, and 30 percent in both hemispheres. Stated otherwise, speech functions are lateralized to the left hemisphere in most adults, regardless of hand preference. Some individuals have speech centers located in the right hemisphere while some have speech centers in both hemispheres.

1 Patients with cerebral lesions: Over 96 percent of adult aphasics with language disorders have brain damage in the left hemisphere.

2 Twin-brain individuals: Studies on these human subjects indicate that the left hemisphere is adapted for linguistic expression through speech and writing whereas the right hemisphere is specialized to sense and appreciate spatial relations.

3 Subjects treated with the short-acting anesthetic agent Amytal (amobarbital): When Amytal is injected into the left carotid artery, the left hemisphere is temporarily anesthetized, whereas the right hemisphere is not affected. On the basis of responses from patients so exposed to Amytal, it can be demonstrated that, in right-handed individuals, the left hemisphere controls handedness, perception of language, and performance

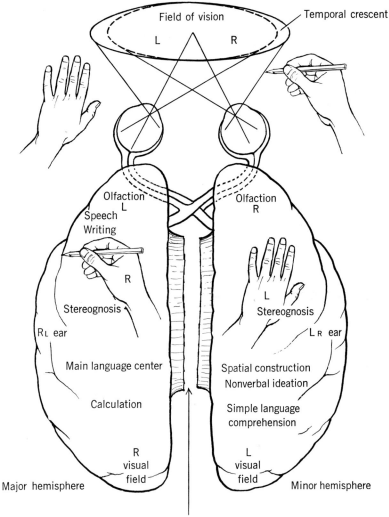

FIGURE 16-16
Some of the roles of the major and minor cerebral hemispheres as established in "twin-brain" man.

General senses from one hand and from one-half of the visual field are projected to the contralateral hemisphere. The olfactory sense is conveyed to the ipsilateral hemisphere. Hearing is largely projected to the contralateral hemisphere. (*Adapted from Sperry.*)

of speech. In some left-handed people (less than half the total), language is controlled by the right hemisphere, while in the remainder language functions reside in the left hemisphere.

On the basis of observations of these subjects, *the left hemisphere has been called the dominant or major hemisphere* and *the right hemisphere has been called the nondominant or minor hemisphere.* The major hemisphere has essential roles in man's verbal and analytic abilities; the minor hemisphere has crucial roles in nonverbal and artistic expressions (see "Twin-Brain Man," further on in this chapter).

The major hemisphere has the substrates and memory traces relevant to thoughts and knowledge expressed and symbolized through language and our highest analytic powers. Through its influence on handedness, the hemisphere is involved in the control of the opposite hand and fingers for precise and delicate grips and movements. By means of this role man has evolved manipulative manual skills, which are often enhanced through the use of tools. There is no known microscopic (ultramicroscopic), neuroanatomic, or neurophysiologic basis for the dominance of this hemisphere in handedness and speech.

Several gross anatomic differences between the hemispheres have been reported; the functional significance of them has been inferred but not demonstrated. The asymmetry between the hemispheres has been demonstrated in the temporal lobes and in the posterior part of the inferior frontal gyrus of a number of brains. The superior surface of the temporal lobe just behind the transverse temporal gyrus of Heschl is larger on the left side in about 65 percent of brains; it is larger on the right side in about 11 percent of brains. This region—called the *planum temporale*—is adjacent to the temporal speech area of Wernicke.

The triangular and opercular portions of the inferior frontal gyrus, which are called Broca's speech area, are apparently larger in about 80 percent of the left cerebral hemispheres. Note that these enlargements do not occur in 98 percent of the brains, as expected from the lateralization of speech in the left hemisphere. The gross asymmetry of these regions is also present in the newborn infant; this occurs before language learning and unimanual preference are expressed behaviorly. According to some investigators, this suggests that the newborn infant may be programmed with the capacity to process speech sounds.

Ontogeny of cerebral dominance The young infant is, to a degree, presumed to be a split-brain individual. This is so because the interhemispheric communication through the fibers of the anterior commissure and corpus callosum is, at the most, slight in the newborn infant. The interhemispheric communication through these commissures increases with age; it is apparently fairly well developed by the second and third year of age. The two hemispheres of the neonate have essentially equipotential capabilities. Cerebral dominance probably develops gradually during childhood and does not become rela-

tively well fixed until the end of the first decade of life. On the basis of the use of hands in manipulatory play it seems that, after the age of 2, the duplication of learning by both hands becomes less frequent and the lateralization of handedness becomes more pronounced. Apparently the language and speech capabilities in young children reside in both sides of the brain, expressing the tendency for each hemisphere to evolve independently as a duplicate of the other. The natural twin-brain of the growing child explains, in part, why a left-handed child can be readily taught to write with the right hand, and why some athletes who have been trained in childhood are ambidextrous. This also explains why a child with a damaged dominant hemisphere can be trained to become left-handed and proficient in language and speech, whereas the older patient with a cerebral infarction of the major hemisphere finds it difficult or impossible to become left-handed and to relearn lost language and speech abilities.

Studies on twin-brain subjects suggest that language learned in early childhood by the minor hemisphere will, during later development, be suppressed and even lost completely. Some skills controlled predominantly by one hemisphere tend to suppress the same skill by the other hemisphere; "excellence in one tends to interfere with top level performance in the other" (Sperry). According to one concept, those individuals who mature into "major hemisphere types" are equipped to function more effectively in a verbal and analytic way, while those who evolve into "minor hemisphere types" will be able to express themselves more effectively nonverbally in many of the creative arts.

Functional role of association fibers and commissural fibers ("split-brain animals")

The interactions of the billions of association and commissural cortical neurons have a significant role in the higher integration of the cerebral cortex. These multitudes of connections suggest that the cortex may function in overall patterns of mass action. This could be a consequence of the continuous spread of impulses through the white matter to other cortical areas.

However, experimental evidence indicates that the interruption of large bundles of association fibers by surgical incisions, especially in the association areas in many regions of the same brain, produces few objective symptoms. Monkeys, dogs, and rats with many association fibers interrupted show slight defects or none in the learning and retention of maze-trained habits. Multiple transections of the cortex and underlying association fibers coming from "motor" areas in a monkey do not essentially alter motor coordination. Any functional depression following such lesions is usually temporary and transient.

The presence of several commissures in the cerebrum—one of them, the massive corpus callosum, with its more than 300 million fibers in man, is the largest fiber tract of the brain—suggests that interhemispheric fiber pathways are of crucial significance to the functioning of the brain. Yet, when the corpus callosum is completely transected surgically, even in man, no functional alterations can be detected, even after careful neurologic and psychologic examinations. Behavior patterns are not noticeably disturbed. Complex activities, such as playing musical instruments (piano, violin, and others), typing, and writing, are performed with the same dexterity as prior to sectioning of the corpus callosum.

An experimental animal with a transected corpus callosum and other commissures (anterior commissure and commissure of the fornix) is, in a way, an animal with two brains; such animals are called "twin-brain" animals or "split-brain" animals. Such cats and monkeys behave normally. These animals are alert and curious and exhibit good muscular coordination. They perceive, learn, and retain learned activities as do ordinary animals. Normal expressions are still observed because the input of complex information from the periphery is apparently projected to both hemispheres and therefore each hemisphere receives sufficient input to operate efficiently by itself.

Experimental animals may be trained in such a way that information may be relayed to only one hemisphere. In this way it is possible to train one of the divided hemispheres with one set of data and the other hemisphere with other data; or one hemisphere with certain information and the other hemisphere without this in-

formation. For example, this can be accomplished by sectioning the optic chiasma in cats and in monkeys so that all decussating fibers from the eye are cut and the nondecussating fibers from the eye are intact. In such animals each eye projects only to its ipsilateral hemisphere. By blindfolding one eye, and training the animal with visual stimuli directed to only one eye, visual information is conveyed to only the ipsilateral hemisphere. This experiment has many variations.

Studies of such split-brain monkeys have been conducted so that the input from the periphery has been projected to only one hemisphere. The memory for the perceptual and motor learning in these animals is confined to the hemisphere to which the sensory information was relayed, and from which the motor output was projected. However, if the corpus callosum was intact this memory is found to be utilized for motor expression by both hemispheres. Apparently the engram, or memory trace, laid down in the directly trained hemisphere is transferred via the callosal fibers to the opposite hemisphere and a second engram is laid down in the contralateral hemisphere. The inference is that the function of the corpus callosum is to transfer information from one hemisphere to the other and to equate the newly acquired engrams of the neocortex of each hemisphere. The corpus callosum may be utilized by the uneducated hemisphere to tap the engram of the trained hemisphere. A double set of engrams is not necessarily always laid down equally in both hemispheres. The lateralization of language functions in the human brain to one hemisphere indicates that some functional expressions are largely confined to one hemisphere. This is in line with the concept of cerebral dominance of one hemisphere.

With training, the split-brain animal can use its two "half-brains" independently or simultaneously to perform different tasks. Each half-brain performs its own perceptual, learning, and memory processes. The animal may have one half-brain trained to respond one way to a specific visual cue from one half-brain and to respond in the opposite way to the same visual cue from the other half-brain. If this cue is visualized simultaneously by both half-brains, hesitancy is displayed by the animal, but marked conflict does not occur. One hemisphere will express itself, and later a shift will occur and the other hemisphere will express itself. A split-brain animal may utilize both half-brains together or in alternation.

The behavioral responses of a split-brain animal with an ablated amygdaloid body are informative. The bilateral removal of the amygdaloid body converts an excitable, temperamental, and wild monkey into a placid and docile animal, whereas the unilateral removal of the amygdaloid body produces little, if any, observable change in a primate (Chap. 15). A split-brain monkey (one with midline transection of the corpus callosum, anterior commissure, and habenular commissure) with a unilateral ablation of the amygdaloid body exhibits interesting behavioral responses. When an aggravating visual stimulus is presented to the eye on the side with the intact amygdaloid body (with the opposite eye blindfolded), the monkey responds in an emotional, aggressive, and belligerent manner. When the same visual stimulus is presented to the eye on the side with the ablated amygdaloid body, the monkey shows no emotional or aggressive responses but remains docile and tame. This is in line with the concept that the commissures act to transfer information from one hemisphere to the other.

"TWIN-BRAIN" MAN

Commissurotomy of the corpus callosum and commissure of the fornix (hippocampal commissure) has been performed in a number of patients in order to prevent the interhemispheric spread of epileptic seizures. The normal behavior of these patients is unaffected by the surgical section. These subjects with "two minds in one head" are alert and curious. They perceive, learn, and retain learned experiences as well as normal people. Careful testing reveals that the two hemispheres are almost completely independent with respect to learning, memory, perception, and ideation. *Language, speech,*

and handedness are almost exclusively lateralized in these subjects to the major hemisphere.

The minor hemisphere can perceive tactile, auditory, and visual information. Although it does think, this mute hemisphere is unable to communicate through verbal language. However, it can respond and communicate by gestures (e.g., pointing) or emotional activity (e.g., fidgeting or blushing). *The minor hemisphere is specialized to appreciate spatial dimensions, to grasp the totality of a scene, and to recognize the faces of people better than the major hemisphere. This mute hemisphere is presumed to have an essential role in creative acts associated with musical, poetic, and imaginative expressions.*

Hemispheric specialization has interesting consequences. The twin-brain subject cannot describe orally an unseen object felt by his left hand because the minor hemisphere, which receives this information, is unable to relay the knowledge to the speech areas of the major hemisphere. On the other hand, he cannot draw accurately with his right hand because the motor centers of the major hemisphere do not receive the critical guidance of spatial knowledge from the minor hemisphere.

Because a visual image is presented to the monocular crescent of the retina of one eye, visual information is projected only to the visual cortex of the ipsilateral hemisphere. This is done by permitting the crescent of the eye to view an object several times tachistoscopically for only from 0.01 to 0.1 sec. Such a quick view prevents other portions of the eye from viewing the object if the eye moves. If a word (e.g., "cat") or an object is so presented to the monocular crescent of the right eye, this information is conveyed to the minor hemisphere. Under appropriate testing conditions, the twin-brain subject will be able to write "cat" with his left hand or identify the object by selecting the correct object from a variety of objects viewed by both eyes. Thus the "mute" hemisphere communicates. The words and objects cannot be named verbally because the minor hemisphere is unable to communicate with the "talking" major hemisphere.

Several basic conclusions concerning the roles of the cerebral hemispheres obtained from studies of "twin-brain" subjects (Fig. 16-16) are

1 perception and memory can be performed independently in both hemispheres, *2* language and speech are almost exclusively the roles of the major hemisphere, *3* the minor hemisphere is superior to the major hemisphere in the recognition and appreciation of spatial dimensions, *4* the primary role of the cerebral commissures is in the bilateral integration of the two hemispheres for linguistic functions, *5* it is through the major hemisphere that man can have thoughts and knowledge expressed through language, and *6* the commissures are essential for maintaining the unity of the higher sensory and motor functions of the cerebrum.

LANGUAGE

The organizational complexities of the neuro-anatomic, neurophysiologic, and psychologic substrates associated with language and speech are, as yet, only slightly known. Much of the current understanding is derived from studies of patients with disturbances of language function resulting from damage to the brain; these disturbances are called aphasias. They are commonly classified as *1 receptive* (*posterior or Wernicke's*) *aphasias*, and *2 expressive* (*anterior or Broca's*) *aphasia*. This simple classification is not accepted by many neurologists because aphasias are known to result also from brain injuries located outside Wernicke's and Broca's areas. *Wernicke's area* is located in the posterior part of the superior temporal gyrus (area 22) adjacent to the auditory cortex (Fig. 16-15). This area is involved in the recognition of the patterns of the spoken language. *Broca's area* is located in the inferior frontal gyrus (orbital and opercular parts) just rostral to that region of the motor cortex with representation for the musculature associated with speech, muscles of the face, tongue, lips, palate, and vocal chords. Speed can be arrested when Broca's area is electrically stimulated in the conscious man.

A patient with a lesion involving Wernicke's area of the dominant hemisphere usually has a *receptive aphasia*, expressed as a failure in understanding both the spoken and the written word. In such a subject the inputs to the cortex from the auditory and visual systems are apparently unimpaired. He speaks rapidly, maintains natural speech rhythms, and has normal nuances of articulation. The conversational output sounds normal, but it is actually devoid of meaningful content. Key words are omitted; they are substituted by empty meaningless words, or replaced by related words (knife for fork), or unrelated words (hammer for book).

In contrast, patients with a lesion presumably in Broca's area have an *expressive aphasia*, which is primarily a failure in the formulation of speech. They have a normal comprehension of language. Speech is labored and crudely articulated. The omission of small words and of the endings of nouns and verbs results in a telegraphic style or delivery. The muscles involved in speech are not paralyzed; this is demonstrated by the fact that many of these patients can often sing a formerly known song rapidly, correctly, and even with feeling.

To explain these aphasias, it is presumed that several areas of the cortex are associated and linked with one another in the following ways. Meaningful sounds are conveyed from the inner ears via auditory pathways to the auditory cortex in the temporal lobe. This processed information is relayed to Wernicke's area, which has a significant role in the conscious recognition of the spoken language. In a sense, spoken words are "understood" in Wernicke's area. The words to be spoken are then projected via association fibers of the arcuate fasciculus to Broca's area, where the articulatory phrases of speech are formulated. This information is relayed to the motor cortex of area 4, which is involved with the control and regulation of the musculature associated with speech. In order to spell a word orally, it must be visualized. This is accomplished by transferring the processed information of a word that is heard and understood in Wernicke's area to the angular gyrus, where the patterns of words are visualized. From the angular gyrus, the information is conveyed successively to Wernicke's area, Broca's area, and the "speech centers" of the primary motor cortex. On the other hand, the processed information obtained from reading written and spoken words is conveyed via the visual pathways to the primary, association, and inferotemporal areas and then to the angular gyrus. The visualized form within the angular gyrus is projected to Wernicke's area for conversion to the auditory form. This is consistent with the concept that *the comprehension of the written word involves the activation of the auditory form within Wernicke's area,* where it is understood.

Following a lesion of the angular gyrus, a patient loses the ability to read (*alexia*) and write (*agraphia*). He can comprehend the spoken language and speak, but to him the written word is meaningless. Patients with alexia and agraphia are unable to recognize words spelled orally to them, nor can they spell aloud and write the spoken word.

In man, speech and language symbolisms of the written and spoken word are lateralized, even though the cortical areas associated with these activities have extensive connections through the corpus callosum. Both the dominant (or "talking") hemisphere and the nondominant ("mute") hemisphere can comprehend, but normally only the dominant hemisphere "talks."

Within the numerous variations of the basic neuronal types in the various regions of the neocortex, there "is a basic constancy in the general organization of the cortical afferents, intracortical neurons and intracortical distribution of the axons. What remains constant is the arrangement of the plexuses of dendritic and axonal branches; i.e., of the synaptic articulations through which nerve impulses are transmitted" (Lorente de Nó).

Bibliography

Colonnier, M. L.: The structural design of the neocortex, in J. C. Eccles (ed.), *Brain and Conscious Experience.* Springer-Verlag, New York, 1966.

Ebner, F. F., and R. Myers: Corpus callosum and the interhemispheric transfer of tactual learning. J. Neurophysiol., 25:380–391, 1962.

Eccles, J. C.: *The Understanding of the Brain.* McGraw-Hill Book Company, New York, 1973.

Gazzaniga, M. S.: *The Bisected Brain.* Appleton-Century-Crofts, Inc., New York, 1970.

Geschwind, N.: The organization of language and the brain. Science, 170:940–944, 1970.

Jouvet, M.: Biogenic amines and the states of sleep. Science, 163:32–41, 1969.

Kandel, E. R., and W. A. Spencer: Cellular neurophysiological approaches to the study of learning. Physiol. Rev., 48:65–134, 1968.

Nauta, W. J. H.: The problem of the frontal lobe: a reinterpretation. J. Psychiat. Res., 8:167–187, 1971.

Pandya, D., P. Dye, and N. Butters: Efferent corticocortical projections of the prefrontal cortex in the rhesus monkey. Brain Res., 31:35–44, 1971.

Penfield, W., and L. Roberts: *Speech and Brain Mechanisms.* Princeton University Press, Princeton, N.J., 1959.

Schaltenbrand, G., and C. N. Woolsey: *Principles of Cerebral Localization and Organization.* University of Wisconsin Press, Madison, 1964.

Scheibel, M. E., and A. B. Scheibel: Elementary processes in selected thalamic and cortical subsystems: The structural substrates, in F. O. Schmitt et al. (eds.), *The Neurosciences—Second Study Program.* Rockefeller University Press, New York, 1970.

Sperry, R. W.: *Mental Unity Following Surgical Disconnection of the Cerebral Hemispheres.* Harvey Lectures, Academic Press, Inc., New York, 1966–1967.

Valenstein, E. S.: *Brain Control: A Critical Examination of Stimulation and Psychosurgery.* John Wiley & Sons, Inc., New York, 1973.

Warren J. M., and K. Akert (eds.): *The Frontal Granular Cortex and Behavior.* McGraw-Hill Book Company, New York, 1964.

ATLAS **1**
THE BRAINSTEM

Transverse sections through the medulla, pons, and midbrain

The *left half* of each figure illustrates the more prominent structures as visualized in Weigert stained preparations. Many of the significant tracts and nuclei are indicated on the *right half* of each figure.

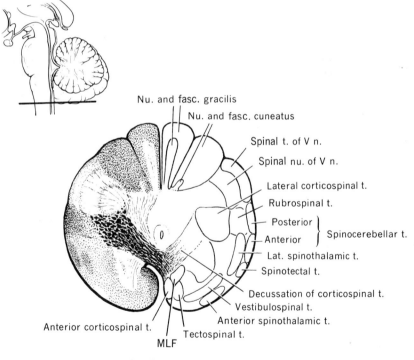

FIGURE A-1
Transverse section of the lower medulla at the middle of the corticospinal (pyramidal) decussation. Refer to Figs. 8-3 and A-12. MLF, medial longitudinal fasciculus; N, nerve; Nu, nucleus; T, tract. (*After Villiger.*)

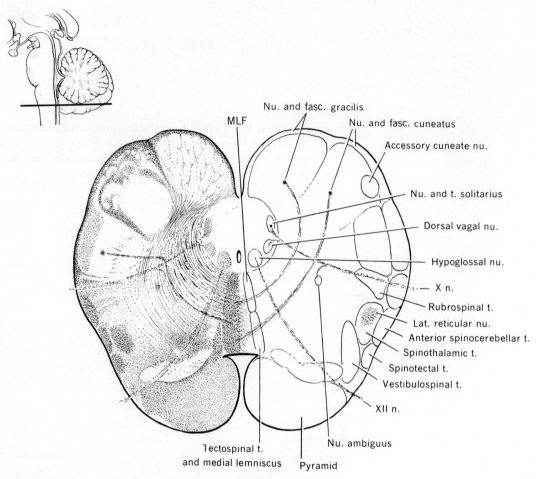

FIGURE A-2
Transverse section of the lower medulla at the level of
the decussation of the medial lemniscus. Refer to Figs.
8-4 and A-14. (*After Villiger.*)

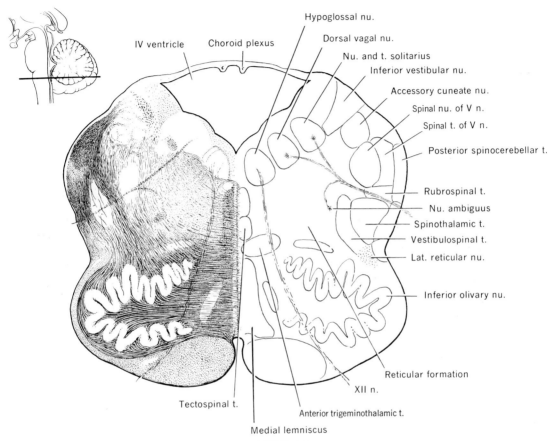

Hypoglossal nu.
Dorsal vagal nu.
Nu. and t. solitarius
Inferior vestibular nu.
Accessory cuneate nu.
Spinal nu. of V n.
Spinal t. of V n.
Posterior spinocerebellar t.
Rubrospinal t.
Nu. ambiguus
Spinothalamic t.
Vestibulospinal t.
Lat. reticular nu.
Inferior olivary nu.
Reticular formation
XII n.
Anterior trigeminothalamic t.
Medial lemniscus
Tectospinal t.
IV ventricle
Choroid plexus

FIGURE A-3
Transverse section of the medulla at the level of the
middle of the olive. Refer to Figs. 8-5 and A-16. (*After
Villiger.*)

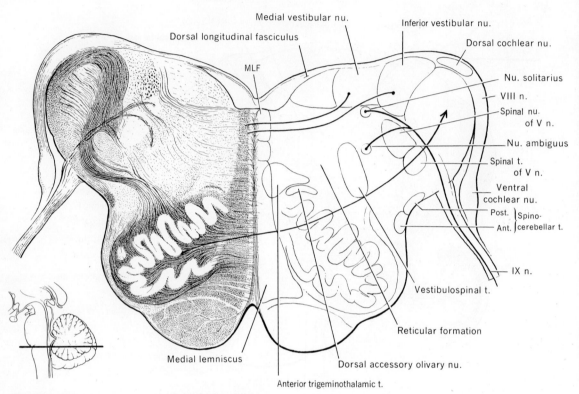

FIGURE A-4
Transverse section of the upper medulla at the level
of the entrance of the cochlear nerve and the
glossopharyngeal nerve. Refer to Figs. 8-6 and A-17.
(*After Villiger.*)

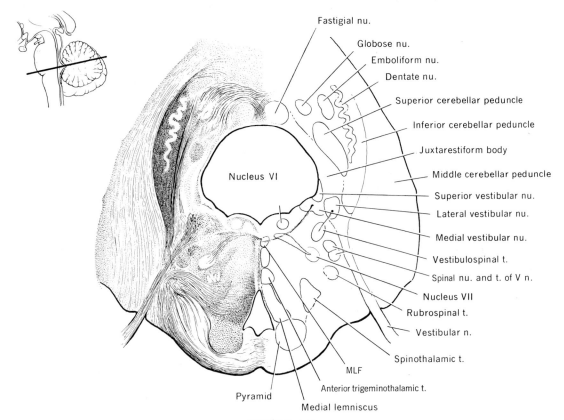

Fastigial nu.
Globose nu.
Emboliform nu.
Dentate nu.
Superior cerebellar peduncle
Inferior cerebellar peduncle
Juxtarestiform body
Middle cerebellar peduncle
Superior vestibular nu.
Lateral vestibular nu.
Medial vestibular nu.
Vestibulospinal t.
Spinal nu. and t. of V n.
Nucleus VII
Rubrospinal t.
Vestibular n.
Spinothalamic t.

Nucleus VI

MLF
Anterior trigeminothalamic t.
Medial lemniscus
Pyramid

FIGURE A-5
Transverse section of the lower pons at the level of the
entrance of the vestibular nerve and of the cerebellum
through the deep cerebellar nuclei. Refer to Fig. A-18.
(*After Villiger.*)

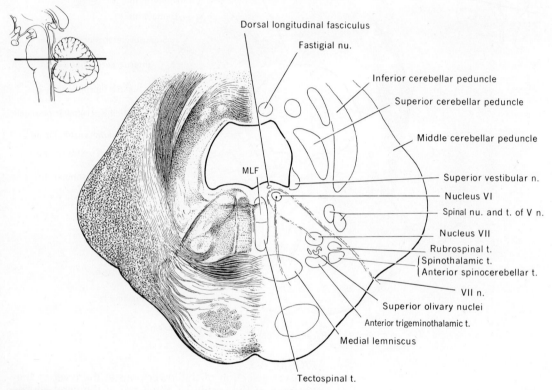

FIGURE A-6
Transverse section of the pons at the level of the facial
colliculus, abducent (VI) nucleus, and the superior
olivary nuclei. Refer to Figs. 8-7 and A-19. (*After
Villiger.*)

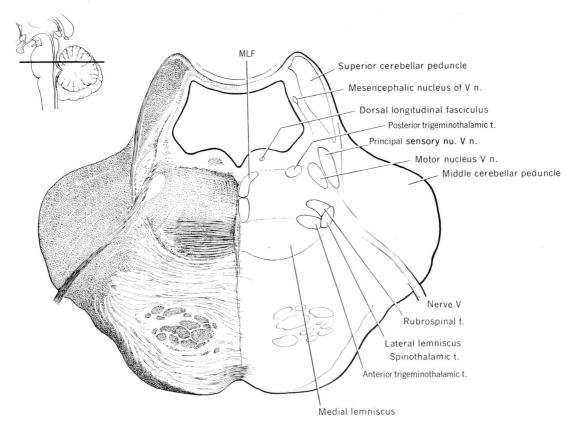

MLF

Superior cerebellar peduncle

Mesencephalic nucleus of V n.

Dorsal longitudinal fasciculus

Posterior trigeminothalamic t.

Principal sensory nu. V n.

Motor nucleus V n.

Middle cerebellar peduncle

Nerve V

Rubrospinal t.

Lateral lemniscus

Spinothalamic t.

Anterior trigeminothalamic t.

Medial lemniscus

FIGURE A-7
Transverse section of the pons at the level of the
entrance of the fifth cranial nerve. Refer to Figs. 8-8 and
A-20. (*After Villiger.*)

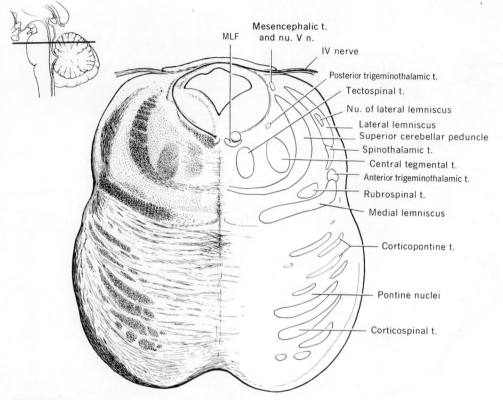

FIGURE A-8
Transverse section of the isthmus region at the level of
the decussation and emergence of the trochlear (IV)
nerve and of the upper pons. Refer to Fig. A-21. (*After
Villiger.*)

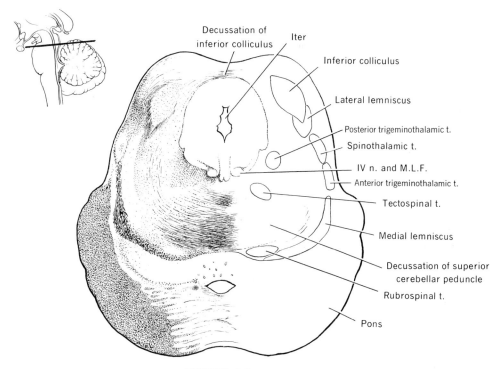

Decussation of
inferior colliculus

Iter

Inferior colliculus

Lateral lemniscus

Posterior trigeminothalamic t.

Spinothalamic t.

IV n. and M.L.F.

Anterior trigeminothalamic t.

Tectospinal t.

Medial lemniscus

Decussation of superior
cerebellar peduncle

Rubrospinal t.

Pons

FIGURE A-9
Transverse section of the lower midbrain at the level of
the inferior colliculus and decussation of the superior
cerebellar peduncle. Refer to Figs. 8-9 and A-22. (*After
Villiger.*)

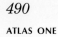

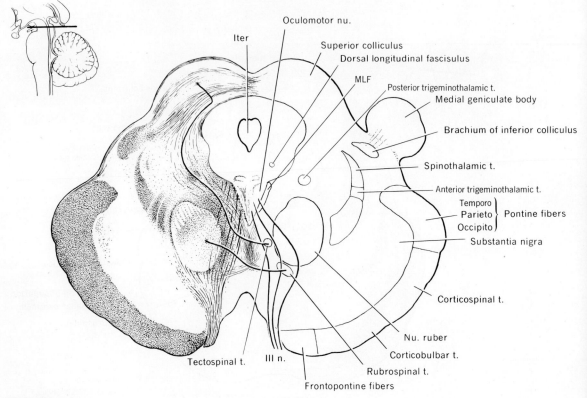

Oculomotor nu.

Iter

Superior colliculus

Dorsal longitudinal fascisulus

MLF

Posterior trigeminothalamic t.

Medial geniculate body

Brachium of inferior colliculus

Spinothalamic t.

Anterior trigeminothalamic t.

Temporo
Parieto } Pontine fibers
Occipito

Substantia nigra

Corticospinal t.

Nu. ruber

Corticobulbar t.

Rubrospinal t.

Frontopontine fibers

III n.

Tectospinal t.

FIGURE A-10
Transverse section of the upper midbrain at the level of
the superior colliculus and the oculomotor (III) nerve.
Refer to Figs. 8-10 and A-24. (*After Villiger.*)

ATLAS 2
THE BRAINSTEM IN
NISSL PREPARATIONS

**Abbreviations used in Figs.
A-11 through A-32:**

A	anterior nucleus of thalamus
AC	anterior commissure
ACN	accessory cuneate nucleus
AL	ansa lenticularis
ALIC	anterior limb of internal capsule
AM	amygdaloid body
AP	area postrema
APS	anterior perforated substance
B	brachium of inferior colliculus
CA	cerebral aqueduct
CC	crus cerebri
CG	cingulate gyrus
Cl	claustrum
CL	central lobe
CM	central median nucleus of thalamus
CN	caudate nucleus
CoC	corpus callosum
CS	corticospinal tract
CTT	central tegmental tract
DC	dorsal cochlear nucleus
DM	dorsal medial nucleus of thalamus
DN	dentate nucleus
DT	dorsal tegmental nucleus
DV	dorsal vagal nucleus
EC	external capsule
EN	emboliform nucleus
ExC	extreme capsule
F	fornix
FC	fasciculus cuneatus
FG	fasciculus gracilis
FN	fastigial nucleus
G	genu of facial nerve
GN	globose nucleus
GP	globus pallidus

H	prerubral field
H₁	thalamic fasciculus } fields of Forel
H₂	lenticular fasciculus
HIT	habenulointerpeduncular tract
HN	habenular nucleus
Hy	hypothalamus
IC	inferior colliculus
ICP	inferior cerebellar peduncle
IL Nu	intralaminar nuclei
IV	inferior vestibular nucleus
LC	lateral column
LD	lateral dorsal nucleus of thalamus
LG	lateral geniculate body
LoC	locus ceruleus
LP	lateral posterior nucleus of thalamus
LR	lateral reticular nucleus
LV	lateral vestibular nucleus
L.Vent	lateral ventricle
MB	mamillary body
MCP	middle cerebellar peduncle
ME V	mesencephalic nucleus of trigeminal nerve
MFB	medial forebrain bundle
MG	medial geniculate body
ML	medial lemniscus
MLF	medial longitudinal fasciculus
Mo V	motor nucleus of trigeminal nerve
MT	mamillothalamic tract
MV	medial vestibular nucleus
NA	nucleus ambiguus
NG	nucleus gracilis
NM	nuclei of midline of thalamus
NPO	nucleus pontis oralis
NR	nucleus ruber
NSO	nucleus of superior olive
NTB	nucleus of trapezoid body
N VI	nucleus of abducent nerve
N VII	nucleus of facial nerve
N XII	nucleus of hypoglossal nerve

VIII   vestibulocochlear nerve
IX   glossopharyngeal nerve
X   vagus nerve

OC   optic chiasm
OT   optic tract

PA   preoptic area of hypothalamus
Pf   parafascicular nucleus
PG   periaqueductal gray matter
Pi   pineal body
PLIC posterior limb of internal capsule
Prt   pretectum
Pr V principal trigeminal nucleus
Pul   pulvinar
Put   putamen
Py   pyramid

R   reticular nucleus of thalamus
RelC retrolenticular portion of internal
      capsule
RT   reticulotegmental nucleus

S   spinal trigeminal tract
SC   superior colliculus
SCN   superior central nucleus
SCP   superior cerebellar peduncle
SMT   stria medullaris thalami
SN   substantia nigra
S Nu septal nuclei
So   nucleus solitarius
SON   supraoptic nucleus
SP   septum pellucidum
ST   stria and vena terminalis
STT   spinothalamic tract
SUB   subthalamic nucleus

TC   tuber cinereum

VA   ventral anterior nucleus of thalamus
VC   ventral cochlear nucleus
VL   ventral lateral nucleus
VLC   ventral lateral nucleus of thalamus,
      pars caudalis
VLo   ventral lateral nucleus of thalamus,
      pars oralis
VM   ventral median nucleus of hypo-
      thalamus
VPL   ventral posterolateral nucleus of
      thalamus
VPM   ventral posteromedial nucleus of
      thalamus
V III third ventricle
V IV   fourth ventricle

ZI   zona incerta

III   oculomotor nerve
VI   abducent nerve
VII   facial nerve

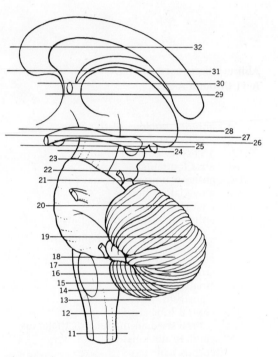

The levels and planes through the brain of
the following sections are indicated in the
diagram.

**The photographs in Figs. A-11 through A-32
were obtained from Dr. Sven O. E. Ebbesson of
the University of Virginia, Charlottesville.**

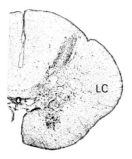

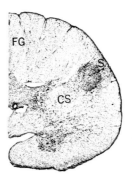

FIGURE A-11
Section of the upper portion of the first
cervical segment (Nissl stain). Refer to Fig. 8-2.

FIGURE A-12
Section of the lower medulla at the level of
the pyramidal (corticospinal) decussation
(Nissl stain). Refer to Figs. 8-3 and A-1.

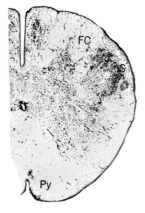

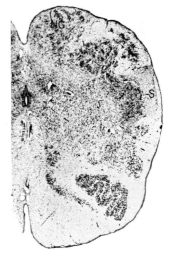

FIGURE A-13
Section of lower medulla at lower level of
decussation of medial lemniscus (Nissl stain).

FIGURE A-14
Section of lower medulla at the level of the
decussation of the medial lemniscus (Nissl
stain). Refer to Figs. 8-4 and A-2.

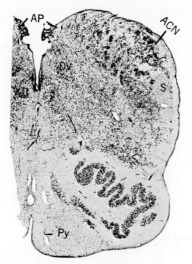

FIGURE A-15
Section of medulla at level of area postrema and rostral to obex (Nissl stain).

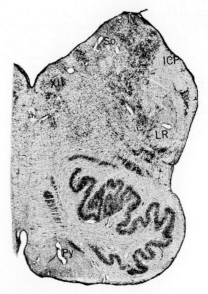

FIGURE A-16
Section of medulla at the level of middle of olive (Nissl stain). Refer to Figs. 8-5 and A-3.

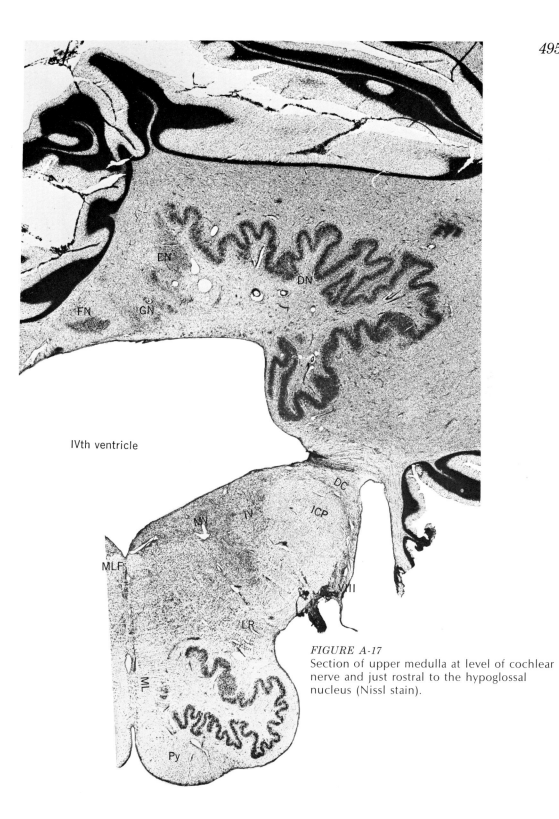

IVth ventricle

FIGURE A-17
Section of upper medulla at level of cochlear nerve and just rostral to the hypoglossal nucleus (Nissl stain).

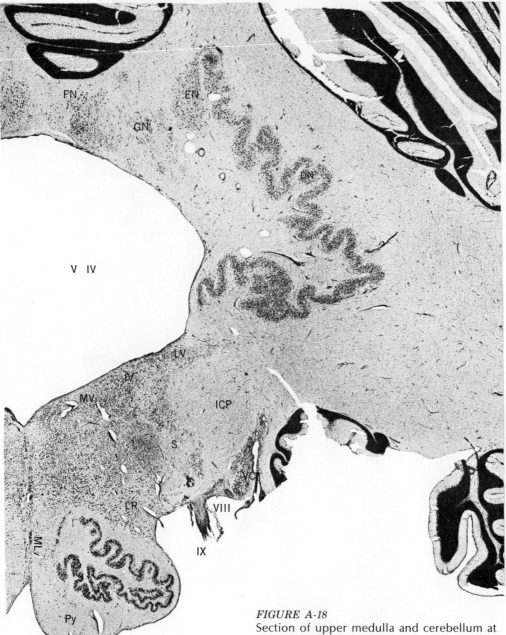

FIGURE A-18
Section of upper medulla and cerebellum at
the level of the glossopharyngeal nerve and
the deep cerebellar nuclei (Nissl stain). Refer
to Figs. 8-6, A-4, and A-5.

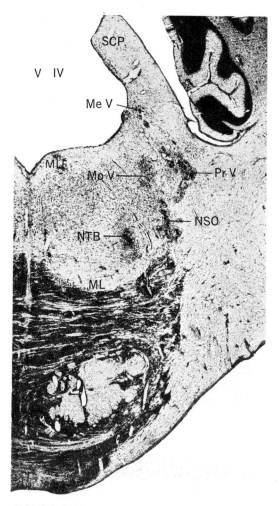

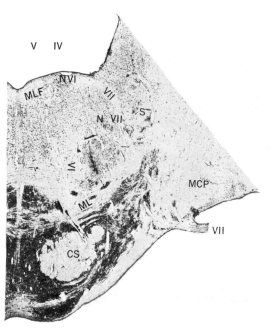

FIGURE A-19
Section of lower pons at level of abducent and facial nerves (Nissl stain). Refer to Figs. 8-7 and A-6.

FIGURE A-20
Section of midpons at level of principal sensory and motor nuclei of the trigeminal nerve (Nissl stain). Refer to Figs. 8-8 and A-7.

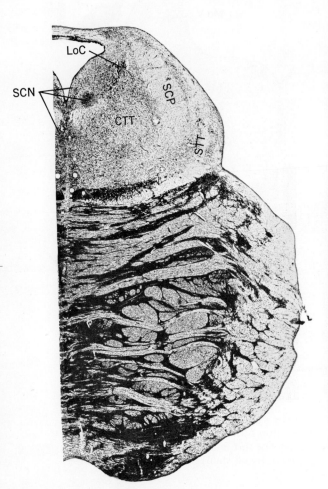

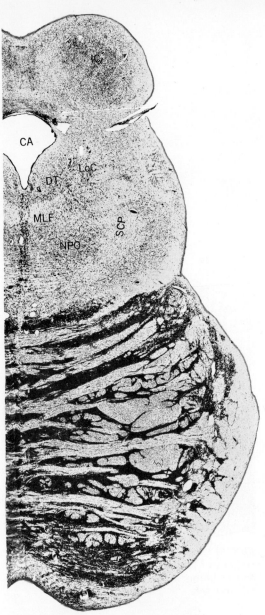

FIGURE A-21
Section of isthmus region of the brainstem
(Nissl stain). Refer to Fig. A-8.

FIGURE A-22
Section of lower midbrain at the level of the
inferior colliculus (Nissl stain). Refer to Figs.
8-9 and A-9.

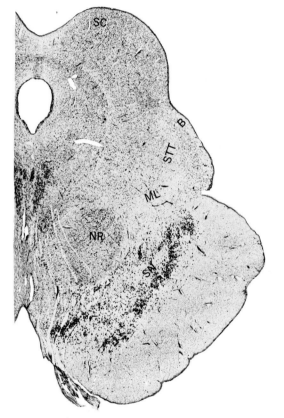

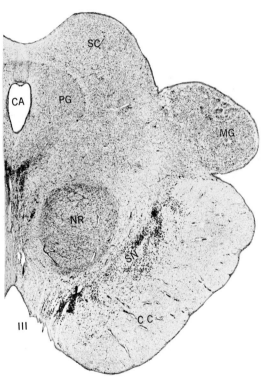

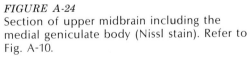

FIGURE A-23
Section of upper midbrain at the level of the superior colliculus (Nissl stain). Refer to Fig. 8-10.

FIGURE A-24
Section of upper midbrain including the medial geniculate body (Nissl stain). Refer to Fig. A-10.

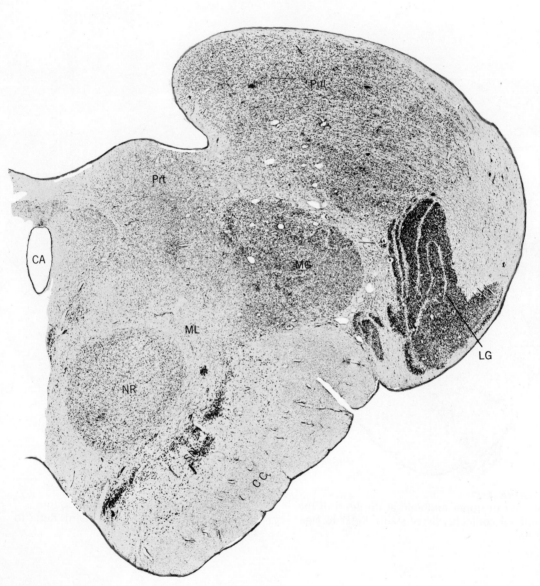

FIGURE A-25
Section at the junction of the upper midbrain and
posterior diencephalon (Nissl stain). Refer to Fig. 8-11.

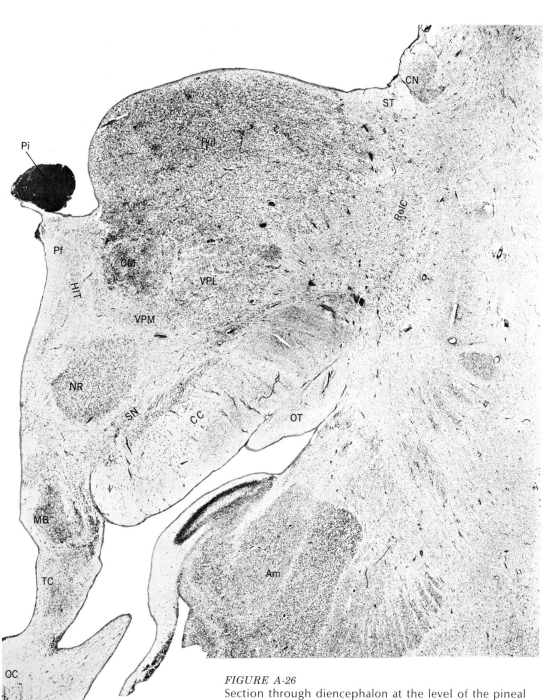

FIGURE A-26
Section through diencephalon at the level of the pineal
body, central median nucleus of thalamus, and
mamillary body (Nissl stain).

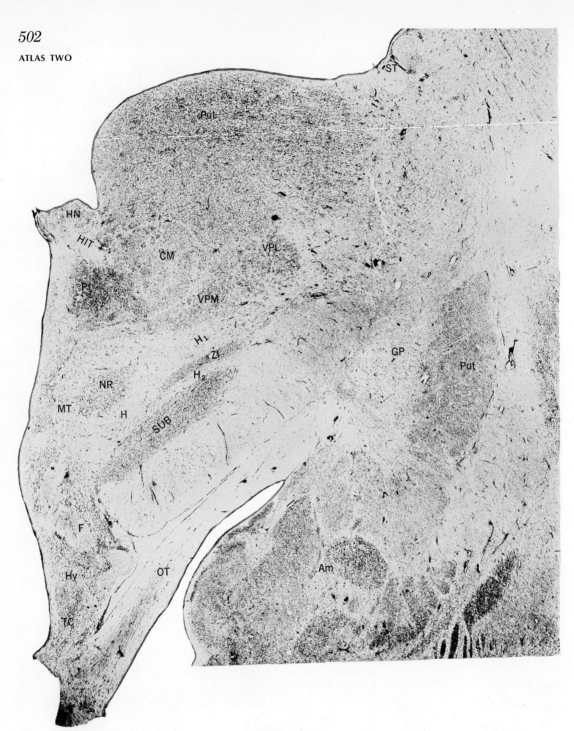

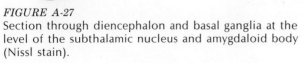

FIGURE A-27
Section through diencephalon and basal ganglia at the
level of the subthalamic nucleus and amygdaloid body
(Nissl stain).

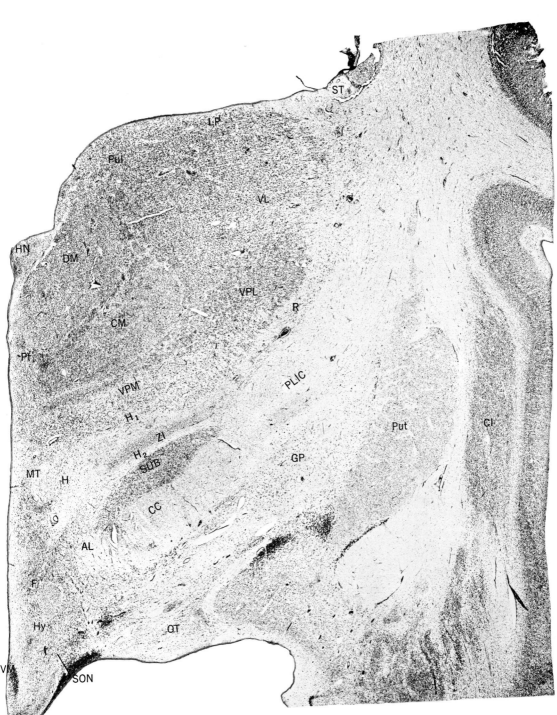

FIGURE A-28
Section through diencephalon and basal ganglia at the
level of ventral lateral thalamic, subthalamic, and
supraoptic nuclei (Nissl stain). Refer to Fig. 1-21.

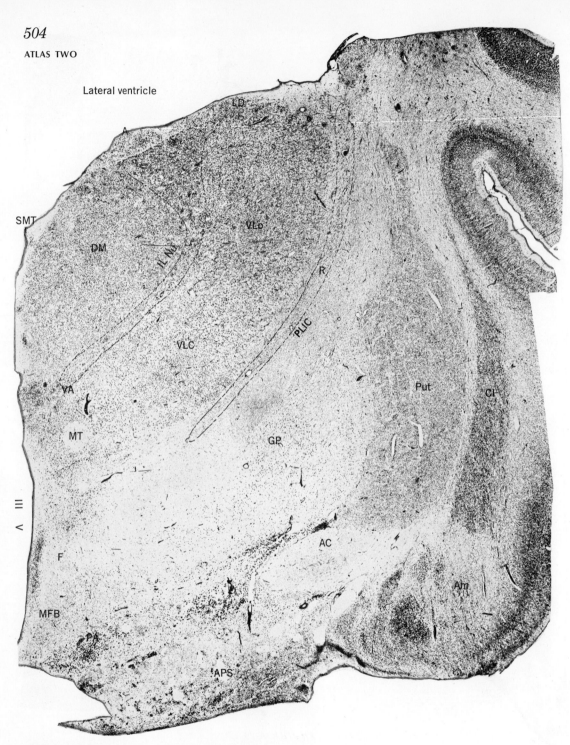

Lateral ventricle

FIGURE A-29
Section through diencephalon and basal ganglia at level
of ventral anterior and ventral lateral thalamic nuclei
and the lateral part of anterior commissure (Nissl stain).

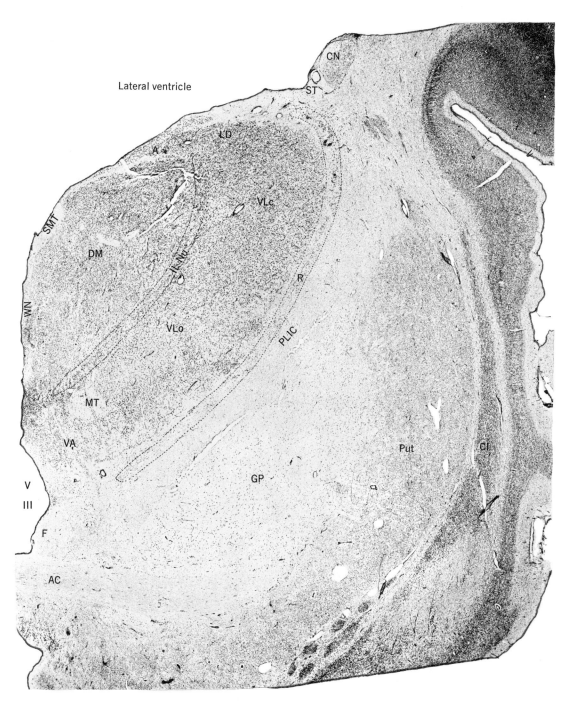

CN

ST

Lateral ventricle

LD

A

SMT

VLc

DM

IL-Nu

R

NN

VLo

PLIC

MT

VA

Put

Cl

V

GP

III

F

AC

FIGURE A-30
Section through diencephalon and basal ganglia at level
of the ventral anterior and ventral lateral thalamic nuclei
and the anterior commissure (Nissl stain). Refer to Fig.
1-20.

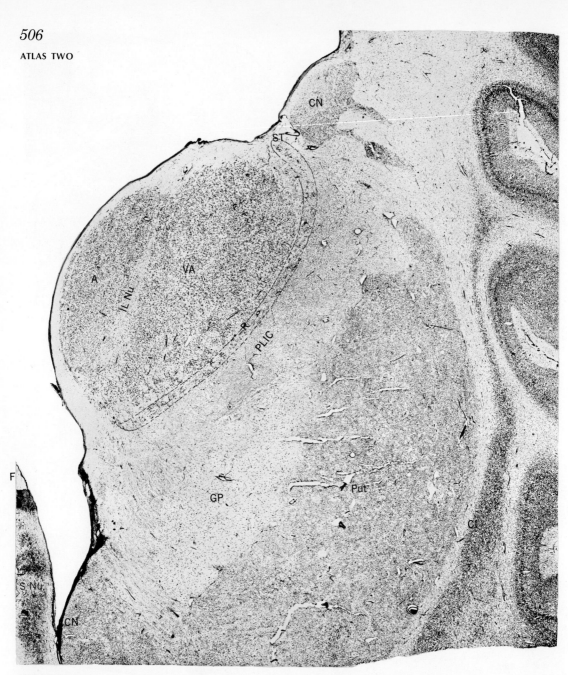

FIGURE A-31
Section through diencephalon and basal ganglia through
rostral thalamus and septal nuclei (Nissl stain).

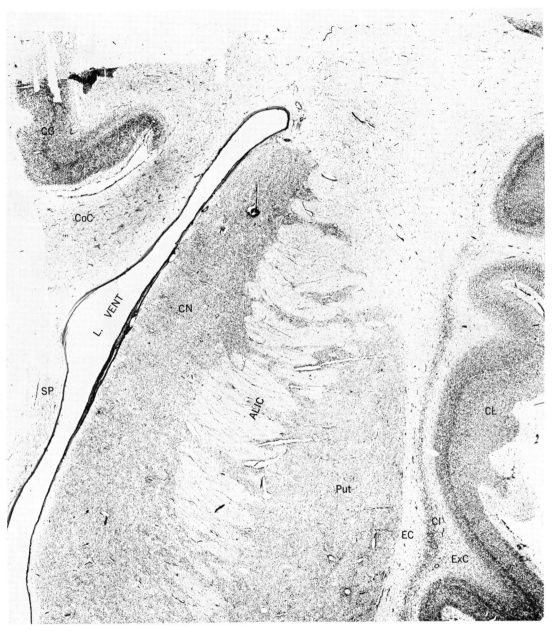

FIGURE A-32
Section through head of the caudate nucleus, anterior
limb of the internal capsule, and the putamen (Nissl
stain). Refer to Fig. 1-18.

INDEX

Page numbers in *italic* indicate illustrations or Atlas.

Abducent (facial) colliculus, 12, *14,* 225, *486*
    nerve, 8, 12, *220, 221,* 224, *225, 226,* 266, 269,
        486
    nucleus, *8, 12, 221, 235,* 251 – 252
Accessory nerve, *8,* 11, *12, 221, 235,* 237
    and root, 243, 245
Accommodation, 204, 224, 349, 377
    convergence, 380
Acetylcholine, 91, 92, 195, 210
    receptors, 87
Acoustic nerve (*see* Vestibulocochlear nerve)
Acoustic tubercle, *14*
Acrania, 130
Action potential, 78, *79,* 81, *90*
    generation of, 78
    propagation of, 80
Active transport (biologic pumping), 78
Adaptation, 96, 264, 268, 363, 389
    light, 363
    at a receptor, 97, 101
Adiadochokinesis (dysdiadochokinesis), 302
Adipsogenital dystrophy, 340
Adrenal (suprarenal) gland, 206
Adrenergic agents, 212
    fibers, 199
    mimetic drugs, 212
    neuron, 199, 200
    neurotransmitters, 212
    palm sweating, 206
    receptor (sites), 212
    system, *194,* 199
Adversive ("orientation") movements, 470
Affect, 437
Afferent fibers, 84, 85
    components of, 138, 218
    endings, 147
Afferent (sensory) input, 148
After-discharge, principle of, 101
Afterimage, 366
Aging:
    of the nervous system, 126, 127
    of neurons, 126
Agnosia, 437, 463
    auditory, 437, 463, 464
    tactile (astereognosis), 463
    visual, 463
Agonistic behavior, 437
Agraphia, 464, 480
Alar (dorsal) plate, 114

Alexia, 464, 480
All-or-none nerve impulse, 83
    response, 78, 90
Alveus, *18*
Amphetamine ("pep" pills), 201
Amphetamine psychosis, 201
Amygdaloid body (amygdaloid complex, amygda-
        loid nucleus, archistriatum, corpus amygda-
        loideum), *6, 8, 18,* 20, *23, 433*
    nuclei and connections, 433, 434
    stimulation and ablation of, 438
Amyotrophic lateral sclerosis, 188
Amytal (amobarbital), 474
Analgesia, 282
Anastomosis of arteries in brain, 29
Anencephalus, 130
Anesthetics (anesthesia):
    effect on lemniscal systems, 390
    effect on reticular system, 390
    in painless childbirth, 37
Annulospiral ending (primary sensory ending), 70,
        71
    (*See also* Neuromuscular spindle)
Anosmia, 223
Ansa lenticularis, *23, 415,* 419, 422
Anterior commissure, 5, 19, 452, 477
Anterior perforated space (substance, olfactory
        tubercle), *8, 9*
Antidiuretic hormone (ADH), 338
Apertures, medial (Magendie) and lateral
        (Luschka), 16, 40
Aphakic, 345
Aphasia, 479
    auditory, 466
    expressive, 474
    sensory (receptive), 464, 473
    visual, 466
Appestat, 336
Appetite, 336
Apraxia, motor, 474
Aqueduct of Sylvius (cerebral aqueduct, iter), 5, 9,
        15, 17, 35, 36
Arachnoid, 1, *30, 35*
    granulations, *35,* 39
    villi, 39
Archicerebellum, *14, 290,* 303, 322
    lesions, 303
Archicortex, 443
Archistriatum (amygdaloid body), *6,* 20, 417, *433*

Area(s):
  association, 445, *465*
  Broca's speech, *465*, 468
  of Brodmann, 445, *446*
  mamillary, 327
  motor, *447, 461*
    primary, *461*, 469
    secondary, *461*, 471
    supplementary, *461*, 471
  parietal, 460
  postrema, *14*, 244, *341*, 343
  premotor, 7, 470
  preoptic, 327, *433, 434*
  sensory (receptive), 445, 460
    for audition, 465
    vestibular, 466
    for vision, 464
  septal (region), *428, 432—435*
  supraoptic, 327
  tuberal, 327
  vestibularis, 12
  Wernicke's, *465*, 476
  [*See also* Cortex (pallium), cerebral]
Argyll-Robertson pupil, 380
Arterial supply to the brain, 25
Artery(ies):
  basilar, 25, *30*
  carotid, internal, 25, 26, 27
  carotid arterial system, 25
  carotid siphon, 27
  central retinal, 27, 223
  cerebellar, 25, *30*
  cerebral: anterior, 28, *30*
    middle (lateral), 28, *30*
    posterior, 26, *30*
  cerebral circle of Willis, 28, *30*
  choroidal, 27
  circumferential, 25
  communicating, 27
  labyrinthine (auditory), 25, *30*
  lenticulostriate, 29
  nutrient, 29
  occlusion or rupture of, 282—284
  ophthalmic, 27, 31
  ophthalmic anastomosis, 27
  paramedian, 25
  penetrating (nutrient), 29
  pontine, 25, *30*
  radicular, 181
  to retina, 27, 258
  spinal, 25, *30*, 181, *182, 183*
  striate, 29, *30*
  superficial (conducting), 29
  vasocorona, 182
  vertebral, 25, *30*, 181
Asphyxia, 236
Asthenia, 302
Astrocytes (astroglia), 41, *56*, 64, 65, *66*, 69
  perivascular foot of (foot plate), *56*, 66
Asynergia, 302
Ataxia (ataxic gait), 302

Athetosis, 424
Atony, 185
Atrophy, 185
Atropine, 212
Auditory agnosia and aphasia, 437
Auditory pathways, *311*, 313—316
  acoustic striae, 314
  cochlear efferent tract, 316
  corticocollicular tract, 315
  corticogeniculate tract, 315
  descending efferent fibers, 315
  geniculocollicular, 315
  inferior colliculus (nucleus), 315
  lateral lemniscus, 315
  medial geniculate body, 315
  olivocochlear bundle, 315, *316*
  primary auditory cortex, 465
  spiral ganglion, 313
  transverse gyri of Heschl, 465
  trapezoid body, 252, 315
  vestibulocochlear anastomosis, 316
Auditory radiation (geniculocortical), 314, *452*
Auditory reflex, 309
Auditory system, 306
  duplex theory, 312
  structural and functional correlations, 317
Augmenting response, 404
Automatic bladder, 207
Automatic control systems, 105
  feedback, 105
  servomechanisms, 105
Autonomic nervous system (involuntary nervous
    system, general visceral efferent system),
    138, 191—216
  adrenergic neuron and synapse, 200
  brain stem and, 208
  catecholamine, life cycle, 200
  cerebellum and, 209
  cerebrum and, 473
  comparisons with somatic nervous system, 191,
    214—215
  concept of, 191
  definition of, 191
  descending pathways, 209—210
  ganglia of, 62, 197, 198
  hypothalamus and, 209
  limbic lobe and, 209
  neurons of, 192, *193, 214—215*
    postganglionic, 192, *199*
    preganglionic, 192, *199*
  neurosecretions of, 200, 201, 203
  optic system and, 204
  organ systems, 204—208
  parasympathetic nervous system, *192, 199,* 201,
    214—215
    cholinergic system, 201, 203
    craniosacral system, 201
  pharmacology of peripheral nervous system, 210
  reflex arc of, 198, *199*
  spinal cord, 208, 209
  sympathetic nervous system, *192, 194,* 196,
    214—215
    adrenergic system, 199
    sympathoadrenal system, 197
    thoracolumbar system, 197
  thalamus and, 210

Axes of the brain, 16
Axis, visual, *346, 347*
Axis cylinder, 43, *60*
Axoaxonic synapse, 53
Axodendritic synapse, 53
Axon, *47, 48,* 49, 50, *60, 61*
  collateral branches of, 52
    recurrent, 52, *447*
    transverse, 52, *447*
  hillock, 50
  initial segment of, 50
  periaxonal space, *61*
  telodendria, *44*
  terminal and preterminal segments, 54
Axoplasmatic (flow) transport, 52
Axosomatic synapse, 53

Babinski reflex (sign), 187
Ballism, 423, 424
Barrier, blood brain, 66, 67
Basal ganglia, 17, 20, 407, 417, 418
  amygdaloid body, 20, 417, 433
  archistriatum, 20, 417
  caudate nucleus, *18 – 19,* 20, *22, 23, 26, 415, 416,* 417
    head and tail of, *18*
  claustrum, 20, 23
  corpus striatum, 20, 417
  functional roles, 423
  globus pallidus (pallidum), 20, *23, 29, 296, 415, 416,* 417, 419, 420
  lenticular (lentiform) nucleus, 20
  neostriatum (striatum), 20, 417
  nuclei and circuits of, 418 – 422
  paleostriatum, 20
  pallidum (globus pallidus), 20, *23, 29, 296, 298, 415, 416*
  putamen, 20, *22, 23, 26, 28, 29, 415, 416*
  role of, 418
  stimulation and ablation of, 423
  striatum (neostriatum), 20, 417, 419
  substantia nigra as, 9, *490*
  subthalamic nucleus as, 9, *24, 415, 416*
  tracts and connections, *414 – 421*
    ansa lenticularis, 422
    bundle H of Forel (prerubal field), *414,* 422
    bundle H$_1$ of Forel (thalamic fasciculus), *414,* 422
    bundle H$_2$ of Forel (lenticular fasciculus), *414,* 422
    extrapyramidal system, 417
      disorders of, 423 – 425
    lenticular fasciculus, *414,* 422
    subthalamic fasciculus, *419,* 422
    thalamic fasciculus, *415,* 419
Basilar portion of brainstem, 9, 24
Behavior and emotion, 437
  consummatory, 339
Bell's palsy, 231, 287
Benedikt syndrome, 286
Biologic "quantum," 86
Biologic transducer, 96
Blood-brain barrier (blood–cerebrospinal fluid barrier, hematoencephalic barrier), 65, *66, 67,* 69

Blood supply of brain, 22
  brainstem, 282
  control, 24
  functional aspects, 24
  hypophyseal portal system, 329, *330*
  spinal cord, 180, *182, 183*
Blood vessels, 205
Body:
  aortic, 195, 283
  carotid, 195, 283
  lateral geniculate, 401
  medial geniculate, 313, 323, 401
  trapezoid, 252, 315
Brachium:
  conjunctivum (superior cerebellar peduncle), 11, *14,* 252, 296, 297, *368*
  of inferior colliculus, 11, *13, 14,* 254, 289, 295, *296, 297,* 313, *490*
  pontis (middle cerebellar peduncle), 11, 273, 289, 295
  of superior colliculus, 11, *13, 14,* 296, 297, *490*
Brain, *23*
  axes of brain, 16, *17*
  blood supply, 25 – 34
  development of (*see* Development of the nervous system)
  gross anatomy, 1
  major subdivisions, 1
  of newborn infant, 125
  solid geometry, *17*
  topographic anatomy, 20
Brain weight, 1
Brainstem, 1, *10,* 11, 12, *13,* 242, 244, 246 – *248, 250, 251, 253, 254, 255*
  autonomic nervous system in, 276
  blood supply of, 25
  cerebellar connections, 273, 274
  descending pathways, 274 – 280
  infratentorial, 1
  levels through brainstem, 243 – 256, *257*
  longitudinal organization, 241
    basilar, 9
    basilar portion, 242 – 243
    roof, 241
    tegmentum, *5,* 241
    ventricular cavities, 241
  major subdivisions, 9 – 11
    medulla, 9 – 11, *244,* 246 – *248, 250*
    midbrain, 9 – 11, *253 – 255, 257*
    pons, 9 – 11, *251, 253*
  reticular formation, *149, 151, 153, 162,* 259, *416,* 421
    input to, 261
    output from, 262, *263*
  reticular system, 257, 260
  supratentorial, 1
  tegmentum, *5,* 241, *263, 322, 416, 435*
Broca's speech area, 2, *3, 7,* 445, *465,* 468, 476, 479
Brown-Séquard syndrome, 187
Bulb, 2

Calcium, 78, 92
Capacitance, 78
Capillaries of brain, 68

Capsule:
  external, 16, *22*
  extreme, 16, *22*
  internal, *6, 10, 12, 13, 20, 21, 153, 452, 453*
    anterior (caudatolenticular) limb, 20, *22, 29, 452,* 453
    components of, 453−455
    genu, 20, *29, 452,* 453
    posterior (thalamolenticular) limb, 22, *24, 452,* 453
    postlenticular (retrolenticular) portion of, 20,
      29, 452, 453
    sublenticular portion of, 20, *24,* 453
Carotid body, 195, 283
Carotid puncture, 31
Carotid reflex, 235
Carotid sinus, 195, 283
Carotid siphon, 27
Cataracts, 350
Cauda equina, *134, 137*
Caudate nucleus (*see* Basal ganglia)
Cavum septum pellucidum, 5
Cell structures associated with nerve:
  axis cylinder, 43, *44, 47, 49, 60*
  axolemma, 43
  axon, 50, *64*
  axon hillock, *47, 48,* 50
  cell body (perikaryon), *42, 43, 44,* 47
  cilia, 49
  dendrite (dendron), *47, 48,* 50, *51, 58*
    apical, 57, *58,* 447
    basilar, 57, *58,* 447
  endoplasmic reticulum, 45, *47, 49*
  Golgi apparatus, 46, *49*
  initial segment, *48,* 50, *98*
  lysosome, 46
  microfilaments, 49
  microtubules, *47, 48, 49*
  mitochondria, 45
  neuraxon, 49
  neurofilament, 46, *49*
  neuroplasm, 45, *78*
  Nissl substance, 45, *47, 48*
  node of Ranvier, *47, 48,* 50, *60, 61, 64, 82*
  nucleolus, 43, *47*
  nucleus, 43
  pigment, 46
  plasma (cell) membrane, 43, *47, 79*
  telodendria, *44, 48,* 52
Cells (in adult) and neurons, 41−52, *56, 66*
  astrocyte (astroglia), *56,* 64, *66*
  of autonomic motor ganglia, 62
  basket, *292, 293*
  Betz, 447
  bipolar, *42,* 57
    olfactory, *428,* 429
    in retina, 356, *357*
    in spiral ganglion, 313
    in vestibular ganglion, 321
  cones, 355, *352−355*
  ependymal, 65, *66*
  ganglion: of dorsal root, 62
    of retina, *351−355,* 356

Cells (in adult) and neurons:
  Golgi type I, 52
  Golgi type II, *42,* 52, 57, *292*
  granule: in cerebellar cortex, *42,* 292, 293
    in cerebral cortex, 446, *447,* 448
    in olfactory bulb, *428,* 429
  hair, in organ of Corti, *308, 309, 310*
  horizontal cells of Cajal, *447,* 448
  horizontal cells in retina, *351,* 357
  interneuron, *42,* 141, 165
  interstitial, 41
  of Martinotti, *313,* 448
  microglia, 63
  mitral, *428,* 429
  multipolar, 57
  neuroglia (glia), 63−69
    astrocyte (astroglia), 64
    microglia, 63
    oligodendrocyte (oligodendroglia), 63
  neurolemma (Schwann), *44,* 59, *60*
  neuron, 41−52
  olfactory receptor, 428
  oligodendrocyte (oligodendroglia), 63
    interfascicular, 63
    perineuronal, 63
  polymorph (multiform), 448
  Purkinje, *42,* 57, *292, 293*
  pyramidal, *42,* 66, *447*
  rods, *352−354,* 355
  satellite, 41, *42, 44,* 62
  Schwann (neurolemma), *44, 47,* 59, *60*
  stellate (granule), 292, 446, *447,* 448
  tufted, *428,* 429
  unipolar, *42,* 57
Center:
  apneustic, 277
  bulbar, 277
    disinhibition, 103
    facilitatory, 102, 277, 408
    inhibitory, 277, 408
  cardiovascular, 277
  control, 106, 107, 413
  drinking, 338
  facilitatory (pools), 408
  feeding, 336
  hunger, 336
  inhibitory (pools), 408
  integration, 107
  modulation, 107
  pleasure (rewarding), 340, 440
  pneumotaxic, 277
  punishing (aversion), 340, 440
  respiratory, 277
  salivatory, 277
  satiety, 336
  sleep, 262, 458
  vomiting, 277
Central canal, 15, *112*
  (*See also* Ventricular system)
Central lobe (insula, island of Reil), 3
Central sulcus of Rolando, 2, 3
Cerebellum, 12−14, 289−304
  anatomy, 12−14, *290, 322*
    gross divisions, subdivisions and fissures, 289, *290*
    hemispheres of, 289, *290*
    vermis of, 290

Cerebellum:
  arbor vitae, 291
  archicerebellum (flocculonodular node), 14,
      290, 291, 322
    lesions, 303
  cells and fibers of: basket cell, 292, 293
    climbing fiber, 292, 293
    Golgi cell, 292, 293
    granule cell, 292, 293
    mossy fiber, 292, 293
    Purkinje cell, 292, 293
    stellate, 292, 293
  corpus medullare, 14
  cortex of: granular layer, 291, 292
    molecular layer, 291, 292
  cytoarchitecture of cortex of, 291, 292
  dysfunction and effects of lesions of, 302
    attenuation of symptoms, 303
    physiologic safety, 303
    release phenomenon, 302
    unilateral lesions, effect of, 303
  flocculonodular lobe, 13, 291, 324
    (See also archicerebellum above)
  flocculus, 14
  folium, 13, 291, 292
  functional aspects of, 301
    role, 301
    servomechanism, 301
    vestibular system, 297, 300, 324
  glomerulus, 292, 293
  lobes, 13, 290
  localization in, 299, 300
    audiovisual area, 299, 300
    auditory, 299, 300
    polysensory, 300
    somatosensory, 299, 300
    tactile, 299, 300
    visual, 299, 300
  loops (feedback): brainstem, cerebellar, 296, 298, 301
    cerebrocerebellar, 296, 297, 300
    intracerebellar, 291, 292, 294, 300
    vestibulo, archicerebellar, 299, 300, 322
  neocerebellum (middle lobe, posterior lobe), 14,
      290, 291
  nucleus(i): dentate 292, 296, 298, 485
    emboliform, 292, 298, 485
    fastigii, 292, 322, 485
    globosus, 292, 298, 485
    interpositus, 292
  paleocerebellum (anterior lobe), 290, 291
  peduncle (brachium, body), 295
    inferior, 289, 296, 298
    juxtarestiform body, 295, 297, 299, 322, 323
    middle (brachium pontis), 10, 289, 296, 298
    superior (brachium conjunctivum), 162, 289, 298
  pyramis, 4
  tracts and fiber connections: afferent, 162, 164,
      295, 296–299
    efferent, 295–300
  uncinate fasciculus (hooked bundle), 297, 299
  vermis, 290
  vestibulocerebellum, 14
  zones of cortex, 290, 300
    intermediate, 290
    lateral, 290
    median, 290

Cerebral aqueduct (iter, aqueduct of Sylvius), 1, 5,
      8, 9, 15, 241, 254, 489, 490
Cerebral cortex, 419, 443, 446, 447
Cerebral dominance, 474, 475
  "mute" hemisphere, 478
  "talking" hemisphere, 478
Cerebral hemispheres, 1, 2
Cerebral ischemic reflex, 25
Cerebral penduncle, 9, 243
Cerebrospinal fluid (CSF), 1, 34, 35, 37, 66, 67
  functional aspects of, 39, 69
  spinal tap, 39
Cerebrum, 1, 3, 210
  lobe(s): central (insula), 2, 3
    frontal, 2. 6, 445
    limbic, 431, 438
    occipital, 2, 445, 464
    parietal, 2, 460
    temporal, 2, 465
    (See also Lobes)
  in neonate, 123
  pole(s): frontal, 2, 17
    occipital, 2, 17
    temporal 2, 17
  (See also Gyrus)
Chemoreceptors, 24, 96, 195, 234, 277
Chloropromazine, 201
Cholinergic fiber, 196, 203
  agents, 211
Cholinesterase, 203
Chordotomy, 155
Chorea, 424
Chorioid plexus and tela chorioidea, 7, 15, 19, 39,
      66, 67, 68
  of fourth ventricle, 5, 15
  of lateral ventricles, 15, 18
  of third ventricle, 15, 18
Chromatolysis, 45, 73, 75
Chronaxie (exitation time), 83, 84
Circuit(s), neuronal:
  closed, 99, 102
    feedback, 99, 102
    multiple chain, 100, 102
    simple chain, 99
  feedback, 99
    negative, 106
    positive, 107
  open, 99, 102
    multiple, 99, 102
    simple three-neuron, 98, 102
    simple two-neuron, 98, 102, 434
Circumventricular organs, 341
Cistern(s), 34, 35, 36
Clasp-knife response, 186
Claustrum, 20, 22, 23, 417
Cleft of Schmidt-Lantermann, 59, 60
Clonus, 186
Coactivation, 180
Cochlea (see Ear)
Coding and processing in nervous system, 385, 386
Cogwheel effect, 424
Cold, 152
Collateral nerve regeneration, 75
Colliculus:
  abducent (facial), 12, 14, 252, 486
  facial (abducens), 12, 14, 352, 486

Colliculus:
  inferior colliculus, *5, 6*, 9, 11, *13*, 241, *298*, 315,
    489
  superior colliculus, *5*, 11, *13, 159, 298, 313,*
    368, 375, 377, 490
Color of eye, 350
Color blindness, 365
Color vision, 360, 365
Coma, 263
Combined system disease, 188
Commissure:
  anterior, *5, 6,* 19, *23, 428,* 452, 477
  corpus callosum, 4, *13,* 19, *23, 27, 29, 432,* 451, 477
  fornical (hippocampal), 19, *26,* 453, 477
  habenular, 5, 453
  hippocampal, 19, *26,* 454, 477
  intercollicular, 9
  posterior, 5, *321, 322,* 376, *377*
  of spinal cord, *143, 152*
Components, functional:
  of cranial nerves, 217–223
  of spinal nerves, 137–139
Conduction:
  antidromic, 86
  cable property, 79, 83
  critical threshold (critical point), 80
  decremental, 83, *98*
  graded, 87
  nondecremental (all-or-none), 78, *79, 80, 98*
  orthodromic, 86
  saltatory, *80, 81, 82*
  speed of, 84
  spike, 78
  unidirectional, 85
  (See *also* Neurophysiology)
Cone (see Visual system)
Confabulation, 439
Congenital defects, 130
Connective tissue elements, 41
  endoneurium, 59, *60*
  epineurium, *60,* 61
  meninges, 34–37
  perineurium, 59, *60*
Contact guidance, 129
Contour sharpening, 362
Control system(s), 105–107, 412, 413
  closed-loop, 106
  feedback: functional significance of negative,
    106, 412
    positive, 107
  open-loop, 105
  servomechanisms, 106, 412
Conus medullaris (terminalis), 133, *134*
Convergence, principle of, 101, *102*
Corona radiata, *10,* 11, *12, 21*
Corpora quadrigemina, 11, 241
Corpus callosum, 4, 6, 10, *22, 23, 27, 29,* 242, 243,
    255, 256
  body (crus), 4, *29*
  functional considerations *475,* 476–479
  genu, 4, *29*

Corpus callosum:
  rostrum, 4, *29*
  splenium, 4, *29*
  tapetum of, 20, *27, 28*
Corpus striatum, 20, 417
Cortex, cerebellar (see Cerebellum cortex)
Cortex (pallium) cerebral:
  areas cytoarchitecturally defined, 456
    agranular, 446
    allocortex, 430, 431, 443
    archicortex (archipallium), 3, 443
    granular, 446
    heterogenetic, 443
    heterotypic, 446
    homogenetic, 443
    homotypic, 446
    isocortex, 443
    juxtallocortex, 445
    koniocortex, 446
    limbic, 431
    mesocortex, 3
    microscopic anatomy, 445
    motor and premotor, 445, *461, 462*
    neocortex (neopallium), 443, 472
    paleocortex (paleopallium), 3
    pallium (cortex), 443
    sensory, 460
  association areas, 463, 465, 466
  autonomic nervous system and, 473
  circuits: cortical, 455, 456
    interhemispheric, 456
    intracortical, 456
    intrahemispheric, 456
  cytoarchitectural laminae of, 445, *446, 447*
    granular, 446, *447*
    molecular, 446, *447*
    multiform, 446, *447*
    plexiform, 445, *447*
    pyramidal, 445, *447*
    spindle, 445, *447*
  cytoarchitectural map, 445, *446*
  descending fibers of, to ascending pathways,
    451, 468
  functional considerations of, *465, 472, 475*
    angular gyrus, 464
    auditory cortex, 465
    Broca's area, *465,* 468
    central lobe (insula), 466
    frontal lobe, 468
    "interpretative" cortex, 445
    limbic lobe, 431
    motor cortex, 469
    neocortex, 6, 443, 445, 472
    occipital lobe, 464
    parietal lobe, 460
    prefrontal (lobe) cortex, 472
    premotor cortex, 470
    "psychical" cortex, 466
    somesthetic cortex, 460, 462, 463
    supramarginal gyrus, 463
    temporal lobe, 466
    visual cortex, 464, 465
    Wernicke's area, 464
  gyrencephalic, 2
  interpretive, 445
  layers of, 445, *446, 447*

Cortex (pallium) cerebral:
  loops and circuits of: intracortical, *447, 456*
    interhemispheric, 456
    intrahemispheric, 456
  motor areas of, 469–472
    functional expression of, *461, 462,* 469–472
    pathways from, 467, 469
    premotor, *461,* 470
    primary, *462,* 469
    secondary, 471
    supplementary, *461,* 471
  neocortical neurons, 445
  neurophysiology, 457
  pyramidal cells, *448*
  sensory areas of, *461, 462*
    auditory (area II), 465
    auditory (primary), 465
    gustatory, 268
  sensory areas of: olfactory, 430
    somesthetic: association, 463
      primary (somatic I), 460, *461*
      secondary (somatic II), *461, 462*
    visual: association, *368,* 465
      primary, *368, 461,* 464
      secondary (visual II), 465
  stripe(s) and line(s): of Baillarger (inner), 456
    of Baillarger (outer), 456
    of Gennari, 456
    of Kaes, 456
Cortically induced movements, 179, 274
Cranial nerves:
  components, 217–223
  functions of, 223–238
  (*See also* Nerves, cranial)
Cretin, 120
Crossed-nerve anastomoses, 76
Crus cerebri (pes pedunculi), 9, 10, *21, 26,* 242,
  243, 255, 256
Curare (*d*-tubocurarine), 211

Dale's law, 86
Deafferented limb, 183
Decerebrate animal, 413
Decerebrate rigidity, 413
Decomposition of movement, 302
Decorticate animal, 414
Decussation:
  of brachium conjunctivum, *297,* 298, *486*
  dorsal tegmental, 256
  of inferior colliculus, *313, 489*
  of medial lemniscus (internal arcuate fibers), *158,*
    160, *482*
  pyramidal (corticospinal), *174, 175,* 280, *481*
  of superior cerebellar peduncle (brachium con-
    junctivum), *296,* 298, *489*
  trochlear nerve, *221,* 254, 255, *488*
  ventral tegmental, 256, 276
Deep sensibility, 146
Defects, developmental, of nervous system, 130,*131*
Degeneration and regeneration, 73, *75*
  in central nervous system, 74
  chromatolysis, 73, *75*
  of nerves, 73, *75*
  primary degeneration, 73, *75*
  secondary (Wallerian degeneration), 73, *75*

Dejà vu, 466
Dendrite (dendron), 49, 50, *51,* 57, 61
Dendritic potential, 95
Dendritic spines, 50
  synapse, 53
Denervation hypersensitivity, 188, 212, 213
  law of denervation, 213
  paradoxical pupillary reaction, 212
Denticulate ligament, 133, *135*
Dermatome, 138, 139, *140,* 182
Descending fibers in ascending pathways, 315
Development of the nervous system, 109–131
  abnormal development, 130
  aging, 126, 127
    atrophic changes, 126
    involuntary changes, 126
    of nervous system, 126
    of neurons, 126
    senescence of neurons, 127
  brain: cerebellar cortex, 116, 122, *123–126*
    cerebral cortex, 115, 121
    postnatal growth, 125, *126*
    prenatal, 122, *123*
    sulci, 123
  cell migration, 114, 120
  concept of initial mass reflex patterned activity,
    127
  concept of initial simple reflex patterned activity,
    127
    congenital defects, 130
    ballooning, 130
    causes of, 119–122
    critical periods, 118
    lip, 130
    of spinal cord (spina bifida), 131
  cortical plate, 114
  critical periods, 118, 125–128
  derivatives of the neural tube: ectodermal, 109
    mesodermal, 118
  embryonic cells and their derivatives, *113, 117*
    germinal (matrix), 111
    glioblast (spongioblast), 111
    matrix (germinal), 111
    mesodermal, 118
    neural ectodermal, 109
    neuroblast, 111, 113, 117
    ventricular (matrix), 113
  embryonic structures: alar (dorsal) plate, *111,*114
    basal (ventral) plate, *111,* 114, 117
    ectoderm, 109
    ependymal (matrix) layer, 110, 113
    ganglionic eminence, 114
    macroglial, 114
    mantle layer, 113
    marginal layer, *111–113*
    matrix (ependymal) layer, 110, *111, 112*
    nasal placode, 109
    neural crest, 110, *111, 112,* 117
    neural fold, 109, *110*
    neural groove, 109, *110, 111*
    neural plate, 109, *111*
      derivatives of, *112*
    neural tube, 109, 110, *111*
      placode, 109
    optic placode, 109, *110*
    optic vesicle, 109, *123*

Development of the nervous system:
   placodes, 109, 110, 115, 116
   rhombic lip, 114, 116, 122, *123*
   somite, *110, 111,* 117
   sulcus limitans, *111,* 114
 environmental factors, 119
 flexures: cervical, 122, *125*
   mesencephalic, 122, *125*
   pontine, 122, *125*
 functional activity during, 127
   components, *117*
   motor, 127
   prenatal and postnatal, 122, 128
   reflex arc, 127
   sensitivity to sex hormones, 120
   sensory, 127
 ganglionic eminence, 120
 genetic code and biochemical guides, 129
 genetic factors, 119
 growth, 125
 hormones, 120
 malformations, 130
 migration, 114
   inside-out, 115
 nutrition, 119
 oxygen and brain damage, 122
 of peripheral nervous system, 117
 plasticity of nervous system, 129
 of spinal cord, *111,* 114, *123*
 vesicles, *110,* 112
   diencephalon (between, twixt-brain), 122, *123*
   mesencephalon (midbrain), 109, *123, 125*
   metencephalon (afterbrain), 122, *123*
   myelencephalon (spinal brain) 122, *123*
   prosencephalon (forebrain), 109, *123*
   rhombencephalon (hindbrain), 109, *123*
   telencephalon (endbrain), 122, *123*
   zones, ventricular, subventricular, intermediate
     and marginal, 113, 114
Diabetes insipidus, 339, 340
Diaphragma sellae, 36
Diencephalon (twixt-brain, between brain), 1, 7,
   122
Disinhibition, 103
Disjunctive movements, 225
Dissociated sensory loss, 183
Divergence, principle of, 100
Dorsal (alar) plate, 114
Down's syndrome (mongolism), 119
Drugs neurotransmitters, and other chemical com-
     pounds:
   acetylcholine, 55, 91, 211
   adrenalin (epinephrine), 200
   adrenergic drugs (agents), 200
     neuron, 200
   amphetamine (pep pill), 201
   anticholinesterase agents, 211
   atrodine, 212
   blocking agents: competitive, 211
     depolarizing, 211
   carbachol, 211

Drugs neurotransmitters, and other chemical
     compounds:
   catecholamines, life cycle of, 200
   catechol-o-methyl transferase (COMT), 201
   chlorpromazine, 201
   cholinergic drugs (agents), 211
   cholinesterase, 211
   cholinesterase inhibitors (anticholinesterase
     agents), 211
   curare (*d*-tubocurarine), 211
   dopamine, 200, 270
   dopamine pathway or system. 273, 420
   dramamine, 326
   epinephrine (adrenaline), 200
   homatropine, 212
   monoamine oxidase (MAO), 201
   muscarine, 211
   muscarinic effect, 211
   nicotine, 211
   nicotinic effect, 211
   norepinephrine (noradrenaline), 55, 200
   parasympathomimetic drug, 210
   pharmacologic agents, mode of action, 210
   physostigmine, 211
   serotonin, 200
   sympathomimetic drug, 210
Dura mater:
   inner and outer, 1, 35
   innervation of, 39
Dural sleeve, 37, 136
Dural (venous) sinuses (*see* Veins)
Dynamic polarization of the neuron, 86
Dysartharia, 287, 303
Dyskinesia, 424
Dysmetria, 302
Dysphagia, 235, 236, 282, 287
Dysphonia, 236

Ear, 305, *306, 307*
   auditory (Eustachian, pharyngotympanic) tube,
     307, 309
   bone conduction, 308
   hearing (*see* Hearing)
   inner (internal), *306–311*
     ampulla, *307,* 317, *319*
     basilar membrane, *307–309,* 312
     bony labyrinth, 305, 307
     cochlea, 305, *306, 307,* 309
     cochlear duct, 305, *307, 308, 319*
     cortilymph, 311
     crista ampulla, 305, 317, 318, *319*
     crista macularis, 305, *321*
     cupula, 318, *321*
     endolymph, 305, *307,* 310, 318
     endolymphatic space, 305, *319*
     hair cells, inner and outer, 309, *310, 311,* 320
     helicotrema, *307,* 309
     Hardesty's membrane, 309, *311*
     Hensen's stripe, 309, *311*
     macula, 305, 317, 319
     membranous labyrinth, 305, *319*
     organ of Corti, 305, 309, *311,* 314, *319*
     otoliths (otoconia, ear dust), 319
     perilymph, 305, *307*
     perilymphatic space, 305, *307, 319*

Ear:
  inner (internal): saccule, 319
    scala media, 305
    scala tympani, 305, *307*
    scala vestibuli, 305, *307*
    semicircular canals, *307*, 317, *319*
    semicircular ducts, 305
    spiral ganglion, *307, 311*, 313
    tectorial membrane, *308*, 309
    utricle, 305, *307*, 319
    vestibular ganglion, *307*, 321
    vestibular (Reissner's) membrane, *307*, 309
  middle, 306, 309
    bone conduction, 308
    ear bones, 307
    ear drum (tympanic membrane), 306
    incus (anvil), *306*, 307
    malleus (hammer), *306, 307*
    oval window (fenestra vestibula), 307
    round window (fenestra cochleae,) *307*, 309
    spiral organ of Corti, 305, 309, 314
    stapedius muscle, 308
    stapes (stirrup), *306, 307*
    tensor tympani muscle, *306*, 308
    tympanic membrane (ear drum), 306, 308
    tympanic tube (Eustachian tube), *306*, 307,
      309
  outer (external), 306
    auricle, 306
    external auditory meatus (canal), 306
    tympanic membrane (ear drum), 306
Ectoderm (neural), 109
Efferent (motor) endings, 73
  of autonomic nervous system, 73
  motor end plate (*see* Motor end plate)
Efferent (motor) fibers:
  alpha, *72*, 73, 84
  gamma, *72*, 73, 84
  general visceral, 73, 218
  somatic, 73, 218
  special visceral, 73, 218
Electroencephalogram (EEG), 404, 457
  alpha, 457
    blocking, 457
  beta, 457
  brain waves (rhythms), 457
  desynchronized (activation) pattern, 273, 457
  K complexes, 459
  role of thalamus in, 403
  "spindling activity," 459
Eminence:
  median, *14*, 327, 341
  trigeminal (eminentia trigemini), 11, 243
Emotion and behavior (terminology):
  affect, 437
  agonistic behavior, 437
  agonistic responses, 437
  emotion, 437
  feeling tone, 437
  hypothalamus and, 339
  motivation, 437
  prefrontal lobe and, 472
  pseudoaffective reflex, 437
  sham rage, 437
  true rage, 437
Encapsulated nerve endings, 69

Encephalon (brain), 1
End bulb of Krause, 71
End feet, 65
End plate potential, 93
Endbrain (telencephalon), 1
Endocrine system, 77
  compared to nervous system, 334
  and nervous system, 77
Endoneurium (sheath of Henle), 59
Engrams, 477
Enlargement:
  cervical, *134*, 139, *141*
  lumbosacral, *134, 141*, 146
Ependyma, 15
Ependymal cells, 65
Ependymal layer, *66*
Epicritic sensation, 160
Epileptic seizures, 439
Epinephrine (adrenaline), 210
Epineurium, 61, *135*
Epidural space, 37
Epiphysis cerebri, 342
Epithalamus, 7
Equilibrium, 317
Excitation, 89
Excitation-contraction coupling (E-C coupling), 93,
  94
Excitation time (chronaxie), 83
Excitatory interneurons, 95
Excitatory postsynaptic potential (EPSP), 89, *90*
Excitatory response, 95
Exocytosis, 206
Exteroceptive, 146, *220*
Extrapyramidal system, 415, 417
  basal ganglia and, 417–422
  disorders in man, 423
    abnormal movements, 425
    athetosis, 4
    ballism, 423
    cog-wheel rigidity, 424
    dyskinesia, 424
    Huntington's chorea, 424
    paralysis agitans (Parkinson's disease), 424
    pathways, 258
    rigidity, 424
    torsion dystonia, 424
    tremors at rest, 424
  physiological aspects, 422
  skilled and voluntary movements and, 422
Eye, 345–351
  anatomy, 345, *346, 347*
    anterior chamber, 346
    aqueous humor, 346, 350
    blind spot (optic disk), 348
    canal of Schlemm, 350
    choroid (uvea), 346, 349
    ciliary body, 346, 349
    cornea, 346, 347, 349, 351
      transplants, 349
    dark adapted, 364
    filtration (iridocorneal) angle, 350
    fovea centralis, 347, 348, 353
    iris diaphragm, 346, 350
    lens, 346, 349, 351
    macula lutea, 318, 343, *348*
    optic cup, *352*

Eye:
  optic disk (blind spot), 347, 348
  optic nerve, *8, 346,* 348, *368,* 369, *370*
  optical axis, *346,* 347
  ora serrata, 349
  pigment epithelium (retina), 353
  posterior chamber, 346
  pupil, 346, 476
  sclera, 346, 347, 349, 351
  uveal tract (uvea), 346
  visual axis, 346
  vitreous (humor), 346, 349, 350
  zonula R fibers, 346
  functional aspects of: accommodation, 337
    aphakic eye, 350
    cataracts, 350
    choked disk, 348
    color or eye, 350
    constriction (miosis) of pupil, 376
    corneal transplant, 349
    dilation (mydriasis) of pupil, 204, 376
    emmetropic (normal) eye, 351
    farsightedness (hypermetropia), 351
    field of vision, 12–13, 367
    glaucoma, 350
    movements of eyes, 323, 380
      conjugate, 225, 379
    near vision, 351
    nearsightedness (myopia), 351
    optic disk, choked, or swollen, 348
    optical axis, 347
    presbyopia, 351
    refraction of light, 351
    visual axis, 347
  pigments (visual) in rods and cones, 356
    chlorolabe, 356
    cyanolabe, 356
    erythrolabe, 356
    rhodopson (visual purple), 356
  retina, *354, 355,* 358
    anatomy of, 352, *354, 355*
    bipolar neuron, *354, 355,* 357
    cone, *352, 353, 355,* 360
    detached, 352
    functional role of, 360
    ganglion cells, *354, 355,* 357
    horizontal neurons, *354, 355,* 357
    intraretinal connections, 356
    layers of, 352, 353, *354, 355*
    organization of, 351, *354, 355,* 358
    pigment epithelium, 353
    rod, *352, 353, 355,* 360

Facial (abducens) colliculus, 12, *14,* 225, 486
Facial (facial-intermediate) nerve, 230, *231,* 252
Facilitation, 102
  recurrent, 104
Facilitatory center, 408
Falx cerebri, 35
Far sightedness (hypermetropia), 351

Fasciculations, 185
Fasciculus, 84
  ansa lenticularis, *23, 415,* 419, 422
  arcuate, 451
  cuneatus, *14, 151,* 160, *242, 244, 246,* 393
  dorsal longitudinal, 209, 276, 329, *435,* 436,
    484, 486, 487, 490
  gracilis, *14, 151, 158,* 160, *242, 244, 246,* 393,
    481, 482
  inferior longitudinal, 451
  inferior occipitofrontal, 451
  interfascicularis, *151,* 172
  lenticular, *414, 415,* 419, 422
  medial longitudinal, *151, 176,* 179, 245, 247,
    321, 322, 323, *481–490*
  retroflexus (habenulopeduncular tract), *434,* 436
  septomarginal, *151,* 172
  spinospinalis (propriospinal), *151,* 172, 245, 258
  subcallosal, 236
  subthalamic, *415, 416,* 422
  thalamic, *414, 415,* 419, 422
  triangularis, *151,* 172
  uncinate, 297, *322,* 451
  vertical occipital, 451
  (*See also* Lemniscal system; Tract)
Fastigium, *5, 9*
Feedback, 99, 105, 160, 287
  loops, 300
  negative (degenerative), 106, 191, 387, 412
  positive (regenerative), 106
  [*See also* Circuit(s); Control systems, loops, feed-
    back in cerebellum]
Feed-forward inhibitory circuit, 294, 387
Feeding center, 336
Feeling tone, 437
Fibers and neurons, 59
  A, B, and C, 84, 85
  adrenergic, *192,* 199
  afferent, 84, 85
  alpha efferent, 149, 167
  arcuate or U, 450
  association, 19, *199,* 448, 450, 476
    intracortical and subcortical, 450
  autonomic, 180
  cholinergic, *194,* 203
  classification of nerve, 83
  climbing, *292,* 293
  cochlear efferent, 315, 389
  collateral: horizontal, 448
    recurrent, 52, 448
  commissural, 19, *58, 388, 389,* 448, *448,* 450,
    476
  corticobulbar (corticoreticular), 179, 274, 278,
    280, 467
  descending centrifugal, to nuclei of ascending
    pathways, 338, 468
  extrafusal, 71
  gamma efferent, 71, *72,* 85, 169
  group I, II, III, and IV nerve, *72,* 85
  intrafusal, 71
  internal arcuate, *158, 159,* 160, 246, *482*
  mossy, *292,* 293
  olfactory efferent, *428,* 430
  pallidofugal (thalamic, subthalamic, tegmental),
    419–422
  postganglionic, *192, 194, 196, 197,* 199

Fibers and neurons:
  preganglionic, *192, 194, 196,* 197, 199
  projection efferent, 19, *446, 448, 450,* 453
  reticuloreticular, 258, 274
  vestibular, 322
  (*See also* Fasciculus; Lemniscal system; Tract)
Filum terminale, *36,* 133
Fissures, 1
  anterior, 135
  of cerebellum, 13, *290*
  horizontal, *290*
  lateral cerebral (of Sylvius), 2, *3*
  longitudinal, *21, 22, 28*
  posterior superior, *290*
  posterolateral, *4*
  prenodular, 14
  prepyramidal, *4*
  primary, 13, *290*
  transverse cerebral, *4, 5*
  secondary, *290*
  ventral (anterior) medial (spinal cord), *135, 143*
Flexor reflex (basic protective reflex) *169,* 170
Flocculonodular lobe (archicerebellum), 13, 14,
  290, 291, 324
Flower-spray ending (secondary sensory ending),
  71, *72*
Focal Act, 423
  focusing effect, 317
Focal seizure, 470
Folia, 13, 291
Foramen (foramina):
  interventricular, of Monro, 5, *15, 17, 18, 29, 33, 36*
  intervertebral, 133
  lateral aperture of Luschka, 40
  medial aperture of Magendie, 40
Forebrain (prosencephalon), 1, 109
Fornix, 5, 6, *18, 19, 23, 24, 29, 433,* 434
  body (crus) of, *18, 24, 29*
  column of, *18, 23, 29*
  fimbria, *18, 26, 29*
  hippocampal commissure of, *26,* 431
  postcommissural, 435
  precommissural, 434
Fossa:
  interpeduncular, *10*
  rhomboid, *14*
Fovea, 245, 361
Frequency coding, 314
Fringe subsequence, 314
Funiculus (column), 142

GABA (gamma aminobutyric acid), 86
Gamma bias and control, 314
Gamma motor neuron, 71, *72,* 85, 165, *168,* 169
  receptor, 89
Ganglion, 58, 62
  autonomic, 62, *194,* 197, 198, *199*
  basal (*see* Basal ganglia)
  ciliary parasympathetic, *196, 221,* 238, *377*
  cell and cell system, 357, 361
  coeliac sympathetic, 198
  cranial nerve, 237
  dorsal (sensory) root, *134, 135, 137, 138*
  ganglionic (trunk) chain, *194,* 197
  Gasserian ganglionic (semilunar), *220,* 227

Ganglion:
  geniculate, *218,* 231
  inferior: of glossopharyngeal nerve, *220,* 234
    of vagus nerve, *220,* 236
  mesenteric sympathetic, 198
  microscopic anatomy of, 62
  otic parasympathetic, *196,* 203, *221,* 238
  parasympathetic, 237
  paravertebral sympathetic chain, *138,* 197, *199*
  prevertebral (collateral) sympathetic, *136, 138,*
    197, 199
  semilunar, 227
  sensory: of cranial nerves, *220,* 237
    of spinal nerve, 237
  sphenopalatine (pterygopalatine) parasympathetic,
    196, 203, *221,* 238
  spiral, *220, 232, 307, 313*
  submaxillary parasympathetic, *196,* 203, *221,* 238
  superior: of glossopharyngeal nerve, *220,* 234
    of vagus nerve, *220,* 236
  terminal, 238
  trigeminal, *220,* 227
  vestibular (Scarpa's) *220, 232, 306, 321*
Ganglionic eminence, 114
Gap junction, 55, 204
Gate-control theory of pain, 155, *156*
Generation of action potential, 78
Genetic code and factors, 119, 120
Geniculate body, *13,* 201, *236, 319, 368*
  (*See also* Thalamic nuclei, geniculate)
Genu:
  of facial nerve, 12, *231*
  of internal capsule, 20, *451, 452,* 453, *454*
Geometry of the brain, 16, *18*
German measles (rubella), 119
Gland, adrenal (suprarenal), *194,* 206
Glaucoma, 350
Glia (neuroglia), 63
  astroglia (astrocyte), *44, 56,* 63, *64,* 66
    fibrous and protoplasmic, 64, *65*
  ependyma, 63, *65*
  macroglia, 63
  microglia, 63, *65*
  oligodendroglia (oligodendrocyte), *44, 56,* 63, *64*
    interfascicular, 63
    perineuronal (satellite), 63
    perivascular, 63
  perivascular foot of astroglia, *56, 65, 66*
  pia-glial membrane, *65, 66*
Glioblast (spongioblast), 111
Globus pallidus (pallidum, paleostriatum), 20, *23,*
  29, 296, 298, 414, *415,* 422
Glomerulus (in olfactory bulb), *428,* 429
Glossopharyngeal nerve, *10,* 11, *12,* 219, *220, 221,*
  233
Glucose (source of energy), 23
Golgi apparatus' 46
Golgi cell, 292, 293
Golgi tendon organ, 71, *72,* 164, *168,* 169
Golgi type I cells, 52
Golgi type II cells, *42,* 52, 57
Gray matter, 142
Growth:
  of brain, 125
  of nervous system, 65
  (*See also* Development)

Gyrus(i), 2
  angular (22), 3, *444, 464, 465*
  cingulate, 3, 6, 431, *432*
  cuneus, 4, 7, *432*
  dentate, 3, *8, 26, 29,* 431, 443
  entorhinal cortex (subiculum), 431
  fasciolar, 3, 6, 431
  frontal, 2, *3,* 6, *432, 444,* 468
    pars opercularis, 2
    pars orbitalis, 2
    pars triangularis, 2
  hippocampal formation, 431
  hippocampus, *18, 29,* 431
  lingual, 4, *6, 7, 8, 432*
  occipital, 3, *4, 444*
  occipital-temporal, 6, 7
  orbital, *3,* 6, *7, 8, 444*
  paracentral lobule, 3, *4, 6, 7,* 469
  parahippocampal, 6, 7, *433, 434*
  parastriate area (18), *367, 372,* 465
  parietal, 2, *3, 444*
  peristriate area (19), *367, 372,* 465
  piriform area, 445
  postcentral, 2, *3, 444,* 460
  precentral, 2, *3,* 6, *7, 444,* 445
  precuneus, *432*
  prepiriform cortex, 432, 445
  rectus, 6, *7, 8, 21*
  striate area (17), *367, 372,* 464
  subcallosal (paraterminal body), 3, 431, *432*
  subiculum, 431
  supramarginal, 3, *444, 463*
  temporal, 3, *432, 444,* 465
  transverse, of Heschl, 3, 7, *313,* 314, 365,
    461
  uncus, 6, 7, 431, *432*

H fields of forel, 422
Habenula, 8
Habenular commissure, 7, 8
  nucleus, *435,* 436
Habituation, 264
Handedness, 474
Hearing:
  audition, levels of consciousness, 317
  auditory pathways, 313–317
  bone conduction, 308
  duplex theory, 312
  focusing effect, 317
  frequency, 312
  functional correlation, 317
  inhibition: lateral, 317
    mutual, 317
  kinocilium, 309, 310, 320
  loudness discrimination, 312
  otosclerosis, 308
  pitch: code, 317
    discrimination, 158
  pitch recognition, 317
  resonator (place) theory of Helmholtz, 312

Hearing:
  sharpening effect, 317
  sound location, 312
  stereocilia, 309, 320
  structural and functional correlations, 317
  telephone (traveling-wave) theory of Rutherford,
    312
  tonotopic organization: within the auditory path-
    ways, 312, 314
    in organ of Corti, 312, 314
Heat:
  conservation of, 336
  production, 336
Hematoencephalic barrier (blood-brain barrier), 65,
  69
Hemiplegia, 186, 189, 284, 285
Hemisphere (dominant and nondominant), 475,
  478, 480
Hemorrhage:
  extradural, 37
  subarachnoid, 37
  subdural, 37
Herpes zoster (shingles), 155, 182
Herring bodies, 334
Hindbrain (rhombencephalon), 1, 109
Hippocampal formation, 3, 6, *433, 434*
  seizures, 439
Hippocampus, *8, 18, 26, 29,* 431, *433,* 434, 435,
  443
  pes, alveus, fimbrae, *18,* 443
Homaropine, 212
Homeostasis, 106, 191
Homeostatic regulation of temperature, 335
Homunculus, 469
  motor, *461, 462,* 469
  sensory, *461, 462*
Hopping reaction, 412
Hormone (humoral agent), 77, 120, 333
  antidiuretic (ADH), 334
  corticotropin, 333
  gonadotropin, 333
  growth, 333
  oxytocin, 334
  prolactin, 333
  releasing, 333, 337
  thyrotropin, 333
  vasopressin, 334
Hyperphagia, 336
Hyperpolarization, 87, *88*
Hyperthermia, 335
  neurogenic, 335
Hypertonus, 186
Hypoglossal nerve, *8, 10,* 11, *12, 225,* 337
Hypophyseal portal system, 329, *330, 331,* 333
Hypophysis (pituitary gland), *5, 8, 10, 328, 330,*
  337, 339
  anterior lobe (adenohypophysis), *328, 330,* 337,
    339
  posterior lobe (neurohypophysis, pars nervosa),
    328, 330, 334, 337, 342
Hypothalamo-hypophyseal pathways, *330,* 333,
  339, 342
Hypothalamo-hypophyseal portal blood vessel,
  329, *330, 331*
Hypothalamus(ic):
  autonomic nervous system and, 335

Hypothalamus(ic):
  clinical considerations, 340
  emotional behavior and, 339
  feeding responses and center, 336
  functional role of (in), 335
    appetite, 326
    emotional behavior, 339
    feeding, 336
    lactation, 339
    objective (consummatory) expressions,
      339
    output, 332, 329
    ovulation, 339
    pituitary hormone-releasing (factors) hor-
      mones, 333, 337
    pituitary hormones, 333, 334
    rage, sham, 340
  heat-conservation region, 336
  heat-dissipating region, 336
  hunger center, 336
  and hypophysis, 336, 339
  input to, 329, 331
  lesions, 340
  mamillary (nucleus) body, 8, 18, 327, 331, 332,
    433
  median eminence, 328, 333, 334, 341
  as a modulation center, 107
  neurohypophyseal system, 337
  neurosecretion and, 330, 339
  neurosecretory neuron, 42, 339
  nuclei of, 327, 328
  pleasure (rewarding) center of, 340
  preoptic area (region) of, 327, 433, 434, 436
  punishing (aversion) center of, 340
  satiety center, 336
  sleep-awake cycle and, 340
  structural aspects of: areas (subdivisions), 327
    basic circuits, 327, 329, 342
    neuroanatomy, 327
    neurohumeral reflex, 334
    nuclei, 327, 328
    reflex arc in, 334
  subjective expressions, 339
  sulcus, 4, 6, 327
  sympathetic tone, 335
  temperature regulation of, 335
  tuber cinereum of, 327, 328, 330, 333
  vagal (parasympathetic) tone, 335
  water balance, 338
Hypotonus, 185, 186, 302
Hypoxia, 122

Impulse nerve, 78, 90
Inferior cerebellar peduncle (restiform body), 11,
  12, 13, 162, 250, 289, 295, 296, 298, 485,
  486
Inferior colliculus, 5, 6, 9, 11, 13, 241, 298, 313,
  315, 489
Infratentorial brainstem, 2, 243
Infundibular stem, 337
Inhibition:
  autogenic, 170, 186
  centers, 408
  lateral (mutual) inhibition, 317, 362
  mutual, 317, 363

Inhibition:
  neurotransmitter substances and, 87
  postsynaptic (IPSP), 89, 389
  presynaptic, 90, 389
  recurrent, 104, 173
Inhibitory postsynaptic potential (IPSP), 88, 89,
  90
  interneurons, 95
  response, 87
Initial segment of the axon, 48, 50, 83, 97
Injuries to the nervous system, 128
"Inside-out" migration, 115
Insula (central lobe, island of Reil), 10, 466
Integration center, 107
  hypothalamus as, 107
  medullary cardiovascular, 107
  neuron as, 94
Intention (action) tremor, 301
Inter (twist) brain (diencephalon), 1, 109
Intercalated disk, 53, 204
Intercolumnar tubercle, 342
Internal capsule, 10, 11, 20, 21, 22, 23, 29, 451,
    452, 453, 454
  anterior (caudata-lenticular) limb, 20, 22, 29,
    451, 453
  genu of, 20, 22, 29, 453
  posterior (thalamo-lenticular) limb, 20, 22, 24,
    29, 451, 453
    postlenticular (retrolenticular) part of, 29, 453,
      454
  sublenticular part of, 20, 22, 24, 453, 454
Internal carotid artery, 33
Interneuron, 165, 172
  commissural, 172
  intersegmental, 172
  spinal, 172
Internode, 59
Interoceptive endings, 70
Interoceptive modality, 147
Interpeduncular cistern, 34
Interpeduncular fossa, 9, 10
Interstitial cells, 41
Interstitial elements, 58
Interstitial fluid, 77
Interthalamic adhesion, 4, 9
Involuntary nervous system (see Autonomic ner-
  vous system)
Iron-containing granules, 46
Isthmus, 6
Iter (cerebral aqueduct, aqueduct of Sylvius), 1, 5,
  9, 343, 489, 490

Jacksonian seizure, 470
Jaw jerk, 228
Junction synaptic, 53
Juxtarestiform body, 295, 297, 322, 323

K complexes, 459
Kinesthetic sense, 157, 159
Kinetic reflex, 411
Kinocilium, 309, 320
Klüver-Bucy syndrome, 437
Korsakoff's syndrome, 439
Kwashiorkor, 119

L-dopa, 424
Labyrinth:
    artery, 26
    bony, 305
    disregard, 423
    loss, 326
    membranous, 305, *307,* 318
        endolymph, 305, 318
        perilymph, 305
    reflexes and reaction, 411, 413
Lamina, definition, 142
Lamina quadrigemina (tectum), 9
    schema of spinal cord, 144
Lamina terminalis, *4, 5*
Language, 474, *475,* 479
Lateral gaze paralysis, 284
Lateral inhibition (mutual), 317, 362
Lateralization of "speech centers," 474
Law of denervation, 213
Law of specific nerve energies, 148
Lemniscal system, 257, 391
    anterolateral column–spinal lemniscal pathway,
        392
    auditory pathways, 313, 394
    concept of, 257
    "efferent," 258
    epicritic pathways, 150
    general statement of, 257, 391, 394
    lateral (auditory), 252, 254, 313, *487–489*
    lateral column–spinal lemnicus, 264, 265
    medial (touch–deep sensibility), *158, 159,* 160,
        245, 251, 265, *269, 482–489*
    neospinothalamic tract (pain and temperature),
        152, *153, 154,* 392
    pain, temperature and light touch pathways, *153,*
        154, 264, 392
    paleospinothalamic pathway, 154
    posterior column—medial lemniscus, 157, *158,*
        159, 393
    protopathic pathways, 150, 264
    roles, 390
    specific system, 257
    spinal lemniscus, 152, 264
    spinothalamic pathways, 152, 154
    touch–deep sensibility pathways, 393
    trigeminal, 264, 329, 392
    visual pathway, 394
    (*See also* Fasciculus; Pathway; Tract)
Lentiform (lenticular) nucleus, *10, 13, 18,* 20, 418,
    452
Leptomeninges, 34
Lesions (effects of, and associated with), 182–189,
    281–287, 302, 303
    of abducens nerve, 226
    of accessory nerve, 237
    adiadochokinesis, 302
    areflexia, 185
    asthenia, 302
    asynergia, 302
    ataxia, 184, 302
    atony, 185

Lesions (effects of, and associated with):
    atrophy, 185
    auditory pathways, 281
    Babinski reflex, 187
    basal ganglia, 423–425
    blood supply, 182, *184,* 282, *283–285*
    of brainstem, 281–287
    Brown-Sequard syndrome, *184,* 187
    of cerebellum, 302
    of cerebral cortex, 463–466, 470–472, 474
    claspknife reflex, 186
    clonus, 186
    collateral regeneration, 74, *75*
    corticobulbar (corticoreticular fibers), 278, 279
    corticospinal (pyramidal) tract, 185, 186, 286
    of cranial nerves, 226, 229, 231, 232, 234–237
    deafferented limb, 183
    decerebrate animal, 413
    decerebrate rigidity, 413
    decomposition of movement, 302
    decorticate animal, 414
    denervation (hyper) sensitivity, 212
    descending tract of fifth cranial nerve, 282
    dissociated sensory loss, 183
    dorsal roots, 183, *184*
    dysmetria, 302
    of extrapyramidal system (*see* Extrapyramidal sys-
        tems, disorders of man)
    of facial nerve, 231, 232, 287
    fasciculations (muscle spasms), 185
    flaccid paralysis, 185, 189
    of glossopharyngeal nerve, 234, 235
    hemiplegia, 186
    herpes zoster (shingles), 155, 182
    Horner's syndrome, *184,* 188
    hyperreflexia (hyperactive reflex), 186
    hypertonia, 186
    of hypoglossal nerve, 237, 286
    hyporeflexia, 185
    hypotonia, 185
    intention tremor, 302
    inverse myotactic reflex, 186
    lateral gaze paralysis, 284
    lateral lemniscus, 281
    lower motor neuron (flaccid) paralysis, 185, 189
    medial lemniscus, 282
    medial longitudinal fasciculus (MLF), 284, 285
    medulla, 282
    "midbrain animal," 413
    midbrain tegmentum, 286
    of nucleus ambiguus, 287
    of oculomotor nerve, 226, 286
    paralysis, 186
    paraplegia, 189
    paresis, 186
    past pointing, 302
    phantom limb, 185
    posterior columns, 182
    prefrontal lobotomy (effect of pain), 472
    quadriplegia, 189
    rebound phenomenon, 303
    reflex bladder, 189
    reflex sweating, 189
    regeneration, 74
    rhizotomy, 182
    spastic paralysis, 185, 186

Lesions (effects of, and associated with):
    spasticity, 186
    of spinal cord, 182
    of spinal nerves, 182, 183
    spinal reflex sweating, 189
    spinal shock, 189
    spinothalamic tract, 187
    thalamic animal, 414
    thalamic syndrome, 405
    tone of muscle, 185
    tremor: intention, 302
      at rest, 424
    of trigeminal nerve, 229, 287
    trigemino-thalamic tracts, 281
    of trochlear nerve, 226, 286
    trophic effects, 212
    upper motor neuron (spastic) paralysis, 185, 186
    of vagus nerve, 236, 237
    vestibular pathways, *176,* 324
    visual pathway, 380, 381
Limbic lobe, 3, *261, 263,* 431, *432–434,* 438
    allocortex, 430, 431, 443
    archicortex, 3, 443
    cingulate cortex, 435
    connections, 435
    core structure, 431
    cortex of, 431
    juxtallocortex, 445
    mesallocortex, 445
    mesocortex, 3, 445
    orbitofrontal, 468
    paleocortex, 3
    paraterminal body (subcallosal gyrus), *432,* 435
    parolfactory area, *432*
    piriform cortex, 432
    prepiriform cortex, 432
    septal area (region), *432,* 434
    stimulation of, 429
    subcallosal gyrus (paraterminal body), *432,* 435
    subicular area, 432
      subiculum (entorhinal cortex), *6,* 431
Limbic system (structural and functional aspects),
    427, 430, *433–435,* 437, 440
    affect, 437
    agonistic behavior, 437
    amygdaloid body (*see* Amygdaloid body)
      anatomy of, 431
    anterior perforated space (substance, olfactory
      tubercle), 9, *30*
    behavior, 437
    circuit of Papez, 436
    core structures of, 431
    emotion, 437
    functional expressions and role of, 437–441
    general circuitry, 433, *434, 435,* 436
    habenular nucleus, *435,* 436
    hippocampal formation, 3, *6, 433, 434*
    hippocampus, *8, 18, 26, 29, 433,* 434, 435, 441,
      443
    isthmus, 431
    Klüver-Bucy syndrome, 437
    limbic lobe (*see* Limbic lobe)
    longitudinal striae, 431, 435
    memory, 439
    midbrain area, 209
    motivation, 437

Limbic system (structural and functional aspects):
    neurotransmitters, 437
    pleasure (rewarding) centers, 340
    prefrontal lobe and, 441
    pseudoaffective reflex, 437
    punishing (aversion) centers, 340
    rage: sham, 437
      true, 437
    relay nuclei, 398
    septal nuclei, 431
    stimulation of, 439
    stria terminalis, *13, 19, 26, 433, 434,* 434
    subjective feelings, 339
    uncinate fits, 440
    visceral brain, 430
Limen insula, 3
Line of Gennari, 456
Linear (progressive) acceleration, 318, 411
Lobes, cerebellum (see cerebellum)
Lobes cerebral, 2, *3*
    central (insula) 2, *10, 22, 23*
    frontal 2, *3, 6,* 445
      hypothalamic connections, 339
      pars opercularis, 2
      pars orbitalis, 2
      pars triangularis, 2
      role, stimulation and ablation of, 469, 470
    limbic, 3, *6,* 431, *433,* 438
      (*See also* Limbic lobe)
    occipital, 2, *3, 5, 6, 7,* 445, 464
      role, stimulation and ablation of, 465
    parietal, 2, *3, 6,* 445, 460
      role, stimulation and ablation of, 462, 463,
        464
    piriform, 432
    prefrontal, *3, 7,* 441, 472
      lobotomy, 472
      role, stimulation and ablation of, 472
    psychical cortex of, 466
    role, stimulation and ablation of, 466
    temporal, 2, *3, 6, 7, 22,* 465
Lobule: paracentral, 3, *4, 6*
    superior and inferior parietal, 2, *3,* 463, 464
Local response (local circuit current), 79
Local static reaction, 410
Locomotor ataxia, 184
Locus ceruleus (nucleus pigmentosus), 253, 255,
    259, *271, 272*
Loops, feedback, in cerebellum:
    brainstem-cerebellar loop, 301
    cerebro-cerebellar loop, *296, 297,* 300
    intracerebellar loops, *292,* 300
    vestibular-archicerebellar loop, *299,* 300, *322*
    (*See also* Circuits; Feedback)
Loudness code, 312
Low tones, 314
Lumbar tap, 35
Lysosomes, 46

Macroglia, 113, 114
Macrophages, 74
Macrosmatic vertebrates, 427
Magnet reaction, 410
Malformations, 130

Malnutrition, 119, 120
Mamillary body, 5, *8, 18, 434, 435*
Mantle layer, 113
Marasmus, 119
Massa intermedia (soft commissure) (*see* interthalamic adhesion)
Matrix (ependymal) layer, 111
Mechanoreceptors, 96
Medial eminence of tuber cinereum, *328,* 341
Medial forebrain bundle, 209, 276, 329, *434,* 436
Medial geniculate body, *13,* 313, 315, *319,* 323, *397, 401, 490*
Medial lemniscus, *158,* 160, 245, 251, 265
Medial longitudinal fasciculus, *151, 176, 179,* 245, 247, 276, 284, 321, 322, *481–490*
Medulla oblongata (myelencephalon), 1, *4,* 9, 241, 243*–*249, *482–484*
Medullary lamina, 15, 142
Meissner's corpuscle (tactile corpuscle), *70,* 71
Melanin, 46
Melanocyte-stimulating hormone, 333
Membrane:
  cell (plasma), 43
    greater, 43
  pia-glial, 34, *66,* 68
  postsynaptic (postjunctional), 54, 91
  presynaptic (prejunctional), 54, 91
  receptor(ive), 83, 386
  subsynaptic, 54, 57
Membranous labyrinth, 305
Memory, 439
Ménière's disease, 326
Meninges and associated structures, 1, *8,* 34
  arachnoid, 1, 34, *35, 36, 66, 67, 135*
  cisterna, 34, *36*
    interpeduncularis, 34, *36*
    lateral cerebral fossa, 35
    lumbar, 34, *36*
    magna (cerebellomedullaris), 34, *36*
    pontis, 34, *36*
    spinal, 35
    superior, 34, *36*
  denticulate ligament, 133, *135*
  diaphragma sellae, 36
  dura mater, 1, 35, *36, 134, 135*
    innervation of, 37, *38,* 136
  dural sleeve, 37, *135,* 136
  epidural space, *36,* 37, *135*
  falx cerebri, 35
  filum terminale, *36,* 133
  innervation of meninges, 37, *38,* 136
  leptomeninges, 34, 66
  pachymeninx, 34
  pia-glial membrane, 34, *66,* 68
  pia mater, 1, 34, *36,* 66
  subarachnoid space, 34, *36*
  subdural space, *36,* 37
  tentorium, 35
  velum interpositum, *24,* 34, *36*
Mental retardation, 121
Merkel's disk, *58,* 70

Mesencephalon (midbrain), 1, *4, 8,* 9, 109, *123,* 241
Mesocortex, 3, 445
Metabolism and blood flow to brain, 24
Metathalamus, 395, 401
Metencephalon (afterbrain, pons), 1, 9, 109, *123*
Microcephalus, 130
Microglia, 41, 65
Microsmatic vertebrates, 427
Microtubules (neurotubules), 46, 48, 49, 52
Midbrain (mesencephalon), 1, *4, 8,* 9, 109, 241
  animal, 413
  cerebral aqueduct, 9, 241
  cerebral peduncle, 9, 10, 241, *247, 452*
  colliculi: inferior, 9, 10, *13,* 241, *298, 489*
    superior, *5,* 9, 10, *13,* 241, *298, 313, 368, 377, 490*
  corpora quadrigemina, 241
  crus cerebri, 9, 10, 241, *252*
  lamina quadrigemina, 9, 10, 241
  pretectum, 9, 10, 241, *377*
  substantia nigra, 9, 10, *26,* 243, *414, 416,* 419, 420, *490*
  tectum, 9, 10, *175,* 241, *377*
  tegmentum, *5,* 9, 10, 241, *261, 266,* 322, *416*
Mitochondria, 45
Modalities, 146, 147, 151
Modulation, frequency, 96
Modulation center, 107
Modulator, 335
Motion sickness, 325, 326
Motivation, 437
Motor area, 468
Motor endings:
  of autonomic nervous system, 73
  of cardiac muscle, 73
  of glands, 73
  of involuntary muscle, 70, 73, 93
  of voluntary muscle, *44,* 73, 91, *92*
Motor endplate, *47, 48,* 73, 91, *92*
  macromotor units, 142
  secondary cleft, *47, 48,* 73
  sole plate, 73
  synaptic gutter (primary synaptic cleft), *47, 48,* 73
  teloglia, 73
  "trail" endings or "en grappe" endings, 71
Motor systems and activities, 128, 466
  cortex, 7, 445, 470, 471, 473
  extrapyramidal system, 415, 417
  focal act, 422
  hopping reaction, 412
  motor (moto) neuron, 141, 165
  motor aphasia (apraxia), 474
  motor (efferent) output, 149
  motor pools, 407
  placing reaction, 412
  postural tonus as a control system, 408, 412
  pyramidal system (concept), 415
  regulation of posture (attitude of body), 409
  segmental levels (general statement), 407
  skilled movements (general statement), 422
  somatic nervous system, 407–417
  voluntary movements (general statement), 422
  walking gait, 410
Motor unit, 69, 141

Movement(s), 407
  of eye, 379
Müllers cell, 356, 357
Multipolar cells, 57
Muscle(s), *92, 93*
  cardiac, 193
  contraction of, 93
  excitation-contraction (E-C) coupling, *92, 93*
  extrafusal, *72, 73,* 91, 93
  intrafusal, *71, 72*
  involuntary (smooth), 93, 204
  multiunit, 94
  neuromuscular linkage, 92
  pilomotor (hair), *70,* 206
  red and white fibers, 164
  sarcolemma, 93
  sarcoplasmic reticulum, 93
  tetany, 78
  transverse (T) tubules, 93
  triads, 93
  voluntary (striated), *92, 93*
Muscle tone, 170, 302
Mutual inhibition, 317, 362, 363
Myelencephalon (medulla oblongata), 1, *4,* 9, 241, *482, 484*
Myelinated (medulated) nerve fiber, 59, *60, 61*
  axon (axis cylinder), 59, *60*
  cleft of Schmidt-Lantermann, 59, *60*
  myelin sheath, 59, *60, 61,* 64
Myopia (nearsightedness), 351

Neocerebellum, 291
Neocortex, 443, 445
  role in "highest order" activities, 472
Neopallium, 443
Neostriatum, 417
Nerve(s), cranial, *8, 10, 12,* 217, *220, 222,* 223, *225, 227, 231, 233, 235,* 280
  abducent (VI), *8, 10,* 12, *220, 221,* 224, *225,* 226, *266,* 269, *486*
  accessory, spinal (XI), *8, 10,* 11, *12, 221,* 235, 237
  acoustic (VIII), *8, 10, 12,* 71, *220,* 305, *313, 321*
  branchiomeric (visceral), 219
  cochlear (VIII), *8, 10, 12,* 220, 305
  components of, 217, *219, 222*
    general somatic afferent (GSA), 138, *219, 220*
    general somatic efferent (GSE), 138, *218,* 219, *220*
    general visceral afferent (GVA), 138, 191, *218, 219, 220*
    general visceral efferent (GVE), 138, *218,* 219, *221*
    special somatic afferent (SSA), *218, 219, 220*
    special visceral afferent (SVA), *218, 219, 220,* 223
    special visceral efferent (SVE), *218, 219, 221*
  facial (VII), *8, 12,* 230, *231,* 252, *484*
    chorda tympani, 268
  ganglia of, *217*
  glossopharyngeal (IX), 233
  hypoglossal (XII), 237, 243
  intermedius, 230, 252
  nuclei, 238, 239
  oculomotor (III) *8, 12, 221,* 224, *225,* 368, *490*

Nerve(s), cranial:
  olfactory (I) *8, 10,* 223, *428*
  optic (II), *8, 10,* 223, 248, *346, 368, 371, 377*
  organization of, 217
  trigeminal (V), *8, 12, 221,* 226, *227, 266*
    mandibular nerve, 228, *266*
    masticator nerve, 226, *266*
    maxillary nerve, 228, *266*
    ophthalmic nerve, 227, *266*
  trochlear (IV), *8, 10, 12, 13, 221,* 224, *225, 488*
  vagus (X), *8, 10, 12,* 220, *221,* 235, *244, 266, 269*
  vestibular (VIII), *8, 12,* 220, *280, 306, 307, 321, 322, 485*
  vestibulocochlear (VIII), auditory, statoacoustic, and acoustic, *8, 12,* 220, *280,* 281, *484*
  visceral arch, 219
    pharyngeal nerve, 223, *266*
    postrematic nerve, 221, *266*
    pretrematic nerve, 221, *266*
    trema, 221
Nerve(s), spinal, 10, 133, *134–136,* 137, *138*
  components, *219*
    general somatic afferent (GSA), 138, *219*
    general somatic efferent (GSE), 138, *219*
    general visceral afferent (GVA), 138, *219*
    general visceral efferent (GVE), 138, *219*
  dorsal (sensory) root ganglia, *134–136,* 137, *138*
  ramus(i): communicantes, 137, *138*
    dorsal (posterior) primary division (ramus), 137, *138*
    recurrent meningeal, 137, *138*
    ventral (anterior) primary division (ramus), 137, *138*
  root: dorsal (sensory), 84, 85, *136, 138*
    neurons, 142, *136, 138,* 140
    ventral (motor), 84, 85
  rootlets of, 133
  splanchnics, pelvic or sacral, 203, 206
Nerve cell, 41, *42,* 51, *99*
  (*See also* Cell; Neuron)
Nerve (secondary) degeneration, 73, *75*
  chromatolysis, 73, *75*
Nerve ending(s), 40, 69, *70,* 147
  annulospiral, 70
  encapsulated, 69
  end bulb of Krause, *70*
  free (nonencapsulated), 69, *70, 72,* 147
  interoceptive, 70
  joint, *70, 72*
  Meissner's corpuscle, *70,* 71
  Merkle, corpuscle of (tactile), 70
  motor end plate, *47, 48, 73,* 91, *92*
  neuroglandular junction, 73
  neuromuscular junction at involuntary muscle, *70,* 73
  neuromuscular spindle, 70, 71, *72,* 164, *167–169, 336*
    intrafusal muscle fibers, *71, 72*
    nuclear bag, *70,* 71, *72*
    nuclear bag fibers, 71, *72*
    nuclear chain fibers, *70, 72*
    primary (annulospiral) sensory ending, 70, *72*
    secondary (flower-spray) sensory ending, 70, *71, 72*
  neuromuscular synapse (junction), *72,* 91

Nerve ending(s):
  neurotendinous endings of Golgi, 71, *72, 168,*
    169
  Pacinian corpuscle, *70,* 71
  plexus around hair follicle, 70
  Ruffini, corpuscle of, *70,* 71
  synaptic gutter (cleft, junctional folds), *47, 48,* 73
  taste, 267
  terminal boutons, end bulbs, 52
Nerve fibers (classification), *72,* 83
  alpha, *72,* 84
  beta, 84
  delta, 84
  gamma, *72,* 84
  groups (A, B, and C), 84
  myelinated, 59
  relation to conduction velocity, 84, 85
  unmyelinated (nonmyelinated), 59
Nerve regeneration, 74
  chromatolysis, 73
  collateral sprout, 74
  functional considerations of, 76
  growth tip, 74
  neurolemma (Schwann) cord (tube), 74
  node of Ranvier in, 75
  terminal sprout, 74
Nervous system:
  autonomic (*see* Autonomic nervous system)
  compared to endocrine system, 77
  development of (*see* Development of the nervous
    system)
Neuralgia:
  glossopharyngeal, 235
  trigeminal, 230
Neurogenic hyperthermia, 336
Neuroglia, 63
Neuronal and neuroglial compartments, 65, 68
Neuronal pool, 142
Neurons, 41, *42, 51,* 99
  adrenergic, *194, 199,* 200, *202*
  afferent, 140, 148
  allodendritic, 50, *51*
  alpha motor (lower motor), *42, 44, 47, 72,* 85,
    141, *158,* 165, *167–169*
  amacrine cell, 357
  anaxonic, 49
  bipolar, *42,* 57
  cholinergic, *192, 202, 203*
  columnar, 144
  efferent, 140, 148
  gamma, *42,* 60, 165, 167, *168*
  Golgi type I and II, *42,* 57
  granule, 293
  idiodendritic, 50, *51*
  as an integrator, 94, *101*
  interneuron (association, intercalated, internun-
    cial), *42,* 165, 172, *389*
    commissural, *145,* 165, 172
    intersegmental, *145,* 165, 172
    intrasegmental, *145,* 165
    spinal, *145,* 165, 172

Neurons:
  isodendritic, 50, *51,* 259, 328, 329
  lower motor (final common pathway), 141, 165
    paralysis, 185
  motor (motoneuron, efferent), 141
  neocortical, 446
  order of: first, 149
    second, 149
    third, 149
  osmoreceptor, 338
  polymorph (multiform), 447, 448
  postganglionic, *42,* 192, *194, 196,* 199
  preganglionic, *42,* 192, *194, 196,* 198, *199*
  Renshaw (interneuron), *101,* 172
  segments: functional, 97
    terminal and preterminal, 50
  sensory (afferent), 140, 148
  serotoninergic, 460
  stellate, 446
  structural and functional concept, 50, 97, *98,*
    99
  unipolar, *42,* 57
  upper motor, 185, 186, 278
    paralysis, 185
  (*See also* Cells; Cortex, cerebellar; Cortex, cere-
    bral; Visual system, retina)
Neurophysiology:
  afterdischarge, principle of, 101
  catecholamine, 200
  conductile segment, 97, *98*
  conduction (nerve), 79, 84
    astroglia, role of, 82
    catechol-o-methyl transferase (COMT), 201
    myelin, role of, 82
    neurolemma cells, role of, 82
    node of Ranvier, role of, 82
  convergence, principle of, 101, *102*
  of cortex, 457
  disinhibition, 103
  divergence, principle of, 100, *102*
  facilitation, 102, *103*
  functional concept of neuron, 97
  general considerations, 77
  generation of action potential, 78
  generator potential, 96
  impulse, 78
  inhibition (*see* Inhibition)
  initial segment (trigger zone, junctional zone),
    97, *98*
  as integration center, 94
  monoamine oxidase (MAO), 201
  neurosecretion, 55, 77, 86, 200, *202*
  neurotransmitter agents, 270
    catecholamines, 200, 270
    storage and release, 92
  occlusion, *103,* 104
  pacemaker, 95, 105, 405
  propagation of action potential, 80
  receptive segment, 97, *100*
  reciprocal innervation, principle of, 170, 171
  recruitment, 104
  refractory period, 82
  resting neuron, 77
  saltatory conduction, 59, 81
  structural and functional concept of neuron, 97
  speed of conduction, 82

Neurophysiology:
  terminal (transmissive, synaptic segment), 97, *98*
  transduction, 386
  transfer of information, 386, 387
  trophic segment, 97, *98*
  summation: spatial, 104
    temporal, 104
  unidirectional conduction, 85, 86
Neuropil, 52
Neuroretina, 351
Neurotropism, 129, 213
Neurotubules, 46, 48, 52
Nexus, 53
Node of Ranvier, 50, 59, 81
Nucleolar satellite, 44
Nucleus(i), 142
  basal ganglia: amygdaloid body (amygdala), *8, 18, 20, 23,* 417, 433
    caudate nucleus, *10, 13, 18,* 20, 22, *23, 414, 415,* 417
    claustrum, 13, 17, *22*
    globus pallidus (pallidum), *23, 29,* 296, *298, 414, 415,* 422
    lentiform (lenticular) nucleus, *10, 13, 18,* 20, 418, *452*
    putamen, 20, *22, 23, 29,* 417, 420, 421
    role of, 418
    striatum, 417
    subthalamic nucleus, 9, *414,* 417, 420, 421
  of brainstem: arcuate, 249
    central reticular, 245, 249
    central superior, 253, 259
    colliculus inferior, 5, 9, 11, 241, 254, *298,* 313, 315, *489*
    colliculus superior, 5, 11, *13, 159,* 298, 313, 368, 375, *377, 490*
    cuneatus, *158, 159,* 246
    cuneatus accessory (lateral, external), 247, *298, 482*
    cuneiform, 256
    of Darkschewitsch, 256, *321,* 323
    giganticocellularis, *176, 179,* 248, 249, *250,* 251, 259
    gracilis, *158, 159,* 245, 246, *481, 482*
    interpeduncular, 256, 259, *435*
    interstitial nucleus of Cajal, 178, 256, *321,* 323
    of lateral lemniscus, *313,* 314, 315, *488*
    lateral reticular, 247, 249
    locus ceruleus (pigmentosus), 253, 255, 259, *271, 272*
    olivary: accessory inferior (paleo-olive), 247, 248, *263, 296, 298, 484, 486*
      main inferior (neo-olive), 247, 248, *263, 296, 298, 483, 484, 486*
      superior, 252, *313,* 314, 315
    pallidus, *250,* 251
    parvicellularis, *250,* 251, 252
    pendunculopontine, *254,* 259
    pontine, *296*
    raphe, *247, 248, 250,* 251–253, 259, 273
    reticular (of reticular formation), 250, 256, 259, *263, 482, 483*
    reticular: lateral (accessory), *247, 248,* 250, 256, 259, *482, 483*
      pontine (oralis and caudalis), *176, 177,* 179, *251,* 252, *253,* 256, 259

Nucleus(i):
  of brainstem: reticulotegmental, 253
    ruber, *175,* 255, 256, 259, *296, 298, 415,* 417, 421, *490*
    supraspinal, 245
    tegmental, 253, 255, 259
    of trapezoid body, 252, *313,* 314, 315
  of cerebellum, 14, 252, 289, 292, *485*
    dentate, *12,* 14, 252, 289, *292, 296,* 485
    emboliform, 14, 252, 289, 292, *296,* 485
    fastigii, 14, 252, 289, *316,* 322, 324, *485*
    globose, 14, 252, 289, 292, *296,* 485
    interpositus, 252, 292
  of cranial nerves, *220, 221,* 245, 251, 252, 280
    abducent nerve, 164, 190, 238, 280, *321,* 486
    accessory oculomotor (Edinger-Westphal), *196, 203, 221,* 224, 239, *321,* 377
    ambiguus, *218,* 234, 239, 246, 281, 287, *482, 484*
    cochlear, *220,* 238, 250, 280, 313, *484*
    columns of, *219–221,* 238
    components, 238
    Edinger-Westphal (*see* accessory oculomotor *above*)
    of facial nerve, *221,* 239, 252, 281, *485*
    gustatorius, 231, 268
    of hypoglossal nerve, *221,* 238, 247, 280, *482, 483*
    of oculomotor nerve, *221,* 224, 238, 255, 280, *321,* 490
    salivatory, inferior and superior, *196, 221,* 234, 239, 249, 252, 281
    solitarius, *220,* 234, 238, 246, 252, *261,* 281, *482*
    of spinal accessory nerve, *221,* 235, 237
    trigeminal: mesencephalic, *220,* 238, *250, 255, 256,* 280, *487*
      motor, *220,* 239, *253,* 280, *487*
      principal (chief, main), *220,* 238, 252, *253*
      spinal (descending), *242, 266,* 281, *298, 481, 483, 485, 486*
    of trochlear nerve, *221,* 238, 254, 280, *321*
    vagal, dorsal, *192, 196, 221,* 239, 246, *482, 483*
    vestibular, 178, *220,* 252, 280, *321, 322, 483–486*
  definition of, 142
  geniculate nuclei (metathalamus) (*see* Thalamic nuclei)
  of hypothalamus, 327, *328, 330*
    of mamillary area, 327
    mamillary body, 327, *328, 434,* 435
    paraventricular, 327, *328, 330,* 338
    of preoptic area, 327, 433
    of supraoptic area, 327
    supraoptic nucleus, 327, *328, 330,* 338
    of tuberal area, 327
  relay (sensory), 397, 398
  schema of, 144
  septal nuclei, 431, *433,* 434
  of spinal cord, *143,* 144, 145, *146*
    commissural, 144
    dorsal (thoracic) of Clarke, *143,* 145, 161, *162*
    intermediolateral, *143, 145, 194, 199*

Nucleus(i):
    intermediomedial, *143*, 145
    lateral cervical, 145, *164*
    motor nuclei of anterior (ventral) horn, *143*,
      146
    pericornualis anterior, *143*
    posteromarginal, *143*, 145
    proper sensory, *143*, 145
    substantia gelatinosa, *143*, 145, *220*
  of thalamus (see Thalamic nuclei)
Nutrition, 119
Nystagmus, 323–325, 412

Obex, 12, *14*, 244, 248
Obligatory contraction, 142
  response, 91
Occlusion, 104
Oculomotor nerve, 221, 225
  nucleus, 224, 256
  system, 379
Odor, 427
Olfactory system and associated structures, *428*,
    430
  allocortex, 430, 431, 443
  amygdaloid body, *8*, *18*, 20, *23*, 417, 433
  anterior olfactory nucleus, *428*
  bulb, olfactory, 9, 429, 430
  cells (neurons): bipolar, *428*, 429
    granule: external, *428*, 429
      internal, *428*, 429
    mitral, *428*, 429
    pyramidal, *428*, 429
    receptor, *428*, 429
    supporting (sustentacular), 429
    tufted, *428*, 429
  cortex, primary olfactory, 430
  efferent fibers, olfactory, *428*
  glomerulus, *428*, 429
  hypothalamus, connections with, 430
  limbic cortex, 430
  nerve, olfactory, 9, 223, *428*
  odorant-receptor interaction, 428
  pathways, 428
  rhinencephalon ("smell" brain), 430
  septal area, 430
  smell, functional aspects, 427, *428*, 430
  striae, *428*, 430
  sustentacular cell, 429
  system, 427
  tracts, *6*, *8*, *21*, *22*, *428*, 430
  tubercle, olfactory (anterior perforated substance
    or space), *428*, 430
  uncus (prepiriform cortex, area), 430
Oligodendroglia (oligodendrocyte), 41, 63
  interfascicular, 63
  perineuronal (satellite), 63
  perivascular, 63
Olivary nucleus:
  inferior, 244, 248, 295
  superior, *251*, 313, 315, 316

Olive, 10, 11, *12*, 244, 295, *483*
  neo (principal nucleus), *248*, 295
  paleo (accessory inferior nucleus), *248*,
    295
Olivocochlear bundle, 315
Ontogeny of sleep, 459
Optic nerve, *8*, *10*, 346, 368, *377*
Optic system (see Visual system)
Organization of cerebral cortex, 443
Organum vasculosum of lamina terminalis, 342
Osmoreceptor cells, 338
Otic ganglion, 234, 238
Otosclerosis, 308
Oxygen demand of brain, 122
  and cerebral palsy, 121
  and perinatal brain damage, 121
Oxytocin, 337

Pacemaker:
  of the heart, 204
  neuronal, 105, 405
Pachymenix, 34
Pacinian corpuscle, 71, *100*
Pain, 151, 393
  gate control theory of, 155, *156*
  intractable, 155
  neural mechanisms associated with, 155
  pathways, *153*, *154*, 264, *266*, 392
  perception, 151
  placebo effect, 393
  prefrontal lobotomy, effect of, 393
  radicular, 182, 188
  referred, 184
  as a thalamic sense, 198
  visceral, 184
Painless childbirth, 37
Paleocerebellum, 14, 291
  lesion of, 303
Paleocortex, 3, 443
Paleo-olive, *248*, 295
Paleostriatum (globus pallidus), 20, 417
Pallidum (globus pallidus), 20, 417
Pallium, 443
Palsy:
  Bell's, 231
  central facial, 274
  facial mimetic, 232, 279
  facial voluntary, 232
  pseudobulbar, 286
Paralysis, 186
  agitans, 423, 424
  flaccid (lower motor neuron), 185
  spastic (upper motor neuron), 186
Paranucleolar body (nucleolar satellite), 44
Paraplegia, 189
Parasympathetic nervous system, 195, *196*, 197,
    201
  cholinergic drugs, 210
  vagal (parasympathetic) tone, 335
Paraterminal body (subcallosal gyrus), 435
Paresis, 186
Paresthesias, 188
Parieto-occipital line, 2
  sulcus, 4
Parkinson's disease, 423, 424

Parolfactory area, 3
Pars opecularis, 2
  orbitalis, 2
  triangularis, 2
Past pointing, 302, 324
Pathway(s):
  anterolateral column–spinal lemniscal pathway,
    144, 149, 151, 392
  ascending from spinal cord, 149, 150
  ascending lemniscal, 264
  auditory, 270, *313*
  cerebellar, 295–301
  corticobulbar, 278, *279*
  corticonuclear, 160, 280, 467
  corticopontocerebellar, 296, 301
  corticoreticular (spinal), 179, 274, *275,*
    278
  corticospinal, 174, *176, 178,* 415, 467
  corticostriate, *414, 415,* 468
  corticothalamic, *397, 415,* 468
  descending autonomic, 276
  descending: to nuclei of ascending pathways,
    173
    to spinal cord, *144, 151,* 173, *174, 176, 275,*
      279
  dopaminergic, *272,* 273
  epicritic, 265
  extrapyramidal, *414,* 415, 417
  hypothalamohypophyseal, 329, *330*
  of the hypothalamus, 329
  lateral column-spinal lemniscal, 264
  lateral pain, 152
  lemniscal, 241
  limbic, *433–435,* 436
  from locus ceruleus, *271,* 272
  monoamine (aminergic) neuronal, 270, *271*
  olfactory, 428
  optic, *367, 368, 369, 370*
  pain and temperature (and light touch), 151,
    153, 154, 156, 159, 266, 392
  posterior column-medial lemniscal, 157, *158,*
    159, 245, 265, 393
  protopathic, 264
  reticulospinal, *176,* 179, *275*
  serotoninergic, 270, *272,* 273, 460
  spinal lemniscus, 152
  spinocerebellar, 161, *162*
  spinocervicothalamic, 163
  spinoreticular thalamic (paleospinothalamic),
    153, 154, 157, *162,* 264
  spinothalamic, 152, *153, 154, 159*
    direct (neo), 152, *153*
    indirect (paleo), *153,* 154
    ventral (anterior), 157, *159*
  supraopticohypophyseal, 169, *330*
  taste (gustatory), 265, *269*
  temperature, 151, *153, 154,* 392
  thalamohypothalamic, 329
  touch–deep sensibility, *145,* 157, *158, 159,* 266,
    393
  trigeminal, 264, *266*
  vestibular, *176,* 324
  vestibulocerebellar, 300, *322,* 324
  vestibulomesencephalic, in median longitudinal
    fasciculus, 276, 321, 323
Pattern theory of sensation, 148

Peduncle (brachium):
  cerebellar, 12
    descending division of superior cerebellar,
      298, 301
    inferior (restiform body), 11, *12, 13, 162,* 250,
      273, *289, 295, 296, 298, 485, 486*
    juxtarestiform body, 297, *322, 323, 485*
    mamillothalamic, *434, 436*
    middle (brachium pontis), *10,* 11, *12, 13,*
      273, *289, 295, 296, 485–487*
    superior (brachium conjunctivum), 11, *12, 13,*
      162, 253, 273, *289, 296, 297, 298, 322,*
      486–488
  of (superior) olive, 315
  cerebral, 9, 243
  of inferior colliculus, 160
Periaxonal space of the internode, 82
Perikaryon (cell body), 43
Perilymph, 305, 310
Perineurium, 59
Peripheral nerves (microscopic anatomy), 58, *60*
  development of, 117
  nervous system, 57
Periventricular gray matter, 241, 242
  zone, 327
Pes hippocampus, *17*
Phantom limb, 185
Phantom sensations, 185
Pharmacology of nervous system, 210
Phenylketonuria (PKU), 119
Phosphenes, 375
Photoneuroendocrine system, 335
Physiology of receptors, 95
Physiology of synapse, 85
Pia-ependymal membrane, 39
Pia-glial membrane, 34, 65, 68
Pia mater, 1, 34
Pigment epithelium, 353
  inclusion, 46
  lipofuscin, 43, 46
  melanin, 46, 420
Pineal body (epiphysis cerebri), 5, *13, 29, 341,* 342
  hormones, 342
Pinocytosis, 68
Pitch coding, 317
Pituitary gland (hypophysis):
  anterior lobe, *328, 330,* 337, 339
  posterior lobe (pars nervosa), *328, 330,* 334, 337,
    342
  (*See also* Hypophysis)
Pituitary hormone–releasing factors, 333, 337
Placode (anlage):
  auditory, 109, 110
  nasal, 109, 110
  neural, 109, 110
  optic, 109, 110
  (*See also* Development)
Planum temporale, 476
Plasma membrane (cell membrane), 43
Plasticity of nervous system, 129
Pleasure (rewarding) center, 340, 440
Plexus:
  nerve, 137
  terminal, 193
Pneumoencephalography, 40
Pole (frontal, occipital, temporal), 2, *3, 17*

Polydipsia, 340
Polysensory input, 300
Polyuria, 340
Pons (metencephalon), 9, 10, *12, 21,* 241, *485–489*
Pontine (cerebellopontine) angle syndrome, 283
Pontomedullary junction, 226
Positive (regeneration) feedback, 106
Posterior:
    column, 160
    perforated substance, 9
    thalamic zone, 155, 401
Postganglionic neuron, 192, 198, 203
Postural reactions, 412
Postural tonus, regulation of, 412
Posture, 407, 408
    reflex, 409
    regulation of, 408, 409
Potassium ions, 77
Potential:
    action (all-or-none), 78, *79,* 81, *90, 100*
    digital pulse, 96
    electric (bioelectric), 77
    excitatory postsynaptic (EPSP), *88, 89, 90,* 457
    generator (receptor), 96, *100,* 386
    graded depolarizing, 83, *90,* 96
    inhibitory postsynaptic (IPSP), *88, 89, 90,* 457
    locus response, 83, 90
    membrane, 77
    miniature end-plate (MEEP), 91
    postsynaptic (PSP), 89
    resting (steady), *77, 78, 79*
    role of glial cells, 98
    slow potential, 83, 90
    standing, 96
    subliminal, 95
"Prechiasmatic gland," 342
Prefrontal "lobe," *7,* 432, 472
Prefrontal lobotomy, functional considerations, 472
Premotor area, 7
    cortex, 470
Prenatal development of brain, 122
Prenatal activity in man, 122, 128
Preoptic area, 327
Prepiriform cortex, 432
Pressure, 148
Presynaptic inhibition, 90
Presynaptic membrane, 54
Presynaptic vesicles, 54, 55, 91
Pretectum, 9, 241, 256, *377*
Principle:
    of afterdischarge, 101
    of convergence, 101
    of divergence, 100
    of reciprocal innervation, 170, 171
Processing, neural, 387, *388, 389*
Proprioception, 147
Prosencephalon (forebrain), 1, 109
Protopathic sensations, 150
Psychial cortex, 465, 466
Psychomotor attacks, 439

Ptosis, 285
Pulvinar, 11, *13, 18, 397,* 402
Punishing (aversion) center, 440
Purkinje effect, 365
Putamen, 20, *23, 26, 29, 414, 415,* 417, 420, 421
Putative transmitters, 86
Pyramid, *8,* 10, *12,* 175, 242, 245, *247, 248*
Pyramidal cell, 57, 447
    apical dendrites, 57, 447
    basilar dendrites, 57, 447
Pyramidal decussation, 10, 244, 245
    system, concept of, 415, 421
Pyramidal tract (corticospinal tract), *140, 174, 176, 261, 416, 452*

Quadriplegia (tetraplegia), 186
Quadrantic homonymous anopsia, 382
Quantal content, 91, 201

Rage:
    sham, 340
    true, 340
Ramus(i):
    communicantes, 137, *138,* 197
    dorsal primary division (ramus), 137, *138*
    gray, communicantes, 137, *138,* 194, 197
    recurrent meningeal, *136,* 137, *138*
    ventral primary division (ramus), 137, *138*
    white, communicantes, 137, *138,* 194, 197
Rebound phenomenon, 302, 303
Receptive aphasia (Wernicke's), 473, 479
Receptor(s):
    adaptation of, 97
    alpha, 88, 212
    alpha blocker, 312
    beta, 88, 212
    beta blocker, 212
    central, 277
    field, 358, 361
    membrane, 83, 87, 386
    nicotinic, 87
    osmoreceptor, 338
    physiology of, 147
    potential, 360, 386
    presso- (baro-), 24, 233, 277
    segment, 97
    sensory (afferent), *70, 72, 147*
    sites, 87
    zones, 49, 50
Reciprocal innervation, *166,* 170
Recruitment, 104, 403
    response, 404
Referred pain, 184
Reflexes, 140
    accelerator, 411
    act, 409
    alpha, loop, 167
    angular (rotatory) acceleration, 411
    arc: with hypothalamic receptor, 334
        with peripheral receptor, 334
    arcs, spinal: three-neuron, 140, *168, 169,* 171
        two-neuron, 140, 165, *167*
    areflexia, 185, 186
    attitudinal, 410

Reflexes:
  auditory, 309
  Babinski, 187
  bladder, 207
  body righting, 414
  cerebral ischemic, 25
  claspknife, 186
  concept, 127
  corneal, 229
  crossed extensor, *166*, 171, 172
  deep tendon (DTR), 165, 188
  extensor (myotactic, stretch), *151*, *167*, 171, 409
  flexor, *169*, 170, 171, 409, 410
  GAG, 234, 235, 283
  gamma, loop, 167, *168*
  general static reaction, 411
  Golgi tendon organ (GTO), role of, 169
  hopping, 412
  hyperreflexia, 188
  hyporeflexia, 185
  of hypothalamus, 334
  inverse myotatic, 186
  jaw, 228
  kinetic, 411
  knee (patellar), 165, 166, *167*, 186
  labyrinthine accelerating reactions, 411
  labyrinthine righting reaction, 413
  lengthening, 186
  light, 376
  linear (progressive) acceleration, 411
  local static reaction, 411
  magnet reaction, 410
  mark time, 171
  monosynaptic, *167*, 171
  myotatic, 165, *167*, 186, 409
  neck-righting, 414
  neural reflex arc utilizing an intrinsic receptor,
      334
  neuro-humeral, 334
  optic-righting, 414
  pharyngeal, 234, 235
  phasic, 169
  placing, 412
  pluck, 410
  postural, 410
  primitive protective, 171, 409
  pseudoaffective, 437
  segmental static, 410
  simple, 140
  spinal, 140, *166*, *167*, *168*, *169*
  static, 410
  stato-kinetic, 411
  stretch, 165, 171, 409, 410
    Hering-Breuer, 277
  sweating, spinal reflex, 189
  tonic (neck), 169, 411
  triple, 189
  two-neuron (monosynaptic), 98
  vestibular labyrinthine righting reflex, 413
  visceral, 195, *199*
  visual, 376
  voiding, 208
  vomiting, 343
Refractory period, 82
  absolute, 82
  relative, 82

Regeneration, 73, 74, *75*
  collateral sprouting, 74–76
  cross-nerve anastomoses, 76
  functional considerations, 76
  primary, 73
  secondary (Wallerian), 73
  terminal, 74
Regenerative process, 78
Reissner's fiber, 343
Release phenomena, 301, 302, 340, 425, 438
Renshaw cell, 172
Respiration centers, 209, 277
Reticular:
  core, 50, 258
  formation (in brainstem), *153*, *158*, 241, 259,
      313, *483*, *484*
    input to, 261, 274
    motor (medial) zone of, *260*, 290
    nuclei, *246–248*, *250*, *251*, *253–255*, *257*, 259,
      263
    isodendritic core, 260
    output from, 262, *263*
    sensory (lateral) zone of, *260*, 290
    of spinal cord, 258, 259
  nuclei, *246*, *247*, *248*, *250*, *251*, *253–255*
Reticular system, 241, 257, 258, 390
  ascending, *149*, *157*, 262, 390
  concept of, 257
  convergence in, 261
  core, 257
  deactivation, 262, 263
  descending, 274, 275
  divergence in, 261
  functional considerations, 262
  input to, 261, 274
  nonspecific, aspecific, and unspecific, 327
  output from, 262, *263*
  searching movements and, 390
  sleep, 262
  tracts and pathways of, *179*, 258, 262, 274, 390
Retina (*see* Visual system)
Rheobase, 83, *84*
Rhinal, 6, *432*
Rhinencephalon, 430
Rhizotomy, 182
Rhombencephalon (hindbrain), 1, 109
Rhombic lip, 114, 116, 122
Rhomboid fossa, 12
Rhythms in the nervous system, 405
Rigidity, 424
Rods of retina, *352*, 355
Role of cortex in "highest order" activities,
    473
Roots, spinal:
  classification, 84, 85
  dorsal (sensory), *135*, *137*, *138*
  ventral (motor), *135*, *137*, *138*
Rosette, 293
Ruffini corpuscle, 70

Saccadic system, 379
Salt, 267
Satellite cell, 41
Scanning speech, 303
Schizophrenia, 201

Schwann cell (neurolemma), 59, 74
Schwann cord (tubes), neurolemmal cord, *61, 74*
Scotoma (blind spot), 380
Sensation(s), sense and modalities, 146, 147, 265, 266
    affective, 403
    auditory, 317
    classification of, 146
    cold, 147
    deep sensibility, 147
    discriminative, 403
    dizziness, 321
    epicritic, 147, 150
    exteroceptive (cutaneous or superficial), 146
    flutter-vibrations, 157
    interoceptive (visceral), 147
    joint, 147
    kinesthetic, 147, 157, 159
    pain, 147, 393
    position, 147
    pressure, 147
    proprioceptive, 147
    protopathic, 147, 150
    smell, 427
    somatic, 147
    tactile, 147
    taste, 265, 268, 462
    temperature, 147
    touch, 147
    touch-pressure, 157
    two-point, 160
    vestibular, 325
    vibratory, 147, 157
    visceral, 147
    visual, 360, 373, 374
    warmth, 147
Sensory (afferent) endings and receptors, 70, *72*, 85, *147*
    annulospiral (primary sensory), 70, *72*
    classification of, *147*
Sensory (afferent) endings and receptors:
    flower-spray (secondary sensory), 71, *72*
    free nerve, 69, *70*
    Golgi, 71, *72, 153*
    Krause's end bulb, *70*, 71
    Meissner's corpuscle, *70*, 71
    Merkle's corpuscle, *70, 147*
    neuromuscular spindle, 70, *72, 151, 153*
    Pacinian, *70*, 71
    pain, 71
    role of, 147
    Ruffini, *70*, 71
    tactile, 71
    thermal, 71
Sensory ganglion, 62
Sensory processing in nervous system, 387
    adaption, 389
        fast, 389
        slow, 389
    apraxia, 474
    cochlear efferent fibers, role of, 316
Sensory processing in nervous system:
    coding, 385
    convergence, 387
    by descending (centrifugal) fibers, 388
    development of sensory activity, 129
    divergence, 387
    environmental energies, 385
    excitatory postsynaptic potentials (EPSP's), 387
    feedback (negative) circuits, 387
    feed-forward circuit, 387
    of information, 386
    inhibition: lateral (mutual), 317, 362, 363
        presynaptic, 90, *389*
    inhibitory circuits, negative feedback, 387
    inhibitory postsynaptic potentials (IPSP's), 89, 387, *389*
    pattern theory of sensation, 148
    receptive membrane, 83, 386
    receptor (generator) potential, 96, 386, *389*
    secondary sensory areas, function of, 460, 462
    sharpening, focusing and contrasting effects, 294, 317
    somatosensory area, 300
    somesthetic association area, 463
    specific nerve energies, doctrine of, 148
    stimulus, 385
    transduction, 386
    transfer of information, 386
    transformation function, 387
    (*See also* Neurophysiology)
Sensory (afferent) systems:
    classification of afferent input, 146
    concept of organization, 150
    general principles, 385
    general statement, 150
    lemniscal system, 391
    reticular system, 390
Sensory unit, 69, 141
Septal region (area), 6, 431, 434
Septum pellucidum, *4, 5, 6, 22, 29,* 431
    cavum, *22*
Serotoninergic pathway, 270, 460
Servomechanisms, negative feedback, 105
    servo-assistance of movements, 180
Sham rage (pseudoaffective), 340, 437
Sharpening effect, 294, 317
Shock, spinal, 189
Silent period of spindle discharge, 167
Sinuses, dural (*see* Dural sinuses; Veins)
Sleep, 457–459
    nightmare attack, 460
    ontogeny, 459
    parodoxic, 270, 273, 458
Sleep center, 262
Sleep-wake cycle, 262, 459
Sleep-wake pattern, 340
Slipped disk, 182
Smell, sense of (*see* Olfactory system and associated structures)
Sodium ions, 77
Sodium pump, 81
Sole plate, 73
Somatic, definition of, 147
Somites, 117
Sour, 267

Space:
  epidural, *36*, 37
    hemorrhage, extradural, 37
  subarachnoid, 34, *36*
    hemorrhage into, 37
  subdural, *36*, 37
    hemorrhage into, 37
Speed of conduction, 84
Spike, 49
Spina bifida, 130, 131
Spinal accessory nerve, *8, 12, 221*, 237, 243, 245, *246*
Spinal cord, *17*, 133–190, 208, 209, *261, 263*
  cauda equina, *134, 137*
  cistern, 35, *36*, 40
  commissures, gray and white, *143*, 144
  conus medullaris (terminalis), *36*, 133, *134*, 137
  cross section anatomy, *141, 143, 144, 151*
  development of, 114
  enlargement: cervical, *134, 139, 141*
    lumbosacral, *134, 141*, 146
  extent during development, 114, 115
  fasciculus: cuneatus, *151, 158*, 160, 265, 393, *481, 482*
    gracilis, *151, 158*, 160, 265, 393, *481, 482*
    interfascicular, *151*, 172
    medial longitudinal, 151, 176, 179, 247, 254, 276, 321, 322, 323, 484–490
    proprius (spinospinal tract), *151*, 172
    septomarginal, *151*, 172
    triangular, of Gombault-Philippe, *151*, 172
  females, 208
  filum terminale, 133, *134*
  functional considerations, 182
  funiculus(i) [column(s)], 142
    anterior (ventral), 142, *143*
    lateral, 142, *143*
    posterior (dorsal), 142, *143*
  horn: anterior (gray), 142, *143*
    lateral, 142
    posterior (gray), 142, *143*
  man, 181, 208
  matter: gray, organization of, 142
    white, 142
  nerves, spinal, 133
    components, 137
    segmental innervation, 138
    [*See also* Nerve(s), spinal]
  nucleus(i) and nuclear column(s): commissural, *143*
    dorsal (thoracic) of Clarke, *138, 143*, 145, *162*
    of dorsal (sensory) horn, *143*
    intermediolateral, *138, 143*, 145, 168
    intermediomedial, *138, 143*, 145, *194, 199*
    pericornualis anterior, *143*
    posteromarginal, *143*, 145
    proper sensory, *143*, 145
    schema of, *143, 146*
    spinal nucleus of trigeminal nerve, 238, 243, 252
    substantia gelatinosa, 145
  nucleus(i) and nuclear column(s) substantia gelatinosa: funiculus, 8
  reflex arcs, 165
    sweating, 165
  reticular formation of (lamina 7), 245

Spinal cord:
  root: dorsal (sensory) spinal, 133, 137, *138*, 148
    ventral (motor) spinal, 133, 137, *138*, 148
  segments, *135, 136, 137, 141*
  tethering of, 131
  tract(s): corticospinal: anterior, *151, 174*, 176
    lateral, *151*, 174, *176*, 245, *261*, 280, *415, 452*, 467
    fasciculus cuneatus, *151, 158*, 160, 265, 393
    fasciculus gracilis, *151, 158*, 160, 265, 393
    medial longitudinal fasciculus, *151, 176, 179*, 245, 247, 276, 321, 322, 323, *481–490*
    posterolateral tract of Lissauer, *151, 152, 153, 159, 220*
    reticulospinal: lateral (medullary), *151, 176, 177, 179*, 248, 258, *263*, 274, 276, 279
      medial (pontine) *151, 176, 177, 179*, 248, 258, *263*, 274, 276, 279
    rubrospinal, *151, 175, 177*, 269, 276, *482–490*
    spinal tract of trigeminal nerve, 243, 246, *266, 481–486*
    spinocerebellar: anterior, *151, 161, 162, 163*, 253, 299, *481–486*
      posterior, *151, 161, 162, 163*, 253, 299, *481–486*
    spinocortical, 163
    spino-olivary, *151*, 295, *298*
    spinopontine, *151*, 164
    spinoreticular, *151*, 164
    spinospinalis (proprius), 145, *151*, 172
    spinotectal, *151, 157, 159, 481, 482*
    spinothalamic: anterior, *151, 157, 159*, 265
      lateral, *151, 153*, 157, *159*, 264, 265, 292, *481–490*
    spinovestibular, *162*, 164
    tectospinal, *151, 175, 178*, 276, *483, 486, 488–490*
    vestibulespinal, *151*, 164, *176*, 178, *179, 255, 321, 322*, 325, *481–485*
  zone, intermediate gray, 142, *143*
Spinal lemniscus, 152, 264
Spinal nerves [*see* Nerve(s), spinal]
Spinal shock, 189
Spinal tap or puncture, 39, 137
Split-brain animal, 476
Spontaneous activity in central nervous system, 105
Strength-duration curve, 83, *84*
  rheobase, 83, *84*
Stria(e):
  acoustic, 314
  longitudinal, medial and lateral, 4, 431, 434, *435*
  medullaris, 14
  medullaris thalami, 8, *433, 435*, 436
  olfactory, 9, *10, 428, 429*, 430
  terminalis, *8, 13, 19, 26, 433*, 434
Striatum (neostriatum), 417
Stripe of Baillarger, 456
Stripe of Kaes, 456
Subcommissural organ, 343
Subiculum, *6*, 432
Subfornical organ, 343
Substance, perforating, *9, 30*
Substantia nigra, pars compacta and reticularis, 9, 26, 243, 255, 256, *415*, 417–421, *490*

534

Subthalamus (ventral thalamus), 8, *24, 26, 414,*
  417, *419,* 420
Sulcus(i), 2
  anterolateral, 135, *143*
  calcarine, 4, 6, *28,* 368
  central, of Rolando, 2
  cingulate, 3, 6
  collateral, 6, *8,* 9
  of corpus callosum, 6
  dorsal median, *14*
  frontal, *2, 3*
  hippocampal, *3, 6*
  hypothalamic, *4, 24,* 327
  interparietal, *2, 3*
  limitans (fovea), *14, 111, 114, 219, 244, 245*
  orbital, 6
  parieto-occipital (line), 2, 4, 6
  postcentral, *2, 3*
  posterior intermediate, *14,* 135, *140*
    lateral, *14,* 135, *143*
    median, 135, *143*
  postolivary, 11
  precentral, *2, 3*
  preoccipital notch, *3*
  preolivary, 11
  rhinal, 6
  temporal, *3, 6, 8*
Summation:
  spatial, 89, 104
  temporal, 89, 104
Superior colliculus, 9, 241, 255, 275
Supraoptic area of hypothalamus, 327
Supraoptico-hypophyseal tract, 33
Supraoptic crest, 342
Sympathetic (ortho) nervous system, *194,* 197
  ophthalmia, 382
  reflex, 198
Sympathetic (thoracolumbar) outflow, 197
Sympathoadrenal system, 206
Sympathomimetic (adrenergic) drugs, 210
Synapses (junctions), *49, 53, 55, 58*
  adrenergic, 55, 200, *202*
  asymmetric, 55
  axoaxonic, 53, *54, 56*
  axodendritic, 53, *54, 56*
    type I, 56, 57, *58*
    type II, 56, 57, *58*
  axon terminal, 50, 52, 97
    boutons terminaux (en passant), 52
    end feet, 52
    synaptic knob, 52
  axo-somatic, 53, *54, 56*
  chemical, 53, *55*
  cholinergic, *202,* 203
  cross-over, 293, 294
  dentritic terminal, 52
    spines, 52
  electrical, 43, *49, 53, 55, 56*
  excitatory, 89, *388, 389*
  fatigability, 86
  gap junction, 43

  inhibitory, *88,* 89, 90, *388, 389*
  junctions, 53
  neuroglandular junction, 53
  neuromuscular, 53, 91
  neurosecretory, 53, *86*
  neurovascular, 338
  nexus, *49,* 53
  physiology of, 85
  receptor sites, 87, 88, *202*
  replacement of, 57
  ribbon, 360
  somatoaxonic, *54*
  somatodendritic, 53, *54*
  somatosomatic, 53
  types I and II, 56
Synaptic:
  cleft, *47, 53, 58, 73, 85,* 86
  delay (latency), 86
  gutter, 73
  junction, 53
  membrane, 53
    postsynaptic, *47, 48, 53, 58, 73,* 86
    presynaptic, *47, 48,* 53
    subsynaptic, *47, 54, 58,* 86
  security, 258
  segments, 50, 52
  vesicles [*see* Vesicles]
Synaptolemma and synatosome, 55
"Synchronized" EEG pattern, 457
Syringomelia, 188
System:
  adrenergic (sympathetic), *194,* 197–201
  auditory, 305, 306
  autonomic nervous (*see* Autonomic nervous
    system)
  cholinergic (parasympathetic), *196,* 201–203
  extrapyramidal, 415, 417
  feed-forward control, 294
  ganglion cell, 361
  general visceral afferent (*see* Autonomic ner-
    vous system)
  hypothalamo-hypophyseal, 329, 337, 339
  lemniscal, 257, 391
  limbic, 427, 430
  motor (somatic), 407
  nigrostriatal (dopaminergic), 273
  olfactory, 427
  parasympathetic, *196,* 201–203
  photoneuroendocrine, 335
  posterior column-medial lemniscal, 157, *158,*
    159, 393
  pyramidal, 415
  reticular, 257
  sensory, 385
  sympathetic, *194,* 197–201
  thalamic reticular, 398, 403, 455
  vestibular, 317
  visual, 345

Tabes dorsalis, 184, 208, 413
Tachycardia, 283
Tactile agnosia (astereognosis), 463
Tactile corpuscle of Merkle, *70, 147*
Tactile sense, 147, 157

Taenia of fourth ventricle, 12, *14*
Tapetum, 20, *27*
Taste, 268, 462
    blindness, 268
    buds, 267, 268
    modalities, 267
    nerves, 267
    pathways, 265, *269*
    role in preservation of life, 268
    sensations, 267
Tectum (lamina quadrigemina), 9, *169*, 241, *377*
Tegmentum of brainstem, 5, 8, 9, 241, 243, 251
Tela choroidea, 15
Telencephalon (endbrain), 1
    median, 5
Telodendria, *44*, 101
Teloglia, 73
Temperature, 147, *153*
Temporal summation, 89, 104
Tentorial incisure, 36
Tentorium, 4, 6, 35, *38*
Terminal tremor, 302
Tethering of spinal cord, 131
Thalamic nucleus(i), 395, 396, *397*
    anterior, *397*, 399, *434*, *452*
    anterior nuclear group, 396, 399
    association, 397, 398
    central lateral, *395*
    central median, *395*
    centrum medianum (central, centromedian),
        396, 399, *414*, *415*, 421
    connection with cerebral cortex, 399, 400, *452*,
        453, 454
    "cortically dependent," 398
    cortical relay, 398
    of dorsal tier, 396
    dorsomedial (medial), *397*, 402, *433*, *452*
    dorsalis oralis, 397
    functional aspects, *388*, 403
    geniculate (metathalamus), *397*, 401
        lateral, body, *10*, *13*, *18*, *26*, *368*, *371*, *397*,
        401
        medial, body, *13*, 313, *319*, 323, 401, *490*
    intralaminar, *153*, *154*, 155, *162*, *263*, 394,
        397, 399, *414*, 421, *434*, *435*
    lateral group, *397*, 401, *446*
        dorsal, 396, *397*, 401
        nuclear group, 399, 401
        posterior, 396, 401
    lateropolaris, 397
    limbic relay, 398
    medial nuclear group, 396, 402
    metathalamus (geniculate bodies, nuclei), 395,
        401
    midline, 395, 399
        parataenial, *395*
        paraventricular, *395*
        reuniens, *395*
        rhomboid, *395*
    motor relay, 398
    nonspecific, 397–399
    paracentral, *395*
    parafascicular, *154*, 396, 399
    posterior thalamic region, *154*, 155
    pulvinar, 396, *397*, 402
    reticular, 395, 399
Thalamic nucleus(i):
    sensory relay, 398
    specific, 397–399
        association, 397
    ventral anterior, *397*, 398, 399, *414*, *415*, *452*
    ventral lateral, *292*, *296*, *397*, 400, *415*
    ventral posterolateral, *153*, *154*, *158*, *159*, 160,
        245, 396, *397*, 400, *452*
    ventral posteromedial, *266*, *269*, 396, *397*,
        400, *452*
    ventral tier, 396, *397*, 399
    ventralis caudalis, 397
        intermedius, 397
        oralis, 397
    ventrobasal complex, 397
Thalamus (dorsal thalamus) (structural and func-
    tional aspects):
    affection sensation, 403
    animal, 414
    closed self-reexciting chain, 406
    discriminative sensation, 403
    electroencephalogram (EEG), 404
    fasciculus, 419, 422
    functional aspects, 403
    generalized thalamocortical system, 398
    input to, *397*
    integrative and synchronizing role, 403
    limbic lobe, 398
    and motor expression, 394, 404
    negative feedback circuit and, 406
    output from, *396*
    peduncle, 402
    prefrontal lobe and, 402
    radiations from, 402
    recruitment response, 403, 404
    release phenomenon, 405
    reticular system in, 398, 399
    rhythms generated in, 405
        roles, 394
        synchronizing roles, 405
    roles of, 394
    syndrome, thalamic, 405
Thermoanesthesia, 282
Tic douloureux, 230
Tidal drainage, 189
Tinnitus, 326
Tone:
    arteriolar, 23
    atony, 185
    hypertonus, 186
    hypotonus, 185
    vascular, 23
Torsion dystonia, 424
Touch:
    light, 265
    tactile discrimination, 157, 159
Tract(s):
    of basal ganglia, associated with central teg-
        mental tract, 249, 251, 258, *261*, 274
    central trigeminal (trigeminothalamic tract,
        trigeminal lemniscus), 256, 265, *266*,
        483–490
    of cerebellum, associated with (see Cerebellum)
    corticobulbar, 243, 278, *279*, 415, *452*, 453,
        467, 490
        and facial nerve, 278

Tract(s):
  corticocollicular, 315, *377*
  corticohypothalamic, 330
  corticonigral, *261, 415, 420, 452*
  "corticonuclear" fibers, 446, 453
  corticopontine, 138, 243, 245, 274, *296, 452,*
      468, 488, 490
  corticopulvinar, *373, 452*
  corticoreticular, *177, 179, 261, 262, 273, 275,*
      415, 452, 453, 467
  corticorubral, 177, *261, 275, 452,* 467
  corticospinal (pyramidal, cerebrospinal), *151,*
      174, 176, 178, 245, *261, 279,* 280, *415,*
      452, 467
  corticostriate, 418, 419, 453, *467,* 468
  corticotectal, *373,* 467
  corticotegmental, *14, 153, 158, 452,* 453, *481,*
      482
  corticothalamic, 468
  cuneocerebellar, 163
  descending fibers to nuclei of ascending sys-
      tems, 280, 315, 394, 453, 468
  habenulopeduncular (fasciculus retro flexus),
      435, 436
  hypothalamohypophyseal, 329, *330*
  hypothalamotegmental, 332, *435,* 437
  interstitiospinal, 178, *313, 487–489*
  lateral lemniscus, 313, 315
  lemniscal, 258
  mamillotegmental, 332, *434,* 436
  mamillothalamic (peduncle), 332, *434,* 436
  median forebrain bundle, *261,* 276, 332, *435,*
      436
  olfactory, *428, 429*
  olivocerebellar, 248, 249, *298,* 301
  optic, 9, *10, 21, 23, 368, 370, 371, 452*
  pontocerebellar, 243, *296, 297,* 301
  posterior column (fasciculus coneatus and grac-
      ilis), 157, *158, 159,* 265, *393*
  posterolateral tract of Lissauer, *151, 152, 153,*
      159, 220
  propriospinal (spinospinalis), *151, 172,* 245,
      258
  pyramidal, 174, 245, 280, 467
  retinohypothalamic, 342
  reticuloreticular (central tegmental tract), 249,
      251, *256, 261, 265,* 274, *435,* 488
  reticulospinal, medullary and pontine, *151,*
      176, 177, 179, 248, 258, *263,* 274, *275,*
      276, 279
  reticulothalamic, *262, 263*
  rubrospinal, *151, 175, 177, 178, 275,* 276,
      481–490
  septopreopticohypothalamic, 329
  solitary (fasciculus), 269, 281, *482, 483*
  spinal lemniscus, 264
  spinal tract of trigeminal nerve, 243, 246, *266,*
      481–485
  spinocerebellar, *151, 161, 162, 163, 164,* 253,
      299, 481–486
  spinocervicothalamic, *164*

Tract(s):
  spinocortical, 163
  spino-olivary, *151,* 249, 295, *298*
  spinopontine, 164
  spinoreticular (spinobulbar), *151,* 156, *162, 164,*
      258
  spinospinalis (propriospinal), *145, 151, 172*
  spinotectal, *151,* 157, *272, 481, 482*
  spinothalamic (spinal lemniscus), *151, 153,* 157,
      159, 264, 265, *392, 481–490*
  spinovestibular, *162,* 164
  supraopticohypophyseal, *330, 333,* 339,
      342
  tectocerebellar, *263,* 295, *298, 322*
  tectoreticular (tectobulbar), *175, 261*
  tectospinal, *151, 175,* 178, 276, *483, 486,*
      488–490
  thalamohypothalamic, 331
  trigeminocerebellar, 295, *298, 322*
  trigeminothalamic, 254, 256, 265, *392*
  tuberohypophyseal, 333
  tuberoinfundibular, 337
  vestibulocerebellar, *162,* 295, *299,* 324
  vestibulomesencephalic, 323
  vestibulospinal, *151, 164, 167, 176,* 178, *179,*
      275, 321, 322, 325, 481–485
  (*See also* Bundle; Fasciculus; Pathways, lemnis-
      cal)
Transport across capillaries, 68
Trema (gill slit), 221
  posttrematic, 221
  pretrematic, 221
Tremor:
  intention (action), 301, 302
  at rest, 124
Triangle of Golbault-Philippe, 172
Trigeminal eminence, 11, *12, 14,* 243
Trigeminal nerve, 8, *12,* 226, 227, 266
  neuralgia, 230
  tract, *266*
  zone, 230
Trigonum hypoglossi, 12, *14,* 237, 244
Trigonum vagi (ala cinerea), 12, *14,* 244
Trochlear nerve, 8, *10,* 11, *12, 13,* 221, 224, 225,
      488
Trophic effects and influences, 213, 215
Trunkal ataxia, 303
Tuber cinereum (hypothalamus), 327, *328, 330,*
      333
Tuberal area (hypothalamus), 327
Tuberculum cinereum (trigeminal eminence), 11,
      243
Tuberculum cuneatus, 11, 12, *14,* 243
Tuberculum gracilis, 11, 12, 14, 243
Twin-brain (man and animal), 474, *475, 477,* 478

Uncinate fasciculus (hooked bundle), 297
  fits, 440
Uncus, 6, *8*
Unidirectional conduction, 85
Unipolar (pseudounipolar) neuron, *42,* 57
Unit:
  macromotor, 142
  motor, 141
  sensory, 141

Unmyelinated (nonmedullated) nerve fiber, 56, 59, 60, 62, 64, 79
Upper motor neuron (spastic) paralysis, 173, 185, 187, 278

Vagus nerve, 8, 10, 12, 220, 221, 266, 269
Vallecula, 14
Vasopressin (ADH), 334, 337
Veins and dural (venous) sinuses, 31–34
    anastomotic vein, 32, 33, 34
    arachnoid granulation (villus), 35, 36, 39
    basal vein, 32, 33
    basilar venous plexus, 33
    caudate vein, 32
    cavernous sinus, 26, 33
    cerebral veins: deep, 31, 32, 33
        internal, 31, 32, 33
        middle, 31, 32, 33
        superficial (external), 31, 32, 33
    choroidal vein, 32, 33
    confluence of sinuses, 32, 33, 36
    drainage of brain, venous, 31, 32
    emissary vein, 34, 35
    great cerebral vein of Galen, 32, 33, 35
    hypophyseal portal vein, 330
    intercavernous sinus, 33
    jugular vein, internal, 31, 32, 33
    longitudinal sinus, superior, 32, 33
    occipital sinus, 32
    ophthalmic vein, 32, 33
    petrosal sinuses, 32, 33
    pharyngeal and pterygoid venous plexus, 33
    sagittal sinus, superior, 32, 33, 35, 36
    sigmoid sinus, 32, 33
    sphenoparietal sinus, 33, 38
    straight sinus, 32, 35, 36
    striate veins, 33
    transverse sinus, 32, 33
    vein of Galen, 32, 33, 35
    vena terminalis, 26, 32, 33
    vertebral venous plexus, 182
Velum interpositum, 6, 33, 34
Ventral thalamus (subthalamus), 6, 9, 417, 420, 421
Ventricle(s) and associated structures, 15
    apertures, medial and lateral, 4, 16, 17, 36, 39, 40
    atrium (trigone), 15, 27
    cavity, 241
    central canal, 15, 36, 143
    cerebral aqueduct (iter, aqueduct of Sylvius), 5, 9, 15, 17, 36
    choroid plexus, 15, 39
        of fourth ventricle, 5, 15, 17, 290, 483
        of lateral ventricles, 15, 18, 19, 24, 26
        of third ventricle, 5, 15, 18, 24
    foramen of Luschka (lateral aperture), 4, 17, 36, 39, 40
    foramen of Magendie (medial aperture), 4, 17, 36, 39, 40
    foramen of Monro (interventricular), 5, 15, 17, 18, 29, 33, 34, 36
    fourth, 5, 15, 17, 29, 36, 244, 483
        lateral recesses of 14, 15, 40
    lateral, 1, 8, 15, 17–19, 20

Ventricle(s) and associated structures:
    anterior horn, 20
    atrium (trigone), 15, 27
    body, 15, 20, 24, 27
    boundaries, 20
        inferior (temporal) horn, 15, 18, 20, 27
        posterior (occipital) horn, 15, 20, 28
    optic, 351
    rhomboid fossa, 12, 14
    third, 15
        recesses of, 15
Ventricular system, 1
Ventricular zone, 113
Ventriculogram, 40
Vermal cortex, 290, 296
Vermis, 13, 290
    nodule of, 14
Vertebral arterial system, 25
Vertebral column, 133
    relation to spinal cord, 134, 136, 137
Vesicles, synaptic, 47–49, 55
    clear centers, 91
    dense core (granular), 55, 200
    flat, 55
    spherical (agranular), 55
Vestibular system, 305, 379
    area in medulla, 14
    connections with cerebellum, 300, 324
    connections with reticular formation, 325
    efferent fibers to labyrinth, 321, 325
    functional considerations, 325
        angular movement, 318
        angular rotation, 318
        antigravity response, 408
        caloric test, 318
        linear acceleration, 317, 318, 411
        linear deceleration, 317, 318, 411
        motion sickness, 325, 326
        movements of body and head, 324
        nystagmus, 323–325
        past pointing, 324
        rotation, 317, 318, 411
        tinnitus, 326
        vertigo, 323, 325
    ganglion (Scarpa's), 321
    hair cells, 320
    medial longitudinal fasciculus, 151, 176, 179, 245, 321, 322, 481–490
    membranous labyrinth, 307, 309
        crista ampulla, 305, 318, 319
        macula of saccule, 319, 411
        macula of utricle, 319, 411
        semicircular duct and canal, 306, 318, 319, 321
    nerve, vestibular, 218, 280, 232, 305, 306, 307, 313, 316, 317, 485
    nuclei, vestibular, 162, 238, 250, 321, 322, 324, 325
    pathways, 176, 178, 248, 270, 276, 321–325
Vestibulocerebellum, 234, 250
Vibratory sense, 157, 159, 312
Visceral:
    afferent system, 195
    definition, 147, 218
Visceral brain, 430

Visual (optic) system, 345–382
  accessory optic, 369
  anatomy and function of, 345–351
  black and white vision, 360, 361
  color, 365
    brightness, 365
    hue or tone, 365
    saturation or purity, 365
  color blindness, 366
  color vision, 365
    theories of, 365
  fields of vision, 367, *368*
    binocular, 373
    fusion of, 373
    monocular, 367
    receptor fields of retina, 359
    vertical median between visual fields, 376
  functional aspects of, 362
    acuity, 364
    adaptation: dark, 363, 364
      light, 363, 364
    afterimages: negative, 366
      positive, 366
  blind spot, 347, 348, 369
  brightness contrast, 362
  broad-band cells, 371
  contour sharpening (simultaneous brightness
    contrast), *60*, 262
  depth perception, 378
  development of visual perception, 129
  diplopia, 285, 369
  duplicity theory of vision, 361
  generator potential, 360
  geniculostriate system, 369
  heteronymous, 381
  homonymous, 382
  lateral (mutual) inhibition, 362, 363
  neurons of visual cortex, 373
  off system (set), 362
  on-off system (set), 362
  on system (set), 362
  perimetry, 367
  Purkinje shift (effect), 365
  response field, 358
  searching movements, 362
  smooth pursuit system, 379
    Snellen chart, 365
  spectrally opponent cells, 360, 371
  stereopsis or solid vision, 378
  tectal system, *367*, 369
  vergence system, 379
  visual cortex, 362, 375
  lesions of the visual pathways, 380, *381*
    blind spot (acotoma), 380
    hemianopsia: binasal, 381
      bitemporal, 381
      homonymous, *381,* 382
    heteronymous, 281
    homonymous, 282
    monocular blindness, 381
    papilledema, 348

Visual (optic) system:
  lesions of the visual pathways: quadrantic
    anopsia, *381,* 382
  pathways, 366–373
    capsule, retrolenticular portion of internal,
      453, 454
    columnar organization of visual cortex, 448,
      449
    cortex, visual (striate), 6, 372, 464
    geniculate body, lateral, *26,* 370, 371
    loop of Meyer, *368,* 466
    neurons of visual cortex, 373, 374
    optic chiasma, *5, 7, 368,* 369, 371
    optic nerve, *5, 8, 9, 10, 346, 351, 352,* 369
    optic radiations, geniculo-calcarine tract, *21,*
      27–29, 372, 451
    optic tract, 9, *10, 21, 23, 368,* 370, 371, *452*
    retinohypothalamic tract, 342
  pigments in rods and cones, 356
    chlorolabe, 356
    cyanolabe, 356
    erythrolabe, 356
    rhodopsin (visual purple), 356
  receptive fields, *359*
  reflex (somatic), 379
    accommodation-convergence, 380
    automatic eye movements, 224, 380
    conjugate movements, 379
    convergence of eyes, 379
    cortical eye fields, *377,* 380
    fixation of eyes, 380
    strabismus, 226
    superior colliculus (functional role), 380
    volitional movements, 380
    voluntary eye field, 380
  reflex (visceral), 376, *377*
    accommodation, 377, 380
    consensual light reflex, 376
    constriction (pupil), 204, 376, *377*
    dialation (pupil), 377
    light reflex, 376, *377*
    paradoxical pupillary reaction, 212
    presbyopia, 351
    pretectum, 380
    pupil, 350
  retina, 351–362
    area: macula (central), 367
      paramacular (paracentral, pericentral), 367
    area: peripheral, 367
    bipolar neurons (midget, flat, rod), *351,*
      357
    cones (blue, green, red), 355, 356
    detached, 352
    fovea, 353
    functional role of, 360
    ganglionic neuron, *351,* 361, 362
    horizontal cell and systems, *351,* 357
    macula lutea, 318, 347
    plexiform layers, *351,* 357
    "private line" system, 364
    receptor fields, 361
    rod, *351, 352,* 355, 356
    synaptic organization of retina, 357
  spectrum, 345
  superior colliculus, 9, 241, 255
  superior colliculus, in act of seeing, 375

Voiding of urine, 207
Voluntary act, 423

Wallerian (secondary) degeneration, 73
Water balance, regulation of, 338
    osmoreceptor, 338
    sense, 267
Weber's syndrome, 285
Wernicke's area, 464, 476, 479, 480

White matter, *21*, 142, 450
Word:
   blindness, 464
   deafness, 466

Zona incerta, *414*, 422
   intermedia, 145
Zone, lateral, 327
Zonular fibers, 346